# HOMOEOPATHY

## "Like cures like"

**English Rendering of Lectures delivered on MTA International**
by

***Hadhrat Mirza Tahir Ahmad***
**Fourth Head of the Worldwide Ahmadiyya Muslim Community**

ہومیوپیتھی یعنی علاج بالمثل
HOMOEOPATHY ("Like cures like")
English Translation from Urdu by:
Dr. Imtiaz Ahmad Chaudhary M.D., F.R.C.S.

First Published in England in 2005



Published by
Islam International Publications Ltd
"Islamabad"
Sheephatch Lane
Tilford, Surrey, GU10 2AQ
United Kingdom

Printed in UK at
Bath Press



ISBN: 1 85372 773 3

# PUBLISHERS NOTE

Upon the instructions of Hadhrat Mirza Tahir Ahmad, Khalifatul Masih IV, this English translation was prepared from the Urdu by Dr. Imtiaz Ahmad Chaudhary M.D.; F.R.C.S. (Edinburgh), with the help of his family, whereas the typing was done by Naureen. Following this, Dr. Mujib-ul-Haq Khan M.B.B.S., B.Sc. reviewed the text with him and Syed Mansoor Ahmad Shah revised the English.

Once the book had reached this stage, Hadhrat Mirza Masroor Ahmad, Khalifatul Masih V, instructed Vakalat-e-Tasneef London to ensure that a thorough proof-reading of the book be carried out. Thus this honour was entrusted to Farina Qureshi, Farida Ahmad, Dr Hamidullah Khan M.B.B.S., M.F.Hom and Munir-ud-Din Shams (Additional Vakil-ut- Tasneef, London). Mahmood Ahmad Malik (Incharge Central Computer Section London) typeset and designed the book. May Allah reward everyone who has helped in the preparation of this book.

We pray to Allah to make this book beneficial to mankind and may Hadhrat Mirza Tahir Ahmad, Khalifatul Masih IV, always be the recipient of its blessings - Amin

Publisher

# CONTENTS

In the name of Allah, the Gracious, Ever Merciful

# PREFACE

The story of my involvement in homoeopathy is very interesting. Soon after the partition of the Indian sub-continent (and our migration from Qadian in India to Rabwah in Pakistan), I started suffering from severe attacks of headache, commonly known as a Migraine. This is usually a one-sided headache associated with nausea, vomiting and restlessness. I used to take Aspirin for relief, but it would adversely affect my stomach and kidneys, and also caused palpitations. My late father had an allopathic medicine called Sandol for his own use, which would give me relief rather promptly. After the partition of the Indian sub-continent, it was not available in Pakistan and had to be imported from Calcutta, (India).

Once during a severe attack of migraine when there was no Sandol available, my late father sent me a homoeopathic remedy. At that time, I had no belief in the usefulness of homoeopathy but I took the medicine in good faith. Suddenly, I realised that my headache had totally disappeared and for no apparent reason, I was lying in bed with my eyes shut. Never before, had I experienced such an astonishingly rapid effect of any medicine.

After that, another incident enhanced my interest in homoeopathy. After I got married, my late wife, Asifa Begum (Allah have mercy on her), told me about her ailment of long-standing. My late father had many books on homoeopathy so I started searching for a remedy for my wife. By good luck, it so happened that I opened up a book and found a discourse on Natrum Mur whose symptoms and signs exactly matched those of my late wife, Asifa Begum. I gave her one high potency dose and she never had the same problem again. This strengthened my faith that homoeopathy was definitely effective, whether I understood it or not.

After that I started a regular study of homoeopathic books in my father's library. Many a time, I studied all night long, and thus acquired knowledge of remedies and their constitution. I diligently learned about the usage and the special features of homoeopathic remedies and then started treating patients.

## Foundation of Homoeopathy

Homoeopathy was founded by Dr. Samuel Christian Friedrich Hahnemann who was born in Saxony in 1755 AD. He loved to learn languages and in fact attained proficiency in eight of them. At the age of 12, he had started teaching Greek. Thus, he became a language teacher at a very young age. He began his medical studies in Leipzig, Austria, and then he went to Vienna and Erlangen. In 1779, he became a medical doctor and started practising in Dresden.

He was a kind-hearted doctor and his income was obviously not much, so he started translating books into other languages in order to supplement it. After eleven years of medical practise, he discovered the homoeopathic system of treatment. For the first six years or so, he mostly experimented on himself and his near relatives. In 1796, for the first time, he informed the medical world about homoeopathic philosophy through the medical journals. In 1810 AD, he published his famous book, *The Organon of Rational Medicine*, also called *Organon of Hahnemann* and then prepared *The Materia Medica* between 1811 and 1821 AD.

Traditional medical doctors of that time strongly opposed him. In 1820 AD, the proponents of the old allopathic system of medicine had his system of homoeopathy declared unlawful by the government, and even they went to the extent of suing him. However, before Homoeopathy was declared unlawful, Hahnemann sent for Prince Karl Schwarzenberg of Austria, and treated him successfully in Leipzig. The Prince being naturally grateful to Dr. Hahnemann recommended to King Friedrich that all restrictions against homoeopathy should be removed and in future none should be re-imposed. Unfortunately for Dr. Hahnemann, the Prince re-indulged himself in a life of ease and resorted to alcoholism. He became seriously sick again and he was treated allopathically but to no avail. When he died, the Austrian government blamed the Prince's death on Dr. Hahnemann. The public was outraged, his books were burnt in the open and Dr. Hahnemann had to run for his life. He took shelter in Cothen, was patronised by the Duke of Cothen and he stayed there for 14 years researching chronic illnesses. He published the first edition of his research in 1828. In 1830, his wife passed away. He married a French lady in 1835 and moved to Paris where he practised homoeopathy till his death in 1843. **The year 1835 is the same historic year in which the Founder of the Ahmadiyya Muslim Community, Mirza Ghulam Ahmad was born in Qadian, India.**

Homoeopathy means "like cures like." This is the method of treating a disease with the materials derived from the toxic and injurious agents causing similar signs and symptoms complex. Before Dr. Hahnemann, this system was evidently outside the established system of allopathic treatment, although some of the treatments offered there worked on the same line as homoeopathy. These, however, were not understood. A few such practices were in vogue on an experimental basis and in a limited controlled way. For example, Ipecac and Opium were given in a diluted tinctured form to relieve nausea and vomiting. In fact, both these medicines are known as strong vomiting and nausea inducers. Dr. Hahnemann had experimented on many such drugs and was surprised to note that not only did they cause a certain illness, yet at the same time they cured that particular illness when administered in diluted form.

During this deep and thoughtful experimentation, Dr. Hahnemann discovered the fantastic defence system of the human body. The physicians believed that the human body had the power of defending itself but were unaware of its magnanimity and the principle of its working. They did not how to utilise the defensive nature of the body against the establishment of the disease. This secret was revealed to Dr. Hahnemann after his constant, thoughtful deep study of the human body's defence system. His observations about the great defensive capability of the human body were astounding and unbelievable, but must be believed because the observations he offered were so clear. In support of this, Dr. Hahnemann further noted that the body reacts naturally to every external attack. Anything alien to the human body, be it an article of food, drug or poison, provokes the body to react against it. External abuse of the body is quickly overcome by the bodily defences. During continuous experimentation and observation, he postulated that if in the past, some disease has been overlooked and not reacted to by the body, then the introduction of a similar symptoms-producing agent in extremely diluted and pacified form would induce defensive body reaction and eliminate the sickness.

So, in principle, homoeopathy is the method of treating an ailment caused by injurious toxic substances with the same or similar substances given in an extremely diluted form. It is absolutely essential that the poison of the like thereof be diluted to the extent that it causes no harm to the body. However, in this imperceptible and chemically ineffective dilution, the body still picks up the message and reacts to it. Most of the time, the dilution of the homoeopathic remedy is such that the original substance is virtually absent i.e. the substance is in abstract form. The more the dilution, the more potently it works, i.e. the potency increases with serial dilutions. This is in total contrast to the quantitative summation of allopathic medicines.

Surprisingly, the minutest dilutions are perceived by the human soul, which in turn directs the body to react with all necessary defence mechanisms. If the soul did not have the capability to perceive the otherwise imperceptible amount of poison and prepare the body for proper defence mechanisms, no homoeopathic medication would have worked beyond the potency 30. However, continuous observation compels us to believe that the homoeopathic remedies in high potencies like CM are indeed very effective.

This system is so superbly delicate that one must come to the belief of the existence of the soul. The homoeopathic "medicines" in serial logarithmic dilutions contain practically no atom of the original substance / poison, yet they work profoundly.

The opponents of homoeopathy cannot even begin to explain the true nature of the system of allergy! In America, doctors experimented on a lady who was allergic to eggs. She was placed in a building where nobody was permitted to keep eggs and for some time, she remained allergy free. One day she came down with a severe allergic attack. The whole building was searched carefully and at last, a nest was found on the topmost floor of the building where a pigeon had laid an egg. The distance between the lady's flat and the nest was 15 to 20 stories. This proves that under the direction of the human mind, the human body can perceive the most delicate effects otherwise undetectable by the most modern and super-sensitive instruments, as in the case here.

It has also been discovered that some allergy patients can predict weather changes even days before some modern and sensitive instruments can do so. For example, some patients are allergic to conditions produced by lightning and thunder. Due to these sudden weather changes, signs and symptoms of allergy begin to manifest themselves in patients prone to such allergies long before science, despite all its sophistication, can perceive these changes. Birds are known to express violent noisy reactions before a change in weather becomes noticed.

The soul perceives and in turn directs the body to react. The body itself does not react per se. In homoeopathic treatment, the remedy is administered in such delicate amounts that there is no chance of adverse effects on the body. It is the soul, the real subtle entity, which is able to perceive the delicate presence of medicines or poisons otherwise undetectable or unperceivable. No wonder the Founder of Ahmadiyyat named this system of medicine, the spiritual system, i.e. the one mediated through the human soul.

## Proving

The characteristic features of different medicines have been investigated for thousands of years. People have repeatedly faced different poisons and have known their nature. Socrates was made to drink Conium 2500 years ago. Although people knew the effects of this poison before this, the personal experience and the moment-by-moment, detailed description of the effects of this poison as given by Socrates had never been known as before. As the poisonous symptoms gradually worsened, he kept describing to his attendants precisely as to what, where and in what order was his body being affected by the poison. Dr. Hahnemann also tried many poisons on himself, in diluted form, and also noted the effects that had been minutely described by Socrates. He also found that when a weakened poison is administered in small doses repeatedly, its unique properties become manifest but do not last forever. This process of registering minute details of the actions of the poison and like substances is called "Proving". Along similar lines to Dr. Hahnemann, many homoeopaths have experimented on themselves with various poisons and noted their detailed effects. In this way, "*homoeopathic Materia Medica*" has steadily expanded. Extended proving cannot be based on one person's experimentation. For proper acceptance, the proving has to be done by many: in different times, weather and localities and on people with different dispositions. Proper registry into the Materia Medica is attained after collective group discussions on the methods and results of proving arrived at individually, as some drugs may work better on obese people and some on thin and lean people. The volunteers of these experiments are not told of what and from what source they have been given a substance. Experimentation is repeated in different seasons and the effects are noted on the body as well as the mind. All studies are carefully scrutinised and determined. Dr. Hahnemann has given the most weight to the effect on the mind. One remedy has a similar effect on two patients with similar mental symptoms, but may not have a similar effect on two patients with similar physical appearance.

## Methods of Preparing Homoeopathic Remedies

Homoeopathic remedies are prepared in two ways:

1. The original substance or extract is mixed in alcohol, stored for a while and then sifted. This is called the Mother Tincture. Many remedies are used in this form such as Carduus Marianus in

liver diseases. Eight to ten drops dissolved in water and taken by mouth are very useful in many liver disorders. The letter Q tells us that the homoeopathic remedy is a Mother Tincture.

2. The Mother Tincture is diluted with alcohol or distilled water in a bottle, one drop in ninety-nine drops of the diluent and shaken vigorously two to four times so that it becomes completely homogeneous. Thus prepared, the potency of the medicine is 1. For example, a drop of Mother Tincture of Aconite shaken well in ninety-nine drops of the diluent, alcohol or distilled water is Aconite potency 1. A drop of Aconite 1 added to ninty-nine drops of alcohol and shaken well will make Aconite 2. A drop of Aconite 2 vigorously shaken in ninety-nine drops of alcohol will make Aconite 3 and so on. If the process is repeated thirty times, we have prepared Aconite 30. Most of the routine homoeopathic remedies are prepared in this way. The letter C written along with the potency indicates that in each dilution, the medicine is diluted one in a hundred.

If the process consists of putting one drop of the Mother Tincture in nine drops of the diluent instead of ninety-nine drops, the medicine prepared would be potency 1D, which means ten. Biochemical medicines are made in this way i.e. serial dilutions of one in ten using a sugar substance Dextrose, prepared from fruit instead of alcohol or distilled water. Some Homoeopaths use the original poison instead of the mother tincture in a very small amount and mix it in 9 grams of the powdered Dextrose. They grind it well, and the medicine thus prepared is 1X. A gram of 1X added to 9 grams of Dextrose well ground will make 2X. Further similar process will make 3X and so on.

In fact, an increase in potency denotes a decrease in the quantity of the poisonous substance or extract. Each time the quantity of the poison is decreased, i.e. one in a hundred, the potency increases by 1. In the biochemical system, as the quantity of poison decreases by one in ten, this is called potency 1. In homoeopathic remedies, the letter C is no longer written. In some countries, however, they still write C or D with the potency of their prepared remedies. In the biochemical system, X is always written as a measure of potency such as 1X, 2X, 3X, 6X or 12X etc. The potency 1000 is sometimes written as 1M, the potency 10,000 is written as 10M and 100,000 is written as CM.

## Usage of Homoeopathic Remedies

It must be remembered that in cases of well-established illnesses of long-standing such as asthma and epilepsy, it is not right to prescribe a casual prescription. Instead, one must see the patient and have a detailed discussion with him or her to find out about the illness as well as the constitution of the person in order to reach the constitutional remedy. Both must match as precisely as possible. In my experience, many a time, the patient did not respond to the standard well known prescription but after a detailed personal examination of the patient, including his state of mind, the prescription given worked wonderfully well. For example, patients of epilepsy experience auras of a different nature before the actual attack. One such patient used to experience loud, unbearable noises and would not go to sleep out of fear. He felt as if his head and mind were squeezed in a vice. Based on his state of mind, I prescribed Cactus and it worked wonders. He started to sleep normally and the epileptic seizures also disappeared. Ironically, Cactus is not mentioned amongst the remedies for epilepsy. It is important that all such patients be observed for at least a few days. If a rush of blood to the head is noted and the blood pressure rises, Cactus would be the ideal medication.

Similarly, one should look for typical signs and symptoms of the illness before prescribing. In diseases of the gall bladder, a number of medications are useful. Once, I tried almost all of them on a gall bladder patient, but none worked. After a personal examination of the patient, I found that he was a nervous, psychic wreck. I gave him Sepia and he got better - the pain totally disappeared!

In all cases of chronic illnesses, the patient should be studied in detail. On another occasion, I gave Aconite and Belladonna to a kidney patient in view of the acute nature of the sickness but it simply did not work. Apparently, I had overlooked the constitution of the patient. Belladonna and Aconite would have worked if heat had been making him worse and if cold offered him relief. However, that particular patient felt worse with cold baths. As soon as I gave him Magnesia Phosphoricum and Colocynth, he immediately got better.

There are no quick fixes in Homoeopathy. One should get into the habit of forgetting the disease for a moment and give due attention to the individual symptoms and constitution of the patient. A list of hot and cold remedies should be kept mind. In a person of hot temperament, the medication designed for a cool-minded person will do harm instead of doing good. Some people tolerate heat better than cold and vice versa. Some like movement, while others like complete rest. All these factors form the constitution of the patient and should be kept in mind while prescribing a remedy. In a busy practice, the experienced homoeopath can prescribe a routine and well tried prescription for a particular ailment and it often works. However in case of chronic, long-standing illnesses, one must spend enough time on a detailed study of the patient as well as the illness.

In general, the homoeopath avoids combining the remedies. I also did the same initially but later on changed my practice. I did not have enough time to be able to arrive at one single remedy. In Rabwah, I was deeply involved in my official duties: in Waqf-e-Jadid, Ansar Ullah and Khuddamul Ahmadiyya etc. I had to be present in committee meetings of Anjuman Ahmadiyya and Tahrik-e-Jadid. Apart from that, I ran a homoeopathic dispensary in the Waqf-e-Jadid office in the evenings and would see up to one hundred patients a day. I had started the dispensary at home during the time between Maghrib and Isha (evening and night prayers). The shortage of time compelled me to devise the compounding of more than one remedy. As I already indicated, I had done an extensive study of homoeopathic remedies and had informally practised homoeopathy for years. On the basis of this knowledge and experience, the compounding of medicines worked very well. In some cases, I had to change the compounds and in certain obstinate cases, I carried out a detailed personal study of the patient's constitution and his disease.

Secondly, more and more remedies are being added to the homoeopathic Materia Medica. New remedies are being found to be more effective. Some ailments are not amenable to just any remedy. Compounding of more than one remedy works like a new medication. Many of the old remedies are already natural compounds themselves, such as Nux Vomica, which is a combination of many natural constituents. While prescribing compounds, my concern is about their final characteristic features. It is not necessary that the total effect of the constituted remedies must be the sum total of all. Some remedies annul some of the effects of the other. Thus at the end, the compound may have a totally different effect.

## <u>Virus</u>

A virus is a rapidly evolving organism. In fact, nothing else changes its shape (or mutates) so quickly. It should be treated properly with homoeopathy. Antibiotics will fight some viruses but the remaining ones will go into mutation, proving extremely dangerous. This may eventually lead to the formation of cancer.

## A General Principle

Generally speaking, chronic illnesses, which have gradually invaded and taken over the body systems over a long period, are amenable only to slow but progressively acting remedies. These remedies should be continued for six to twelve months. One should start with low potency 30 and when it stops working, advance to the next potency of 200 once a day for seven to ten days. After that, potency, 1000 is to be given every fortnight a few times. The last dose should be in potency CM to be repeated after six months or one year. Throughout this time, one should carefully observe the slowly evolving effects of the homoeopathic treatment.

## Potency

With regards to the topic of potency, there has been extensive scientific research as to what kind of patients should receive which medications, administered in what potency. In the diseases of the stomach, low potencies work well. For neurological disorders, usually potency 200 or higher is useful. In profound mental illnesses, higher potencies are required. In some kinds of cancer, much higher potencies are needed. However, in some cases, if the patient is too sick, a higher potency medication may prove dangerous. In such cases, the physical strength should be restored first with supplements of food and vitamins. When general health has improved enough to tolerate the reaction, remedies should be given in gradually increasing potencies such as from 30 to 200 and 1000, as already indicated. Two entirely opposite remedies should never be given together. Would you drop ice cream into a hot cup of tea? There is no sense in it.

Dr. Kent has warned against using some remedies in CM potency, especially Silicea, but in my experience of many years Silicea in a potency of anything less than CM has not worked in patients of AIDS and some cancers.

In homoeopathy, if an administered remedy does not show its desired effect, then there are two possible ways to proceed. It may either be repeated a few times, or its potency may be increased gradually. The other method is that the potency may be maintained and another remedy may be used in between the treatment for the enhancement of the body defences.

Tuberculosis patient must never be treated with Sulphur in high potency. Rather, the treatment should always be started in low potency.

**Dosage of Homoeopathic Remedies:**

I am often asked about the frequency and how much of the remedy should be taken. There is no consensus of opinion on this. Every prescriber has his own way, based on experience. In this book, I have suggested the practical useful potencies based upon my own experience. I have also referred to the dosage prescribed by some well-known homoeopaths. The matter has been left to the discretion of the individual practitioners. The potencies I have observed to be effective in my experience will, God-willing, also benefit the user, with some exceptions where the potencies used are not suitable for the patient.

The quantity of the homoeopathic remedy, per se, is not that important. The patient may take a few pellets or a lot of them - it does not matter. It is the frequency that makes the difference. Every time the remedy is taken, it 'strikes' the body to respond. Taking a homoeopathic remedy once is called one strike. The effect of the remedy starts as soon as it is put in the mouth. Every time it is taken, it repeats the strike.

Some homoeopaths insist that the medicine should not be touched with the hand. Instead, to preserve its effectiveness, it should be taken on paper. However, hands are much cleaner than the mouth, contains so many impurities, layer upon layer, yet it can and does react to the presence of the remedy. What difference would the use of the hand make? Paper itself is not free from contamination. Natrum Mur is the homoeopathic potency of the common table salt but the mouth is full of salt. So taking a dose of Natrum Mur is like pouring a drop of salt water in the salt mine. Yet, it works. The reason is that the homoeopathic effect of Natrum Mur is not related to the material particles. In the preparation of the homoeopathic remedy, the original substance disappears completely. It only exists in the form of a memory which is capable of showing its effect through the blood and body fluids. The command is perceived by the soul. This is a unique indelible divine system of memory, mediated through the soul, which is, in a way, related to physical matter also.

**When to take the Remedy**

It is important to take the remedy at least half an hour before or at least half an hour after taking food for a better effect. It will still show some effect if taken during this period, though not optimal. It is better to take the remedy on an empty stomach i.e. first thing in the morning or two to four hours after dinner. In emergency situations, it may be used at any time.

**Diet of the Patient**

In homoeopathy, there is no restriction regarding the diet. Homoeopathic remedies work irrespective of the kind of food taken by the patient. Yet, the patient must refrain from consuming foods that aggravate his symptoms or do not suit him. The patient can decide this for himself better than the doctor.

**Preservation of the Homoeopathic Remedies**

In general, homoeopathic remedies last a long time. They may not even expire in a hundred years or more. In general, they should be kept in a dry temperate place with the covers of the bottles tightly closed. The temperature as such does not alter the effectiveness of the medicine, but, if the cover is not airtight, the remedy will evaporate. If the bottle has completely dried out, the remedy should be made afresh. If even a drop remains, it may be made up again by adding more of the diluent. In this way, the potency will increase by one, such as from 30 to 31 or from 200 to 201. This however, does not reduce the effectiveness of the remedy.

As a caution, homoeopathic remedies should not be placed in direct sunlight. The rays of the sun may make the remedy ineffective. Empty bottles should be thoroughly cleaned, boiled in water and dried in the sun in order to destroy any residual effects.

As a rule, all homoeopathic remedies must be kept in separate bottles but some remedies may be mixed without losing their individual effectiveness. Incompatible remedies should always be kept separately. It is better that the mixture be prepared fresh, when required.

Homoeopathic remedies must be kept away from strong perfumes, especially Camphor. Camphor destroys the effectiveness of most homoeopathic remedies. One should also refrain from opening the bottle in a room sprayed with strong antiseptic or perfume.

## Electrolytes

The fluid part of the blood (i.e. plasma/serum), in which the red and white blood cells are suspended, contains electrolytes. These are twelve salts. According to one school of thought (biochemy), it is the imbalance of these salts which causes disease and every kind of illness can be controlled by maintaining the balance of these salts in the body. In my opinion, this is only partly true.

## The Difference between Homoeopathy and Biochemic Remedies

Biochemy is also called the twelve-tissue remedies. According to this view, there are twelve important chemicals in the blood, which when not properly balanced result in sickness. For perfect health, all the twelve must remain in balance or the person will become ill.

On the other hand, it is well known that certain serious illnesses do not result from an imbalance of the salts, but due to the foreign invasion of killer germs. The diseases, in turn, disturb the balance of the salts which if left uncorrected may prove fatal.

In biochemy, a lot of research has been done as to the diseases treatable with these biochemicals. For example, psychological diseases seem to benefit from Kali Phos and spasmodic conditions from Mag Phos.

"Bio" means life and "chemic" stands for chemicals i.e. the chemicals essential for the maintenance of life. Silicea is one of them, and although it is not derived from any chemical compound, it is formed from Silicon, a universal constituent of the earth. Everywhere, Silicea alerts the body to react against every kind of foreign invasion. Many homoeopathic remedies are prepared from it in high potencies. In addition to Silicea, all the biochemic medicines are now being routinely and successfully used in potency X and C.

Some physicians believe that they can treat all ailments while remaining within the biochemic field and have formed a separate branch of homoeopathy, while most of the homoeopaths also use biochemic medicines

However, it is not essential that the twelve chemicals be out of their normal balance for an illness to be contracted. There are thousands of diseases which develop irrespective of these salts being in balance or otherwise. For example, typhoid and polio attack a person with normal electrolytic balance in the blood. Their treatment with appropriate homoeopathic remedy can cure them as long as the body has some residual strength with which to react.

## A Warning

I must caution all physicians that continued indiscriminate use of biochemic medicines can severely disturb the electrolyte balance. Therefore, the electrolytes in the blood must be checked every now and then. There are cases on record that some children developed incurable leukaemia (blood cancer) by use of biochemic tonics. The risk is obviously too high to take.

## A Misunderstanding Corrected

It is not true that all homoeopathic remedies are completely harmless. Like a fast car, built to the highest standards of safety, it may still prove very dangerous in the hands of an untrained and inexperienced driver.

The allopathic doctors, no matter how intelligent they may be, are helpless in this respect. Their medicines cure an ailment, but in doing so create another.

***Mirza Tahir Ahmad***

# Some Important Points Concerning this New Edition

When I first started the Homoeopathic Class in the UK, my main purpose was to promote Homoeopathy throughout the world, with the gradual expansion of Muslim Television Ahmadiyya (MTA) International.

In the beginning, some among the students present in the studio were allopathic and homoeopathic doctors, but these numbered only a few. The majority among them were pupils who did not even have an elementary knowledge of medicine, let alone homoeopathy. Most of them were not familiar with science either. It was a great challenge for me to teach them in such a way that I could make them understand, step by step, the philosophy of homoeopathy, the effects of various homoeopathic remedies, as well as the proper recognition of the patient and the sickness.

Accepting this challenge, the plan which came to my mind was that while repeatedly explaining a remedy in detail, I would also mention similar remedies in the same place. Similarly, I would expand on the nature of the patients, and some quick-fix remedies for various illnesses. In this way, a beginner in homoeopathy might benefit from them in his day to day use.

As a consequence, this would also increase my pupils' faith in homoeopathy. Adopting this method of teaching, while speaking of one remedy, I also detailed other remedies producing similar symptoms along with various kinds of illnesses that could be treated with these remedies. Furthermore, I explained in detail the nature of all the remedies. In short, while describing each remedy, I mentioned other illnesses and remedies with such repetition, that I made the novice pupils drink "pulverised" Homoeopathy. As lectures, this method proved very useful and successful, but in book form this repetition was not appropriate.

I had personally corrected the text of the first edition of this book, although there were still some typographic errors. But I could not read that edition of the book from the perspective of as to how this repetition would affect the reader. When I read the book from this angle, I found it very nerve-racking. An inexperienced reader would only perceive that the author of the book may have a very weak memory, as he had been repeating things already mentioned in previous chapters. Since I intend to publish this book in English and in other major languages of the world, and to distribute it widely, therefore this new edition is being prepared with utmost care and, as far as possible the repetition is kept to a level which would not be burdensome to the reader. Instead, it would serve only as a reminder. Besides, remedies which are akin to each other are described with their corresponding diseases. In that case only the names have been retained. At some places, the reader has been directed to refer to the relevant chapters. Consequently, the size of the book has been significantly reduced, and rather than decreasing the beneficial effect, it has enhanced it.

The contents of this book have been prepared anew including the remedies contained in the second volume in alphabetical order. For this reason it was necessary to prepare a new contents list. It is gratifying that despite the inclusion of the contents of the second volume, the size of this book has decreased rather than increased.

A few coloured plates showing the pictures of plants, herbs and other elements from which remedies are prepared, have also been included in this book.

Finally, my submission to the readers is that they forgive me for any error due to human imperfection and any other mistakes usually attributed to the author. I pray to God Almighty that, despite these few mistakes, He forgives me and makes my humble effort the source of great benefit for mankind. Ameen.

**Wassalam,**
***Mirza Tahir Ahmad***

# MATERIA MEDICA

# Abrotanum

The name Abrotanum brings to one's mind the subject of transfer of a disease from one organ to another. In English, this process is known as **metastasis**. It means that the disease shifts from one part of the body to another. For instance, in the case of mumps, the parotid glands (situated below the ear) swell, and when the disease becomes suppressed at this place, it transfers itself to the reproductive organs. There are many reasons for it being suppressed, for example it could be due to the use of antibiotics, or through local application of poultices. Sometimes it could be due to sudden exposure to cold in high fever. Among all medicines used in the migrating type of ailments, Abrotanum is one of the most salient ones.

Sometimes, by the suppression of diarrhoea, the patient experiences sudden severe pain in the joints and at other times, the heart may be affected. Similarly, sudden cessation of menstruation may result in mental or other ailments.

We shall continue talking about the migration of a disease from one place to another in the context of different remedies so that one may be able to understand well, the indication and usage of remedies for shifting the illness back to where it started.

If a patient suffers from gout or rheumatism, yet at the same time experiences restlessness as if the blood through the heart seems to be scraping the heart, and also he has Epistaxis or blood in the urine, then he is very likely to get cured by the use of Abrotanum.

The basic nature of the Abrotanum patient is that loose frequent stools (diarrhoea) give him relief by excreting the harmful products that would have otherwise involved the joints. In such a patient, Abrotanum will also gradually cure **diarrhoea** as well as joint pains. If the joint pains are suppressed by using some remedies, or by local heat application and the patient contracts pleurisy instead of diarrhoea, then it becomes imperative for the Homoeopath to retrace the course of sickness back to its origin. If the joint pains had preceded the development of **pleurisy** (inflammation of the outer lining of the lung which causes pain on deep breathing and much more so on coughing), then surely the remedy in this case would be Abrotanum. Abrotanum will cure the pleurisy but may initially cause the recurrence of joint pains, which will eventually be cured by continued use of Abrotanum, Insha Allah.

Abrotanum is also very useful in the generalised wasting disease of the children (**marasmus**) when its basic features are also present. For the treatment of marasmus in children, Aethusa, Natrum Mur and Calcaria Carb are also well known remedies. In Calcaria Carb, the wasting affects the legs, while in Abrotanum it starts at the legs but extends to the upper body. This symptom alone is sufficient to suggest that Abrotanum is the remedy to be given in potency 30, three times a day. This could bring complete cure, by the Grace of God.

If the **joint pains** get better but the heart becomes affected, one should not ignore Abrotanum in addition to the other remedies for the heart.

Sometimes on the sudden cessation of diarrhoea, joint pains and **bleeding piles** develop, Abrotanum would still be the right choice. Such a patient feels excessive cold. His symptoms aggravate in cold and humid weather. He often complains of **backache** worsening at night. The backache of Abrotanum always worsens at night irrespective of any specific time, but the backache of Kali Carb is specific for late night or very early morning hours around 3-4 am. In such a patient, if we find the core symptom of 'amelioration by onset of diarrhoea', then the back pain will also be cured by Abrotanum. The general improvement of symptoms with the onset of diarrhoea is also present in Natrum Sulph and Zinc, but to make proper diagnosis, their salient features should also be present in a patient.

Abrotanum pains are sometimes of cutting or piercing nature, which can involve the ovaries, in addition to the joints. A patient having pains at the ovaries and the joints and backache, aggravated at night, the symptoms subsiding with the onset of diarrhoea, will also immensely benefit from Abrotanum as the cure for her **infertility**.

| | |
|---|---|
| **Potency:** | 30 |

# ABSINTHIUM
## (Common Worm Wood)

The main action of Absinthium is on the brain. It is very useful in **epilepsy**. In the epilepsy associated with bluing of the body (Cyanosis) and violent twisting of the hands and feet (as in Cuprum), Absinthium may also be indicated. Before the epileptic fit, there is intense nervousness, restlessness, nausea, visual hallucinations and delusions. The body trembles and the tongue may be caught between the teeth. There is froth at the mouth and then the patient becomes unconscious. In addition to the mental anxiety, there is loss of sleep. Hysteria may also ensue. The clinical picture of Absinthium epilepsy is similar to that of having ingested poisonous mushrooms. One should be very careful in picking mushrooms from the fields because many of them are very poisonous. Only the experts can properly recognise them.

The Absinthium patient is afraid of going into the open and being at high altitudes. He feels **dizzy** and may fall backwards. His **memory is weak** and he is very superstitious. He becomes indifferent to everything. His mind is confused. The pupils are unequal in size and move in different directions. The vision is blurred and there is **pain at the nape of the neck** (as in Gelsemium).

The Absinthium patient also exhibits **gastric symptoms** such as loss of appetite, indigestion, belching, nausea, vomiting, fullness of the stomach and intense flatulence. The patient is usually **constipated**. There is frequent urination and the urine is deep coloured and has a foul, pungent odour. Sometimes, the tongue becomes swollen and protrudes out of the mouth. It trembles and speech is difficult. There are symptoms of numbness and weakness.

Women who go into **menopause** prematurely will benefit from Absinthium. It will reinstate their menstrual cycle if other basic features of Absinthium are also present.

There is a **heaviness in the chest** over the area of the heart. The heartbeat is rapid but irregular. The throat feels scalded, sore and swollen, and the person feels as if a ball is stuck in the throat. The feet are very cold, the back and shoulders hurt, the muscles quiver and there may be **tonic convulsions.**

| | |
|---|---|
| **Potency:** | 30 or more, or less according to the experience of the homoeopath. |

# ACETIC ACIDUM
## Acetic acid
## (Vinegar- an acidic solution)

Acetic acid is considered useful in (the treatment of) **cancer of the stomach**. The Acetic acid patient suffers from a severe cutting type of pain in the stomach, associated with intense thirst, nausea and burning in the stomach. Generally, burning and swelling of the body is common to all acids.

If the patient becomes gravely ill after surgery and feels very weak, the administration of Acetic acid may be very helpful in restoring his condition. In such cases, Strontium Carb and Carbo Veg are also very useful. It is stated that the Acetic acid 1X applied on the stomach can dissolve the cancerous mass of the stomach. Acetic acid 1X has the capability of softening the tumour and converting it into pus. Dr. Owens is of the opinion that in epithelial cancers, Acetic acid should be administered internally as well as externally. Typically, severe burning in the stomach and the chest, followed by cold sweats on the forehead, are salient features of Acetic acid.

The Acetic acid patient suffers from debilitating **diarrhoea**. Acetic acid is considered useful in **diabetes** also. If there is marked weakness associated with frequent fainting fits due to lack of blood (anaemia) and there is difficulty in breathing, Acetic acid will be found very effective to relieve these symptoms. Specifically, in Acetic acid, the patient sweats during high fever, red spots appear on the left cheek, but there is no thirst.

Another special characteristic of the Acetic acid is backache which gets better only by lying on the stomach (prone position).

**Potency:** 3 to 30, should not be repeated too frequently.

# ACONITUM NAPELLUS
## (Monks Hood)

Once the art of homoeopathic treatment is fully understood, day-to-day ailments can often be controlled at the outset and complications can be avoided. In the early stages of all ailments, Aconite is at the top of the list. Its full name is Aconitum Napellus, though it is commonly called Aconite.

Aconite is a poison which affects different parts of the body. In the traditional books on medicine, there is some mention of it among other poisons. However, the minutely detailed account of Aconite is based on proving of Aconite done by Dr. Hanneman and other experienced Homoeopaths on themselves.

In the process of proving, Aconite, or any other poison, is not used in pure form. Instead, as Dr. Hanneman suggested, by example of Aconite, the poison is diluted to the extent that it virtually loses its harmful effect on the body. However, if given repeatedly to a healthy person, it will overwhelm the body and produce its injurious effects in a mild form. These effects are temporary but noticeable enough for the nature of the poison to be studied in minute detail. Through this proving technique, the characteristic features of the Aconite were revealed. These are great fear, suddenness, and severity of illness. The sickness comes on suddenly and the patient thinks that he will not be able to survive.

Aconite is usually considered to be the remedy of dry and cold weather because the diseases related to it are contracted in such weather, though not necessarily so. In general, any **sudden, severe illness of any weather associated with intense fear of death** should be treated with Aconite.

Aconite given along with Rhus Tox at the onset of a severe illness becomes more widely effective. In my opinion, it is a substitute for Aspirin and a very good one. In all such ailments in which there is **restlessness and fever** with a feeling of something untoward in the offing, Aconite 200 and Rhus Tox 200, two or three doses given in the early stage of disease, offer almost immediate relief.

Once my security officer, (Retired Major Mahmood Ahmad), accompanied us for cycling. It was pouring with rain and the weather was very cold, we were all soaking wet. The next morning, he was caught up by high fever and severe body aches. He was given Aconite 200 combined with Rhus Tox 200 and Arnica 200 combined with Bryonia 200 alternatively, every half hour. In a few hours, there was no trace of the ailment left, and Major Mahmood Ahmad Sahib healthily returned to his duty. However, after getting wet in the rain in cold weather, one should not rely only on Aconite and Rhus Tox, but Arnica combined with Bryonia should also be given alternatively.

I discovered this prescription, after long experience. It acts on the diseases of the intestines, lungs, and in **typhoid fever**, as well as on **malaria** and **dysentery** promptly. Many a time, the disease is not completely controllable with this combination, and the analogous remedy will be required for complete recovery. In influenza, this combination formula may not work at all, unless given right at the onset of symptoms. If treatment is delayed, then other indicated remedies would be required.

Diseases may be divided into two categories according to their duration. Regarding their duration, the diseases can be:

1. <u>Acute</u> i.e. the ones which come on with sudden severity and disappear just as fast.
2. <u>Chronic</u> i.e. the ones which gradually establish themselves in the body over a long period. Some of them stay for a relatively short period such as typhoid, while others linger on for a long time, such as tuberculosis, asthma and chronic enlargement of the glands sometimes leading to a transformation into cancer.

Aconite is the topmost remedy in acute diseases.

**Kidney pain** (renal colic) immediately responds to the administration of two doses of Aconite 1000 and Belladona 1000 repeated every fifteen minutes, in most patients. However, if the colicky pain is relieved by heat, the above combination will not work as it works only where heat aggravates. In such cases, one dose of Colocynth CM will offer immediate relief, or Mag Phos 6X dissolved in water and sipped, will relieve this spasmodic pain. But Aconite and Belladona will work well if the colicky pain is relieved by cold application.

Aconite will work immediately in **sudden, severe dysentery** if associated with an element of fear. There is no match for Aconite in **acute dysentery of dry, hot weather**. Aconite is useful in **heart disease** also. My late father, a well-experienced homoeopath, used to prescribe Aconite and Crataegus together in Mother Tincture form. The combination of these two works like a tonic for the heart muscle. Eight to ten drops of Crataegus Q and only one to two drops of Aconite Q are mixed in water. Aconite being a strong poison should not be used in a larger quantity. Large amounts could be dangerous.

Aconite is useful in a patient with a **rapid heartbeat**. Unusually rapid heart and lack of sleep may be secondary to distension of the stomach with gas or mental anxiety. Fear, bad news or apprehension for an examination or some other worry may also cause palpitations of the heart. Aconite 30 or 200 will promptly restore the heartbeat to normality and the mind will be set at peace.

Aconite is of great use in some **mental illnesses** too. When a sudden calamity or depression causes mental shock, or there is an unreasonable sense of fear from everything, Aconite at the outset of symptoms will benefit significantly. Once the disease has already established, other remedies should be given. In this respect, Sulphur is the most salient. Sulphur carries on the action of Aconite on a long-term basis, while Aconite exhibits the same symptoms in the short term.

Aconite is very useful in common diseases like bacterial food poisoning after the ingestion of stale rotting food, resulting in **sudden severe diarrhoea** or dysentery. **Blood-mixed dysentery** of the rainy season associated with fear is well controlled by Aconite.

In some illnesses, the patient **violently screams with fear**, and feels dizzy. For example, in case a dog suddenly jumps on somebody along the way and they feel terrified and dizzy. Aconite will promptly benefit in this situation.

Aconite and Belladona together are very good in the **sudden inflammation of the eyes**. They are complementary to each other, and should be started right away without waiting for further symptoms. However, where the signs and symptoms evidently pertain to either of the two, only that one should be used. It will work precisely and for long time.

Aconite is good in **sudden severe earache** due to exposure to cold. Typically, every pain or ache of Aconite is associated with a throbbing sensation. The patient cannot tolerate noise or loud music.

Aconite is similar to Pulsatilla in that the **feverishness** and discomfort is more evident on one side of the face. One cheek may be red and the other pale. This is common in children. Early administration of Aconite will offer prompt cure. In case the delay has already occurred, Pulsatilla, Lycopodium or Natrum Mur should be tried.
If due to cold, there is **severe toothache** or soreness in the throat, Aconite would definitely be needed. If there is congestion of a part of a body due to the increased blood flow and pressure, spontaneous bleeding may start internally or externally. Whatever the reason of this sudden episode associated with sense of fear, Aconite should be administrated without any reservation.

If due to a sudden mental shock, there is a stoppage of **urine**, Aconite should be given. The prompt use of Aconite in the case of bad news of somebody's death or financial loss will save the person from delayed deleterious effects. Some doctors believe that Aconite is more useful in women than in men. The internal diseases of the women and **inflammation of the uterus** can be controlled if Aconite is given at the beginning of the disease. The Aconite illnesses subside in open air, but get worse at night in a warm room or if there is dry, cold air.

| | |
|---|---|
| **Adjuvants:** | Sulphur, Coffea, Arnica, Belladonna, Bryonia, Phosphorus, Spongia |
| **Antidotes:** | Nux Vomica and Sulphur |
| **Potency:** | Mother Tincture or usually 30, 200, 1000 or CM, depending upon the situation and the experience of the homoeopath. |

# Actaea Racemosa
## (Black Snake - Root)

This remedy is also called Cimicifuga. It is extraordinarily effective in **women's diseases**, especially those complicating pregnancy. Normally, if during menstruation copious bleeding occurs, most menstrual complaints cease automatically. But in the case of Actaea Racemosa, the more the bleeding, the more is the pain and associated discomfort. Sometimes, the symptoms continue even after the cessation of the menstrual period.

Actaea Racemosa is very useful for **joint pains**. The tissues hurt like an abscess. There is a lightning type of **pain in the muscles of the neck and back**, spreading in all directions. Rest relieves the discomfort, while movement makes it worse. Cold and humidity relieve the symptoms. In Actaea Racemosa, there is also **shifting of the disease** from one part of the body to another, like Abrotinum. Generally, the physical illnesses transform into mental illnesses. If the physical illnesses in children are suppressed by some kind of treatment, mental symptoms appear and can produce conditions like **hysteria**. A sensitive girl of a touchy disposition will become totally silent. If called in a loud voice, she will simply start crying. She would be indifferent to the rest of the world, and seem totally lost in herself. In such a case, Actaea Racemosa is the best possible remedy.

This remedy is deeply related to sadness. Grief **and sorrow** can result in physical illnesses. **Mental shock in sensitive women can result in irregularity of the menstruation, joint pains or other physical illnesses**. **Mental shock** will make them fearful and superstitious. They will not even like to take any medicine in case it is mixed with poison. If there is preponderance of suspicion in addition to other symptoms, two doses of Actaea Racemosa can clear the symptom of suspicion and make the patient well again.

In Actaea Racemosa, there are symptoms of two apparently opposing remedies. In some aspects, it is like Bryonia, and in another aspect, like Rhus Tox. In Bryonia, it is movement, and in Rhus Tox, it is rest which aggravates the discomfort. In Actaea Racemosa, the person will feel discomfort on whatever side he or she lies. There would be twitching of the muscles. The **headache** is mostly behind the eyeballs and the back of the head, which is relieved by pressure, but movement makes the headache worse. The person feels **dizzy** and there is heaviness in the head. The vision becomes dim. Engrossed deep in studies, worry and bladder symptoms cause headache.

Like Abrotinum, in Actaea Racemosa, **constipation and diarrhoea** alternate with each other. There is severe pain in the stomach, which gets better on bending forward. Due to pressure on the backbone and over the reproductive organs, there is a tendency towards **nausea and vomiting**. Young girls experience severe vomiting during their first pregnancy, which does not seem to be relieved by any medicine. In such a case, one should study carefully the temperament of the patient and the symptoms of the ailment before prescribing any remedy. If the patient is of Actaea Racemosa type, then she would definitely get better with Actaea Racemosa.

In feeble-minded women, at the time of **delivery**, the labour pains, instead of pushing down to facilitate the childbirth, scatter right and left, causing spasms over the hips. This is the main feature of Actaea Racemosa. Actaea Racemosa, when given in time, will normalise the direction of labour pains and facilitate the childbirth. Caulophyllum is another very important remedy at the time of child delivery. In Caulophyllum, instead of pains bearing down, they scatter down inside of the thighs and the mouth of the uterus does not open. Sometimes, physicians and midwives try to alleviate this problem by using ergot but instead this closes the mouth of the uterus tightly and makes the woman suffer further. Unfortunately, some women die in such circumstances. Once, while I was in Anwarabad, Sindh (Larkana), in a convention, a person came to me and very humbly submitted that his wife was in the process of labour but the mouth of the uterus was tightly closed, and there was a danger that his wife might die. I took Colophylum out of my travel bag and gave it to him to give to his wife. Within ten to fifteen minutes, a healthy baby boy was born normally. Homoeopathic medicines should not be taken lightly. Their timely use can save from potentially serious complications.

Women with weak uterine muscles and associated organs abort repeatedly or conceive after great difficulty. Colophylum may be very useful in such women. At the time of labour, Gelsemium should also be kept in mind, like Actaea Racemosa and Colophylum. If during **labour**, the pains remain localized at the back and after bearing down return to the back, then Gelsemium would be very useful in such a case. In Kali Carb, instead of bearing down, the labour pains scatter to the outer side of the thighs. In Pulsatilla, due to nervous disability or fear, the labour pains are very weak and rare.

In Actaea Racemosa, the **periods are irregular or delayed**. There is severe spasmodic **pain at the uterus and in the back**. The organs feel heavy. A typical Actaea Racemosa woman is very lazy, sad and confused. Her mind is clouded. She observes dreadful dreams, speaks constantly but does not concentrate on anything. She becomes easily frightened; especially the **fear of death** prevails in her mind. This reminds one of Aconite.

In Actaea Racemosa, there is irritation of the throat, a **dry cough** is very bothersome at night and becomes worse on talking. The heartbeat is fast while the pulse is weak and irregular. There are symptoms of angina, like numbness of left arm, which is typical of Actaea Racemosa. The **muscles and bones of the back hurt** a lot. The neck and the upper part of the back are very stiff. There is sense of discomfort and restlessness of the arms and legs. The person feels itching, and there is **jerking of the limbs**. There is lack of sleep and the mind remains perturbed and undulating. The person feels as if his head has grown bigger in size. The ears are very sensitive to noise. The symptoms of Actaea Racemosa are aggravated in the morning and in cold weather, except the headache, which gets better in hot weather and by taking food.

| | |
|---|---|
| **Antidotes:** | Aconite, Baptisia |
| **Potency:** | 30 to CM |

# ADRENALIN
## (Epinephrin)

Adrenalin is the secretion of the glands situated above the kidneys called the Suprarenal Glands. It keeps the function of other glands in balance. All Adrenalin patients exhibit symptoms resulting from anger, fear and terror. The heart beats faster and the blood pressure rises. There is a feeling of suffocation and tightness. The peristaltic movements of the intestines become sluggish and the mouth is dry. It has the property of constricting the muscles in the walls of the arteries. In Homoeopathy, it is used to **stop any kind of bleeding**, whether it be in the lungs, nose, intestines, uterus or somewhere else. In case the signs and symptoms do not point to one particular medicine, Adrenalin should be used right away. It has been especially found useful in the control of bleeding from the nose. Some **surgeons use it before an operation to decrease the blood loss.**

One expert physician has described it to be useful in **angina** and similar symptoms, like pain over the heart area and behind the sternum (chest-bone), which gets worse on walking. Adrenalin is also useful in the suffocating **tightness of the chest**. **High blood pressure**, secondary to contraction of the arteries can also be treated with Adrenalin in Homoeopathic potency. This is not my own observation; I have just presented the opinion of other physicians. Adrenalin should be put to use with extreme care, after careful evaluation of the patient.

I have certainly found it useful in some illnesses like **blood in the urine,** or if the urination is frequent and plentiful and associated with scalding before and after passing the urine. These symptoms are also found in Natrum Mur.

Adrenalin is very useful in **corns of the toes**. The Adrenalin patient complains of tiredness at the legs and feels pain and cramps in the calves.

| | |
|---|---|
| **Potency:** | 30 to 200 |

# Aesculus Hippocastanum
## (Horse Chestnut)

The most salient feature of Aesculus Hippocastanum is mental confusion. Physical and mental fatigue can naturally result in some sort of mental confusion and restlessness but in Aesculus, the mental confusion is aggravated by sleep. On waking up in the morning, the patient is confused and disorientated as to where he is and what is going on around him. A healthy person can also feel lost in a strange place following a journey, but this confusion is very short-lived. In the Aesculus patient, the mental confusion is very prolonged. The **memory is weak**, and there is feeling of anger or grief along with a dislike for every kind of activity.

The Aesculus children have **poor memory**. They are angry by nature and if they are startled in sleep, and if treated harshly, they can go into mental shock and become **unconscious**. Sometimes, it can lead to epilepsy. Aesculus is not only for children, but it can be used in patients of all ages.

**Congestion of the eyes** is a very salient sign of Aesculus Hippocastanum. This is due to the weakness of the blood vessels of the eyes. The eyes become red on slight increase of pressure. Some Homoeopaths call it the piles of the eyes. The eyes feel heavy and watery. The eyelids and the area below the left eye exhibit twitching of the small muscles and the eyeballs hurt.

An Aesculus patient generally feels cold. Pain is alleviated by heat application. **Pains fleet around the whole body,** as in Pulsatilla. However, the Pulsatilla symptoms however are aggravated by heat, and cold relieves them. The Pulsatilla patient has the tendency to remain grieved, but with a mild temperament. The Aesculus patient also inclines to be in a state of grief, but is hot-tempered and feels better by heat.

In an Aesculus patient, the **back constantly feels weak and tired**. The **backbone also is weak**. The patient staggers on walking due to the **weakness of the back and legs**. He finds it difficult to stand up after sitting down. There is pain between the shoulders and back of the neck. The **pain in the right shoulder and the chest** gets worse on deep inbreathing. Hands and feet burn and hands become red on washing them. There is a fleeting type of stiffness and aching of the joints. There are lightning spells of a piercing type of pain, which get better with heat application. All these symptoms are in the domain of Aesculus Hippocastanum.

In Aesculus, there is a unique kind of **piles** consisting of large, bluish warts, like bunches of grapes, associated with severe burning. The pain becomes worse on standing and walking. There is burning at the anus and dryness and a feeling as if some small sticks are lodged in the rectum. Stools are hard, dry and are passed with difficulty and after defecation, there is intense pain.

In Aesculus, **kidney pain** is also very evident especially in the left kidney. Urination is frequent, scanty and associated with burning. Urine is dark-coloured.
Women experience severe **backache**, weakness during the menses and a feeling of sagging of the uterus that is typical in Aesculus. Leucorrhoea is dark yellow coloured and thick and sticky.

In Aesculus, there are **symptoms related to the heart** also, such as burning pain over the heart, rapid heartbeat, pulsating blood vessels, and a feeling of heat over the chest.

Other features of Aesculus are a feeling of constant discomfort, burning and severe nausea after food intake. **Digestion is weak.** A heavy feeling of the stomach as if there is a weight on it, food turning acidic, excessive sour belching, a metallic taste in the mouth, copious sticky sputum and a thick yellowish-white coating on the tongue are all characteristics of Aesculus Hippocastanum. The **throat feels hot,** dry and sore. While swallowing, the pain goes to the ears. In Aesculus Hippocastanum, the symptoms aggravate with cold, walking around, after eating and on getting up after sleep. The discomfort of piles also gets worse in cold weather. Lying down in the open, and rest relieve the symptoms.

Aesculus Hippocastanum is also very useful in **varicose veins. Varicose veins commonly occur in women during pregnancy in**

**the form of blue spider webs** and distended tortuous veins which can be really bothersome.

| | |
|---|---|
| **Antidote:** | Nux Vomica |
| **Potency:** | 30 to 200 |

# Aethusa Cynapium
## (Fool's Parsley)

Aethusa Cynapium, if truly analogous to the disease complex, works wonders. In allopathy, there is no match for this Homoeopathic remedy. This is the best remedy for **wasting disease of the children (marasmus).** The child cannot digest milk; he throws up as soon as he drinks milk. The **vomiting** renders him very weak. He feels hungry, takes milk-feed and immediately vomits again. The **constipation** is severe. If **diarrhoea** ensues, the stools are small. Firstly, they are yellowish in colour and then, turn greenish (bile-coloured). There is intense griping in the abdomen. In addition to diarrhoea, there is a tendency to repeated vomiting of clotted milk.

The majority of the children are severely constipated. Diarrhoea is rare. The child is usually drowsy and steadily goes on getting weaker. Once a marasmic child was brought to me who looked terrible. His head was large, his face drawn and shrivelled, and his body was just a bony skeleton. His parents told me that they had tried many medicines but to no avail, since the child was constipated for over a month, and threw up after every milk feed. I gave him Aethusa. Soon his constipation was relieved, he could digest milk and his condition started improving. Within a week, the child became hale and hearty.

Marasmus is also found in Abrotanum. In Abrotanum, the wasting begins in the legs and then spreads upwards towards the chest and neck. In Aethusa, wasting involves the entire body simultaneously. Another sign of Aethusa is that with heat, the sickness migrates towards the head. For a child with some **mental deficiency** and a **tendency to throw up milk immediately after feed,** Aethusa is the remedy. Aethusa will cure his mental as well as abdominal problem. With conventional allopathic treatment, if the child is treated for his abdominal problem, he will become mentally ill, even insane. Clear-cut symptoms of Aethusa warrant the use of Aethusa alone.

In Aethusa Cynapium, the illness comes on with full force followed by **mental and physical exhaustion, drowsiness and delirium**. The patient is extremely superstitious and hallucinates about cats, dogs and mice. He lacks concentration. He is sad and feels uneasy. The head feels tied up in a vice. There is **pain at the back of the head**, which radiates down the neck, shoulders and upper back. This pain is relieved by pressure or lying down, as well as after passing stools and wind (flatus). Hairs feel stretched. There is drowsiness, dizziness and palpitation. When dizziness ends, the head starts feeling warm.

The **eyes are very sensitive to light. The margins of the eyelids swell**. The eyeballs roll around during sleep. The eyes are drawn downwards. Things appear larger than their actual size. The **ears ache**, with a feeling of discharge of warm fluid with hissing sounds. Thick nasal secretions causes blockage of the nose. The tip of the nose feels sore. An ineffective desire to sneeze is typical of Aethusa. Red marks appear on the face. The jaws hurt and feel stiff. The tongue is dry and feels too long. **Burning and blisters of the throat** make swallowing difficult. At times, due to difficulty in breathing and feeling suffocated, the patient may not even speak. The chest feels tight.

Aethusa is very useful in **diseases of the women**. During **menstruation**, if there is excessive watery bleeding and painful swelling of the breasts, uterine discomfort and sluggish intestinal movements (peristalsis), vomiting soon after eating without nausea, along with some other peculiar symptoms of Aethusa Cynapium, they will all respond to Aethusa.

The symptoms of Aethusa intensify early in the morning, at about 3 to 4 a.m., with cold water and in warm bedding. All the symptoms, except mental, subside in the open air. Aethusa is very good in **teething diarrhoea of children**. In Aethusa patients, there may also be numbness of the arms and feet, and developing cramp. The elbows are spastic. Fingers and thumbs clench. There is numbness in the hands and the feet. Aethusa is useful in **epilepsy** too. The limbs feel cold and tight along with frothing from the mouth. The child cannot hold the head up, vomits immediately after milk feed and then demands milk soon after.

Aethusa is considered useful by some homoeopaths for students who get confused and very apprehensive in the examination hall. One dose of Aethusa Cynapium 200 taken on the morning of the exam is found very useful.

| | |
|---|---|
| **Adjuvant:** | Calcaria Carb. |
| **Potency:** | 30 to 200 |

# Agaricus Muscarius
## (Fly Fungus)

The most salient sign of Agaricus Muscarius is shaking of the body, secondary to **mental stress** and weakness of the muscles. The hands are tremulous, the limbs display jerky movements and the whole body quivers.

**Jerky movements** are also a characteristic of Actea Racemosa (Cimicifuga), with the difference that the violent movements are on the same side as one lies on, while in Agaricus, the whole body quivers. **Tremors and spasms** both exist. The eyes also shake and sway. The eyesight is not focussed. I once happened to see a young man suffering from this ailment which was progressing with age. Agaricus Muscarius significantly benefited him to the extent that he could do his regular work normally.

In Agaricus, **eye symptoms** are very prominent, such as double vision, black spots dancing before the eyes, **squinting, burning and irritation of the eyes** and a feeling of fatigue. It is difficult to focus the eye on one particular point. Reading becomes difficult, the eyeballs swing like a pendulum, and the discharge of the eye is yellowish and sticky. The mind becomes weak. Concentrated studies and mental work cause fatigue. Such children are very stubborn in nature, irritable and sensitive. **If checked harshly**, they may go into mental shock and become unconscious (more so in the case of Aesculus). Agaricus should be given to children even if rolling movements of the eyeballs are absent. Some children are basically mentally weak, more so in the morning. They cannot understand any new idea. They are sluggish, physically as well as mentally. As the day passes, they become mentally alert, normal and cheerful by the end of the day. These symptoms are very similar in Agaricus and Aesculus, except for their timing.

In Agaricus, weakness of nerves can induce **deafness**. Exposure to cold causes **earache**, with redness and burning of the skin. The feet burn, itch and become red. Sometimes in extreme cold, if one enters a heated room, hands and feet start to itch and become red and swollen. This condition is called Chillblain. Any condition in which the blood accumulates in one particular part of the body causing distension, redness, **itching** and pain, will be relieved by Agaricus Muscarius. Similar conditions can be found in some **allergies** (for example, during the treatment of malaria). If associated with other symptoms and signs of Agaricus, Agaricus Muscarius will cure these without the help of any other anti-allergic treatment. One or at the most two doses will suffice (by the grace of Allah). Sometimes, Phosphorus may also be helpful in such a situation. Some children happen to stammer. **Stammering** is in fact due to some kind of fear. It should be treated psychologically also. In general, Stramonium is very useful in deep mental and neurological conditions, but has not been found sufficiently effective in the treatment of stammers. So one must carefully scrutinize the cause of the illness before suggesting any remedy. Agaricus may be one possible remedy for stammering.

In Agaricus Muscarius, the illness has **fleeting tendency**. Sometimes women, during their nursing period, may have been subjected to mental shock (due to some severe accident, grief or mental pressure), causing the **milk production (lactation) to be suppressed**. If the milk is insufficient due to the mental shock, Agaricus can be very useful. Pulsatilla will be the right medication for Pulsatilla type patient. Other remedies used for normalizing lactation are:

| | |
|---|---|
| Agnus Castus | Aconite |
| Bryonia | Asafoetida |
| Causticum | Calcarea Carbonica |
| Lac Defloratum | Chamomilla |
| Phytolacca | Phosphoric Acid |
| Silicea | Secale |
| | Urtica |

In Agaricus, like Aesculus, the pains tend to radiate downwards. Being related to the nerves, the pains are not dull and localised; instead, they may radiate to one side and then to the other. In such a case, Agaricus is more effective

In Agaricus Muscarius, the **abdomen is full of wind** (or gas) due to sluggish intestinal movements. In such cases, Nux Vomica is also very promptly effective. It restores the intestinal mobility in transient as well as established condition. Sulphur works for prolonged periods and Aconite works temporarily. Nux Vomica is between the two.

The Agaricus patient is usually very quiet. Typically the facial muscles twitch. The intestinal muscles also fasciculate, but do not have the propulsive power. In such a case, Agaricus is the remedy.

In Agaricus Muscarius, one experiences **hallucinations** as a result of blood poisoning due to the toxins produced inside the uterus. If the uterus does not expel the placental membranes after the childbirth, it can affect the mind. In this condition, Pulsatilla is a good general remedy for the **natural cleaning of the uterus**. If the infection sets in the uterus and Puerperel fever develops, Sulphur 200 and Pyrogenium 200 should be given. If there are hallucinations and milk formation in the breast is decreased, Agaricus Muscarius will be very advantageous. In the case of infection, Silicia, Kali Mur, Ferrum Phos and Kali Phos, all six 6X, should be mixed and given in addition to Sulphur and Pyrogenium.

In Agaricus, we see **eczema** also. It is recognised by the blisters containing yellow exudate, which develop along the course of the nerves. It is often seen that the neurological conditions can transform into eczema. In some other conditions, vesicles develop along the course of the peripheral nerves, such as in herpes. But Agaricus is not the remedy for herpes.

**Herpes** of different kinds is a very painful disease. It should be clearly recognised and treated timely to avoid dangerous complications. Previously, I used to prescribe Silicia, Kali Phos and Kali Mur for herpes which helped to some extent. Later on, I found that the best treatment for herpes was that as for snakebite, i.e. Arnica 200, Ledum 200 and Arsenic 200. This combination offered unusually quick cure (when I used this formula on late Aftab Ahmad Khan Sahib during a **severe attack of herpes**). Due to the frequent mutation of the herpes virus and changing pattern of the disease, in my knowledge there is no one standard remedy which would be of use all the time.

The Agaricus patient does not have full control on his limbs. **Things drop out of his hands**. Crockery frequently falls and breaks. His grip is not strong enough. Severe muscle pains and spasms occur in the limbs. Hands and feet twist violently.

In Agaricus, the symptoms aggravate after taking food, in the open and in cold weather. Sleep fails to improve the symptoms. The patient feels drowsy all day. Itching and burning are conspicuously present.

| | |
|---|---|
| **Antidotes:** | Cinthium, Coffea, Camphor |
| **Potency:** | 30 to 200 |

# Agnus Castus
## (The Chaste Tree)

Agnus Castus is mostly related to diseases of women. After **childbirth**, the **muscles become weak, stretched and flabby**. They do not revert to their original tone and physical status. (This is just like a stretched out piece of rubber which loses its elasticity.) The uterus feels like it is sagging downwards. **Menses are scanty. Infertility** and **hatred towards conjugal relationship** develops. **Leucorrhoeal** discharge is yellow. The woman feels uneasy, sad and depressed. She is usually sad and sallow. She may develop **hysteria**. The uterus remains inflamed. The nose bleeds. Agnus Castus is a treatment of choice in this symptom complex.

The Agnus Castus patient thinks of committing **suicide** and is indifferent to the world around her. She prepares herself for impending death. In Arum Mur, the tendency to commit suicide and **depression** are prominent features which become part of the patient's temperament. But in Agnus Castus, such tendency is transient and short-lived.

The patient has a weak **memory**, she is absent-minded and neurotic, she lacks courage and lacks determination. She feels pain on the temporal areas and forehead, aggravated by movement.

The patient is **hypersensitive to light** (as in many other remedies) and develops headache due to light-hypersensitivity. In case the headache is already present, it becomes unbearable in light, so much so that the eyes cannot be opened. Graphites is good in isolated light-sensitivity without the symptoms of Agnus Castus.
The **bony bridge of the nose is painful** but feels better with pressure. The patient can be unusually sensitive to certain kinds of fragrance. The cheeks itch and tingle, this is specific in Agnus Castus.

There is wind in the tummy. The stomach rumbles. The intestines seem to be falling downwards, and the patient holds on to the drooping belly.

Agnus Castus is useful in certain **male sexual disorders**, such as sexual weakness and impotence, secondary to the pubertal misconduct. It also relieves **nervous disorders** (like Kali Phos).

| | |
|---|---|
| **Adjuvants:** | Caladium, Selenium |
| **Antidotes:** | Camphor, Nux Vomica |
| **Potency:** | 30 to CM |

# ALLIUM CEPA
## (Red Onion)

Allium Cepa is prepared from the red onion and is very helpful in **nasal catarrh** of the winter season. Its symptoms resemble those caused during the peeling of onions. The **throat becomes hoarse**, nasal secretions are watery and acidic. The eyes water, but do not get red or irritated. (Euphrasia causes watering from the eyes with burning type of itch and redness.) The other point of difference in Allium Cepa is that there is a persistent cough day and night. **In Euphrasia**, as the nasal secretions pour out of the eyes during the day the cough is less frequent, but at night the cough gets aggravated due to the dripping of the nasal secretions in the throat or into the lungs. The patient wakes up and experiences severe **bouts of coughing**. The cough steadily starts easing off in the morning. The eyes start watering and redness occurs.

Allium Cepa does not produce redness in the eyes, instead it involves the ears which ache, discharge and become partially deaf. If it happens as the result of a nasal cold, it can respond favourably to Allium Cepa, or other remedies like Chamomilla, Pulsatilla and Ammonium Carb should be sought as indicated.

In Allium Cepa, the **symptoms tend to migrate from the right to the left**. This also happens in Lachesis, where the symptoms start on the left side, and as the body defence responds, they migrate to the right side. The venom of the majority of the snakes mostly affects the left side of the body. It is strange but interesting to know that snakes hate onions. In the Sindh province of Pakistan, people spread onions around their beds to keep the snakes at bay and this method works.

In Allium Cepa, the symptoms of illness are aggravated by rest and relieved by movement. At night, the symptoms worsen. One catches cold in cold and damp weather, and feels relieved in open air. Along with the cold, there is **headache**, especially on the right temporal area to the forehead. The **cold affects the left nostril** before the right.

Allium Cepa is very helpful in **whooping cough** and **chicken pox**. Allium Cepa is very good in vomiting, indigestion and the passing of foul gas in the early course of chicken pox. It is also good in the **abdominal pain** of children.

In Allium Cepa, abdominal pain causes an urge to pass urine with **burning pain at the bladder**. The **urine is reddish** in color. Along with cold symptoms there is frequent urination. The voice is hoarse, the throat is irritated and the windpipe hurts. There is severe coughing and repeated sneezing. The back of the neck hurts. The patient feels chills from the back downwards at night. Consequently, the patient has to pass urine frequently.

Sometimes along with the nasal catarrh, tiny little red pimples appear with a piercing sensation. Some areas of the body feel burning hot. Allium Cepa is useful in **neuralgic pains** especially of the face, teeth, head and neck.

| | |
|---|---|
| **Adjuvant:** | Phosphorus, Thuja, Pulsatilla |
| **Antidotes:** | Arnica, Chamomilla, Veratrum Album |
| **Potency:** | 30 to 200 |

# ALOE
## (Socotrine – Aloes)

This medicine is prepared from a plant called *Kanwar Gandal* in Urdu. Its main characteristics are flatulence, diarrhoea and the tendency to vomit. Hundreds of medicines can be used in this kind of symptom complex, but they have their own additional, distinctive features as well. In Aloe and Lycopodium, typically, one gets diarrhoea after ingesting oysters. Aloe should also be considered along with Lycopodium wherever a patient suffers from diarrhoea after eating seafood. In the patients of Aloe and Lycopodium, the abdomen is bloated in the right lower part. Generally, homoeopaths suggest one of the three remedies for distension of the abdomen: Carbo Veg for the fullness and distension in the upper part, Lycopodium for the distension of the right lower abdomen and China when the whole of abdomen is tense. However, distension of the abdomen is also a symptom of other homoeopathic medicines, which will need to be used as indicated. The above three have been mentioned in most homoeopathic books as quick fixes for immediate use. Prolonged abdominal distension may lead to colicky pains. In emergency situations, especially if the condition of the patient is deteriorating fast, the standard formula as detailed above should be adopted. Nevertheless, real, lasting relief will only be offered by a proper constitutional remedy.

Nux Vomica is very useful when the **intestinal movement is sluggish**. Carbo Veg will be more appropriate if the patient passes offensive wind. In the Carbo Veg patient, there is a **spasm at the pyloric end of the stomach due to hyperacidity**. The food becomes stagnant and decays. The stomach becomes distended with foul smelling gas.

China is useful in abdominal distension only where other signs of China are also present, i.e., patient has dryness in constitution and generally displays signs of the ill effects of Malaria. Sometimes, the wind or gas becomes trapped in the intestines due to a lack of digestive secretions from the stomach, liver, pancreas and the intestines. China is especially useful in this kind of distension.

Returning to the main subject of Aloe, **ingestion of seafood, especially oysters, is immediately followed by diarrhoea**. Along with **nausea and vomiting**, the patient suffers from **headache**, starting from the forehead. The eyes are red, heavy and difficult to open. The lips are dry. Chewing produces an audible noise in the ears. Sometimes, Aloe patients bleed from the nose as they wake up in the morning. The mouth tastes bitter. Typically, there is pain under the ribs on the right side. Loose motions are associated with gripe. The **piles** hang in bunches and feel burning hot. Cold applications offer relief. If the patient is **constipated** instead of having loose motions, the lower part of the abdomen feels severely tense. Meat does not bother the patient of Aloe, yet the patient does not like to eat it.

Aloe women experience **aggravation of their symptoms during their menstruation** period. Walking and standing becomes difficult. The uterus feels full and heavy due to pelvic congestion. The **periods appear earlier than usual and are excessive** (Menorrhagia).

Another sign of Aloe is irritation of the throat and coughing. The joints ache. The symptoms are worse in the morning, more so in the hot, dry weather. The cold weather and open air offer relief. Mostly the symptoms start or intensify after food intake.

**Adjuvant:** Sulphur
**Antidotes:** Sulphur, Opium
**Potency:** 30

# Alumen
## (Common Potash Alum)

Alumen is the common alum, which is used to control bleeding from any wound. It is famous for clumping together the suspended particles in a solution (colloids). However, it cannot clump suspended matter in air or in gas. The venom of several kinds of snakes acts similarly on the blood. The clots/clumps thus formed, precipitate heart attack by blocking the blood vessels of the heart.

If Alumen is directly added to the blood, it will clump the red and white cells, but the fluid part of the blood i.e. serum, which contains the 12 salts in a properly balanced form, is not affected by it. The alum is also used to clean dirty water. The dust particles in colloidal form precipitate to the bottom of the container and the clean water comes to the surface. In this process, a slight amount of alum remains in the water. Therefore, Alumen symptoms are not uncommon in areas such as the Sindh province in Pakistan.

In Alumen, the patients develop deep **ulcers** or abscesses. The abscesses may gradually progress to cancer formation. Chronic ulcers, as well as cancer of the tongue and throat can develop. The lymph glands become swollen and indurate. The tonsils enlarge and become firm. Hard nodules develop in the uterus, as well as in the mammary glands (the breast).

Like Sulphur, there is a feeling of heat and pressure on the scalp. Being very sensitive, the patient of Sulphur cannot tolerate the pressure of the hand or even the touch of a cloth, while the patient of Alumen feels comfort with pressure.

In Alumen, the **muscles are very weak** as in Plumbum. In other words, the **paralytic features** of Alumen and Plumbum are very much similar.

All these ill effects of Alumen, as already mentioned, are amenable to the homoeopathic potency of Alumen, irrespective of the cause of the symptoms. If these symptoms and signs are of Alumen and the constitution of the patient is also of Alumen, then Alumen will offer cure. In addition, **prolapsed uterus due to weaker pelvic muscles** will also get better with Alumen.

One of the salient features of Alumen is **persistent hoarseness of the voice**. Transient hoarseness is treatable with Borax, Coca or Arsenic. However, as a matter of principle, one should not merely depend upon hoarseness of the voice to establish the diagnosis. Other relevant features of these remedies should also be sought. The illnesses of the throat will benefit from this proper constitutional remedy. Persistent hoarseness is the nature of Alumen.

Alumen acts profoundly and for long time. Nevertheless it can also cure acute illnesses. It is very useful in **diseases of the intestines**, **obstinate constipation** and intractable bleeding tendency. It is of great use in the breathing problems of the elderly. It is also very beneficial in relieving the tightness of the air passages, difficulty of swallowing liquids and the indurate glands under the tongue.
A severe **headache** associated with heaviness of the head is also a symptom of Alumen. Pressure applied locally offers comfort. All the muscles feel weak. The cold weather aggravates all the symptoms except the headache, which the cold relieves.

| | |
|---|---|
| **Antidotes:** | Chamomilla, Nux Vomica, Sulphur, Ipecac |
| **Potency:** | 30 – 200 |

# ALUMINA
## (Oxide of Aluminium – Argilla)

The chemical compound Alumina is prepared from aluminium, a metal from which numerous utensils are made. Most cooking pots and bathroom appliances are made from it. Early on, this metal was very costly, only the rich and the elite could afford aluminium pots. Now, due to industrial development, this metal is vastly available and is quite cheap with the poor tending to use these utensils the most.

Modern research has indicated that the prolonged use of aluminium pots for cooking produces a very harmful effect on the health of the users. This poison affects slowly, but becomes a permanent part of the human body. The aluminium constricts the walls of blood vessels. Cholesterol starts depositing itself inside the blood vessels. Progressive narrowing or even total blockage can ensue. Thus, cholesterol can cause a heart attack due to the blockage of the arteries leading to the heart. Similarly, it affects the blood vessels going to the brain. This process of progressive hardening and narrowing of the arteries is called “Arteriosclerosis". The ageing process starts to manifest itself fast. The memory becomes weak. The blood pressure fluctuates. Mental and physical deterioration sets in. Alumina, being a slow acting remedy, should be used for long periods extending over years. To achieve permanent cure, one should use Alumina in high potency at long intervals, such as 1000 or 10,000 given once in a month. A potency 200 will have to be given every ten days, extending over many months or years. In the beginning of the treatment, no beneficial effect will be noticed. Once the improvement begins, the dead and dying fibres of the circular muscles start reverting to life. The patient must be told to continue the treatment for at least a year or two without fail in order to get relief from this long-established disease.

The Alumina **itch** does not exhibit lumps or bumps. At first, the itching begins on apparently clean, healthy-looking skin. Itching leads to inflammation which leads to formation of pimples or, on scratching intensely, blister formation. One may bleed as a result of scratching. The affected part becomes insensitive and subject to infection and further complication. In general, (unlike Alumina), in most of the remedies, the bumps over the skin appear first and the itching comes on later.

The **eyelids swell** and become thick and heavy. The eyelashes fall. The vision becomes blurred. The eyes are very sensitive to light, especially in the morning. The eyelids are sticky and the objects look pale or yellow.

The stomach fails to function. There is a complete loss of appetite and dislike for meat. The patient craves to eat indigestible things like clay and coal. The stomach becomes inflamed and goes into spasms. One of the main features is marked acidity. Nothing tastes right. There is frequent acidic belching. Alumina is useful in all these symptoms. The dysfunction of the stomach is due to the narrowing and thickening of its blood vessels.

Alumina is very useful in acute **hyperacidity**, as well as the chronic illnesses of the stomach. It relieves long-standing **haemorrhoids**. It also relieves acidity in both men and women. It is particularly useful in the leucorrhoea associated with acidic discharge. This discharge is so acidic, that it may lead to other illnesses. Normally, women do not get constipated during pregnancy, in Alumina however, they do. **Constipation associated with pregnancy**, which is transient or of long-standing, will respond to Alumina administration.

Alumina is very important in a **chronic cough** originating from the lungs, as are Bacillinum, Phosphorus, Arsenic, Iodide and Kali Carb. If the other symptoms of Alumina are also present, this would be the most appropriate remedy.

In Alumina, typically, **reasoning and decision-making** deteriorate. One may not easily decide one way or the other. The mind becomes cloudy and suspicious. Whatever the patient sees or hears, it appears to him as if somebody else is seeing or hearing it. He loses his self-identity. Sometimes, he wishes to occupy someone else's mind so that he may observe things better. This slowly progressive trend of his drives him insane. However, he is not dangerous to others, he simply gets lost in himself.

Mentally, the patient shows impatience. For him, time stands still, but he likes it to pass quickly. At the sight of sharp weapons, he is afraid, lest he may hurt himself. Such patients frighten others by pretending to commit suicide, though actually they do not do so. Sometimes, people look down from a height and others get terrified, in case they may leap to their death.

The Alumina patient is very sad and sallow. He has the desire to distance himself from his surroundings. He worries that he may be going insane. Such negative thoughts are at their climax in the morning.

Sometimes, the alumina affects the **throat muscles**, resulting in difficulty in swallowing. Due to weakness of these muscles, the food may enter the windpipe or nose.

Paralysis may affect the sphincter muscles of the bladder and the rectum, resulting in difficulty in passing urine and stools. The patient has to strain his abdominal muscles, even if the stools are soft. Urinary symptoms resemble those of enlarged prostate gland. Many a time, the stools resemble the droppings of a goat, camel and horse, in the shape of small or large balls, which stick to each other. The stools may be soft or thick but are difficult to pass.

In Graphites and Plumbum too, stools are similar. The urine may leak unknowingly due to the paralysis of the muscles of the neck of the bladder. Involuntary defeacation can also occur due to weakness of the sphincter muscles at the anus.

The Alumina patient experiences dizziness and imbalance during walking. The feet tend to be numb. Pain radiates from one point to all directions, like the spokes of a wheel. When all these symptoms are together, Alumina is the remedy.

The movements of the limbs, lower as well as upper, may not remain under voluntary control, thus resulting in a staggering gait. In this situation, long term use of Alumina is beneficial.

In Alumina, **catarrhal and skin symptoms** are very frequent. The patient has chronic catarrh, which is full of dry encrustations with long strings. The catarrh may result in the dimness of the eyesight. The inner linings (mucus membranes) of the stomach, intestines and kidneys become inflamed. Headache also, is common with the cold.

Like the mucus membranes, the skin also becomes subjected to many ailments. As a result of intense itching, the skin becomes thick and sore and may even ulcerate. As in Sulphur, the warmth of the bed intensifies the itching. The face feels as if a cobweb is spread over it. The tip of the nose shows cuts. The eyes burn and trachoma may develop. Alumina affects both flexor as well as extensor muscles (the flexor muscles bend the joints, while the extensors stretch the joints).

Salt, alcohol, vinegar, chillies, potatoes, and fizzy drinks aggravate the symptoms of Alumina. **Piles and anal fissuring** are typical of Alumina.

Male sexual impotence and **nocturnal emission** are common. The **prostate gland enlarges** along with the feeling of heaviness and fullness around it. Sexual organs become partially paralyzed. The man becomes sexually impotent in spite of being in good general health.

As a result of prolonged catarrh the women develop chronic **leucorrhoea**. The uterus tends to sag downwards, much more so on standing and walking. If **gonorrhoea** has merely been suppressed by some kind of treatment, but not cured, the residual inflammation of the pelvic organs results in the sensation of heat and discomfort. Alumina may be of use in this situation.

The cough of Alumina may be associated with sneezing and the throat feels as if it is being gently tickled with feathers. In Alumina, at the point of backache, the patient feels intense heat, as if a hot iron has been placed on the numbed part. The soles of the feet become soft, swollen and tender. The side the patient sits or lies on becomes numb. The legs tend to be numb also. The patient feels cold and likes to wrap himself well, but he likes the face to be exposed to the cool breeze. The patient likes the warmth of the bed for a while, but intense itching begins when the bed becomes too warm. The hands usually remain cold and warm up slowly on retiring to bed. The skin is dry and sweats only sparingly, or not at all.

| | |
|---|---|
| **Adjuvant:** | Bryonia |
| **Antidotes:** | Ipecac, Chamomilla |

# Ambra Grisea
## (Ambergis – A morbid secretion of the whale)

Ambra Grisea is a useful homoeopathic remedy for thin, lean, short-tempered, irritable and easily provoked children as well as adults. Over-sensitivity is its peculiar feature. Vertigo and loss of balance can manifest in early age, which normally happen in old age. So this remedy can also be very useful in common old age ailments.

The Ambra Grisea patient is usually very **sad**, even if there is no specific underlying cause. Ambra Grisea is the correct treatment of the patients who remain sad, like to sit aloof in the dark, become depressed over trivial matters, lose all zeal to live, show total indifference to their surroundings and start showing physical signs of ageing prematurely. They feel **dizzy**. The head and the stomach feel weak. The forehead feels heavy and the head hurts with variable intensity. There is drowsiness too. The **memory is weak**. The hairs on the scalp fall easily. When bleeding from the nose and gums occurs, it is copious. Gas accumulates in the stomach. Belching is sour, but the feeling it produces in the stomach is that of soothing, rather than burning.

In Ambra Grisea, a **lack of concentration** is natural. The head feels numb and this feeling spreads over the whole body.

Ambra Grisea ailments tend to remain localized only on one side like in Bryonia, Belladona and Spigelia. They are present and remain strictly either on right or left side.

Typically, the Ambra Grisea patient **cannot tolerate music**. The music intensifies the headaches, mental anguish as well as the physical symptoms. In other words, instead of comforting the person, the music provokes mental and physical commotion.

In Ambra Grisea, symptoms of old age, such as **numbness of the hands and feet**, palpitation and flabby muscles creep in rapidly. Ambra Grisea is very useful in minimizing the effects of sudden shock. I have often used Ambra Grisea on women who have been

**deeply grieved** due to sudden emotional shock. In transient emotional shock, however, Ignatia is the best.

| | |
|---|---|
| **Antidotes:** | Camphor, Coffea, Nux Vomica, Pulsatilla, Staphysagria |
| **Potency:** | 30 to 200 |

# Ammonium Carb
## (Carbonate of Ammonia)

This is a profoundly effective medicine, which works on blood circulation. Its effect resembles several kinds of snake venom. Ammonium Carb has been successfully used in the Sindh province of Pakistan by eminent homoeopaths, for the treatment of snakebites. The resulting bleeding is thin and dark. The dark colour signifies that the inner lining of the nose, mouth, pharynx, stomach and intestines are no longer intact, they have either ulcerated or ruptured. The same also happens following a snakebite. The blood that comes out is dark and thin. Ammonium Carb is extremely useful in combating such conditions. In some diseases, the lining of the blood vessels becomes permeable and cannot retain the red cells. For such diseases, there are other useful remedies described elsewhere in this book. Dark blood is usually indicative of a severe illness, which may lead to death, unless treated promptly. There are also other remedies for the dark bloody discharge, as mentioned in other places of this book. The dark bloody discharge occurs in in serious illnesses. This requires urgent treatment otherwise the patient's life will be in danger. To distinguish between different remedies, one has to keep the differences of different remedies in mind. Otherwise, only the mere presence of this symptom will not help. For example, the dark blue bleeding of piles is a result of failure of the portal venous system, rather than the effect on the inner lining. This system of circulation is related to the liver and the veins of the intestines draining into the liver. The veins contain dark blood. Portal system dysfunction may be treated with Sulphur or Hamamelis. However, if the dark blood is exuding from the broken **down lining of the kidneys or intestines**, Ammonium Carb is the ideal remedy in this critically serious condition.

In snakebites, the blood may either clot or flow freely. Bleeding is from the junctional area (i.e. where the outer skin and the inner lining meet), such as the roots of the nail, lips, and other natural orifices. Whenever there is such bleeding, this is a sign of snake venom and similarly that of Ammonium Carb.

Female Ammonium Carb patients may become hysterical. Their symptoms aggravate with sleep (as in Lachesis). Puerperal fever or other fevers due to blood poisoning (toxaemia or Septicaemia) can influence the mind. The patient experiences strange, dreadful dreams. Detailed analysis of such dreams can help in making a proper diagnosis. If the patient sees snakes in his dreams, it indicates Natrum Mur, although, snake venom is Lachesis, rather than Natrum Mur. If the patient sleep walks, it indicates Silicea. Such patients may walk long distances and then come back to their bed. One such patient got up during her sleep and picked up the bedding and took it to another house. Finding the door of that house locked, she dropped the bedding there, returned home and lay back on the bed devoid of bedding. In the morning, she did not remember anything about it at all!

Restlessness during sleep, or non-satisfying sleep should be properly looked into, so that a diagnosis may be established and correct treatment offered for natural relief.

An **offensive discharge from the ear** should lead the homoeopath towards Ammonium Carb. Ammonium Carb is very useful in chronic illnesses of the ears associated with putrid discharge. In a chronic illness, the patient may be on the verge of death. The affected tissues start decaying and dying. The deadly odourous discharge from the ear results from the destruction of the inner lining of the ear. Ammonium Carb should be used in these patients on a permanent basis.

Pulsatilla will offer immediate relief in case of a **sudden, severe earache** associated with restlessness, provided the patient is of mild nature and has the sobbing tendency. Chamomilla would be the best remedy if the patient suffering from earache is also irritable. Allium Cepa is good if the earache is secondary to a nasal cold. If there is lots of blood congestion of the ears associated with a reddish glow on the face, one should also add Belladonna 30 to Pulsatilla.

Ammonium Carb is useful in **diseases of the glands and chronic diseases of the lungs**. Sometimes the lymph glands of the neck enlarge, become firm and then harden due to chronic inflammation and may resemble cancerous glands. So Ammonium Carb is also useful in cancerous conditions of the lymph glands. When the skin diseases are suppressed due to some kind of treatment, the diseases settle in the lymph nodes making them hard and subject to cancerous transformation. Even if cancerous, such lymph adenopathy is very amenable to Ammonium Carb.

| | |
|---|---|
| **Antidotes** | Arnica, Camphor |
| **Potency:** | 30 or as high as needed |

# ANTHRACINUM

Anthracinum is prepared from the putrefied matter taken from the spleen of sick sheep. It is a first-rate treatment for **ulcers and bleeding**. Most homoeopaths use it sparingly but I have found it to be very useful in my practice. Abscesses developing in inflamed glands are hard and bundled together. They exhibit an ugly, bluish discolouration and are painful, but do not progress to softening and pus formation. For such boils, Anthracinum is a sure-shot homoeopathic remedy, resulting in cure within a month or two.

Chronic wounds and ulcers of the internal organs, which exude blood and have a tendency to turn into cancer, can possibly be treated with Anthracinum. Anthracinum is also very useful in the treatment of deep wounds, which rip the skin apart and bleed. In view of this symptom, I am of the opinion that Anthracinum would also be beneficial in **Ulcerative Colitis** (in which, the lining of the large gut disintegrates, ulcerates and bleeds). In the allopathic system of treatment, there is no definite cure for this disease. The medicines used only temporarily control the disease, and have side effects. Only the surgical removal of the diseased part of the colon offers cure. When a disease has been merely suppressed by inappropriate medication, this may lead to Ulcerative Colitis. I have found Anthracinum to be very useful in such medically induced colitis.

Anthracinum not only has the capability of curing chronic sores and abscesses, but also prevents their recurrence. Anthracinum can be useful in combating the persistent, dark bleeding from any part of the body.

| | |
|---|---|
| **Antidotes:** | Apis, Camphor, Carbo Veg, Kreosote, Silicea, Rhus Tox |
| **Potency:** | 30 to 200 |

# ANTHRAKOKALI

Anthrakokali is very useful in **skin conditions associated with itching**, dryness, fissuring and blister formation, as well as in cracking at the nostrils and the nails, followed by the formation of sores. Typically, the mouth and the throat are very dry. Excessive bile formation leads to vomiting, the abdomen distends with wind, the thirst is intense and there is copious urination.

| | |
|---|---|
| **Potency :** | 30 |

# ANTIMONIUM CRUDUM

The salient feature of Antimonium Crudum is that the gastric function is badly affected. There is a coating on the tongue, which is essentially thick and white unless altered by the colour of food taken, e.g. the coating can obviously turn brown after eating chocolate or drinking tea. The Antimonium Crudum patient eats a lot and constantly so, until the sudden functional failure of the stomach sets in.

Antimonium Crudum is a profound and widely effective medicine. It stops the **vomiting following excessive eating**. It is very useful in deep warts and corns of the feet. Sometimes, streaks on nails or their irregularity may be a sign of deep-seated disease. In the Antimonium Crudum patient, raised warts develop near finger nails. The nails either become loose or shrivel and streaks appear on them. The same happens on the feet. The gums swell and recede from the teeth and the teeth decay. If this is a prominent feature, then it is diagnostic of Antimonium Crudum. In Antimonium Crudum and Antimonium tart, the toothache may be of neuralgic nature.
In Antimonium Crudum, the stools are formed and the blood is only smeared on the outside. In dysentery, the stools are mixed with blood.

Antimonium Crudum patient suffers from the pain at the heels. Along with the dysfunction of the stomach, various skin conditions can also develop. The Antimonium Crudum symptoms are relieved in the open air and hot, humid weather. However, the patient cannot tolerate heat, especially direct sunlight. The classical signs of Antimonium Crudum are gastric dysfunction, nausea and its effects on the lungs, involvement of the nails, peeling of the tip of the nose and lips, and dry eczema.

| | |
|---|---|
| **Adjutant:** | Sulphur |
| **Antidote:** | Hepar Sulph |
| **Potency:** | 30 |

# Apis Mellifica
## (The Honey Bee)

Medicinally, bee venom is used in several diseases. In ancient times, it was used to treat insect bites and stings. Apis is especially useful in the illnesses caused by honeybee stings and like ailments.

The typical pain of the Apis patient is fraught with burning and piercing sensation. Cold application relieves the pain while heat aggravates it. The symptoms usually begin on the right side and then spread to the left. The skin feels sore and cannot tolerate any pressure. Even the touch of cloth is unbearable. The patient feels intense heat in the blood and is relieved by exposure to the open air. He is worse for heat (feeling heat). Apis is very useful in every kind of **inflammation and swelling** aggravated by exposure to heat or heat application. This is the best remedy for **Meningitis** also. When used promptly, it also prevents the subsequent development of epilepsy whereas even if Meningitis is cured by conventional treatment, some long-term complications persist, one of which is epilepsy. If cold, rather than warmth, worsens the symptoms, Apocynum should be used instead.

In the later part of **pregnancy**, some women develop **convulsions** (Eclampsia). The general perception is that in such a condition, a patient gets relief from a hot bath. However, if the patient's constitution is that of Apis, a hot bath leads to severe convulsions to the extent that due to constriction of the cervix, the baby can die in utero. If not treated immediately, the mother may also die. Similarly, small children, of Apis temperament, can also fall into a state of convulsions with a hot bath and these convulsions can result in their death. It is extremely important to know if the symptoms worsen with heat or cold. If heat aggravates the symptoms, Belladonna 1000 and Aconite 1000 should also be added to Apis and repeated 2 to 3 times within 15 minutes. If the condition is aggravated by cold, Mag Phos should be administered.

Apocynum is the ideal remedy for a cool disposition and Apis, that of a hot disposition. If a child does not like to be covered but kicks the cloth off, this shows that he does not like heat.

The salient sign of Apis is that the **affected area swells and throbs** (as after a bee sting). Apocynum does not exhibit this feature. Sometimes, the swelling of Apis appears in the outer lining of the brain. Typically, the patient feels worse in the heat and feels severe throbbing. A young child cannot express himself and suddenly screams loudly. The doctor should take immediate notice of this sign and administer Apis.

Apis also affects the membranous coverings of the heart, lungs and liver. In other words, it works mostly on the coverings rather than these organs themselves. Apocynum, like Apis, also affects the coverings. Both these remedies affect the secretory membranes of the abdomen like those of the intestines or kidneys, which filter the blood and produce urine. In both, the body swelling is soft and pits on pressure. In Apocynum, the swelling (Oedema) may become rather hard.

The Apis patient with a kidney disease will show soft baggy swelling below the eyes. If along with this, the **kidneys** have a throbbing pain, or there is a sign of worsening of symptoms by heat, this is a clear indication of Apis.

The affected eyes show severe swelling of the eyelids and Conjuctiva, along with **bright redness,** a **piercing pain in the eye** and aggravation of the symptoms by heat. Such a patient will not be able to open his eyes in bright sunlight. In Apis, some signs and symptoms manifest themselves on the right side. On hearing bad news or out of jealousy or sheer dislike, the **right side of the body may be paralysed**. However, the ailments of the eye and throat begin on the left side and then migrate to the right side (like Lachesis). In Apis, cold water gargles, instead of warm water, relieve the throat discomfort.

In Apis, the **abdomen (belly) becomes markedly distended with wind or gas**, causing **spasms** below the ribs on the right side and then possibly on the left side also, like a vice. Pressure on the affected area of the belly relieves the discomfort. Apis is the sure-shot remedy if the symptoms aggravate with heat. Apis shows its beneficial effects in ten to fifteen days, however, it starts relieving the distension and spasm of the abdomen immediately after use. In an hour or two, the effect is well evident. It works fairly fast in Meningitis, unless it is associated with **Hydrocephalus**. Apis will relieve the swelling of the membranes of Meningitis, but the cure of Hydrocephalus will not be achieved without Silicea, which is the correct treatment for this condition. Silicea should be started in small potency and then advanced steadily to very high potency. In abdominal distension, Apis gives immediate relief. However, in some chronic intestinal problems, it has to be used over a long period.

As a matter of principle, in slowly progressive illnesses, the treatment will also be effective gradually, whereas, in sudden acute illnesses, the response to the medication is also prompt. In kidney disease, when Apis has to be used over a long period, this does not mean that the appearance of its beneficial effect will also take that long. If Apis starts working in kidney disease, the kidneys start forming urine within seven to ten days, which is a clear indication of its effect, although complete recovery will take time. In such a situation, the potency should be increased gradually with longer intervals in between. This way of administration is called rising potency and is described in detail in the chapter on Tuberculinum and Bacillinum.

| | |
|---|---|
| **Adjutant:** | Natrum Mur |
| **Antidotes:** | Cantharis, Ipecac, Lachesis, Ledum, Natrum Mur |
| **Potency:** | 30 to 200 |

# Argentum Metallicum
## (Metallic silver)

Argentum Metallicum is the other name for silver. Pure silver cannot be absorbed into the body. However, when silver is combined with other elements, the body is able to absorb its compounds. In Greek medicine, it was used in the form of silver foil as a tonic, but pure silver cannot become a part of the body tissue. Unfortunately, these days lead is beaten into the form of a foil and sold as silver even though lead is very harmful to the health of a person.

As far as homoeopathy is concerned, any metal which comes into contact with the lining of the skin or the inner lining of the gut is absorbed into the body, although it may not be detectable by any sophisticated gauges.

The main effect of the Argentum Metallicum is on the **elastic cartilage bones**, which become thick and hard. The thickened nasal bone can cause difficulty in breathing. Small bones of the ears develop nodular thickening. This process of progressive thickening of the bone can lead to cancer formation.

Argentum Metallicum works profoundly on the brain cells. The cells start melting away slowly, and premature senility sets in. The capability to comprehend deteriorates. This weakness starts in the central part of the brain and then spreads gradually to other organs of the body. Mental faculties start failing. Hands and feet start to bend. The **memory becomes weak** to the extent that the patient goes out of his senses and talks nonsense. The **ability to think decreases**. Serious thinking causes **dizziness**. This is a danger signal and indicates the degeneration of brain cells. In such cases, Argentum Metallicum in high potency should be administered without delay and repeated every fifteen to twenty days or monthly. The inhaler used by asthmatic patients also contains a poisonous substance which, like Argentum Metallicum, makes the brain tissue shrink and then degenerate.

Argentum Metallicum resembles Lachesis in the way that the symptoms aggravate during sleep, especially the nervous exhaustion leading to generalized physical fatigue.

Argentum Metallicum works deeply on the muscles of the limbs. **Neuralgic pains** mostly affect both **the legs and the feet**. The nerve fibres feel as though they are being torn apart. These **neuralgic pains** aggravate during sleep and in cold and wet weather. (Rheumatic aches and pains also get worse in stormy and humid weather). In the rainy season, they also get worse before and after the rain. There is no associated swelling of the limbs, but the patient is definitely very restless. Light movements lessen the joint pains while rapid motions intensify them. The discomfort is not due to the sleep itself, but the rest offered by sleep. The pains are worse at night as in Rhus Tox. The difference is that in Rhus Tox, there is a severe physical uneasiness and the person spends the night tossing about.

Argentum Metallicum is very useful in **the cancers of the skin and mucus membranes**. **Cancer at the uterine neck,** which most doctors label as incurable, is very amenable to Argentum Metallicum, even curable. In case the cure is not achieved, the patient can still remain comfortable for a long time. Tarentula Hispania, Helonias and Carbo Animalis are also very useful in cancer of the cervix of the uterus.

In Argentum Metallicum, there are widespread ulcerations on the body. The **ulcers** over the cartilage bones respond very well to Argentum Metallicum. It is also associated with the lining of veins. A very special feature of Argentum Metallicum is that it affects the internal organs of women strictly on the left side, and the internal organs of men strictly on the right side. Usually it is not difficult to differentiate the remedies specific for the right or the left and upper or lower part of the body. This remedy, however, particularly differentiates the ailments of right and left in men and women respectively. In women, the ovary swells into a form of a large cyst. Accumulation of different materials makes it large and more thick. The uterus also expands and loses its elasticity. Once expanded, it does not return to its original condition. This problem aggravates after every delivery and sometimes the uterus descends down. Argentum Metallicum is extremely useful in such women, offering cure. The **uterus becoming hard and the cervix stiff,** in association with a putrid discharge, indicate the presence of a deep serious problem. Administered early on, Argentum Metallicum can abort the disease.

If **the legs hurt** but the real cause is not known, Argentum Metallicum is worth a trial. It can be very useful in post-menopausal bleeding. Argentum Metallicum is generally, though not necessarily, indicated in women of thin, lean build with long slender hands. It may be useful in obese women also.

Some people feel sudden **jerks on retiring to sleep or during sleep.** This is quite troublesome. Grindelia is ideal in such cases. Arsenic may also be useful. Argentum Metallicum is indicated if such **jerks of violent motion** are secondary to severe physical fatigue. Generally, Grindelia is good enough in most such patients. One single dose may work for many weeks, and does not need to be repeated.

Argentum Metallicum symptoms are at the climax exactly at midday. The patient feels dizzy. The **headache** is localised to the forehead and face or sometimes on any one side of the head, but mostly on the right side. It intensifies gradually, but then subsides rapidly. This pain is related to facial neuralgia, because basically this is a neuralgic remedy and headache is also related to nerves.

**Severe itching,** limited to one ear and leading to the injury and thickening of the ears, is indicative of Argentum Metallicum. Thickening of both ears is an early sign of leprosy. Leprosy, a very slowly progressive disease, can best be controlled by early use of Hydrocotyle.

Argentum Metallicum is extremely useful in **diabetics** and patients passing albumin in the urine. Provided its other signs are also present, it can be completely cured. Argentum Metallicum is also very beneficial in inflammation of the inner lining of the kidneys (Nephritis).

In Argentum Metallicum, two signs are shown in urine. If it is **dark coloured**, this indicates passage of albumin in the urine. If it is **cloudy and copious**, this indicates the presence of sugar, as is in juvenile diabetes. Argentum Metallicum would only be useful if other constitutional symptoms are also present. Argentum Metallicum would be useful in **diabetics** with failing kidneys **who wet their beds at night.**

In Argentum Metallicum there is a feeling of extremely unusual weakness and lethargy and the body feels lifeless. Argentum Metallicum is the treatment for this extreme fatigue. Argentum Metallicum is a remedy of speakers and singers. It is well known for the treatment of **hoarseness of the voice** following excessive speaking and singing. Hoarseness is known in other homoeopathic remedies too, such as in Rhus Tox, however, it is not difficult to differentiate between them. In Rhus Tox, the patient feels a hoarseness of the voice at the outset, which gradually gets clearer and better gradually on continued talking. If the voice becomes worse on talking, Borax can be used. However, if the overall symptoms are of Argentum Metallicum, this will prove better than Borax.

In Argentum Metallicum, the **trachea swells up and is very painful**. The cough becomes aggravated by laughing (as in Phosphorus). Argentum Metallicum patients develop **cold** on exposure to the cold which can lead to irritation of the throat, and discomfort at the upper part of the chest. The fever comes on in the afternoon. There is severe weakness in the chest and pain on the left ribs. Argentum Metallicum is of good use in **diseases of the lungs**. Stanum is better than Argentum Metallicum in diseases associated with a lot of sputum/expectoration, unless the overall picture resembles that of Argentum Metallicum. There is **premature ageing** in Argentum Metallicum. Even at the age of 20 to 25 years, the face appears full of wrinkles. Sarsaparilla is the best remedy for premature ageing. Chinisum Ars is good in ageing which is secondary to deep illnesses of long-standing. The liver and spleen fail. In Sarsaparilla the skin shrivels.

In Argentum Metallicum, if the patient lies flat on his back, **watery fluid accumulates in the lung,** causing palpitations and difficulty in breathing. On sitting up and standing, the upper part of the lung becomes clear of the fluid, and the person can breathe easily. Argentum Metallicum is very advantageous in pregnant women experiencing **sudden or severe palpitations of the heart.** Typically, the symptoms of Argentum Metallicum aggravate by touch and at midday. Sleeping in the open air at night lessens the severity of the cough, but other physical ailments get worse.

| | |
|---|---|
| **Antidote:** | Merc Sol, Pulsatilla |
| **Potency:** | 30 to CM |

# Argentum Nitricum

## (Nitrate of silver)

Argentum Nitricum has previously been used in treating epilepsy. It relieves epileptic fits but causes itching of the skin. Traditionally, it has been used in eye diseases.

People who wear silver jewellery may develop symptoms of silver poisoning. Similarly, prolonged allopathic use of silver can have a negative effect on mental faculties. When **the mind becomes slow** and **creative skills decline**, Argentum Nitricum must be kept in mind. The **memory is weak**, and reasoning is flawed. Superstitions, visual hallucinations and delusions prevail. The patient is afraid of visiting some particular places. Such children should be accompanied to such spots and told that there is nothing to be afraid of. Argentum Nitricum is not only capable of curing these symptoms, but is also effective against some other deep-seated illnesses. The Argentum Nitricum patient is afraid of heights lest he may leap off. Argentum Nitricum patients are afraid of even looking up at a very tall building or a building with a high ceiling, in case it may fall on them. Most homoeopaths have not stressed these symptoms: they have only mentioned fear of heights and epileptic fit. However, when I personally analysed the symptoms of my patients after closely observing them, the above mentioned symptoms became clearly evident. Such a patient is afraid of jumping into the river while crossing a bridge. In advanced illness, there is a strong desire to jump from the bridge. Such patient trembles with fear and also feels weak.

Some people have **loose motions** prior to an exam or an important interview. Some may feel agitated and angry.

Extraordinary **mental fatigue** and gastric hyperacidity adversely **affect the memory**. Transient loss of recent memory can also occur as a result of narrowing of the arteries going to the brain (due to arterial thickening or just because of spasms of the artery). If the tendency to spasm is frequent, the patient loses his memory permanently. This is not related to transient stomach upset or mental fatigue. Argentum Nitricum also shows these signs, however, loss of memory appears as a permanent sign. Alumina is also useful in this disease; but has to be used for a long period.

In Argentum Nitricum, the **heart becomes weak**. There is bluish discolouration of the body as in Cuprum and Carbo Animalis. In Cuprum, the cyanosis is due to the spasm of the blood vessels. In Carbo Animalis it is due to lack of oxygen and disorder of the blood. The blueness of Argentum Nitricum resembles that of Carbo Animalis. In both these remedies, blueness appears all over the body as if somebody has been suffocated. In Cuprum, there may be violent spasms of the hands and feet, along with cyanosis of the face and the lips. In Argentum Nitricum, there is a tendency to form sores. In allopathy, silver nitrate was used in many eye conditions. In homoeopathy also, silver nitrate in a well-diluted form can benefit many eye conditions, especially corneal ulcers. The eyes are hypersensitive to light. The eyes ache and feel tired. Argentum Nitricum is good in **persistently sore eyes** with purulent discharge. The eyelids are swollen. Their inner linings are inflamed and form red circles. This condition (which is called purulent Conjunctivitis) is very common in the Indo-Pak sub-continent during summer.

Argentum Nitricum is very useful in **diseases of the women**, like abdominal discomfort and discharging sores at the mouth of the uterus before the onset of periods. The periods become frequent, but are scanty. If other symptoms of Argentum Nitricum are also present, this remedy can cure other internal diseases of uterus as well.

The wounds tend to bleed. There is a tendency of vomiting containing blood. Argentum Nitricum may be used in chronic resistant ulcers of the stomach. The peptic ulcer of the stomach can be treated with ground liquorice. Unripe banana, dried and powdered, taken two to three times a day, is also very useful in such ulcers. The powder coats the ulcer, as well as inducing healing. This treatment has been described in a scientific magazine and I have often used it very successfully.

Argentum Nitricum patients with chronic ulcers tend to have anaemia. They crave sweets. This craving for sweets is also found in other homoeopathic remedies. Some people can eat a lot of sweets but this does not bother them, whereas in a patient of Argentum Nitricum, sweets do not suit him: on ingestion, the stomach becomes upset and other symptoms also aggravate. In an Argentum Nitricum patient, **the desire to eat sweets, if associated with wind and abdominal distension,** is very typical. The patient cannot sleep on his right side. This symptom is also found in Naja. On lying on the right side, the pulse becomes rapid. The symptom of a rapid pulse is common to Kalmia, Spongia, Kali Nitrate, Alumen, Platina, Lilium Tigrum also. A distinction among these remedies can be made by keeping their respective characteristic features in mind.

The symptoms of Argentum Nitricum aggravate in a warm room or sitting near the fire. The perspiration on the face is very prominent. It appears as if water is erupting out. The face is sallow and bluish. The eyes are drawn in and are without lustre. Like in Thuja, there is tendency to develop warts. **Blisters form in the throat.** The throat feels as if something is stuck in it, like Hepar Sulph, but any attempt to cough it out makes the sensation worse. In fact, there is nothing inside the throat; it is just a feeling and it is typical in Nitric Acid also. The person feels as if something is poking him on his body. If touched by hand anywhere on the body, the person feels pain.

In case of Argentum Nitricum, the symptoms of lactating mothers are exhibited in their children. If the mother eats too many sweets, the child develops diarrhoea. In case of Argentum Nitricum, the **vomiting and diarrhoea start concurrently**. The stools are green. The ingested food passes out of the system quickly. Such children are generally dehydrated and marasmic. However, the marasmus of the children may not always be the result of suckling Argentum Nitricum mothers. They can be patients of Argentum Nitricum per se. The stools are green; vomiting and diarrhoea can alternate or be present at the same time. With the stools, the child passes a lot of mucus.

In Argentum Nitricum there is pain in the deep organs of the body. The liver, spleen or stomach may hurt. The discomfort may not be felt spread throughout the abdomen.

In Argentum Nitricum, one may involuntarily pass urine. Children may wet their beds at night. Another sign is that one may have the desire to urinate, but is unable to pass urine easily. There may be pain, swelling or itching in the urethra. This is also one of the best remedies for **gonorrhoea**.

Argentum Nitricum is very useful in **many problems associated with pregnancy**. The patient feels a weakness of the heart which worsens due to the additional load of pregnancy. The feeling of weakness of the heart by physical exertion or mental anguish continues throughout the pregnancy. The patient may have nightmares.

In the morning, as the person gets up, the legs feel as if they have been beaten. Walking is uncomfortable. The legs feel weak and the upper arms feel numb. The back hurts and the backbone area is very sensitive. The backache is worse at night. In Argentum Nitricum, there can be **paralysis of the lower half of the body**, and stiffness and tightness at the tissues surrounding the backbone. The symptoms aggravate in the heat and after food. The open air and the cold relieve the symptoms.

In epilepsy, fear of heights, and the tendency to see dreadful dreams, a very high potency should be given.

| | |
|---|---|
| **Adjuvants:** | Merc Sol, Pulsatilla |
| **Antidotes:** | Natrum Mur, Arsenic, Phosphorus |
| **Potency:** | 30 to 200 |

# Arnica Montana

Arnica has a special place in homoeopathy. It is prepared from tobacco grown on the mountains, and has long since been used in the treatment of blunt injuries. To fall and get hurt is common in hilly areas, no wonder that the Gracious God has provided the appropriate remedy right there!

In homoeopathy, Arnica is used in the treatment of new as well as old injuries. Its main symptom is the clotting of blood (resembling Alumen); thus, it is an essential ingredient in the treatment of heart diseases. Arnica, in homoeopathic form, liquefies the clotted blood. Yet, unlike allopathic medicine, it does not make the blood too thin to clot when needed. In the case of **heart attack**, Arnica is given in combination with Lachesis. Lachesis is a remedy for snake venom, which causes the blood to clot in the arteries supplying the heart and causes heart attack.

Some snake venoms affect the nervous system instead of the blood. Naja is one such example. Its venom affects the heart musculature. Arnica and Lachesis, both are closely related to the coagulation of blood. They must be given together, and not one after the other, so that their action does not conflict with each other. Administration of two to three medicines, together or in sequence, demands a special skill based on deep knowledge and long experience about the nature of the medications to be used. I usually give Arnica and Lachesis together or just one of the two. If the heart attack has been precipitated due to coagulation of the blood, Arnica will adequately dilute the blood, and re-establish its flow.

Arnica is the best remedy for accidents and **blunt injuries**, causing the injured part to turn blue or black due to the accumulation of clotted blood. Once, a patient had been badly beaten with a club and his entire body was black and blue. His condition was critically serious and I thought he would not survive. I gave him sufficient supply of Arnica and prayed for him. By the next evening, I was very worried because I had received no information about his condition. On inquiry, I was told that he had become well enough that night and he was even up and about by then. Alhamdolillah.

Arnica 200 given along with Aconite 200 is much better and faster in action than Arnica 200 alone. If the injured area is flushed and swollen due to increased local circulation, Belladonna should also be given along with Arnica for better response. Increased blood flow to the injured part is a natural response to the physical insult. In Arnica alone, local blood flow is not enhanced and there is no unusual swelling. In the case of increased swelling, Belladonna or Aconite should also be administered. This general prescription may be used without any hesitation or fear of harm. It can simply work to one's advantage.

Arnica works equally well in low as well as high potencies. However, in deep-established illnesses, it should be administered in high potency. Once an army officer, Major Mumtaz, slipped off the snow-covered cliff during military exercises and landed in an abyss 75 feet deep in the Himalayas. He was seriously hurt with no apparent hope of survival. I gave him Arnica 1000 and Natrum Sulph 1000 twice on the first day and then once a day. By God's grace, he recovered astonishingly well.

One of my patients had been badly hurt and his backbone had also fractured. The doctors told him that he would not survive, if he luckily survived, he would be bed-ridden or bound to a wheelchair for life. I prescribed him Arnica, Ruta, Hypericum, Calcarea Phos and Symphytum, all in potency 30 to be taken 3 to 4 times a day. After some time, he showed up in my office in London walking on his own, without any support. I failed to recognize him, although I remembered his face. It was unbelievable to see him walking independently. He smiled and told me that he had used the homoeopathic prescription suggested by me and that I had prayed for him, and given him hope. His recovery was indeed miraculous. Hence, this prescription is the best remedy in all injuries causing swelling, inflammation, pain and stiffness. In the first patient, I had also included Natrum Sulph 1000, which in my opinion is the best for injuries of the nape of the neck. Over many years of practice, I have found a triad of homoeopathic medicines that are very effective in the treatment of broken bones. This consists of Symphytum, Ruta and Calcarea Phos. It virtually doubles the speed of healing of a broken bone, even when there is a gap due to the loss of bone. The bone starts growing from both ends of the fracture to fill up the gap.

Apart from physical trauma, Arnica is also very useful for **fatigue and discomfort following physical exertion**. If the aching is severe, Arnica and Bryonia together will offer sure relief. Arnica is very useful in various women's diseases. At the time of **childbirth, unusual straining can tear apart the pelvic muscles and tissues**, resulting in chronic pain. Arnica 1000 given a few days before childbirth will prevent against such happening. The **puerperal sepsis** and fever are very amenable to Sulphur and Pyrogenium. Prophylactic use of Arnica 1000 will most probably preclude their use or Arnica can be given also with Sulphur and Bryonia.

As a matter of principle, the more medicines are mixed, the less their individual beneficial affect would be. The medicines similar in action but not analogous to the illness will lose, rather than gain any beneficial effect. I personally resort to mixed prescription due to the shortage of time at my disposal. I have used them over the years and found them uniformly effective in all the patients. The rigid types of homoeopaths still stick to the practice of using only one remedy for a particular illness, I do not agree with them. I would rather advise the use of well-tried and tested combination prescriptions rather than letting the patient remain untreated and suffer. One, if not more, of the combinations may happen to be a truly analogous remedy.

The Arnica patient does not usually fear during the day but has nightmares during sleep. The pregnant women feel lower abdominal pain due to the foetal movements, which intensify as the pregnancy progresses. At night, the pain being suppressed by sleep expresses itself in the form of scary dreams. In the case of chronic, deep-seated illnesses, the Arnica patient may also develop a **fear of death**. In Opium, the person experiences such fear irrespective of the severity of the illness or timing of the day and night. In Arnica, however, he does not fear much in the absence of severe illness. The bleeding is dark and smelly. The Arnica patient exhibits the early symptoms of malaria and typhoid i.e. the body aches. The skin feels raw and uncomfortable and the skin is very sensitive, even to touch. So are the joint pains of Arnica.

Arnica given in high potency cures **the sprain and the strain of the ankle** effectively. In spite of being given repeatedly, low potency will not be very effective. Even soft bedding feels unbearably hard to Arnica patients. They change side frequently to get relief, but in vain.

In Arsenic and Rhus Tox, tossing about in bed is secondary to restlessness.

Arnica resembles other homoeopathic medicines also. Like Belladonna, the head is warm but the body is cold. The fever suppressed inside the body can be dangerous. One dose of Arnica high potency will induce gradual warming up of the body and the suppressed symptoms of the disease will start manifesting externally and thus give time for the appropriate treatment. In case the diagnosis is already made, the appropriate analogous remedy can be administered without the intermediary use of Arnica.

Once, a lady suffered from severe sprain of the ankle and was unable to walk. She took homoeopathic remedies but at the same time continued massageing the injured ankle. I gave her Arnica, Bryonia and Causticum and strictly forbade her from doing massage, because the massage caused recurrent injury to the tissues. She got better in a week. The other remedies were combined with Arnica because sometimes it is not a superficial injury, rather some muscle has also become weak. Bryonia is effective for the deep muscular injuries and is also a muscle tonic. In Causticum, the muscles are flabby and may predispose to hernia.

If the symptoms are on the **right side**, a combination of Arnica, Belladonna and Bryonia will do the job, while the symptoms on the **left side** respond better to a combination of Arnica, Ledum and Lachesis.

Arnica is the best remedy when the **joints** get **twisted and sprained** badly during a fall or an accident. It will offer visible relief in a few hours.

When the **back** gets **sprained or strained** as a result of jerky movements, it can settle down after a while. Sometimes, it becomes chronic. The previously damaged muscles and ligaments become weak and stiff or flabby further. Arnica is quite helpful in such a condition; although it does not have a direct effect on the muscles. Cimicifuga is more appropriate for deep-seated muscular conditions. If the backache becomes chronic, initially Arnica should be combined with Bryonia. However, if the relief is only temporary, Arnica should be combined with Rhus Tox. Rhus Tox is very effective in deep-seated muscular ailments. Rhus Tox is very beneficial is cases of **muscular paralysis**. It strengthens and invigorates the muscles. It is useful in case of a dilated heart also. In chronic paralyses, it is given along with Sulphur. Calcarea Carb, being chronic of Sulphur and Rhus Tox, may also be indicated to prolong their useful effects.

Arnica is very useful in **herpes**. The common kind of herpes is related to the nervous weakness or infection. The other kind is related to venereal diseases and is very resistant to treatment. Herpes due to nervous weakness responds well to Arnica, which is more effective when combined with Arsenic and Ledum. The triad of Arsenica, Arsenic and Ledum offers cure in all kinds of poisonous insects/animal bites. In Arnica, the inner lining of the gut is as irritable as the skin is in malaria and typhoid. There is a tendency to **bleed from the ruptured small vessels**. If there is bleeding in the vomiting, stools or sputum and the appropriate analogous remedy cannot be thought of, Arnica may well be tried. If the disease has advanced, the mucous membranes of the intestines may disintegrate, leading to offensive smelling, **blood mixed stools**. The specific analogous remedy has to be sought after in such a case, since Arnica alone will not be of much use. The patient of Arnica sometimes presents with the offensive breath and sweat, smelling like that of Baptisia.

When the disease becomes severe, the Arnica patient, like that of Arsenic, becomes fearful of death. His head feels warm. He wants his body to be warmed up but not his head. The Arsenic patient likes the head to be cooled and the body warmed. Being constantly cold, the Arsenic patient resembles that of Psorinum, though in Psorinum, the patient is cold from head to toe. Lachesis is very useful, especially if the feet are cold after going to sleep. The feet are cold on and off and not all the time. The excreta or the discharges are not offensive smelling, unlike Psorinum. The Psorinum patient smells terrible, and feels intense cold. Sometimes the **skin is covered with ugly-looking, thin scales** like Arsenic. If the scales and scabs smell awful, Arsenic and Psorinum should be given together.

If the fever prolongs, the Arnica patient may involuntarily pass urine, as well as stools, in their sleep. The urine is deep coloured and **contains blood**. The bladder feels full and tense, the kidneys ache. There is tendency of chills, nausea and vomiting. The stools are dark and reddish in colour and frequent. The **frequency of stools** is associated with severe griping pain in the intestines. The patient feels progressively weak after every motion and likes to retire.

Arnica is a good remedy for **whooping cough** also. The child screams before or after the bout of cough. Excessive straining can rupture the small capillaries and cause them to bleed. If Arnica is not given, the patient may go blind due to bleeding in the eyes. The whole body feels badly beaten up due to increased internal pressure. Arnica is not a cure, but offers sufficient relief of symptoms so that the serious after-effects of **whooping cough** can be minimized. Drosera is very effective in whooping cough and similar coughs. One dose of potency 30 taken at night, works extraordinarily well.

The Arnica patient is irritable, sad and distressed only during the ailment, even though he is not of this nature. When the symptoms progress, the pain is ameliorated and the drowsiness prevails. The mind, however, remains clear. On questioning the patient will respond clearly. In the heart diseases associated with Arnica, the heart feels as if squeezed into a vice. The patient's heart beats out of fear. The pulse is irregular. The heartbeat becomes fast in response to physical exertion and exercise, and slows down with rest. The patient wants to **move to a new place**, hoping that he may feel better. Arnica combined with Bryonia and Iris Tenax is very useful in Appendicitis. Arnica 1000 given prior to a surgery or childbirth prevents many complications.

| | |
|---|---|
| **Adjuvants:** | Aconite, Ipecac |
| **Antidote:** | Camphor |
| **Potency:** | 30 to CM. |

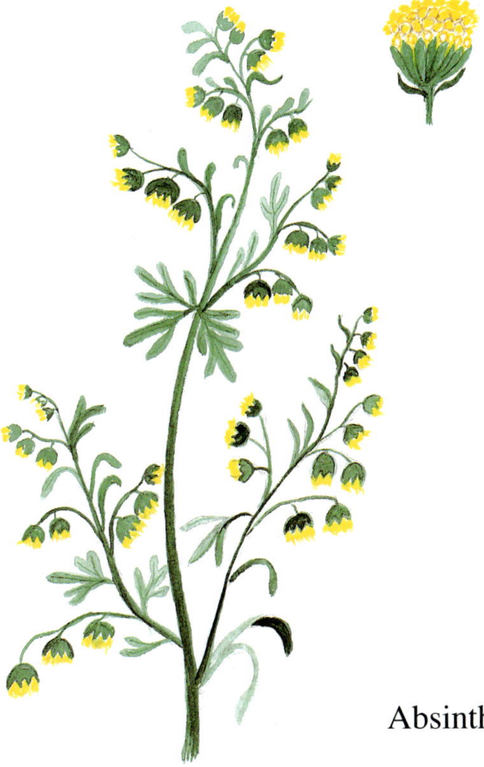

Absinthium

Aconitum Napellus

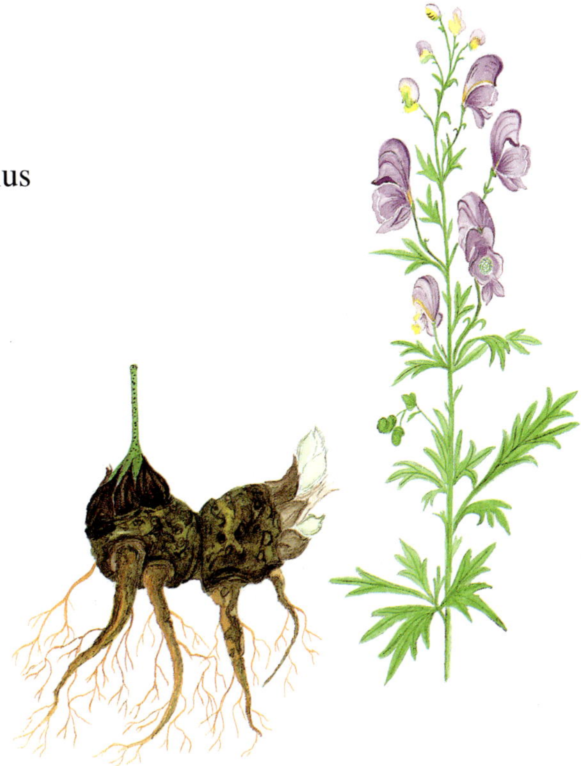

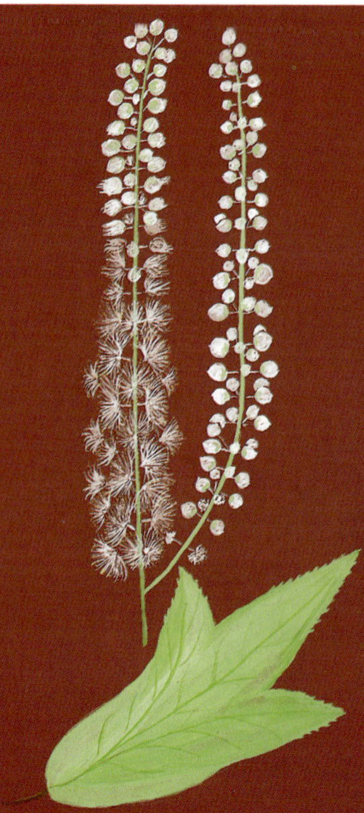

Actaea Racemosa

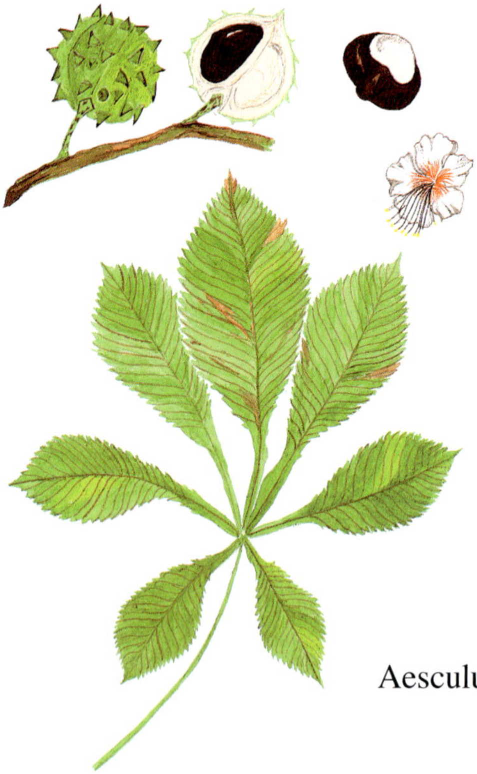

Aesculus Hippocastanum

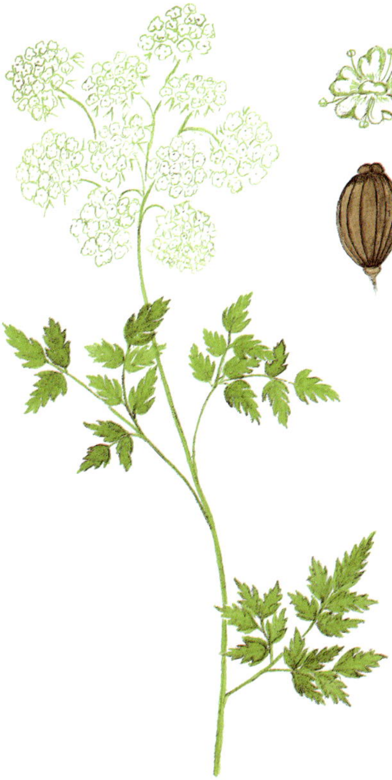

Aethusa Cynapium

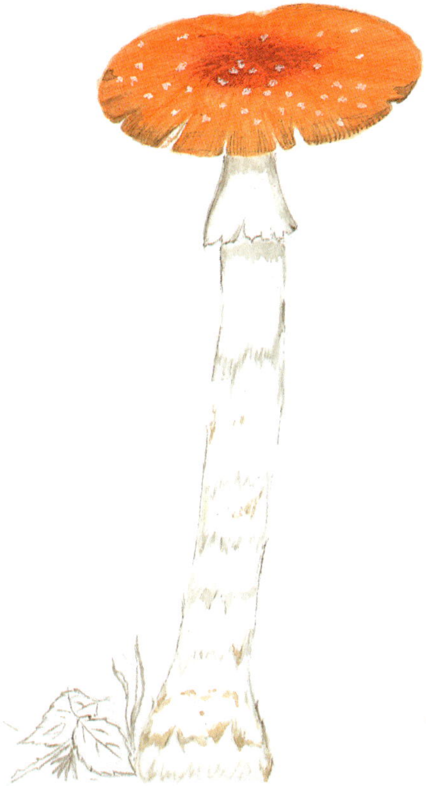

Agaricus Muscarius

Agnus Castus

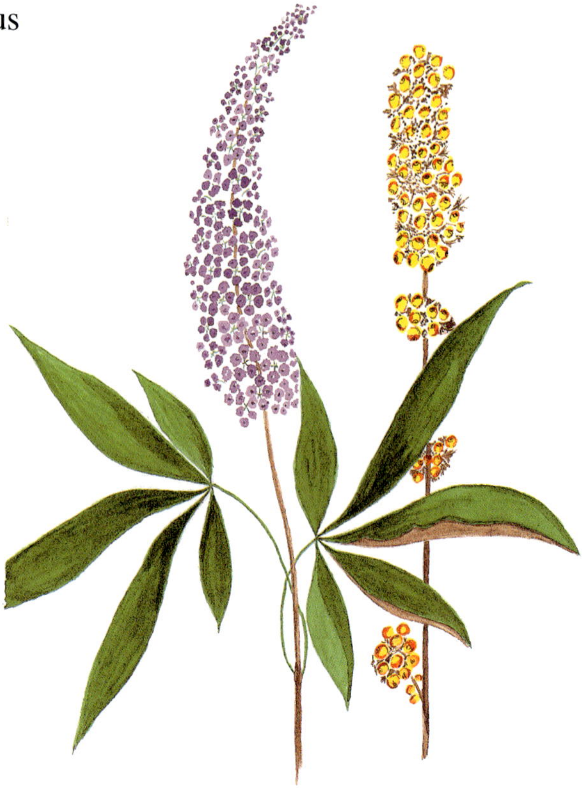

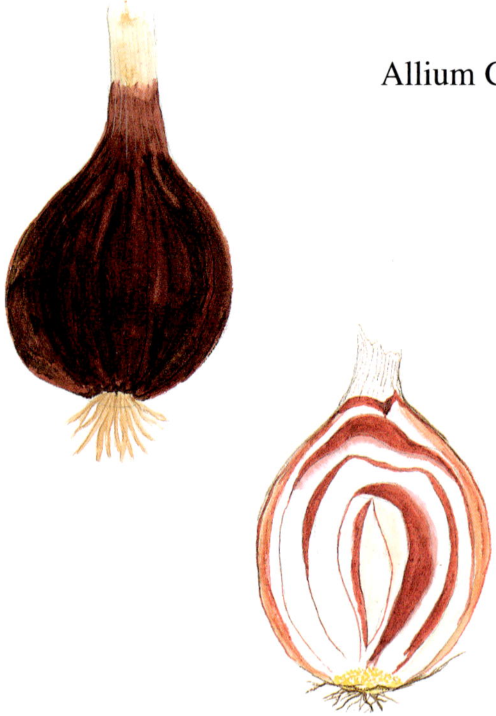

Allium Cepa

loe

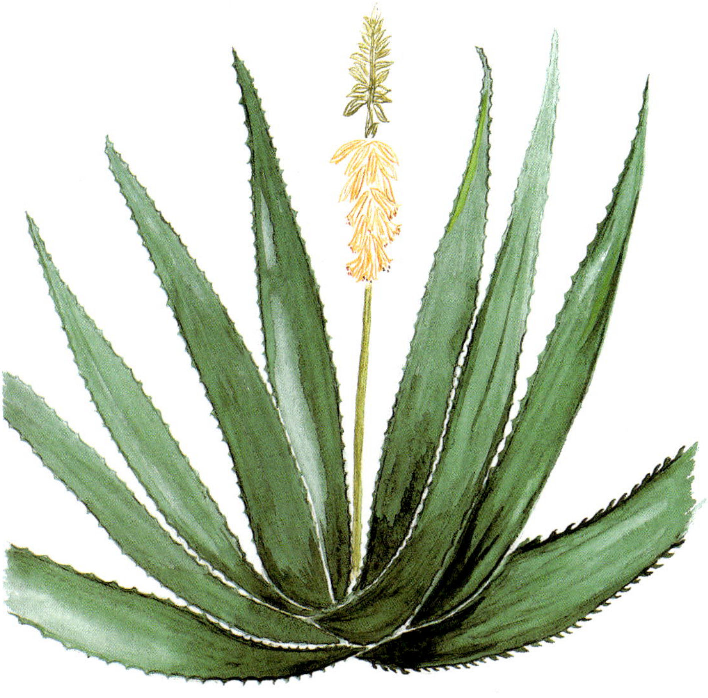

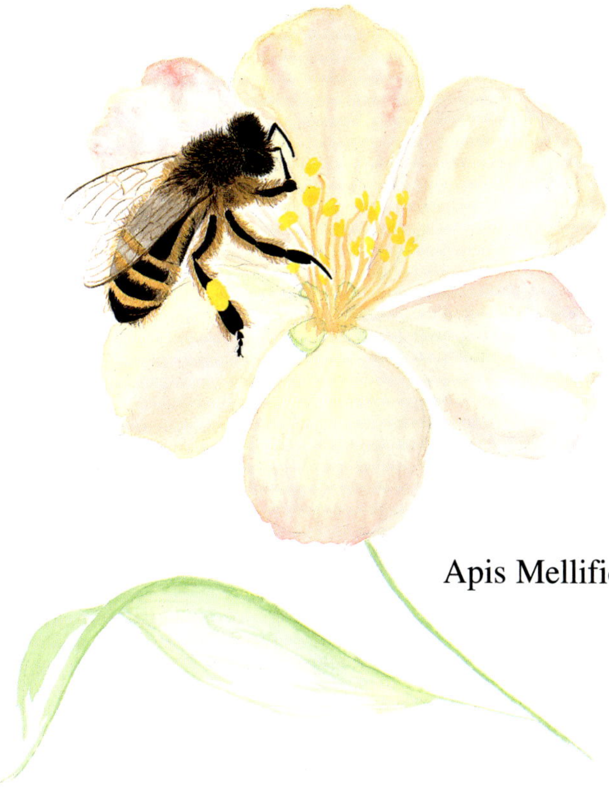

Apis Mellifica

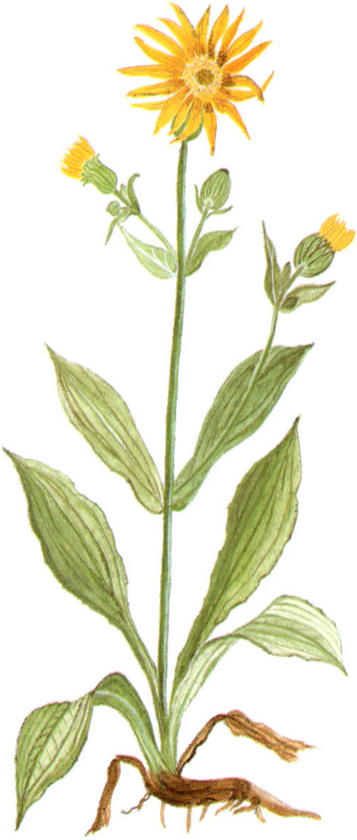

Arnica

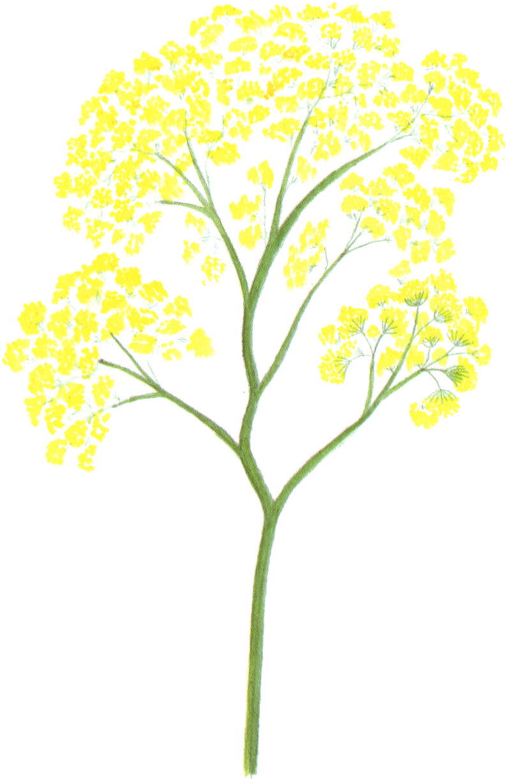

Asafotida

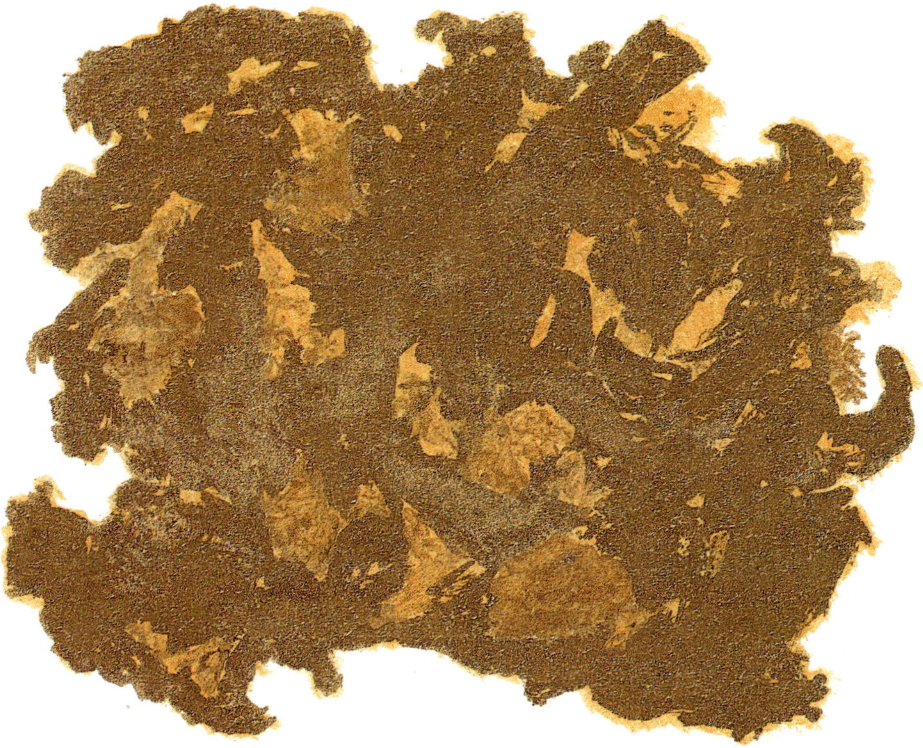

Aurum Metallicum

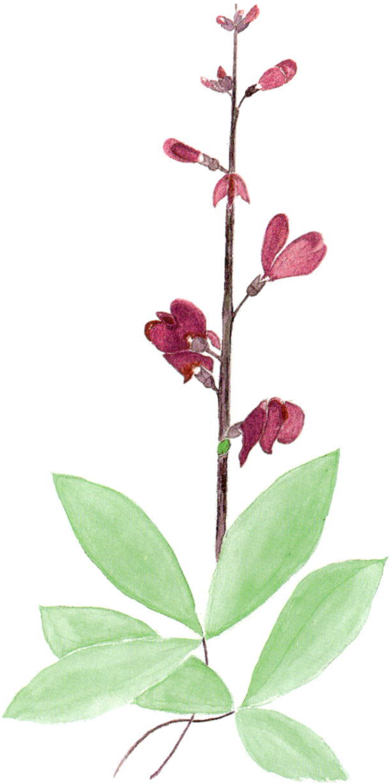

Baptisia

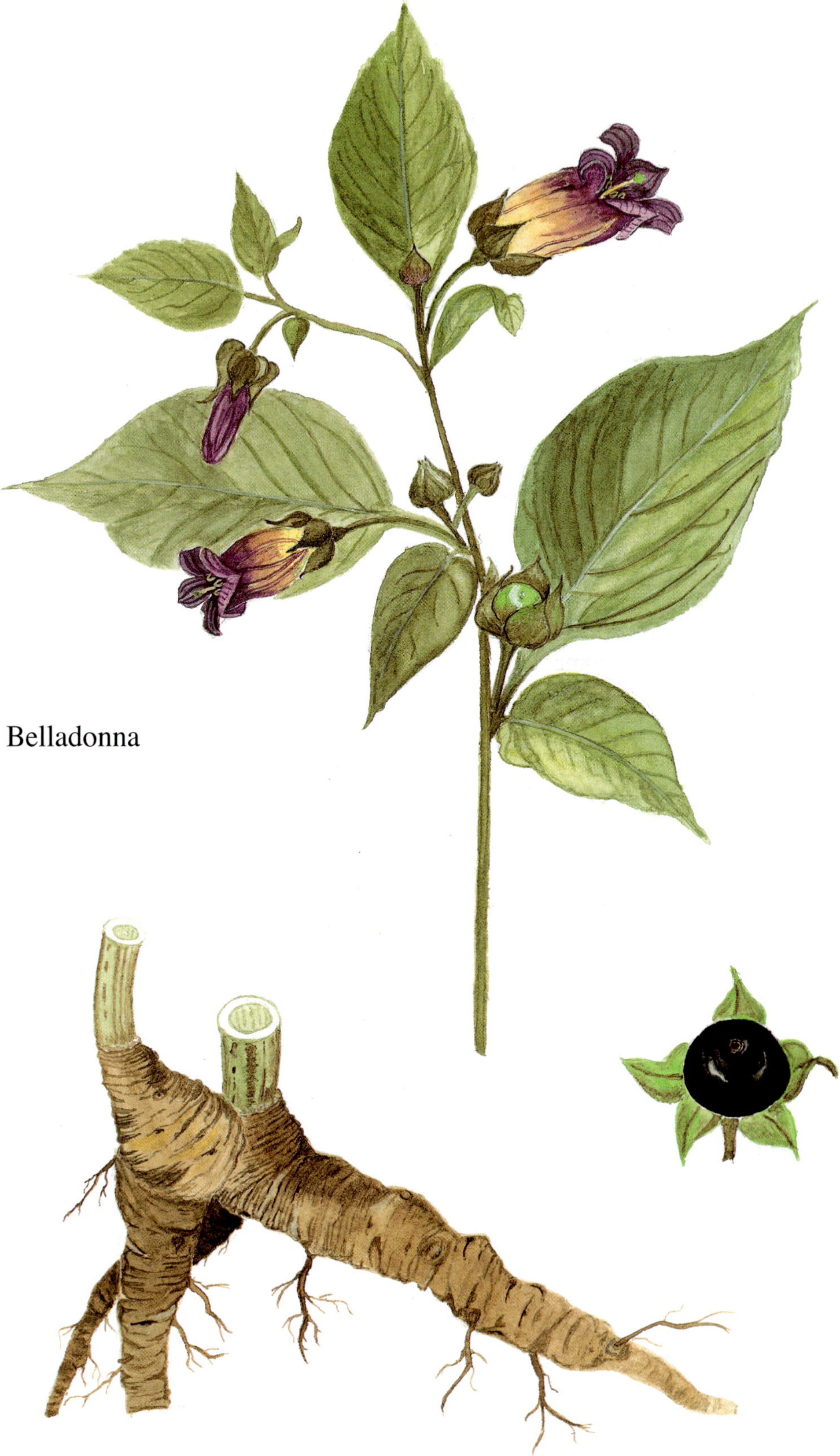

Belladonna

# Arsenicum Album
## (Arsenious Acid) – Arsenic Trioxide

Arsenic alb is a deadly poison. It is said that once it enters the body, it gets absorbed into the bones and hair permanently.

**Restlessness and anxiety** are the main feature. The restlessness is mental rather than physical as in Rhus Tox.

**Fear of death** with anxiety and restlessness. Some women become very anxious following emotional shock or septic fevers.

**Tidiness** - the Arsenic patient is tidily dressed. He keeps his room tidy and in order and soon gets upset if things are disturbed in his room.

**Diarrhoea** - stools are frequent, black and offensive. The patient is restless and can have convulsions, as toxins gets absorbed from the inflamed gut. Prompt treatment with Arsenic Alb will soon restore the inflamed bowel.

**Thirsty** - increased thirst for small and frequent drinks is due to anxiety. Anxiety causes dryness of mouth that leads to increased thirst. In chronic cases he becomes less thirsty despite having dryness of mouth, but anxiety persists. He tosses and turns in bed resembling Gelsemium. The main difference is that there is no restlessness in Gelsemium, while the arsenic patient is constantly restless in bed with increased frequency of urine. Anxiety and restlessness with throat or bladder illness indicates that the patient may be suffering from cancer. Arsenic Alb will relieve the symptoms but one should treat the case constitutionally.

**Restlessness** with anxiety can be helped by high potency of Arsenic Alb in cases of terminal cancer. Restlessness also acts as a stimulant for natural body defenses. I once gave it to a lady with a terminal illness, whose doctors had stopped administering her painkillers. It greatly helped and she was peaceful.

**Kidney diseases** - Arsenic Alb is closely related to renal diseases. Its patient has **albuminuria with inflamed kidneys**. Anxiety and restlessness can also result from mental overwork causing increased sensitivity of the kidneys. In cases of diseases of the bladder, prostate and kidneys, where Arsenic alone is indicated but does not help, the addition of Phosphorus will help when given separately. This combination of Arsenic and Phosphorus is also useful in the cancer of the prostate. In my experience this also helped in a case of terminal cancer with limited life expectancy - the patient was helped by the grace of God and lived peacefully for another year.

**Chilliness** – the Arsenic patient is very chilly and feels cold. The patient feels better for heat (feeling of heat) except for stomach ailments and headaches which is better for cold (feeling of cold). Headache is better with the application of pressure.

**Nausea and vomiting** - Arsenic Alb patients can have severe nausea and vomiting.

**Periodicity of symptoms** - the relapse of symptoms at a particular time, such as in migraine, recurs every seven to fourteen days. The headache is better with cold applications. If acute headache is not treated properly in the Arsenic individual it can become chronic and move to the joints.

**Aggravation after midnight** - the symptoms are worse at night. The patient is afraid of being alone and is anxious. When the disease progresses the patient will not find any relief even in company.

**Menorrhagia and menstrual problems** - many a time uterine ailments can change into mental symptoms of anxiety and restlessness, with fear of death and depression. If menses are stopped suddenly with medicine and the mental symptoms appear this is not a good sign. The symptoms become chronic with offensive vaginal discharges with blood clots. The patients have mental symptoms of restlessness as well as general body pains. Arsenic will relieve all symptoms if indicated and gets rid of toxins from the body. In these cases Kali Iodide and Arsenic Iodide combined or given separately are also of benefit. In addition, Sulphur and Pyrogenium 200 given together is very effective in such cases. It will clear the infection and associated symptoms.

**Arsenic and Secale Corn have many similarities**. Secale is useful for offensive and dark colored discharges The Secale patient feels hot while Arsenic Alb is chilly. Secale, even though he feels hot, feels better with external heat while the Arsenic Alb patient has offensive discharges, with fear of dying and increased thirst for small drinks.

**Dry cough and asthma** – the patients have nasal obstruction with itchy nose, sneezing, clear runny nose and swollen neck glands as in hay fever.

Arsenic* is useful in dry asthma and chronic cardiac asthma. In cardiac asthma the pulse is weak and rapid but palpable. In the Aconite and Belladonna patient, the pulse is palpable. In a Carbo Veg patient, the pulse is weak but not palpable. It disappears under the finger. Arsenic is helpful in other cardiac diseases. The patient gets breathless on climbing uphill and also when flying. Such cases will benefit from Arsenic given before, during and after the journey.

**Gangerine and Arsenic Alb** - Arsenic is a very useful remedy in gangerine. In gangerine the afflicted part gets ischemic and infected. In my experience, Arsenic has proved life saving in many cases. In some cases where surgery seemed unavoidable the patient, by the grace of God, was completely cured with timely use of Arsenic Alb 200. In another case, a young man had his arm crushed in a machine, the wound became infected and amputation was advised. I treated him with Arsenic Alb in CM to be repeated weekly over a few weeks. By the grace of God the arm of the patient soon started regaining normal color and the black colouration disappeared, thus surgery was avoided. If the case does not respond to Arsenic Alb one should try other remedies like Silicia or Sulphur in high potency before surgery, otherwise it is better to have surgery to save the patient's life. In deep ischemic ulcers Kali Iodide and Arsenic Iodide can be helpful.

*Arsenic on its own always means Arsenic Album.

**Arsenic Alb and eyes** - the whole eye is inflamed. In Kali Carb the inflammation is confined to the upper eyelid, while in Apis it is the lower eyelid.

**Premature ageing** - the patient can have symptoms of ageing in Arsenic, but it is more marked in Sarsaparilla and Chinumum Ars.

**Arsenic alb and depression** - there is anxiety with depression. The patient has suicidal tendencies and thinks he is beyond redemption.

**Malaria and Arsenic Alb** - as in malaria periodicity is also found in Arsenic Alb, the relapse of symptoms every fourth, seventh or fourteenth day. Arsenic Alb given in high potency is also effective as a preventative in malaria. Arsenic should be given during remission of fever and not during the attack. Natrum Mur is also useful in malaria but one should avoid its use in rising fever. I have also found Arnica in high potency of great help in the treatment of malaria. Chinumum Ars is reported to be useful in malaria but this is not so in my experience. In fact, I have found that Arsenic Alb and Arnica are much better than Chinumum Ars. Bryonia and Rhus Tox is useful for general bodyache in the beginning of fevers generally.

The success of treatment in malaria is judged by the fact that the fever will not return or will be of less severity or if the fever relapse is early or delayed. These are good signs and indicate that the treatment is effective. Otherwise, one should change the treatment or start allopathoic treatment.

**Retention of urine after labour** - the best treatment is Causticum, but if it is ineffective Arsenic Alb can be useful.

**Hoarseness** – Arsenic Alb is beneficial when the throat is hoarse. Also, if the patient has earache with offensive catarrh and burning in eyes and nose.

Arsenic symptoms are worse in damp weather, after midnight, at the seaside, after cold food, with heat and worse for hot drinks.

| | |
|---|---|
| **Adjuvants:** | Rhus Tox, Carbo Veg, Phosphorus and Thuja |
| **Antidote:** | Opium, Carbo Veg, China, Hepar Sulph, Nux Vomica |
| **Potency:** | 30 to CM. |

# ARSENIC IODATUM
## (Iodide of Arsenic)

Arsenic Iodide is very closely related to Arsenic Album. Arsenic Iodide is the best prevention against the **sores** becoming chronic state or turning **gangrenous**. It is very effective against abscess in the lower part of the lungs and the large air passages in the lungs (bronchi). In Arsenic Iodide, there may be multiple kinds of disease manifestations (indistinguishable from Arsenic Album).

Contrary to Arsenic (in which the patient always feels very cold), the Arsenic Iodide patient feels hot and manifests his restlessness by way of quick movements and walking fast. An overactive, uncontrollable child, eating a lot and staying thin, indicates the nature of Iodine. So also may be the condition in Arsenic Iodide. The patient of Arsenic Iodide shows contrasting clinical pictures of Arsenic and sometimes of Iodine. However, these two remedies, have opposing symptoms. So diagnosis needs to be carefully established.

Arsenic Iodide is a very wide-ranging homoeopathic remedy. Its discharges are abrasive in nature and make the exiting orifice red and inflamed with burning. The inner lining of the nose becomes swollen and rather indurate. Inflammation of the ear-tubes (Eustachian tubes) leading into the ear can cause deafness.

Arsenic Iodide is extremely effective in **all kinds of diseases of the lungs**, including the lung cavities. For this reason, it is very commonly used in tuberculosis and chronic bronchitis associated with **abundant expectoration**.

It is also very useful in **Lupus** and skin cancer. It also, very **effectively stops the growth of ovarian cancer** though it may not eradicate it. Dr. Kent is of the opinion that Arsenic Iodide is very useful in stopping the growth of **any kind of cancer**. The author has found it more effective when combined with Suchi Bootie (a herbal medicine).

Arsenic Iodide works very well on **eczemas** in which the skin is dry and scaly but under the thick scales is rather raw, abrased and moist.

Arsenic Iodide is useful against **Psoriasis**, though the apparent cure is incomplete and short-lived. According to the traditional western medicine, when diseases of the glands are treated, a violent skin reaction takes place in the form of wide spread, psoriatic condition and when the skin condition is suppressed by a drug, yet another kind of ailment may ensue. So far, there is no known remedy for the control of both skin and glandular pathology. However, Sulphur 1000 and Psorinum 1000, given alternatively, benefit to some extent. Hydrocotyle is also quite useful. It is also very useful in **leprosy**. Arsenic is also a psoric remedy, capable of controlling the mucous membranes (the inner linings of the viscera) as well as the skin. Some remedies are good for inflammatory conditions of the intestines and skin, while others are good in diseases of the uterus and skin. Sulphur and Mercury are saliently effective against the diseases of the skin and glands. Arsenic Iodide may be indicated in different stages of syphilis.

In Arsenic Iodide, the **pain is in the nape of the neck** and there is a burning sensation at the back. A cold chill and numbness radiates down the left leg. The **wrist aches on writing**. The patient feels cold though he sweats at the same time.

When symptoms of Arsenic Iodide are aggravated, the patient feels nauseous and very thirsty. After drinking water he throws up (as in Phosphorus) soon after. There is **intense pain in the stomach** which is relieved by bending over forward as in Colocynth. **Frequent stools** that start early in the morning are associated with severe gripe inflammation. The stomach becomes bloated with gas. The appetite is strong but the body does not thrive.

| | |
|---|---|
| **Potency:** | 30 to 200 |

# ARSENICUM SULPHURATUM FLAVUM

Arsenicum Sulphuratum Flavum is very commonly used in leprosy. It has been found very effective in **all kinds of itching, leprosy and skin lesions associated with syphilis**. Its salient features are flashes of piercing pain emitting from inside the chest and a stinging sensation on the forehead on the right side and behind the ear. The pain is like being jabbed with a needle and tends to shift its position. **Ants seem to be creeping** all over the body. Spasms and twitching of the body are not uncommon. The feeling of being hot is accompanied by a rapid irregular pulse that becomes worse on walking or running. The pain is intense and unbearable.

The Arsenic Sulphuratum Flavum patient is very easily provoked. Irritability is apparent right at the dawn of the day. Prevalent in vertigo is the fear of falling on the right side. The head feels cold. The eyes are red and sticky due to reddish yellow exudates. The discharge from the ears smells very offensive. In case of cold, the nasal secretions are copious. The person feels weak and debilitated.

Arsenic Sulphuratum Flavum is particularly famous for its use in skin diseases. It is widely used in white skin spots of **leprosy**; eczema, acne and wide spread pimples and moles. It is worth a trial for the cure of **non-healing ulcers** associated with burning and severe discomfort. The symptoms of the Arsenic Sulphuratum Flavum patient aggravate in the morning and in the evening. The patient does not like open air, which aggravates the symptoms further.

**Potency:** 30 to 200

# ARUM TRIPHYLLUM
## (Indian Turnip)

Aurum Triphylum is prepared from a vegetable that resembles a gourd and turnip and grows abundantly in the forest. Its poison causes intense irritation and tingling on contact with the body. The homoeopathic form has been found very affective against intense nasal irritation at the tip of the nose. Children who pick their nose and cause ulceration respond well to Aurum Triphylum.

During catarrhal conditions, when the eyes itch and water and the upper eyelids feel tremulous, Aurum Triphylum may offer relief. The symptoms of **cold** are very intense, and associated with copious, watery discharge and severe itching. The brain feels drained out. Prolonged Irritation and tingling of the throat may result in numbness and lack of sensitivity. Swallowing may be impaired due to the weakness of the appropriate muscles of the throat. A person may choke with the fluids or food, if not careful. The **tonsils swell** and the mouth feels raw and burns with the feeling of suffocation at the throat. The **tongue is red with a burning** and tingling sensation. This condition is called strawberry tongue. There is **painful blistering of the mouth cavity** causing difficulty in even swallowing water. Aurum Triphylum has an extraordinary effect in such cases. The voice waves and wanes. Too much talking and cold suppresses the voice, which occasionally becomes loud.

There is loss of appetite, however, to relieve the headache one has to eat. The **diarrhoeal stools** are as in typhoid fever (pea soup appearance).

The lungs hurt. The inner lining becomes itchy or painful due to irritation. If not treated in time, the viscera (internal organs) become paralysed. Intestinal movements may not stop completely but they definitely become sluggish. Symptoms of Aurum Triphylum are more pronounced on the left side of the head, face and nose. When the chest is badly affected, urination becomes scanty and deep coloured. The administration of Aurum Triphylum will restore normal, clear urination. (In Gelsemium, urine is clear and copious.) The skin develops specks like measles. The skin feels raw and starts oozing on mild scratching. The headache becomes worse by drinking hot fluids or wrapping oneself in warm clothing.

| | |
|---|---|
| **Antidotes:** | Acetic Acid, Pulsatilla |
| **Potency:** | 30 |

# ASAFOETIDA

Asafoetida is often used as a seasoning spice and to promote digestion of food. The homoeopathic form of Asafoetida is very useful for the **spasmodic contraction of the stomach and the oesophagus (gullet).** Its salient feature is a numbing headache mostly on the surface, though it may be felt deep inside the head. (In Hydrocyanic Acid, Tarentula Hispania and Conium, there is a generalised sensation of numbness.) Asafoetida patients are of very sensitive nature. The symptoms are worse at night. They ameliorate in the open air, by movement and local pressure.

Brittle porous bones are well within the range of this homoeopathic remedy. As in syphilis, where the bones of the nose die and rot resulting in persistently malodorous discharge.

| | |
|---|---|
| **Antidote:** | China, Mercury |
| **Potency:** | 30 |

# AURUM METALLICUM

Aurum Metallicum is mostly related to the mental aptitude of a person. Its illnesses are secondary to mental strains and stresses. Repeated mental trauma leads to physical illnesses. The main characteristic of Aurum Metallicum is that the patient **loses self-confidence**. He constantly scolds himself and considers himself to be a totally useless person and a burden on society. He becomes suicidal and in fact **attempts to commit suicide**.

The Aurum Metallicum patient is apparently calm, quiet, depressed and withdrawn, but when provoked, may rather jump to kill somebody else (against his usual suicidal tendency). The constant self-denial, indifference to others and others mistreating him, all make him introverted. He may suddenly explode violently, often to harm himself. If bothered too much, he may prove extremely dangerous and avenge his anger on others. One should better avoid bothering the Aurum Metallicum patient or indulging him in argument. In the Aurum Metallicum patient, the madness is born out of prolonged emotional suppression. When the patient's self-prestige is very low, hopelessness prevails around him and he considers himself to be a total failure. His mental anguish and emotional torment can drive him mad permanently. In the early stage, however, he can think and comprehend clearly.

In Aurum Metallicum, the main physical effect of the disease is on the **liver** and then on the heart also. The heart muscle becomes weak and the liver fails. The heart and lung ailments go hand in hand. There is inflammation of the inner lining of the heart, causing chest pain. The heart dilates leading to accumulation of water in the lungs.

Aches and pains like rheumatism are common. The joints are inflamed. The membranous covering of the bones are badly affected, resulting in the bones becoming weak and carious. The inner lacework of the bones trabeculae become rigid, though structurally weak (as in a Argentum Nitricum). There is a feeling of stabbing pain in the bones. The joints become stiff and difficult to move, like in a frozen shoulder. Many a time, the shoulder becomes stiff as a result of injury. Aurum Metallicum is the best remedy, provided the stiffness of the shoulder is due to rheumatism.

In Aurum Metallicum, **the veins become dilated** and the blood starts clotting within them. The arteries pulsate and feel warm. There are microscopic bleedings into the joints, causing them to hurt. Due to the ailments of the heart and the liver, there is swelling in some parts of the body and the glands all over the body enlarge. Swelling of the legs and ankles is very common in women. Their leg veins have remained congested because they have to carry heavy weight during pregnancy. In addition to Aurum Metallicum, other remedies can also work in such a condition, provided their particular symptoms are also present.

In Aurum Metallicum, there is **severe headache** and there is feeling of air rustling over the head. The face is swollen and shines due to the skin being taut and tense.

The **hair on the scalp tends to fall** leading to **baldness** (Acid Phos is also very useful in falling hair). If a specific remedy is not known, then the general formula of Alopecia may be used, such as Bacilinium 200 + Natrum Mur 30 + Teucrium Marum 30 and Picric Acid 30, to significant effect. Alopecia is a form of localized baldness. I have found the above formula quite effective in general baldness also, especially when the face shows signs of ringworm infestation. If other constitutional symptoms are also present (in addition to baldness), then Graphites and Phosphorus may also be very effective. In case of syphilis baldness, the combination of Natrum Mur 200 and Bacilinium 200 has also been found to be effective. In the books, Aurum Metallicum has also been quoted to be effective in baldness, secondary to suppressed syphilis. To augment the useful affect of Aurum Metallicum, one should administer Syphlinum CM and repeat it after two months before resorting to Aurum Metallicum and follow with Natrum Mur and Bacilinium.

In Aurum Metallicum, the **eyes are extremely sensitive to light**. Strong light of gas lamps is very troublesome. Flashing light perturbs the patient. The moonlight, however, is soothing to the eye, though this is not the leading feature of Aurum Metallicum.

**The patient eludes the stars as falling downwards**, while in Calcaria the illusion is upwards. This sign is typical of Aurum Metallicum.

Sometimes, **the eyes swell and protrude out**. In allopathic medicine, the only treatment for this condition is surgery. Swollen protruding eyes may be due to diseases of the glands or some other chronic debilitating illness in which tuberculous matter is found. Aurum Metallicum has been found very useful in combating this condition irrespective of its cause. I have also found Natrum Mur and Bacilinium useful in this condition. If the pressure inside the eye is elevated, Belladonna and Arnica must also be used. The important point again is to keep in view the natural aptitude of the patient and find the appropriate match from the homoeopathic armamentarium. If the symptoms are mixed up, the above combination may be employed. At least, I have found it very beneficial.

Aurum Metallicum is very useful against the **deep wounds of the ears,** in which the bony structure of the ear becomes rotten, resulting in discharge of extremely putrid material.

The **nasal cold** of Aurum Metallicum patient is of chronic type. The cause is not the inflammation of the mucosal lining, but the involvement of the cartilaginous bones of the nose. The nasal catarrh of Natrum Mur is related to the inflammation of the lining of the nose and not the bones. Administration of Natrum Mur first aggravates the symptoms resulting in copious secretions, and then makes them disappear.

In homoeopathic literature, Aurum has been mentioned in relation to the treatment of suppressed syphilis. Recent studies of AIDS patients in America have shown that severely sick patients of AIDS exhibited symptoms of syphilis also. This is attributed to have been acquired from their ancestors who had syphilis, were treated and apparently were cured.

One characteristic sign of Aurum Metallicum is the **formation of spider webs on the nose** and the tendency of the blood to clot in these little veins like varicose veins. The lips also look bluish.

In the Aurum patient, the liver becomes stone hard and nodules form. Aurum Metallicum is also useful in Inguinal Hernia, an inflamed hardened uterus associated with widely spaced, scanty menses. In Natrum Mur also, similar symptoms develop, with the difference that there is a lot of pain in the back and the condition is mostly prominent in unmarried girls. One dose of Natrum Mur may often provide cure. In Aurum Metallicum, the associated ache is of a floating nature.

Most of the symptoms of Aurum resemble those of Argentum Metallicum. But there are certain differences. For example, in Argentum, the symptoms are relieved through rest and slow movement. In Aurum, the symptoms worsen on walking fast especially, which also raises the blood pressure and causes tightness of the chest and suffocation. In Argentum, the situation is just the opposite.

| | |
|---|---|
| **Adjuncts:** | Aurum Mur, Asafoetida, Kali Iodide, Phosphorus |
| **Antidotes:** | Belladonna, Cuprum, China |
| **Potency:** | 30 to 1000. |

# AURUM MURIATICUM

Aurum Muriaticum is prepared from a salt of gold (Sodium Chloraurate). The ailments related to it revolve around the heart, and like Aurum Metallicum, affect the liver and heart together. **The patient passes urea in the urine**. The blood urea is also high. It is also found effective against glandular diseases. On that basis, it is used in **cancers of the glands**. If the symptoms present are specific for Aurum Muriaticum, this particular remedy can offer cure even in dangerous cancer.

The typical symptom of Aurum Muriaticum is the **pain** which, wherever it manifests, will be **associated with a burning sensation**. **Symptoms ameliorate in cold, damp environment**, but intensify in hot muggy weather. There is a **tendency towards committing suicide** like Aurum Metallicum but the patient does not like to be aloof and is ill-tempered, irritable, and rather quarrelsome.

Throbbing is a sign of Aurum Muriaticum ailments. Aurum Muriaticum is useful in syphilis-like symptoms of the eyes, associated with **decay and destruction of the bones**. The vision is decreased in artificial lighting. Thus Aurum Muriaticum would significantly improve eyesight which, although otherwise normal, is blurred in the nightlight.

In Aurum Mur patients, **music particularly relieves the ear symptoms**. At night, the skin behind the ears burns and itches. Aurum Mur is also very affective against the chronic nasal problems and old nasal catarrh.

In Aurum Muriaticum patient, if the thick scabs in the nose are attempted to be removed, bleeding ensues. The discharge is yellowish-green. Aurum Mur is also reported to be useful in **Lupus-like conditions at the margin of the nostrils.**

In Aurum Mur, the stools are either greenish or clay coloured. This indicates liver dysfunction. Many a time, the stools are whitish. Stools are more frequent at night, and so is the urination. There may even be bed-wetting at night. Salivation from the mouth is excessive.

Aurum Mur is very effective in the **enlargement of the uterus associated with hardening**, especially the cervical part of the uterus. Carbo Animalis, Tarentula-Hispania, Lapis Albus are also very useful in cervical problems. When sleeplessness is secondary to mental anguish and associated with a throbbing sensation, Aurum Muriaticum may also be useful (in addition to other Homoeopathic remedies for this condition). Such a patient experiences sadistic or sorrowful dreams. He usually experiences the dream relating to his own ailment. When the disease is too advanced, the dreams are of extreme horror while sorrowful dreams indicate that the illness is in the early stage, and that recovery may be expected soon. Many homoeopaths believe that Pulsatilla and Kali Sulph are similar to Aurum Muriaticum but this is not true.

During early pregnancy, especially if detected on the first day, a single dose of Aurum Mur CM, by Allah's grace, usually brings about **the birth of a son**. Delayed use of Aurum Mur is much less predictable. Nevertheless, this is not a sure formula. I have noticed some women have delivered baby girls even after taking Aurum Muriaticum the next morning of the pregnancy, but whose next children were male-born. In my experience, some women who take Aurum Muriaticum CM may not even conceive sometimes. When they do, their chances of having a baby boy born to them are 80% or even more. Aurum Muriaticum is well-known in this aspect. I receive scores of letters every year to that effect. For instance, a lady wrote to me from Lahore, Pakistan. She and her two sisters-in-law had no male issue. All three used the prescription from the book and each was blessed with a baby boy.

| **Potency:** | 30 to CM |
|---|---|

# Baptisia

Baptisia is a well-known, tested remedy for day-to-day ailments. It is related to decay and fetidness. For example, the diarrhoea of typhoid fever in which **the stools smell awfully putrid** will best respond to Baptisia. Typhoid diarrhoea is not that severe, but the stools are pasty and smell foul.

Baptisia is very useful in the **infectious conditions of the throat**. The throat is commonly involved in infections which may not be painful as yet, however, the tonsils exhibit the grievous state of infection. Baptisia is the most effective homoeopathic remedy for such a throat condition with offensive odour, even if there is no associated pain.

In cases of uterine sepsis and infections of other parts of the body associated with putrefaction, Baptisia is very useful, but the best remedy would still be Sulphur 200 and Pyrogenium 200 given together. However, if the specific symptoms of Baptisia are manifest; Baptisia 30 may also be administered for added advantage.

In **typhoid fever**, if the signs and symptoms of Baptisia are present, administration of Baptisia is a must. The combined use of Typhoidinum 200 and Pyrogenium 200 will enhance its effectiveness. In typhoid, the distension of the abdomen is much more compared to the degree of fever. The entire body is being melted gradually, while the belly becomes puffed up. In this condition, if Baptisia symptoms are also present, then the following regimen should be implied:

1. Until the fever subsides completely i.e. no fever in the morning and evening, Typhodinum and Pyrogenium should be administered three times a day and Baptisia 30 five to six times a day.
2. After the fever has subsided, Pyrogenium and Typhoidinum should be administered once a day and Baptisia 30 three times a day, for at least one week.
3. In the third week, Pyrogenium and Typhoidinum should be administered twice a week and Baptisia 30 three times a day.

If the above regimen is continued for at least 21 days then there will be no fear of recurrence of typhoid and, by Allah's grace, no residual bad affects will remain.

In case there are no associated symptoms of Baptisia and the patient is rather constipated, Kali Phos and Ferrum Phos 6X should be used along with Typhoidinum and Pyrogenium (instead of Baptisia).

One homoeopathic doctor has written in his book about a patient who went blind due to typhoid and regained his eyesight during a fever he contracted after taking some other medicine. Such astounding events do take place, although rarely. According to allopathy, neurologists claim that once dead the nerves cannot rejuvenate. One thing is definitely certain that typhoid is a very dangerous disease. Its ill effects on the brain can result in insanity for the rest of ones life. Such an afflicted patient exhibits signs of Stramonium and Hyoscyamus (both these remedies are also useful in typhoid). They ameliorate the symptoms but do not provide a cure.

Baptisia is also useful in **dental diseases** especially when the **gums are inflamed,** produce stinking pus and recede from the teeth.

One typical sign of Baptisia is that the patient is drowsy or semi-conscious. He feels as if his limbs are not connected together. His personality is also similarly divided. The organs of his body are lethargic. Even on being awakened, he is drowsy, trying to concert his efforts. He sometimes talks to his limbs. At times, he feels as if one of his legs is actually talking to the other. He has to be aroused to answer a question, yet he will fall asleep while still trying to find an answer. Baptisia is the best remedy in such a state of mental confusion, provided the other symptoms of Baptisia are also present.

In Baptisia, the stools are clay-coloured, yellowish or sometimes greyish and are pasty in nature. At times there are beads of cold sweat on the forehead showing that the body strength is dwindling. In this condition, the tongue becomes dry and stiff, ulcers form around the teeth which stink. Even in this grave condition, if given promptly, Baptisia may restore life.

In Baptisia ulcers in the mouth can become gangrenous (Cancrumoris). They are not painful though there is an extremely bad taste in the mouth. The tissues around the ulcers become numb and demarcated or separated. At this stage, the Homoeopathic remedy cannot reach the affected tissues. So it is important that the condition be diagnosed in good time in order to avert this grave situation.

In Baptisia, involvement of the throat permits the swallowing of the liquids but causes great **difficulty in swallowing solid food**. If the patient forces himself to swallow the solid food, he may choke himself.

In Baptisia, some ailments manifest weakness due to paralysis. On the same basis the intestinal paralysis causes distension of the abdomen. In Homoeopathy, it is vital to know the basic nature of the remedy. A characteristic feature is that the afflicted part of the body is only partially paralysed and there is decreased sensitivity of that part to the pain. By remembering this particular feature, Baptisia will hopefully be put to use in a timely fashion.

| | |
|---|---|
| **Adjuvants:** | Bryonia, Arsenic, Arnica, Pyrogenium, Sulphur, Typhoidinum |
| **Potency:** | 30 to 200 |

# Baryta Carb

Some homoeopaths describe the nature of Baryta Carb in one word i.e. **dwarfism**. Not only is the stature of the person small but he may also be mentally retarded. Both physical and mental deficiencies go hand in hand. In my experience, Baryta Carb works very well even in just a physical short stature. It is not right to associate every case of physical dwarfism with mental deficiency. In my hand, by God's grace, Baryta Carb has worked equally well in dwarfs of average intelligence and great thinkers alike. Combined use of Silicea 6X and Calcaria Flour 6X is the best prescription for increasing height.

Baryta Carb also works in dwarfs who are mentally deficient. It has also been found very effective in paralysis of long-standing, especially in the **paralysis following typhoid and polio**. Baryta Carb used alternatively with Sulphur or Rhus Tox has been found to produce wonderful results. However, so far, there is no known remedy for typhoid-stricken nervous system. The toxins produced in the typhoid kill the nerves and there is no cure for death. If the paralytic effects of typhoid/polio are on the muscles while the nerves are only partially afflicted, Homoeopathy can offer an effective treatment. Baryta Carb (in addition to the other known remedies) has been found significantly effective in the paralysis of the limbs following typhoid and polio. The effect is more evident in polio than in typhoid. Baryta Carb may not offer cure, but the patient definitely feels much improved. The wasted legs start gaining mass and strength. The stiff paralysed hands start reverting towards normal use. However, every patient does not find that kind of improvement.

The children of the nature of Baryta Carb tend to be very shy. At school, they are typical backbenchers. They hide themselves on the sight of strangers. When associated with some physical weakness, such children should be treated with Baryta Carb. Baryta Carb and Calcaria Carb are both famous for the treatment of **weak-legged children.** The main difference is that in Calcaria Carb, the legs are not only weak but they also look weak due to the underdevelopment of the bones. The belly of such children bulges forward and the head is prominently big. In Baryta Carb, the legs of the child may apparently look normal but are weak. Their walking is delayed. The weakness of the legs and **delayed walking** is also found in Borax and

Natrum Mur. In Natrum Mur, there is delay in both learning to walk and to talk. In case there is only a **delay in learning to talk** but not in walking, Kali Phos would be very useful. In my experience combination of Kali Phos 6X and Natrum Mur is the best remedy for the delayed onset of walking and talking in children.

Baryta Carb is very useful in the treatment of **delayed onset of puberty** in some girls. Baryta Carb mainly works on the glands, especially on the **lymph glands** in the upper part of the neck, which get chronically inflamed. With every episode of an illness, their swelling increases. Similarly, **fatty lumps** (lipomas) form on the body particularly at the back. (Multiple small nodules may also be found in conditions other than Baryta Carb). In Baryta Carb, once the glands become enlarged, they do not decrease in size nor does the potbelly become small, even if the rest of the body is visibly wasted. In such a situation, Baryta Carb can safely be used repeatedly, in high potency.

Baryta Carb lowers the **systolic blood pressure,** though it does not affect the diastolic blood pressure. During the prolonged use of Baryta Carb, one should regularly check the blood pressure to ensure that the systolic blood pressure has not fallen too much. If so, Baryta Carb should be temporarily stopped and then restarted as necessary.

Baryta Carb is very important in the treatment of **Cerebral Arteriosclerosis** i.e. the thickening and narrowing of the arteries of the brain. Continued use of Crataegus by the patient also proves very beneficial. Remember that Arteriosclerosis is a very slowly progressive disease and so its treatment would also be slowly effective. Baryta Carb will have to be administered at least for a year or two to show its good effects. Thus, for most old folks, it is their best friend. In fact, Baryta Carb is mostly used in the **two extreme ages** i.e. the childhood and old age.

Many a time, diseases come and go but they may leave bad effects. Baryta Carb is very useful in alleviating these aftereffects. According to Dr. Kent, Baryta Carb is also very useful in **malaria**. I have no experience of that, though I have found it effective in treating the **aftereffects of malaria.**

Dr. Kent has written in his book that Baryta Carb is effective in fatty lumps, tumours and enlarged glands, Lupus and **tuberculous abscesses**. I personally have no such experience. I have used Baryta Carb in patients who had ugly bumps and lumps on their body to no avail, maybe their lumps were not of fatty nature. Baryta Carb does, however, specifically cure the tumours of fatty origin. I have also found Baryta Carb ineffective in the treatment of Lupus. Dr. Kent is of the opinion that when indicated, Baryta Carb must be used in all potencies. Some deep-seated illnesses do not respond to low potencies. Therefore, Baryta Carb must be used in increasing potencies of 1000, 10,000, 50,000 and CM with suitable intervals. When Baryta Carb is found effective at the outset of the illness, it may well cure the condition for good.

The Baryta Carb patient has a constant fear of unknown dangers. On that basis, Baryta Carb is specifically helpful in alleviating certain kinds of **hallucinations and delusions**. Some patients feel as if their brain is also vibrating along with the movement of their head. This is a typical symptom of Baryta Carb. **Epilepsy** resulting from temporary blockage of circulation to the brain, as happens in Meningitis, can be cured by prolonged, regular use of Baryta Carb.

In case of **bleeding,** which is red in colour (from ruptured arteries), Baryta Carb may be used besides Phosphorus.

In certain **eye ailments** particular to Baryta Carb, the eyelids become swollen and stay swollen due to the retention of their internal secretions. The same kind of obstinate swelling also affects the lymph glands of the upper part of the neck i.e. they do not diminish in size.

Baryta Carb is also a treatment for **falling hair, as well as the the dryness and baldness** of the scalp. Dryness of the skin and eczema is also found in other drugs. In Baryta Carb, the weakness of the hair may possibly be due to the accumulation of waste materials in the hair follicles (causing weakness of the hair). Baryta Carb is also useful in correcting **failing eyesight**. The long-term, regular use of Baryta Carb is not only safe but in fact may improve the eyesight of advancing age. Sometimes, the eyesight becomes weak due to **high cholesterol** in the blood (causing arteriosclerosis of the artery to the eye). Combined use of Cholestrinum 30, Phytolacca 30 and Phosphorus 30 will benefit this condition. Phosphorus 30, however, should not be used continuously over a long period for fear of increasing the thickness of the blood and its coagulability.

Baryta Carb is also useful in **corneal conditions**, as well as the formation of **sties**. Baryta Carb is very useful in the treatment of **swollen neck glands** and possibly in **mumps**.

The **paralysis of the tongue in old age** is deeply related to Baryta Carb. Baryta Carb must be used in older patients who are unable to bring out their sputum, once other medicines have proven ineffective. Similarly, Senega and Ammonium Carb are also very useful in chronic lung problems of the aged.

Baryta Carb is also linked to **earache**. When the earache becomes chronic and the ears feel full and heavy, even if there is no associated nasal discharge, Baryta Carb will be very beneficial in relieving the congestion of the ears and the earache.

In Baryta Carb, the **stools** are like hard balls sticking together. As in Nux Vomica, the person does not feel fully relieved after passing stools. There is also aching of the abdomen.

Baryta Carb is also useful in treating **sexual weakness in men as well as women**. The potency should be gradually increased, since very high potency of Baryta Carb at the outset may in fact increase sexual weakness. Along with sexual weakness, the women may also be **infertile**. Their ovaries shrink in size (instead of getting bigger). In such a condition, Baryta Carb must be administered promptly to avert possible transformation into cancer.

In Baryta Carb, the **paralysis of throat and legs** is a very prominent feature. When the paralysis affects only one side of the body, the main remedies would be Sulphur, Causticum, Rhus Tox, Gelsemium, Lachesis or Cadmium Sulph as indicated by the symptoms. Baryta Carb is extremely useful in **paralysis of the lower half of the body**. Besides this, Cocculus is also very effective for the treatment of the paralysis of the lower part of the body, but in high potency.

A typically strange characteristic of the Baryta Carb **cough** is that when the patient lies prone on the stomach, the cough is suppressed. Any change of side and posture will provoke coughing. In Baryta

Carb, abundant **warts** form on the body. The **feet are smelly** and malodorous. Severe low-back pain may be the precursor of impending paralysis of the lower half of the body. Baryta Carb may prevent this.

I know of a child whose legs were badly afflicted by **polio** and were badly bent. He was given Sulphur and Baryta Carb, which resulted in significant improvement. He walks around and leads a pretty independent life, though not completely cured. The doctors had told him that his weakness of the legs would worsen with age. Thus homoeopathic remedies may look simple and insignificant but show far-reaching profound affects, when used properly.

| | |
|---|---|
| **Adjuvants:** | Dulcamara, Silicea, Psorinum |
| **Antidotes:** | Camphor, Antimony Tart, Belladonna, Zincum |
| **Potency to be used:** | 30 to CM |

# Belladonna
## (Deadly Night Shade)

The Belladonna plant grows in dense, shady areas, in most of Europe. It blossoms in July and by September bears a red-coloured fruit. Belladonna is a very poisonous plant. Herbalists use it in the treatment of many diseases. The ointment made out of it is applied to wounds. During its full bloom season, the extract is made out of the whole plant for Homoeopathic use.

Belladonna acts on the **circulatory system** as well as on the heart, lungs, brain and nervous system. Like Aconite, a **sudden onset of the disease** typifies Belladonna, though the disease process is more prolonged. The salient feature of Belladonna is the inflammation especially affecting the brain, lungs, heart and intestines.

Although the acuteness of the symptoms is like that of Aconite, there is no associated fear. The patient expresses his suffering in the form of a groan or remains silent. He does not like to talk much except for crying out on having a nightmare during sleep. He usually remains quiet with the body covered. The slightest sound of somebody walking, and light also, intensify his suffering. His skin is so sensitive that even the touch of a cloth at the site of pain is unbearable. The afflicted part is red, with a severe **burning sensation.** Due to the rise of blood pressure, the patient may experience **spasms or convulsions**. Jerky movements of the body during sleep, secondary to stomach upset or disorder of the nervous system, are very responsive to Grindelia. In Grindelia, the jerky movements do not affect the whole body, though may be perceived as the jerking sensation at the heart. In Belladonna, the **whole body gets jolted** waking the person up. This happens repeatedly and the patient is unable to sleep. A single dose of Belladonna may relieve the symptoms in no time. **Photophobia** associated with the diseases of the eye or headache, is also a Belladonna symptom.

When Belladonna symptoms and the symptoms of the patient match exactly, Belladonna works instantaneously. In fact, the patient is amazed with the prompt efficacy of the treatment rendered.

In Belladonna, the symptoms pertaining to the **nervous system** are much more pronounced than in Aconite. Belladonna affects the mind and may even cause **severe frenzy**. When an insane person gets too excited and is ready to kill somebody or himself, if he is extremely enraged and starts hitting even his carer, then Belladonna should be administered at once. If the condition becomes chronic, then Belladonna will not work. Belladonna is certainly effective in sudden cases of insanity such as in **Meningitis** and other delirious states, but Sulphur and Stramonium are more effective in chronic insanity. A severe state of frenzy requiring the patient to be chained typifies Belladonna. After Belladonna has relieved the acute problem, one should look for an appropriate, long-acting constitutional remedy to prevent recurrence of insanity. Aconite and Belladonna are not long-acting remedies. Sometimes, the attack of madness is only short-lived. However, a chronic form of madness, despite having subsided temporarily, can recur again and again. Stramonium works for a much longer period than Belladonna.

In **typhoid** too, sometimes the symptoms may be similar to those of Belladonna. High fever affects the mind causing **delirium**. Belladonna may temporarily relieve the symptoms, but its effect will not be long lasting because typhoid and Belladonna are not alike in their characteristics. Stramonium is relatively more similar to typhoid and it works for a relatively longer duration. Thus, it may not only control the delirium of typhoid, but it will also cure the typhoid. Stramonium and Sulphur are very beneficial in mental patients, whether the madness is due to typhoid or something else. Sometimes an insane person is not only aggressive but may also talk obscenely. This is due to inflammation of the internal reproductive organs, and will also need to be attended to. Some people may become insane due to an old calamity affecting their mind, while others become insane due to intense grief or a big financial loss. Proper diagnosis of insanity needs an in-depth study of the case. Unfortunately, physicians do not always have enough time to go into details and thus make use of the everyday prescription of Stramonium and Sulphur to some benefit at least.

One peculiar feature of Belladonna is that its fever is a continuous one. Once it is down, it does not recur. On the contrary, the typhoid fever is high at night and relatively low in the morning. It returns the following day higher than on the previous day. Sometimes it is so high that it may even kill the patient. The Belladonna fever typically comes down suddenly. A fever that is suppressed by some strong medication and then recurs suddenly may very well be controlled by Belladonna. However, Belladonna is not the remedy for fevers which come on slowly.

In Belladonna patients, pimples and affected lymph glands show visible sign of inflammation. The **throat gets swollen** suddenly due to severe inflammation causing difficulty in swallowing. Belladonna is very useful for this condition. Another characteristic feature is that red spots form over the surface of inflamed glands. The redness lasts a while, and then becomes discoloured. The joint pains are associated with redness and swelling. The red spots also appear on the joints, which later discolour, but do not lead to pus formation.

Belladonna can also offer instant relief from a severe, **acute pain of the gall bladder,** if the pain gets worse by application of heat. After that, Sulphur, Natrum Sulph, Lycopodium and Chelidonium can be used for permanent cure.

Belladonna is also very useful in the colicky **pain of the kidneys** in addition to gall bladder colic (Biliary colic). Belladonna along with Aconite will work better still. Both Belladonna and Aconite 1000 should be given together every ten to fifteen minutes for two to three doses. If still ineffective and the pain seems to be getting better by heat, Colocynthis CM or Mag Phos 6X mixed in water should be administered repeatedly. The spasmodicity of the pain may apparently be the same, but the constitutional difference dictates the type of remedy required.

Swelling is a manifestation of Belladonna. When Belladonna is combined with Arnica for the treatment of **injuries**, it enhances its effect. In the case of an injury, the blood is rushed to the affected part for which doctors usually prescribe cold packs. Belladonna is more effective than cold packs and also fast acting. Belladonna given with Arnica is the best initial treatment for any kind of **injury**. Belladonna ailments get worse with heat but cold compresses, applied locally, offer relief. If liver and the gut are inflamed, the body becomes cold. In this condition, even if the patient is of Belladonna nature, external application of heat offers relief.

In Belladonna, each affected part of the body pulsates. Sometimes the whole body throbs. Belladonna will relieve any acute pain of a **spasmodic nature** with associated throbbing, which gets worse with jolting and noise, and is associated with the sensation of warmth.

Belladonna acts on the small circular fibres in the walls of the blood vessels (veins and arteries). Whenever these fibres contract violently due to heat, Belladonna will relieve this spasm. Belladonna works instantaneously in **spasmodic tightness of the mouth of the uterus at the time of labour,** provided other symptoms of Belladonna are also present. Otherwise, Colophylum has the capability of relieving this severe spasm. Calcaria Carb is the long-term remedy for the diseases of children who have initially responded well to Belladonna. Any **convulsions which get worse on the movement of the body or jolting**, will respond to Belladonna.

One strange feature of Belladonna is that during the illness, the patient feels better by taking food. Even if the patient is in a state of madness, he will calm down if fed. This symptom is also found in Phosphorus and Psorinum. An insane person feels hungry but he does not ask for food. If he is provided with some food his desire to eat, and the anguish will subside while the Phosphorus patient is usually very hungry and feels hungry soon after having food.

When the blood circulation towards the brain increases, the patient will envision demons and ghosts. Nightmares where objects are on fire disturb the patient during sleep. If such a patient is given Belladonna, he will stop dreaming about fire. In Belladonna, there is a tendency of **deep unconsciousness**. One pupil of the eye gets dilated. This particular symptom makes it similar to Opium, however Opium is different from Belladonna in other symptoms.

Belladonna should be the first medicine to be given when a **child has high fever** affecting mostly his head, but his feet are ice cold. It is a dangerous situation when, during a **fever**, the body becomes cold but the head is very hot. The mothers may believe that the fever has subsided but actually, it is the fever caused by the severity of the disease. If a proper homoeopathic remedy is administered, the body will start warming up. Otherwise, dangerous illnesses like meningitis and epilepsy can develop. In such conditions, Belladonna is one of those remedies which will work promptly. If the proper remedy is not provided, the child may die.

Belladonna will offer immediate relief when the patient has **severe vertigo** and is restless. This symptom is also present in Phosphorus. When there is a **headache**, the scalp starts hurting. Combing the hair or even touching it with the hand is very bothersome. The **hypersensitivity of the scalp** is also found in Hepar Sulph, which is so saliently present that some women may actually become unconscious. When there is lack of sleep due to preoccupation of thoughts and restlessness, Belladonna, Coffea and Phosphorus are all useful. When the **sleeplessness** is due to the mental perturbance, any slight noise or bump against the bed becomes unbearable and the ailment becomes aggravated at once. In Nux Vomica also, noise makes the symptoms worse. Many symptoms of Nux Vomica resemble those of Belladonna because Belladonna is a natural element of Nux Vomica.

Some patients react to the treatment very slowly and will likewise respond to slow acting remedies, but the patients whose symptoms progress rapidly will find the faster acting remedies work better. Some patients are very sensitive in reacting to the treatment. In such patients, instead of improving the patient's condition, the Homoeopathic remedies can actually produce the poisonous effects of the substance from which they are derived. Whatever medicine is given, it will produce corresponding symptoms. For this reason, one should prescribe the medicine with great care and should give it in low potency. At the same time, it is important that the hypersensitivity of the patient should also be treated.

There are three possible remedies to decrease hypersensitivity: Belladonna, Nux Vomica and Zincum Metallicum. Zincum Metallicum is the most sensitive type of medication. It can be so sensitive that the patient may not even tolerate a low potency. For this reason, such a patient should first be given Zinc which will then make the body react to other medicines in a proper way. Zinc should be started in a low potency of 30.

One symptom of Belladonna is similar to Gelsemium. The **headache** becomes better when the head is tilted backwards but if the head is tilted forwards, it makes the headache worse, (there are certain exceptions however). Such a patient should be treated with Belladonna or Gelsemium. Many a time when discharges accumulate in the nose or in the sinuses, the headache becomes worse when the head is tilted forwards.

Generally, Belladonna is a treatment of sudden short-lived illnesses. An ailment which comes on suddenly will also disappear suddenly. But sometimes, when the headache disappears, it may leave a heaviness of the head for many days along with the sensation of being tired. In Belladonna, having the **hair cut or getting the beard shaved** can provoke headache.

In Belladonna ailments, rest brings about relief, but movement exaggerates the symptoms. Most of the ailments of Belladonna start in the upper part of the body and migrate downwards. When the headache becomes better, the joints and the muscles start hurting starting from the upper part of the body to the lower part. Ledum is famous for the treatment of diseases that start in the lower part of the body and migrate upwards.

Belladonna is also very useful in the **diseases of the eye**. The eyes are unusually red, and the **eyelids are swollen**. The patient experiences flashes of light before their eyes. One peculiar sign is that the eyes remain completely dry while in Euphrasia, the eyes water in addition to the redness. In Belladonna and Euphrasia, the symptoms of redness and the intensity are similar. In Euphrasia, the redness is not that pronounced, but the eyes water a lot.

Belladonna is very useful in **glaucoma** (the rise of pressure inside the eye). There was a patient who had severe glaucoma who the doctors had labelled as incurable. The patient was told that due to the high pressure in the eye, the interior of the eye could burst open which might result in permanent blindness. The prescription that I gave to the patient mainly contained Belladonna. Surprisingly, within a week, the pressure inside the eye started returning to normal and the patient completely recovered. Gelsemium is also useful in decreasing the intra-ocular pressure in **glaucoma**. It is better to give Calcaria Phos 6X also.

Nux Vomica and Belladonna both have the element of Cuprum and Cuprum is one of the best remedies for **convulsive** states.

When the body becomes tremulous or blood pressure rises due to **mental irritability**, Belladonna will lower the pressure very effectively and quickly. The **thirst** associated with Belladonna ailment resembles that of Bryonia. The thirst is intense but is not relieved by drinking water. Sometimes the patient's mouth is dry as in Arsenic and the patient frequently sips water to quench his thirst. Arsenic and Bryonia have different symptoms of their own, but regarding the dryness of the mouth, all three, i.e. Bryonia, Arsenic and Belladonna are similar.

The women of the Belladonna type love to eat **sour things**. Diarrhoea of Belladonna is characterized by frequent, scanty stools.

In Belladonna, the patient also develops **piles**. Belladonna is very useful in frequent urination if it is due to the infection of kidneys or the bladder. Otherwise, frequent urination is not a typical symptom of Belladonna.

If the urethra is injured by the passage of broken stones due to some medication, Belladonna will relieve the inflammation of the urinary passage. Belladonna will also offer immediate relief of the **spasms of the uterus**, especially if the condition worsens by heat.

At the time of delivery, Belladonna is a very good treatment if the bleeding becomes severe. The trouble is mostly on the right side, and gets worse by heat. Belladonna can be very useful in preventing an abortion or miscarriage in those pregnant women who are very sensitive in nature, to the extent that they cannot tolerate noise or even the sound of footsteps. The sound of cough of the Belladonna patient is usually very forceful. Belladonna is a temporary initial treatment but if administered at the outset of making a proper diagnosis, it prevents further complications.

One of the symptoms of Belladonna is **cramping of the calf muscles**. During a convulsion, the head is pushed backwards. In Apis, like Belladonna, there is an element of excessive heat and swelling. The difference between Belladonna and Apis is that in Belladonna, the body is cold except for the affected part. Therefore, the patient wants to be kept warm and likes to wrap himself in warm clothing. In Apis, the entire body feels burning hot, and no external heat can be tolerated. In fact, if such a patient is made to sit close to fire, he may go into a state of convulsion.

In Belladonna and Apis both, the patient develops urticaria due to exposure to heat. This also happens in Pulsatilla. In such a condition, Pulsatilla and Belladonna given together are useful. Sometimes, the urticaria can be due to gastric upset. For this, Pulsatilla and Nux Vomica are more useful.

In Belladonna, **red spots** and pustules develop on the skin. There is also inflammation, as in Apis. The appearance of pimples and **blisters** on the skin can help in diagnosis, though the presence of other additional symptoms is also helpful. Aurum Triphyllum is also very useful in the treatment for urticaria. In Aurum Triphyllum however, the itching is at the nose and around the lips.

Belladonna is also related to Calcaria Carb, especially in sub-acute diseases. Calcaria Carb proves very useful where Belladonna has failed. Sometimes the symptoms of Belladonna transform into those of Sulphur, which in turn produces the symptom complex of Calcaria Carb. Calcaria Carb is a meeting point of many Homoeopathic remedies but Sulphur should not be administered after having given Calcaria Carb. If so desired, Lycopodium will have to be given in between. However, Calcaria Carb can be given directly after having used Sulphur.

Belladonna symptoms get worse on touch, jolting, noise and the passing of wind (emitting gas). The patient feels better when lying half-stretched.

| | |
|---|---|
| **Adjuncts:** | Calcaria Carb, Aconite, Sulphur |
| **Antidotes:** | Camphor, Coffea, Opium, Aconite |
| **Potency:** | 30 to CM |

# Bellis Perennis

Bellis Perennis offers the best treatment for **sprains of the ankle, muscle pains and collection of blood in the soft tissues** resulting from a blunt injury. Although, it is not used as often as Arnica and Ruta, it is very important in the treatment of such conditions. The sprain of the ankle is a very troublesome condition and can linger on for life, but Bellis can gradually cure even an old sprain of the ankle and its associated pain. Many a time, while walking, the ankle can turn inwards and cause severe pain. Arnica gives temporary relief, but after some time the pain returns. The possible chronicity of the condition can be obviated by using Bellis. The symptoms of Bellis intensify on exposure to cold air. Bellis is the best remedy for the **physical fatigue** and **aching muscles** of hard-working farmers and labourers. Bellis also benefits joints which tend to fail as a result of long, strenuous use.

During pregnancy, women often develop prominent swelling of the veins on the legs (varicose veins). Bellis is a very useful remedy in this condition. However, most homoeopathic physicians forget to use Bellis and resort to other remedies instead. Bellis is very beneficial for the treatment of pain and discomfort of the muscles of the abdominal wall. There may be pain in the muscles of the uterus and the muscles of the abdomen, which can make it difficult for some women to stand up without support. Bellis is also very useful for them.

Bellis Perennis is deeply related to the **muscles around the backbone**. The weakened muscles make the vertebrae unsupported and unstable. Bellis is most beneficial in strengthening the muscles of the back. Sometimes, the pain at just one particular vertebra of the back can make walking difficult. Bellis significantly benefits this condition. Bellis is very useful in the treatment of injury to the backbone and inflammation of the nerves.

Hypericum is the very special remedy for treating pain at the coccyx (coccalgia). When given with Bellis or Arnica, its beneficial effect becomes more pronounced. The symptoms of Bellis intensify by taking a cold shower or on exposure to cold air.

| | |
|---|---|
| **Adjuvants:** | Arnica, Arsenic, Staphysagria, Bryonia |
| **Potency:** | 30 to 200 |

# Benzoicum Acidum
## (Benzoic Acid)

The most salient feature of Benzoic Acid is extremely **foul smelling urine**, resembling the smell of a horse's urine, which is difficult to get rid off. The smell is unusually foul and is so strong that it remains in the clothes even after washing. If in such a house the clothes are not washed regularly, the whole house will smell of this strong odour. If the Benzoic Acid child wets his bed, the repugnance is doubled. The stained clothes do not get clean even on washing. The urine is deep and dark in colour. If such patients have **excess uric acid in the blood**, they will benefit from Benzoic Acid. Uric acid causes pain in the kidneys and also decreases their functional capability. Usually, the urination is normal. If the urine becomes sparse, it will cause pain in the joints.

The Benzoic Acid patient **omits words while writing**. Occasionally, this kind of omission can be due to mental confusion. Some people's minds work much faster than their hands; the hands cannot keep up with the mind. This symptom may be present in other homoeopathic medicines, so it should not be related to any particular one. Whenever there is omission or substitution of words during writing, it indicates that the person is looking deeply into the meanings rather than the wording of his idea and it becomes difficult to balance both at the same time. However, one should not simply label one whose thinking is much faster than his writing as a patient of Benzoic Acid. If there is mental confusion and the urinary symptoms of Benzoic Acid as well, then certainly the person will respond to Benzoic Acid.

In Benzoic Acid, there is **vertigo** and fear of falling on one side. The headache becomes worse with a draft of cold air, exposure to cold, or on exposing the head. There is sense of warmth in the temple areas, leading to a pitting type of swelling around the ears. Along with the **headache**, there is tendency of **nausea and vomiting**, cold sweats on the head and chilling of the hands. There is irritation and pain at the nose, with a decreased sense of smell. The eyes burn and feel warm. The eye symptoms become worse in the open air and the tube light. The headache starts at the nape of the neck.

In Benzoic Acid, the **red spots appear on the face** indicating the state of being unhealthy. This commonly happens in women. One side of the face feels warm and burning. Sometimes, small blisters develop on the face. The facial symptoms are relieved in a warm climate and by applying local pressure.

In Benzoic Acid, the person **sweats while eating food.** The stomach feels tight and under pressure. Over the liver area, the person feels a piercing sensation and pain. The **stools are frothy, offensive** and thin in consistency. The patient passes a lot of gas.

In Benzoic Acid, **the voice is hoarse** in the morning. The sputum is greenish. The **cough** becomes worse at night. The pains become intensified during sleep. At about midnight, severe palpitation and the sensation of heat wakes the patient up.

In most books, it is written regarding Benzoic Acid that the attack of gout originates from the stomach. Commonly, **stomachache is due to an ulcer or indigestion**, but it could also be due to the gout. I do not know exactly how the gout affects the stomach. Possibly, the foul acidic contents of the stomach also contain uric acids, which cause the symptoms of gout. I have no firm knowledge about the production of Benzoic Acid in the stomach. It is likely that when the Benzoic Acid causes inflammation of the linings of the joints (synovial lining), it may very well affect the muscles by way of blood and start the symptoms of gout. It may be so or not, but most homoeopaths describe it as a symptom of Benzoic Acid.

Excess of Benzoic Acid can cause **swelling and pain at the joints of the wrist, knees, especially the big toes, etc**. Similarly, the feeling of pressure and chills in the backbone along with the **swelling of the tongue** are also the symptoms of Benzoic Acid. These also exist in Picric Acid as well as Mercury.

| | |
|---|---|
| **Potency:** | 30 to 200 |

# BERBERIS VULGARIS
## (Bar Berry)

The plant of Berberis Vulgaris grows in hilly areas. Its fresh leaves are used in the treatment of typhoid fever. Berberis is normally used in the form of Mother Tincture and most homoeopath physicians use it in the treatment of kidney problems. However, it is a very effective remedy for **gall bladder stones and deeply-rooted illnesses of the liver**. When liver dysfunction has affected the heart also, Berberis Vulgaris will be useful, though by itself it is not a tonic for the heart. Primarily, it is a remedy for liver dysfunction. The ailment of the heart, secondary to the liver failure would certainly be responsive to Berberis Vulgaris.

Berberis is also very effective for **joint pains**. Its use promotes the excretion of injurious acidic substances through the urine and the body feels relieved. The joint pains decrease. The Berberis patient feels irritation and itching as if something is creeping inside the nose. Often, the cold settles in the left nostril and becomes chronic. The mouth is dry and the tongue sticks due to dryness. It feels burnt and abrased. Sometimes, there is frothy sputum at the mouth with the consistency of thrashed cotton which does not, however, make the mouth moist. Sometimes blisters develop on the tongue.

In men, there is undulating pain along the course of the spermatic cord, which becomes worse during infection of the kidney and the bladder. The patient cannot empty his bladder completely and keeps on straining to evacuate himself fully. Sometimes the urine contains pus or mucus and sometimes, also red cells. The urine smells extremely foul. The undulating type of pain at the shoulders, arms, hands, legs, feet and the nails, associated with generalised weakness, are the special symptoms of Berberis Vulgaris.

The typical sign of Berberis pain is that it starts at one point and spreads out, radiating like the spokes of a bicycle wheel. The kidney pain also behaves in the same way. The throbbing pain radiates downwards towards the bladder and upwards towards the back and the liver. The pain radiating downwards reaches the testicles through the nerves. Often, the patient feels intense desire to pass urine when he stands or walks, and the urge is uncontrollable. At the urinal, when one passes urine, although a major portion is passed, the weak stream of urine is never-ending. It appears as if the kidney is continuously making urine.

Regarding the urinary symptoms of Berberis, either the urine is plenty and dilute or sparse but thick and smelly due to an excess of waste products. The frequency or relative infrequency of urination are both present in Berberis Vulgaris. When the urination is copius, the kidneys are washed out and the bad smell of the urine dissipates. When the urine becomes less in quantity, it becomes deep-coloured and offensive. When the quantity of the urine is decreased, the patient feels a burning sensation along the urethra.

The kidney pain of Pareira Brava usually radiates only in one direction and that is often from the kidney down into the thigh. In Berberis Vulgaris, however, the pain from the kidney or the gall bladder radiates in all directions. In this particular symptom pertaining to the **gall bladder pain**, Berberis is very effective. In a week to ten days, the stones of the gall bladder start breaking and are excreted in the stools.

In Berberis Vulgaris, the joint pains resemble gout in that they affect the small joints of the hands and the feet much more, as compared to the joint pains involving the big joints (in Rheumatism). The pains in the hands and the fingers, like Benzoic Acid, are deeply related to Berberis Vulgaris. The pain at the hip or the leg starts as soon as the person stands up and worsens after walking a short distance. The feet also hurt, especially the heels and the soles. In gouty pains, Benzoic Acid may prove to be the best substitute of Berberis Vulgaris. Both may also be used alternately.

Experienced homoeopaths believe that when **the heart becomes weak secondary to liver failure**, Berberis first corrects the state of the liver and as a result, the heart becomes normalized automatically. When there is a retention of acidic products and urea in the body, Berberis Vulgaris mobilizes them from there and redirects them to the blood. They are then excreted through the kidneys. When acidic matters increase in the blood, they can affect the heart. The heart will not improve unless these acidic waste products are excreted. Otherwise, Berberis Vulgaris does not have any direct effect on the condition of the heart. If during the use of Berberis Vulgaris, the heart is adversely affected, the patient should be made to drink a lot of water so that the amount of urine increases. The waste products and acidic matter can be washed out of the body rapidly thus preventing them from affecting the heart again. During a severe cramp, the Berberis Vulgaris patient cries uncontrollably. The gouty pains of Berberis become worse on movement. The patient walks very slowly and guardedly. The symptoms take time to disappear.

The patient feels as if the head is wrapped in something. In Glonoine also, there is a feeling of the head being tied up in a bandage. A cap and buttoned-up collars are unbearable. But in Berberis Vulgaris, even if there is nothing covering the head, the person feels as if something is holding tight. As in Psorinum, the patient also feels bouts of hunger pains. One symptom of Berberis is that the person feels as if he has been stabbed in his liver and gall bladder with a knife. The pain radiates like fireworks in all directions from the affected part of the body.

In Berberis, the patient is **jaundiced** and the stools become clay-coloured. In this condition, Carduus Marianus may also be given along with Berberis Vulgaris to enhance its beneficial effect. These two remedies work as adjuvants to each other. In the case **of liver diseases**, I give Berberis Vulgaris in the form of mother tincture, while in kidney troubles and gout, I use it in potency 30. Berberis Vulgaris and Carduus Marianus have similar constitutions.

Berberis Vulgaris is useful in the treatment of severe **kidney pain as well as kidney stones**, but it has to be used over a long period so that the stones gradually dissolve and are excreted. Berberis Vulgaris has no affect on the Oxalic Acid stones. The oxalate stones are very hard, and they are treatable by using ultrasound rays. In my experience, Silicea and Calcarea Flour 6X given together for some time, dissolve and then expel the oxalate stone.

In Berberis Vulgaris, one of the symptoms is that the mouth feels sticky due to thick, sticky sputum. **Small spots develop on the tongue** that feels raw. In the morning, one feels nauseated and has a burning sensation in the chest. In Berberis, with movement and on standing, the legs start hurting, and the urinary symptoms intensify.

|  |  |
|---|---|
| **Antidotes:** | Camphor, Belladonna |
| **Potency:** | Mother Tincture (Q) |

# Bismuthum

In olden days, Bismuth was used by allopathic doctors for the treatment of diarrhoea. Although it controls the diarrhoea it does not cure the disease of the intestine causing diarrhoea. The pain stays nonetheless. In homoeopathy, the **mental symptoms** of Bismuth are more pronounced. The patient does not like to be alone for even a moment. He must have somebody nearby. In old age, many such patients need somebody by their side at all times. They want to relate their story to them.

Bismuth is useful in **toothache**. The **gums are swollen**; the **tongue** is whitish and swollen. On its margins are darkish ulcers, resembling those of gangrene.

The Bismuth patient has **poor digestion**, and like Phosphorus and Aethusa, the stomach does not accept water. As soon as the fluid becomes warm, the patient vomits. However, the patient does not vomit after solid food. The patient **belches** out foul gas. The pain in the abdomen resembles that of dioscorea. The patient bends backwards. The nature of the pain in the abdomen is different from ordinary pain but the patient cannot explain it. During diarrhoea, there is no pain in the abdomen. When, after administration of Bismuth the diarrhoea stops, the pain in the abdomen returns. The stomach feels inflamed.

Bismuth is also useful in the treatment of **angina**. In the case of Bismuth, the chest pain starts at the left side of the heart and radiates to the shoulder and down to the fingertips, instead of the pain normally starting from the sternum. Many a time, chest pain can be due to **ulcers in the stomach or inflammation of the stomach**. In both conditions, Bismuth can be used.

In Bismuth, as in Hyoscyamus, there is a tendency of experiencing **violent sexual dreams**. It seems as if there is some kind of injurious material in the diarrhoea of Bismuth, which after being absorbed from the intestines into the blood affects the mind, as a result of which the person experiences strange dreams.

| | |
|---|---|
| **Adjuvants:** | Arsenic, Belladonna, Kreosotum |
| **Antidotes:** | Nux Vomica, Capsicum |
| **Potency:** | 30 to 200 |

# Borax

In allopathic medicine, Borax is used in the treatment of eye diseases. In addition to this, it is also used mixed with honey in the treatment of a sore throat. In the homoeopathic system of treatment, Borax is a vastly effective medicine that works tremendously well in deep-seated, serious illnesses of women. Borax is the best remedy to treat **ulcers in the mouth of lactating women** when their children also suffer from the same condition. In Borax, there is a tendency to develop sores and blisters. Red painful blisters develop on the tongue. The women of Borax nature suffer from **leucorrhoea**, in which the discharge is plentiful, hot and burning in nature. Women suffering from such leucorrhoea are mostly infertile. Unless they are treated with Borax, they cannot conceive. This symptom must be kept in mind when treating women for **infertility**. Borax is a unique remedy in this connection. The periods of Borax patient occur before time and are copious in amount. During the periods, there is intense pain in the abdomen which radiates towards the back.

Borax is a useful medicine for **whooping cough** also. It works very effectively on all spasmodic types of cough. The bout of coughing is very severe and there is a rattling sound inside the chest. The chest hurts along with the sensation of pins and needles. The pins and needles are also felt on the soles of the feet.

The special characteristic of Borax is that the **person feels scared on descent.** If the child is lowered into the bed, he feels scared and screams out of fright. The symptom may be present in grown-ups too. The person gets terrified while coming down the elevator or when the car is descending down a sloping road. The person is oversensitive to noise and loud talking. He gets startled on hearing a sudden noise or blast. In Borax, there is a **tendency of hoarseness of voice**. The excretions or discharges of Borax patients have the nature of heat. The tears are also warm but they do not cause any burning. Instead they are catarrhal in nature. Borax is useful in trachoma. The discharge from the nose dries up and turns greenish.

In Borax, when the stomach is upset, it feels bloated with gas. The patient has the tendency of vomiting which, once it begins, does not stop. The vomit is greenish in colour and sour in taste. Due to nervous exhaustion, the person sweats at night. Borax is very useful when there is sexual weakness resulting from a severe illness.

Regarding **pleurisy**, the symptoms of Borax resemble those of Bryonia. If Bryonia does not work or stops working further, Borax will take its action further. Borax is also considered useful in the treatment of epilepsy. The symptoms of Borax worsen in a hot climate.

| | |
|---|---|
| **Adjuvants:** | Bryonia, Sulphur, Calcarea Carb |
| **Antidotes:** | Chamomilla, Coffea |
| **Non-compatible:** | Acetic Acid, Vinegar, Alcohol |
| **Potency:** | 30 |

# BOVISTA

In everyday English, Bovista is also known as Puff-Ball. It has been used for treating the **eczema of children**. It is an excellent treatment for patients who have eczema and also have a tendency to bleed and **stammer**. Compared to normal people, Bovista patients feel more suffocation in the presence of smoke from burning wood. When the wood is partially burnt, its smoke contains carbon monoxide which can be absorbed into the bloodstream of every person and may put one to deep sleep. This sleep is not healthy due to the poisonous effects of carbon monoxide. If the person is not treated immediately and taken out into the fresh air, his apparently calm sleep may lead him to death. The skin becomes blue. Its immediate effective treatment is Arnica and Carbo Veg 30 mixed together. But in some books, Bovista has also been mentioned to be a good treatment for this condition.

In Bovista, **ulcers form at the opening of the mouth and the nose**. The sores become covered with a layer of thick crust. This symptom is also present in Natrum Mur, but its sores rather feel raw and do not form scabs. In Bovista, like in Coccus, the catarrhal discharge is thready. The nose and the gums bleed. There is itching of the scalp, along with the sensation of faint headache. In Bovista the person feels uncomfortable in tight clothes. In fact, any kind of tight fit is bothersome. This symptom is also present in Lachesis.

In Bovista, sometimes the patient gets **diarrhoea between two menstrual periods**. The bleeding is before time and plentiful. This can also be followed by thick greenish leucorrhoea. Sometimes there is light inter-menstrual bleeding or spotting. The pain is at around the navel and feels relieved on bending forwards. Sometimes, during a colicky abdominal pain, the urine may become red in appearance. One peculiar sign of Bovista is that food somewhat relieves the **colicky pain**.

In Bovista, there is **sweating of the armpits, smelling of onion**. There is eczema on the back of the hands. The skin symptoms are aggravated by excitement and mental anguish. In Bovista, when the skin is pressed, the skin pits and stays for some time. The skin symptoms become worse with heat.

For a chronic type of **urticaria** that does not respond to Rhus Tox, Bovista may offer a complete cure. Its effect may be compared with Calcarea, Rhus Tox, Sepia and Cieuta. This comparison will help the treating physician to better diagnose and treat. Some books mention the use of potency 3 to 6 but experience shows that potency 30 is the best in daily situations. The Bovista patient may feel itchiness at the anus even in the absence of any eczematous symptoms. Pimples form on the entire body. The urticaria develops in the morning and taking a shower proves harmful. Bovista is said to be the best antidote for Coal tar.

# Bromium

Bromium was once considered to be the special treatment for **Diphtheria**. For a long time this was the favourite of new homoeopaths. In the West preventive vaccination has almost eliminated Diphtheria, but in poor countries this disease may still spring up as an epidemic, from time to time. In treating Diphtheria, compared to Bromium, Muriatic Acid Kali Mur and Diphterinum prove much more effective.

In Bromium, when compared with Diphtheria, **other throat conditions** are more common. The glands at the neck swell, harden and and keep on growing in size, they do not disappear by suppuration (pus formation). Bromium is deeply related to all kinds of **inflammation of the glands** but most homoeopaths do not use it. It is very useful in the treatment of all thyroid conditions. Bromium must be remembered if the glands become very hard, and keep on gradually increasing in size when other remedies are not effective. Bromium has the capability of gradually softening the hardened lymph glands but it must be used in increasing potencies over a long period of time. It should be started in potency 30, then it should be increased to 200, and then after some time, it should be given in 1000 and then in still higher potency, and then stopped.

In Bromium, **ulcers often develop in the stomach**. Bromium is extremely useful when the vomitus is of ground coffee colour and there is an ulcer in the stomach with the tendency of enlargement of the glands. In fact, it is very important for the treatment of **cancer of the stomach**. Bromium is also very useful for the treatment of **laryngitis**, as it has a tendency towards ulcer formation. Even if such patients become asthmatic they would favourably respond to Bromium. The burning sensation and pain at the sternum is also a sign of Bromium. Convulsions also occur. It is useful for the treatment of suffocation. Bromium patients feel very relieved at the seaside but their symptoms aggravate when they move away from the sea to dry areas.

| | |
|---|---|
| **Adjuvants:** | Conium, Spongea, Iodum, Argentum Nitricum |
| **Antidotes:** | Ammonium Carb, Camphor |
| **Potency:** | 30 to CM |

# BRYONIA ALBA

Bryonia Alba is a wild creeper plant, found on forest trees and bushes. Its root is very poisonous and bitter. The root is ground in the form of a powder and then homoeopathic potencies are made from it. Bryonia is related to most of the vital organs of the body including the lungs, liver and heart. It acts more effectively over the outer linings of these organs (pleura and pericardium) but its effect on the **liver** is much more pronounced. Similarly, it proves very effective in the treatment of deep-seated illnesses of the lungs like **pneumonia** and its aftereffects. Although it is not of much use in the treatment of **tuberculosis** and other chronic illnesses of the lungs, it enhances the action of other profoundly acting remedies.

In addition to its effects on the muscles, it also works on the lining of the intestines. A Bryonia patient is generally **constipated**, but sometimes blood-mixed **dysentery** also occurs. Due to the dryness of the intestines, the lining ulcerates leading to a painful type of severe dysentery. Bryonia will be immediately effective in this type of **dysentery,** provided other signs and symptoms of Bryonia are present.

Some homoeopathic doctors believe that Bryonia Alba is the homoeopathic remedy of flail, flaccid and easily fatigable muscles, but this is not right. In fact, Bryonia is also the best remedy for strong and toned-up muscles. For the proper functioning of Bryonia, the weakness of the muscle fibres is not a precondition. In Bryonia, **generalised body ache** is, as in malaria, a salient feature.

Some people are afflicted with such illnesses that as a result they do not have the strength to move around. The weakness is not generalised. But after walking for some time, the body starts feeling heavy and this heaviness turns into severe pain. The **legs become lifeless**. Bryonia is very useful in such patients, but it has to be given over a long period. Before going for a long walk or resorting to intense physical activity, administration of Bryonia 200 combined with Arnica proves to be very beneficial.

Some women develop swelling of the leg after childbirth called **white leg.** This is probably due to clotting of the blood and slowing down of the circulation. When the condition becomes chronic and disables them, and blue and black spots develop on the legs along with the development of varicose veins, it is already too late for the treatment of this condition with Arnica and Bryonia. However if in addition, Aesculus 30 is administered, a better response will be expected. If the condition affects the left side, Arnica 200 should be combined with Lachesis 200 as well as Aesculus 30.

When given alternately with long-acting remedies such as Sulphur and Lycopodium, Bryonia can cure chronic illnesses as well. In the **deep intrinsic illnesses of the liver**, the following formula is very effective: Bryonia 200 once or twice a day, Sulphur 30 three times a day and a few drops of Mother Tincture of Carduus Marianus mixed in water, three times a day.

This prescription has proven very effective in **Hepatitis B**, as well as in **cancer of the liver**. In my experience, I have seen patients with cancer of the liver who, following treatment with radiation and other medicines, the doctors had declared untreatable. Thinking that the patient's end is very near, they had discharged the patient home. When the particular prescription mentioned above was used, instead of dying in three days, the patient started showing signs of recovery to health. The first hopeful sign noted in such patients was that the thirst and appetite that had completely disappeared returned. Many other patients of liver diseases have also benefited from this treatment and are still alive.

Sometimes the liver diseases shift to the spleen, especially in **chronic malaria**. First, there is liver disorder and then the **spleen enlarges**. Such patients should be given Carduus Marianus as well as Ceanothus in the form of Mother Tincture. Ceanothus is the best treatment for the spleen. Sometimes these patients develop distension of the abdomen. **There is painful swelling and induration over the spleen and the liver**. When treated with the above combination and Ceanothus, such patients recover remarkably in a period of two to three months, so much so that their abdomen reverts to normal size and there is no pain on pressure. In areas where malaria is common and such ailments prevail, this prescription must be put to use.

The development of **pain on every movement** and worsening of the affected part of the body is typical of Bryonia. This resembles Rhus Tox somewhat. Commonly, it is thought that rest increases the pain of

Rhus Tox and movement relieves it; this is not exactly right. In Rhus Tox, when the patient walks, this increases his pain which gets somewhat better after walking a little. However, the pain never disappears completely. In fact, it becomes worse when one stops walking or resorts to rest. The Bryonia patient feels much relieved on resting for a few days continuously, but the pain of a Rhus Tox patient becomes worse on resting.

For most conditions that develop in the beginning of the summer after the winter is over, Bryonia is of great use. In this changing weather, **pneumonia** is very common. With the sudden onset of hot weather, the outer body feels discomfort but the inside of the body is not ready for this change. Therefore when the warm clothes are taken off, various kinds of ailments overtake which are not the direct result of the heat but are due to exposure to the cold in warm weather. For this kind of **seasonal pneumonia**, Bryonia is the best. The kind of pneumonia that occurs in Bryonia usually affects the right lung and does not shift from the right to the left. The pneumonia in Lycopodium starts on the right side and then also affects the left where it settles. In Bryonia, the symptoms travel from above downwards and gradually settle in the lower part of the lungs. Bryonia is not a chronic remedy as such. Therefore, in such an illness other remedies need to be given. Kali Carb is an important remedy in this condition, acting on the lower part of the lungs. Arsenic Iodide and Kali Iodide are also useful.

**If due to tuberculosis, spots and cavities develop in the lungs**, the combination of Merc sol and Kali Carb is very useful. Once a woman had developed cavities in the lungs and in the view of the doctors it was incurable. When she was treated with Merc sol 200 and Kali Carb 30, she completely recovered within a few months. When the x-rays on the chest were done in the hospital, no cavities were found. The doctors did not believe that the x-rays belonged to the same patient who previously had the cavities in their lungs!

Homoeopathic remedies can work miraculously, showing that Allah Almighty has blessed our body with great defensive power that the doctors of today do not fully understand in spite of their extensive research. This great defensive power is deeply related to the chemistry of the body. For example, the liver is given a message to produce an appropriate chemical for a particular ailment and so it happens. This can never happen due to a blind evolutionary type of reaction. How is it possible that this profound mechanism could develop by sheer chance, as a result of long evolutionary process in the form of a strong interrelated defence mechanism of the body and then work with such precision, and this effect remain in the body indelibly? If the general health of a person is good, there is no need for any kind of formal treatment because the defence mechanism of the body will automatically overcome the illnesses, but when the body defences are at fault they have to be activated by homoeopathic treatment. Simple, hard-working people usually do not suffer from the complicated illnesses of the rich, because their body has a sound defence system against those diseases. This is in spite of the fact that they live in the same environment and area where other people are overcome by many diseases. The defence system of the body points vividly to the existence of God and His magnificence. This system must be well remembered by homoeopathic physicians. It is this system which makes the working of homoeopathic remedies more conspicuous, bringing it to the limelight.

The joint pains of the Bryonia patient subside by heat. The **cough** becomes aggravated generally by movement and noise, resembling Belladonna with one difference, that in Bryonia there is no suddenness of the symptoms. The Bryonia symptoms start gradually and then become more and more severe, till every **movement sound and noise becomes troublesome**, so much so that the patient does not even like people visiting him, and in fact is vexed on their arrival. The reason for the anger and vexation is that every movement bothers him. The movement of his own lips to talk also bothers him and he does not like to speak. He feels weak. If such a patient develops pneumonia or headache, he should not even be asked to talk. He remains in the state of drowsiness. When the ailment prolongs, he may become permanently unconscious. Movement and speaking are of no avail to him at all.

The **headache** of a Bryonia patient feels better in cold. The headache is usually on the back of the head or on the forehead. **Intense thirst** is a characteristic symptom of Bryonia. The patient likes to have very cold water as it offers him relief. Soon afterwards he feels awfully thirsty again. Intense thirst reminds one of Bryonia. But in certain situations, the thirst may be totally absent. The stomach gets inflamed, the mouth becomes dry and the tongue is dry hard, but there is no thirst. There are yellow deposits on the tongue. Primarily, this is the particular symptom of Gelsemium, which occasionally may appear in Bryonia. In his book, Dr. Kent has also written that in Bryonia, sometimes the thirst may be totally absent.

**Feeling dizzy in a Bryonia patient may be due to some problem in the ear or with movement**. Dizziness and associated nausea are commonly present in motion sickness, in a motor car or a ship. For such patients, some ready prescriptions may be put into use and are very useful. Generally, it is not possible to ask everybody individually about the symptoms. This prescription includes Bryonia, Cocculus, Nux Vomica and Ipecac. Cocculus is also related to the vertigo associated with ear problems. In fact, this is the most effective remedy for this purpose. As a matter of fact, Bryonia and Cocculus are very similar in this respect. In the tubes of the middle ear (semi-circular canals), there is a fluid. When one's head is tilted, it sends an impulse through the nerve giving the sensation of balance or imbalance. Rapid change in the position can cause vertigo. When the vertigo is due to rapid movement or an ailment of the ear causing hypersensitivity of the internal ear, this can be treated with Bryonia and Cocculus. There is a slight difference. In Bryonia, it is the inflammation of the ears that causes vertigo, whereas in Cocculus, it is the irritability of the nerves that causes vertigo. When there is vertigo but no apparent problem in the ear, Cocculus is useful. In the case where there is infection of the ear causing **vertigo**, Bryonia would be better.

Bryonia is also useful in the treatment of **glaucoma,** but if there is no associated thirst, Gelsemium would be the most appropriate treatment. Gelsemium is also a good remedy for vertigo due to irritation of the nerves. But Bryonia is more widely effective, as it is able to work on the internal membrane of the ear as well as the nerves. Glaucoma is mostly related to the nerves. When Calcaria Phos 6X and Kali Phos 6X are given along with Bryonia and Gelsemium, the effect is more pronounced. Sometimes after the administration of Bryonia, the thirst disappears. At that time Gelsemium may be given and both Bryonia and Gelsemium may be used alternatively. These remedies are good for **headaches** also. A Gelsemium headache gets worse in cold air and a Bryonia headache feels relieved in the cold. However, the effect of cold or heat does not always hold good in Gelsemium, because when the headache becomes severe, neither cold nor heat has any effect. A Bryonia headache essentially settles in the nape, forehead or the eyes. When it **settles in the eyes**, the **headache becomes very severe in the form of waves and undulations**. Sometimes, when joint pains are controlled with a strong medication, the eyes may become the centre of severe pain. The slightest movement of the eye feels as if somebody is being poked with a knife. This particular feeling may be related to Bryonia as well as Berberis. Gelsemium headaches radiate down the back of the head, in addition to the entire head, neck and then along the arms. Gelsemium **headaches** may also be related to a change in the daily routine of a person. If the planning for retiring to bed or taking the food gets disturbed, the person develops headache which will respond to Gelsemium. A Bryonia headache is more closely related to the generalised joint pains, stomach upset or fever.

Bryonia is very effective in the treatment of both **malaria and typhoid**. In Bryonia, when the body hurts headache must also be present. In the state of fever, sometimes the headache may lead to **delirium** and the patient becomes absurd and meaningless in his conversation. Otherwise, the Bryonia patient does not talk much in simple delirium i.e. without fever. The delirium associated with Hyoscyamus, Stramonium, Sulphur and Belladonna is much more severe and results from the toxic or poisonous products of the feverish conditions. By making a proper diagnosis of the headache, one may easily diagnose the nature of the sickness. The Belladonna kind of headache caused by typhoid or some other sickness would be of sudden onset. In addition to the headache, the face would be flushed, even if the patient were anaemic. The **patient is not frightened but tends to be aggressive instead**. In spite of physical weakness, the patient reacts with unusual strength and it becomes difficult to control him. In Hyoscyamus, when the patient is delirious, his talk is so obviously obscene that not only the family but also the doctor feels embarrassed. This does not reflect immorality on the part of the patient but is simply due to the inflammation of the sexual organs which disturbs the mind also. All these symptoms together produce a state of severe delirium. Another point of recognition for the Hyoscyamus patient is that he keeps on pinching his body and picking his clothes. This does not happen in the case of Bryonia.

One sign of Bryonia is that there **is fissuring at the corners of the mouth**, scabs form on the lips which when attempted to be removed by the patient, start bleeding. This also happens in Natrum Mur. Natrum Mur is chronic of Bryonia.

When the excretions or discharges of a Bryonia patient get blocked, they cause significant discomfort. The sweating becomes a source of blessing to the patient. In the Bryonia cough, the **expectoration is very dry, sticky and difficult to expel**. To help get rid of dry and sticky sputum, Hepar Sulph and Coccus are also very important remedies in addition to Bryonia and Ipecac. In Bryonia, when the lungs get diseased, the inner linings of the lungs tear and ulcerate causing light bleeding, which mixes up in the sputum. The sputum appears rusty. This is typical of Bryonia. Bryonia works as a useful adjuvant to Phosphorus in the treatment of cancer of the bone. It should be used in potency 30, alternating with Phosphorus.

In women, Bryonia can be useful in the **treatment of diseases of the right ovary**. For the **lumps** in the breast glands which are firm and hurt on movement, due to cancer or otherwise, the first remedy to be used should be Bryonia. The Bryonia patient with pneumonia of the right lung usually sleeps on the right side, because lying down on the same side helps minimise the movement of the chest wall during breathing.

Sometimes **during sleep, the patient wakes up with sudden jerking of the body**. In homoeopathy, there are three terms used for fever, as follows:

1. Continuous fever which once it starts, will either prove fatal, or when it subsides will never return.
2. Remittent fever is the one which shows peaks. Sometimes it is low and sometimes high, but does not subside completely.
3. Intermittent fever which can totally subside but returns. Malaria is one such example.

Typhoid fever is of remittent type which may subside but does not go. Bryonia may be useful in the treatment of remittent and intermittent fevers but not in continuous fever. Often it is needed in the treatment of **malaria** but is also useful in the treatment of **typhoid**.

The **diseases of the glands** in Bryonia begin very slowly and then intensify to become chronic, like in Causticum. In Causticum too, the illnesses progress gradually but continuously, and involve the fibrous and glandular tissues. The toxic material settles in the glands. When the glands become chronically inflamed and their appearance changes, Bryonia may be the remedy. Bryonia should be remembered in relation to Arnica as well.

In regard to the **diseases of the glands**, Bryonia also resembles Phytolacca. In both, the glands swell. Phytolacca should be used if Bryonia does not work to satisfaction. In the chronic diseases of the glands, the effective prescription is Kali Mur, Silicea, Ferrum Phos, Calcarea Phos, Calcarea Flour, etc., mixed together and given repeatedly. An **infectious fever** originating from the **infection of the throat** may prove to be very chronic and dangerous because the infection settles in the deeper part of the glands not effectively accessible to the blood circulation, so the protective materials cannot reach the affected part either. If the above combination does not show beneficial effect in the first two to three days of the sickness, more effective, appropriate remedies should be considered.

Sometimes, there is high fever due to infection of the tonsils and it keeps on increasing everyday, and in particular shows a high peak in the latter part of the night. One should not take its relative subsiding in the morning as a sign of recovery. The family or the doctor would become somewhat carefree towards the treatment. The next evening, the fever becomes still more elevated and so on. Two to three such episodes of high fever may even prove fatal. Therefore, the high fever of infection of the tonsils must not be taken lightly. The allopaths commonly prescribe antibiotics for it. The fever subsides but tends to recur again and again. In fact, a new bout of fever sets in right after the previous one subsides. More and much stronger antibiotics have to be used. These destroy the liver function, resulting in the loss of appetite. The sick child becomes a skeleton devoid of flesh. The tonsils enlarge in size with every successive episode of fever. As a word of caution, antibiotics should be avoided as much and as long as safely possible. Sulphur and Pyrogenium 200 are **generally very beneficial in controlling infection**. Similarly, Silicea in high potency may also prove very useful at times. If all these prove ineffective, a combination of Belladonna, Phytolacca, Calcarea Flour, Ferrum Phos and Baptisia in potency 30 repeated frequently may control the sickness in one night. In addition, the mixture of Ferrum Phos, Silicea, Kali Mur, Calcarea Phos, Mag Phos 6X may be administered

6 to 7 times a day to a significant benefit. The fever will gradually subside in two to three nights if not on the first.

Like Nux Vomica, if Bryonia is used more than necessary, it causes headaches. The antidote for both is Gelsemium. In Bryonia, the illness presents two patterns. Firstly, when the discharges or sweating stop, the suffering worsens. With the treatment the excretions begin again. The inner linings of the organ become moist and the normal perspiration starts from the skin. Secondly, when there is **cessation of periods in women, they suffer nosebleeds**. By administering Bryonia, the condition is relieved.

The thick sticky expectoration may block the main air passages temporarily causing **a state of asthma**. Repeated coughing is needed to expel it out of the air passages. If the sputum is like a thread, Coccus definitely is the best remedy. If the cold deteriorates and deep infection sets in, the expectoration becomes greenish, showing further deterioration.

In Bryonia, the symptoms progress gradually but it does not mean that they take many days to become evident. If the Bryonia patient is exposed to cold in the morning, by the evening he will start showing symptoms of cold, and by the next morning the sickness is in full swing. The pain in the joints and muscles becomes severe and chronic. Bryonia behaves the same way in acute illnesses also. The Bryonia symptoms become more intense by 9 o'clock in the evening and persist all night. The symptoms of Chamomilla and Natrum Mur are at their peak at 9 o'clock in the morning. There is no definite explanation of the periodicity and punctuality of these symptoms, but this is how it has been designed by nature.

Like Chelidonium, Bryonia is the remedy for the illnesses of the right side. It is deeply related to **liver disorders**. Its discharges are yellowish in colour, including the sputum from the lung. In Chelidonium, the liver pain radiates towards the back like the pain of the gall bladder, getting worse on movement. When a **pregnant woman becomes exhausted or there is danger of aborting following heat stroke**, Bryonia should be administered. If combined with Arnica 200, this will also prevent against the aftereffects of physical exhaustion. In the case of trauma, Bryonia and Arnica together prevent the danger of abortion. It is very useful for this purpose and should be administered at once and better still with Aconite.

| | |
|---|---|
| **Adjuvants:** | Rhus Tox, Alumina |
| **Antidotes:** | Aconite, Chamomilla, Nux Vomica |
| **Potency:** | 30 to 1000 |

# BUFO

Bufo is prepared from the secretions of toad neck glands. Its main function is on the **mental faculties and the mind**. Its patients suffer from a **loss of memory**. The mind is cloudy and there is a feeling of severe mental fatigue. Bufo is the best remedy for **neurosis**. Neurosis, the **feeling of numbness, and muscular convulsions** are benefited with Bufo. The small muscles exhibit paralytic condition. Twitching of the eye or some other parts of the body is typical of Bufo.

In Bufo, **sores tend to develop on the skin**. Many homoeopathic experts use it in the treatment of sexual diseases but rarely use it for the treatment of skin diseases and violent muscle cramps. Bufo is the ideal treatment for a young man who becomes involved in sexual misconduct. It prevents one from **self-abuse** and its bad consequences. Some young men, who have wronged themselves and contracted **epilepsy**, will significantly benefit from Bufo. Such an epileptic should first be treated with Bufo. In case it fails, other remedies should be sought.

In Bufo, also like Sarsaparilla, **premature ageing** is found. This is also a symptom of Baryta Carb. In Bufo, the premature ageing is not in the physical form of skin tightness and wrinkles but it relates to the mental functions. The patient does not become crazy but simply looks naive. Bufo should also be used for a sixty-year old mature person behaving like a teenager. If such a person is not treated on time, he will become insane. He becomes incapable of communicating with others and making people understand what he means to say.

In Bufo, there are contradictions. The patient likes to be alone and away from others, but at the same time feels frightened when alone. This makes him angry, and he shows his anger by way of biting things. He expresses his helplessness but does not harm others. He laughs, cries and jumps around like a child. The conduct of a Bufo patient is of innocence and childishness. Occasionally, this state may progress to insanity. Bufo works profoundly and continuously in this condition for a very long period.

In Bufo, there is tendency towards **partial paralysis**. As a result of paralysis of various organs, the overlying skin becomes numb.

In Bufo, **violent muscle cramps** are common. Before epileptic seizure, the mouth opens wide due to muscular spasm. Blood pours out of the mouth and the tongue or lips get caught between the teeth, causing severe discomfort. Along with this comes headache, the pupils of the eye get dilated and fixed. The patient cannot tolerate light. Sores and ulcers develop on the skin. The eye becomes congested with blood. Ulcers form on the cornea of eye. **Blisters also form on the eye** and various parts of the body in the form of clusters. Antimonium Crude and Antimonium Tart are also described to be useful in the treatment of such blisters. Other symptoms also being present, Bufo is useful in the treatment of all **skin conditions**. As in Ambra Grisea, the Bufo patient hates music. The patient, gradually **tends to stutter and stammer**, making it difficult to understand him, and this upsets him. Use of Bufo is ideal to treat a patient who suddenly becomes drawn and mute. His eyes are bewildered and completely indifferent to his surroundings, even if he does not exhibit the complete picture of epilepsy. This condition is only temporary. When the patient regains consciousness, he has no knowledge of what had happened to him.

Being also related to sexual impotence, some Bufo patients may develop **epileptic fits during sexual intercourse**. The Bufo women patients either have their period before time or their periods cease all together. There is burning sensation and cramps in the uterus with the formation of blisters inside, emitting foul **leucorrheol discharge** mixed with pus or blood, resembling offensive gangrene-like discharge. Bufo proves to be very effective in the treatment of this condition.

Bufo is also very useful in the treatment of **breast cancer**. It does not cure the cancer but does offer relief from suffering and works as adjuvant for other remedies.

The **cough** of a Bufo patient is very bothersome. The blood mixes with sputum along with a significant burning sensation. Bufo sicknesses come on rapidly and spread fast, leading the patient towards his end. Its symptoms aggravate in a warm room and on waking up from sleep while taking a bath and soaking the feet in warm water offers relief.

| | |
|---|---|
| **Adjuvants:** | Baryta Carb |
| **Antidotes:** | Lachesis, Senega |
| **Potency:** | 30 to 200 or higher |

# CACTUS GRANDIFLORUS
## (Night-Blooming Cereus)

The Cactus plant grows in the desert. Although it is considered as an unattractive plant, in the desert it exhibits its own unique beauty. Blooming in full all around, it is pleasing to the eye. The fruit of the Cactus is very nice and looks good too, while its juice is also quite tasty, though it leaves an unpleasant odour. Excessive use of its fruit affects the kidneys adversely. **Urination becomes very painful**. A **burning sensation** is also associated with cramping of the bladder. In Cantharis also, there is severe burning sensation on passing urine. The urine dribbles with severe scalding. In Cactus, along with the burning sensation, there is also cramping at the bladder. The special feature of the cactus is that wherever there is pain, there must be **spasms/cramps** also.

Cactus adversely affects the circular muscle fibres and valves. Its ailments come on suddenly. The **heart also gets afflicted suddenly** as if somebody has been caught in a powerful vice. Cactus proves to be very effective in the treatment of those diseases of the heart in which there is dilatation of the muscles and the damage to the valves. The **spasm of the muscles at the throat** can cause the sensation of tightness. The blood tends to accumulate everywhere. The congestion of the heart, kidneys, intestines and face with accumulation of blood is also found in Belladonna. Palpitations and cramps are also present in both. But in Cactus, there is no fever. In Belladonna, the affected part of the body becomes warm. Warmth is a special sign of Belladonna. In Cactus, the affected part gets congested with blood, but there is no feeling of warmth and there is no fever. Cactus patients become extremely terrified with **sudden attacks** of the disease, and symptoms resembling those of Aconite appear. In view of the sudden onset of the illness and the specific nature of Cactus, it is only natural to have a **fear of death**. The severe **muscular cramps of the affected part of the body** resembles the feeling of being tied up in steel wires. There is feeling of tightness and generalized suffocation. The patient cannot even tolerate a buttoned-up collar. This symptom, to some extent, is also found in Lachesis and Glonoine. In Cactus, the affected part becomes badly hurt due to severe muscular contraction. A similar situation develops **inside the**

**uterus**. Cactus is a very important remedy for the treatment in newly wed women for severe pain due to spasm (Vaginismus). The feeling of tightness and cramps in that part of the body which does not usually suffer from actual cramps, is a salient feature of Cactus. Violent muscle spasms are well known in rheumatoid arthritis and rheumatism. Blood accumulates locally. In Colchicum and Benzoic Acid, the big toe swells but does not show any cramping. In Cactus such an afflicted part also has cramps.

Cactus will be of use for the heart. If the ailment is confined to the heart and there is the **feeling of tightness,** the pain over the central bone of the chest called sternum, is **angina**. When the **heart becomes enlarged** and beats irregularly, there is a piercing pain in the chest, along with hissing. Such a patient is not only relieved by Cactus but by the grace of God can be cured permanently.

When the **diseases of the kidneys** become chronic, soft pitting edema develops in the body, especially at the feet and the legs. If other symptoms of Cactus are also evident, Cactus can offer cure of the whole body by God's grace. Sometimes, even if the salient symptoms of Cactus are not present, sudden tightness and its extreme severity may be indicative enough of Cactus. In these kinds of symptoms, Cactus should be administered without any hesitation. If the symptoms of the patient match that of Cactus, the relief will be prompt and if the patient is not of Cactus, no harm will be done. So Cactus should always be kept in the emergency kit for use.

**Rheumatic pains** indicative of Cactus do not present signs of tightness and spasms in the arm and thigh muscles because Cactus is related only to circular (smooth) muscle fibres. It does not have an effect on long (skeletal) muscles. Colocynth is an important remedy which works on the long muscles. Belladonna also is useful whereas Cactus has no effect on the long muscle fibres. In Belladonna, when there is an excessive flow of blood towards the brain, there will be a feeling of severe tightness at the head as in Cuprum. But in the case of Cactus, there is no such feeling at the brain because there are no circular muscle fibres within the brain substance. In Cactus, when the brain is afflicted, the patient becomes unconscious or semi-conscious but exhibits no convulsions. In Belladonna, the tension in the brain can show its effect and even reach the big toe which may present severe cramps or spasms. In Cactus, giddiness is very common which gets worse with physical labour and fatigue, and is relieved by rest. Movement makes it worse. The **headache is on the right side**, and is aggravated by noise and bright light. In Cactus, palpitation is also present. Sometimes, the entire body throbs. This also happens in Belladonna, where the body is warm and feverish, but is absent in Cactus.

The tendency of **numbness of the left arm** along with the feeling of pull demands the use of Cactus. These symptoms sometimes develop in the beginning of a heart problem. However, it is not necessary that the pain in the left arm should always be due to a heart ailment. This can be caused by acidity of the stomach. In case there is tightness and sensation of suffocation (as if somebody has strongly squeezed the chest) or there is palpitation and numbness, the obvious treatment should be Cactus.

In Cactus, if at all there is fever, it starts at 11 o' clock in the morning. Before noon, the patient feels severe chill. Along with thirst, headache and the feeling of warmth at the time of contracting fever, there is difficulty in breathing. The feeling of warmth on the head on mental exertion is a characteristic of Cactus. The head feels as if caught in a vice. There is a fear of having apoplexy. The eyes are red. The hearing is affected due to congestion of ears with blood. The feeling of warmth and buzzing in the ear, spasm at the gullet (oesophagus), dryness of the tongue and difficulty in swallowing food without water, the feeling of **tightness and twitching of the stomach**, with the sensation of heaviness, **blood-mixed vomiting**, hard and dark stools, morning **diarrhoea**, painful **swelling of piles** and heaviness at the anal verge, are all the symptoms of Cactus. In malarial fever, as well as during heart trouble, the intestines may also bleed.

In Cactus, there is contraction of the bladder neck, causing **difficulty in passing urine**. Sometimes, there is bleeding in the bladder and the blood may clot in the urethra, making the suffering still more grave. **Swollen hands and feet**, soft ice-cold hands and the feeling of feet being big, with restlessness in the legs, are all symptoms of Cactus which aggravate at night and on lying on the left side, along with noise light heat sun and hard work.

| | |
|---|---|
| Antidotes: | Camphor, Aconite, China |
| Potency: | 30 |

# CADMIUM SULPH

Cadmium Sulph is a profoundly effective homoeopathic remedy. Its patients do not like to do any physical or mental work. They hate doing anything. Sulphur patients are also lethargic. They keep planning to become rich but do nothing to attain their goals. The Opium patient also remains in his imaginary world and thinks about the same way, but does not want to move himself or do any kind of work.

The salient features of Cadmium Sulph are **anguish and restlessness**. In this way it resembles Arsenic, but an Arsenic patient has one typical feature opposite to Cadmium Sulph. An Arsenic patient cannot tolerate any irregularity in his day-to-day life. He keeps everything in its proper order and is not afraid of hard work, while the patient of Cadmium Sulph is lazy, like a Sulphur patient, and his things are in great disarray.

Cadmium Sulph acts on the stomach like Arsenic. There is **irritation inside the stomach** that sometimes may not even let the patient sleep. Cadmium Sulph is a good treatment for this condition. Another distinguishing feature is that the Arsenic patient keeps on turning sides and cannot lie in one position for long, while the Cadmium patient feels pain on movement. Even if he is restless, his tiredness and laziness are more pronounced. He does not like to move at all. His expression of restlessness is merely verbal. In Cadmium Sulph, like Zinc, there is cramping of the muscles. The Zinc patient keeps on moving the affected part of body, placing his one foot on the other, or keeps on shaking his legs. Unlike Zinc, the Cadmium Sulph patient feels restlessness all over, yet does not make any movement at all.

Cadmium Sulph is useful in the **diseases of the eye**. It is very useful for swollen eyelids, pain in the eye, as well as sores and ulcers of the eye. It is also useful in the treatment of drooping eyelids (ptosis). It is useful for invigorating the nerve fibres of the eye, in addition to working on external eye conditions. Cadmium Sulph is mostly indicated in the treatment of diseases affecting one side. I have mostly found it useful in the treatment of strokes affecting the **left side of the body.** The paralysis affects one eye or one side of the body. If apoplexy leaves behind the weakness of one arm or one leg, Phosphorus may also be beneficial.

In the Cadmium Sulph patient, numbness of the skin is well known but it should not be overlooked that, before the actual numbness sets in the skin has been oversensitive for some time. Over the affected parts of the body, there is aching and a feeling of pins and needles. Some parts of the body become numb, such as the nose or ears only. One big problem is that swallowing becomes weak and **swallowing food becomes difficult**. Many a time, swallowing becomes weak, as the person ages, and the food may choke the air passage, which proves very dangerous. In such patients, Cadmium Sulph is not only useful but it becomes absolutely necessary to administer. Some children may also exhibit similar symptoms.

Cadmium Sulph also works on the bones. When the cold in a Cadmium Sulph patient becomes chronic, the bones of the nose start decaying. Like Cadmium Sulph, this is also a symptom of Mercury.

In Cadmium Sulph, **minute spots form on the skin** as in goose skin. These can be compared to the skin of a waterfowl, after its feathers have been plucked. In English, it is known as goose flesh. This is also present in Capsicum.

Cadmium Sulph is very useful for the proper functioning of the stomach. It proves very effective to **treat the failing stomach**, indigestion or rotting of the food inside the stomach, foul-smelling belches and severe nausea and vomiting. It is also useful in the treatment of **cancer** of the stomach. It does not cure but offers significant relief of the ailment. Cadmium Sulph restores the strength of a patient whose **muscles start wasting**, leading to progressive weakness.

In Cadmium Sulph, movement and sleep both aggravate the symptoms. Resting after taking food offers relief. The patient feels hungry constantly. The hunger remains strong even if the digestive system of the stomach has significantly failed. Cadmium Sulph has the capability of reviving a seriously sick patient who has strong appetite, throws up dark vomit and whose condition is so grave as if he is about to die. In such a grave situation, Cadmium Sulph rather than Carbo Veg will virtually revive the patient, unless destiny so prevails.

| | |
|---|---|
| **Potency:** | **30** |

# CALADIUM
## (A type of turnip growing in America)

Caladium is commonly used for the treatment of **tobacco addiction** and this is what it is famous for. However, it is not just for this limited use. It has many more prominent features. Its mental manifestations are unique. Caladium poison adversely affects the **memory** of a person. He forgets as soon as he has done something. Caladium could be used for the treatment of **epilepsy**. It is also related to the **hardening of the arteries** (arteriosclerosis) but it is not a specific treatment for arteriosclerosis.

After having done a task, a Caladium patient will typically keep wondering whether he did it or not. He cannot recall if he said what he had to, or did not say it, or in fact did write a letter to somebody, or not. In short, he is very unsure in his day-to-day life, but this symptom does not relate to his eating and drinking. For example, he will not forget having taken breakfast. Routine things are forgotten because a person usually remains lost in his own thoughts and cannot remember if he has done what he had to. It is correct to think that a Caladium patient is under great mental pressure. His mind is occupied by two kinds of activities. One is the routine activity and the other is being mentally preoccupied. This is the reason why a Caladium patient is absent-minded, like the philosophers who also tend to forget things. Such patients get mentally fatigued and cannot perform any literary work.

Caladium is also the treatment for **sexual weakness, secondary to tobacco addiction**. In this respect, it is similar to Picric Acid and Selenium. The Caladium patient is in a state of **constant fear**; fear of darkness, fear of future, so much so that he becomes even scared of his own shadow.

The Caladium patient suffers from **vertigo** that worsens on closing the eyes. In contrast, the vertigo gets in Conicum worse on opening the eyes. The patient feels dizzy even on lying down and moving the eyes. In this kind of vertigo, Conium alone is not effective, but becomes a powerful treatment when given with Cocculus. In both Caladium and Conium, movement intensifies the symptoms.

Caladium symptoms intensify with heat. Hot weather or a heated room aggravate the symptoms, while cooling relieves them. Although the stomach symptoms aggravate by taking cold things, it is the opposite of Phosphorus. In Phosphorus, the stomach feels relief by taking cold drinks. A Caladium patient's sleep is disturbed even with the slightest noise. Once awakened it is extremely difficult for him to go back to sleep.

In Caladium, the **skin feels a tingling** sensation, as if some insect is creeping on it. The sweat has a sweet smell that attracts flies. The skin is very itchy for no specific reason. When the creeping sensation intensifies, the entire body starts itching all the time. There is no rash or eczema. Some women may suffer from internal itching which can cause severe irritability.

Caladium symptoms intensify on movement and are relieved by sweating and with sleep.

| | |
|---|---|
| Adjuvant: | Nitric Acid |
| Antidote: | Aurum Triphylum |
| Potency: | 30 |

# Calcarea Arsenica

No doubt, Calcarea Sulph is well known for the treatment of **epilepsy**, but Calcarea Ars is also an important remedy. It comes next to Calcarea Sulph. About Calcarea Ars, Dr. Kent is of the opinion that it can cure epilepsy completely. In my opinion, every kind of epilepsy is not curable. Epilepsy which is secondary to the structural deformity of the head needs to be treated surgically.

In Calcarea Ars, there is a **tendency towards twitching of the muscles**, as well as paralytic weakness. In fact, calcium causes profound weakness even if slightly imbalanced in the body. The **blood pressure** is also affected and sometimes the patient can suddenly collapse. These kinds of symptoms are very common in cattle. Due to calcium imbalance in their body, they collapse suddenly. Usually the day-to-day weakness of the patient is not related to the imbalance of Calcarea, but the sudden weakening may very well be due to the hyperacidity in the stomach. The condition is scary and frightful but not fatal. Sometimes these patients may become unconscious, but it is not epilepsy per se. The fits of weakness and unconsciousness due to epilepsy are for life. But sudden episodes of unconsciousness are not necessarily due to epilepsy.

The epilepsy secondary to congenital abnormality can adversely affect the rational thinking of a person. The patient's forehead reflects his mental abnormality i.e. he is mentally not at par. His eyes express an idiotic look or, if the patient happens to be oversensitive, he keeps on pondering over trivial things. He is incapable of thinking wisely and seriously.

Some opponents of Islam viciously criticise the Holy Prophet[sa] of Islam and other Prophets, peace be on them all, saying that they did not receive any revelation from God but that they suffered from epilepsy. When the great achievements of Prophets are pondered upon, there remains no room for raising any such absurd objections at all. Even under very heavy pressure, the Prophets did not suffer from any kind of serious ailments. Whereas, when somebody is under that much pressure, epilepsy must ensue. It is said about the great Roman monarch Caesar, that when he used to address his people under great mental pressure, he used to faint and fall unconscious. In contrast, the Holy Prophet of Islam, peace and blessings of Allah be upon him, was ever so ready and alert, rather much more so in the face of dangerous situations. The rocky hillock of Uhad and the battlefield of Hunain are evidence enough to make these wretched opponents feel ashamed. The thought of the dozing and slumber which is present at the time of revelation from God, is no way close to an epileptic seizure.

**Mental overload and acidity of the stomach** can sometimes create a state of extreme **physical weakness**, so much so that the person may not be able to even move his finger. I have gone through this situation myself and felt during the physical exhaustion that I used to have, as if I was about to die. For many days I could not even get out of bed. This condition is temporary. When the acidity of the stomach is properly treated, the condition of this kind of serious weakness will leave forever.

The weakness that is observed in Calcarea Ars is not necessarily a sign of epilepsy. Arsenic is a part of the compound of Calcarea Ars. It has the tendency to **produce an excessive amount of acid in the stomach**. However, for the treatment of this kind of weakness, Nux Vomica is a better remedy than Arsenic. Calcarea Ars is different from Nux Vomica and other medicines. In Calcarea Ars patients, the paralytic tendency is a permanent feature while mere hyperacidity of the stomach does not cause paralysis. In Calcarea Ars, the hands start to shake and the entire body trembles before the onset of paralysis.

In medical terms, the word *aura* is used by doctors to describe the sensation of twinkling or tingling before the onset of epilepsy. In some patients, the aura starts at the stomach, while in others it starts at the heart. For example, the heart has a sinking feeling with a sensation of fright. In Calcarea Ars, the aura always starts at the heart. So if the patient notices something strange happening over the heart and the fit is like that of epilepsy, Calcarea Ars has the capability to completely cure this condition. Another sign of Calcarea Ars is that before the epileptic fit, the voice subsides and the person cannot speak.

Calcarea Ars is useful in the treatment of **shortness of breath while going up the stairs**. Its diseases tend to affect the left side of the body. In Calcarea Ars and in Staphysagria, neurological diseases develop as a result of anger, dislike and displeasure. The patient imagines ghosts and suffers from other kinds of hallucinations and delusions. Sometimes its patient sees fire in the dreams. This also happens in Natrum Mur, in which the patient **sees fire and snakes in his dreams**. If along with these symptoms, permanent insanity seems to be developing, Calcarea Ars would prove to be a good remedy for such insanity.

Calcarea Ars is also useful for the treatment of vertigo, imbalance and convulsions secondary to the excessive rush of blood towards the head. Calcarea Ars can be of use in old and chronic types of **headache**. It is worth a try if everything else has failed to relieve the headache. The headache in Calcarea Ars is just the reverse of the headache in Cimicifuga. In Cimicifuga, the pain becomes intense on lying on the affected side. In fact, local pressure on the affected side may provoke twitching of the muscles. In Calcarea Ars, the person will feel pain on the side opposite to the one he lies on. If he **lies on the right side, his headache would be on the left side**, and vice-versa. This is typical of Calcarea Ars. Any chronic headache showing this kind of pattern will be most responsive to Calcarea Ars. Other than this, there is no other specific sign of the headache in Calcarea Ars.

**Eczema develops on the skin of the face and the scalp**. The **kidneys** hurt, the pain being the result of inflammation rather than of a stone in the kidneys. In Calcarea Ars, the leucorrhoeal discharge is yellowish and is corrosive like acid. Sometimes, this type of **leucorrhoea** can also cause psychiatric complications. In the treatment of this kind of leucorrhoea, Kali Phos and Arsenic are also useful remedies. In fact, these are the true antidotes for foul smelling discharge resulting from internal inflammation.

Calcarea Ars is very useful in the treatment of the constant oozing of the blood-mixed, acidic, foul-smelling discharge due to **cancer of the uterus**.

| | |
|---|---|
| Antidotes: | Carbo Veg, Glonoine, Pulsatilla |
| Potency: | 30 to 1000 |

# CALCAREA CARBONICA

Calcium Carbonate is a basic component of milk. In the development of bones, sclera and some other parts of the body Calcaria Carb is needed. In milk, a wholesome food, Calcium plays a very important role. The Imbalance of Calcium in the body results in various diseases, especially those of the bones. Calcaria Carb has its role on the glands, skin and the bones. The Calcarea Carbonica patient is very sensitive to cold. The feet sometimes feel very cold and sometimes hot. The chest feels tied up. The **cough is dry at night** but usually **phlegmatic during the day**. The sputum is yellowish, smelly and difficult to expel. In children, the cough that develops during teething and does not subside easily often responds to Calcarea Carb. The patients of Calcarea Carbonica constitution have listless faces. The skin is oily and yellowish. Sometimes they feel exhausted while talking and also suffer from lack of blood. Mental exercise further weakens them. They sweat profusely and may experience difficulty in breathing. They dislike cold and humidity. They hate the fresh air and chill. On being wet, like Rhus Tox, their ailments appear suddenly.

Calcarea Carb has a significant effect on **anaemia**. This anaemia is due to lack of the intrinsic factor from the lining of the stomach, as a result of which vitamin B12 cannot be absorbed. Vitamin B12 alone cannot cure this kind of anaemia, although it needs to be constantly administered to prevent against the associated bad effects. Vitamin B12 cannot be absorbed in the stomach so it needs to be given by injection for life. In such patients, if Calcarea Carb is given in homoeopathic potency, this obviates the necessity for supplementation with vitamin B12, and the body itself starts making blood.

In Calcarea Carb, the **muscles feel flaccid**. The disarrayed body associated with flail muscles and obesity will benefit from Calcarea Carb if given over a period of time. Calcium deficiency in the body can be treated by homoeopathic potencies of Calcarea Carb. In Calcarea Carb patients, sometimes on standing up suddenly, their leg muscles cannot bear the weight of the body and they fall down. In the case of low blood pressure also, it is difficult for a person to stand up suddenly. Calcarea Carb is useful for the treatment of weak muscles due to lack of calcium. The profoundly active constitutional remedies which are necessary for the physical development of human beings, when given with suitable intervals on a long term basis, will effectively treat these ailments resulting in the cure of the patient as a whole. Undoubtedly it is time-consuming.

It must be remembered that if Sulphur needs to be given after Calcarea Carb, Lycopodium should be instituted first, and then Sulphur. Hidden diseases made manifest by the use of Sulphur, for example piles, often respond to Nux Vomica. But Calcarea Carb is also useful in the treatment of **piles**. There are other homoeopathic remedies resembling Calcarea Carb, such as Aesculus for the treatment of bleeding piles and the infection thereof.

Calcarea Carbonica is very valuable to prevent the **tendency of developing cancer** if it matches the constitution of the patient, otherwise it will not be of use. In some conditions, an incision needs to be made, but Calcarea Carb obviates such a need. Calcarea Carb is a very effective treatment of deep-seated **abscesses**, even better than Silicea. The abscess either dissipates or produces only a small amount of pus. The abscess disappears without much discomfort and throbbing. It will be of timely use for such a condition.

The patient of Calcarea Carb can be easily recognized. He is rather obese and of yellowish complexion. The head is relatively big and there is a tendency to sweat a lot. The body is sometimes cold and sometimes hot. If all the systems of the body are slow, it becomes the general description of a Calcarea Carb patient. However, each and every symptom does not have to be present to make the diagnosis. Nor is there one unique symptom of Calcarea Carb. Some children have a large head from birth; this does not necessarily make them Calcarea Carb patients, although some may be. Sometimes the symptoms of Calcarea Carb develop over the passage of time.

The Calcarea Carb patient has his **nose stuffed with dried mucus** and may have difficulty in breathing through the nose. With the use of Calcarea Carb, this material becomes easily expelled without the need of any operation. Due to the imbalance of Calcium, sometimes **bones develop spurs at their ends** and bony prominences of Calcium develop at the **knee joints**, which are very painful. Calcarea Carb can cure this problem. Calcarea Carb is the right treatment for a child who, due to the weakness of the muscles, has **delayed walking**. If there is **delay in speaking**, then Baryta Carb is the best remedy. Natrum Mur will be useful when delays in both walking and speaking are present in a child.

When there is a sodium imbalance in the body, it can adversely affect the mental faculties. The legs become weak and the **patient becomes rather wasted**. The special feature of Natrum Mur is the wasting of the legs as well as the upper part of the body. The tongue also is affected. Consequently the child starts walking and talking rather late. In Calcarea Carb, the tongue is not affected and the child learns to talk normally. However, he is late in learning to walk. Being **short-statured** is also a symptom of Calcarea Carb. Physical weakness and mental deficiency are symptoms of Baryta Carb. Calcarea Carb gradually produces clear improvement of unsightly **bending of the bones** if the patient is that of Calcarea Carb constitution.

The patient feels cold inside but sometimes his hands and feet may feel burning. The symptoms aggravate before the onset of a storm such as a dust-storm. An asthma patient will start exhibiting signs of allergy to the dust many hours before the storm comes. Calcarea Carb is one of the remedies indicated for such patients. The patient who gets mentally fatigued, and various parts of his body shows signs of weakness will respond to Calcaria Carb. Calcarea Carb gives him relief and his restlessness does not last long. **When extremely excited**, a Calcarea Carb patient starts visualising pointed objects, and the pictures and bodies will appear to be dancing. Similarly, he visualises inanimate objects, nails, wires, piercing and cutting instruments. Calcarea Carb is a sure shot remedy, with rare exception, whenever these symptoms are present in children.

Calcarea Carb is also indicated whena person feels generally tired, is chilly and experiences the burning of hands and feet. The Calcarea patient afflicted mentally keeps on pinching with his hands and has hallucinations about various faces before going to sleep but has no fear of death. The **skin peels off at the nails** causing great discomfort. This symptom is also present in Petroleum. The skin becomes dry as in dry eczema and recedes from the nails.

In general, **grief and dejection** are more amenable to treatment with Sodium compounds. These include Natrum Mur, Aurum Mur, and

Gratiola. Ambra Gresea and Arnica may be useful in the treatment of a patient who is very sad and becomes indifferent towards his life. A peculiar sign of Calcarea Carb, which does not exist in any other remedy, is depression. For example, a little girl who should normally be playing around becomes sad and indifferent to everything. The depression developing in the girls before puberty, needs to be attended promptly or the patient may **commit suicide**. The patient is not aggressive nor is there any evident cause of her sadness. The patient cannot seriously think much. Routine normal worries can make the patient feel mentally as well as physically fatigued. Calcarea Carb in homoeopathic potency, given along with allopathic Calcium tablets, is very good for the treatment of this kind of fatigue.

The Calcarea Carb patient experiences **scary dreams** and is scared of ghosts in the dark. In the dream he often finds himself hurt in an accident or due to fire. Any form of headache may be present in a Calcarea Carb patient. For distinction, its headache becomes worse with light and is worse during the day than at night. A Graphites **headache also aggravates with light** because Calcarea Carb as well as Graphites both contain an element of carbon. It is also found in Carbo Veg. Cold packs or cold sponging relieves the headache.

When the **head of a child starts growing bigger**, the reaction of the pupils becomes sluggish, and the child screams at night; generally surgical treatment is required. Yet the chances of cure are rare. The child becomes semi-insane. Timely use of Calcarea Carb, and more so of Silicea, will be needed. With these, the excessive fluid from the brain discharges by way of the eyes or sometimes the ears. Excessive leakage of water from the eye or the ear on one side will make the pillow wet and the head on that side will start getting smaller in size. After a few days similar effects will occur on the other side. In this condition, called Hydrocephalus, I have often treated many children with Silicea and Calcarea Carb. When the disease is far advanced Calcarea Carb in high potency may be useful but not necessarily.

A white material may form on the **cornea of the eye** which then gradually starts to flow. If the infection is old, the discharge becomes yellowish. In this condition, Calcarea Carb can also be used in addition to other appropriate remedies. If the discharge from the ear is yellow, Calcarea Carb is more likely to be the remedy. The weakness of the eardrums or **slowly progressive deafness** of the ears, need to be treated with Calcarea Carb. Some other remedies like Chenopodium may also benefit. Calcarea Carb is of benefit for the **weakness of the eyes due to** their being **tired and the increased pressure** in them. However, Onosmodium is more effective than Calcarea Carb in tired eyes. Along with the tiredness of the eyes there is constant headache which is not very severe. A combination of Onosmodium along with Gelsemium 200 will be extraordinarily more effective. Sometimes the **change of weather brings in the sadness and lethargy**. Due to some change in the atmosphere, the body temporarily feels weak. Calcarea Carb, being of long acting type, is useful in the treatment of prolonged illnesses. In these illnesses the recovery is slow and the medicine has to be administered at intervals over a long period.

Calcarea Carb patients have an **intense desire to eat eggs**. In addition, the child would also eat certain **indigestible things like clay and paper**. Many of these children happen to suffer from chronic indigestion. The patient feels heaviness on the top of the head. With the headache, the hands and feet become cold. Mental work aggravates the headache. There is itching on the scalp, and the eyes are very sensitive to light.

Calcarea Carb is also useful in the treatment of **chronic constipation**. Silicea and Veratrum Album are also good remedies for constipation. Generally, Veratrum Album is used for the treatment of **severe diarrhoea**. In fact, it is very useful in the treatment of the obstinate type of constipation, yet most homoeopaths do not use it for the this. Silicea can relieve the chronic constipation of children. If ineffective, Veratrum Album must be used. If other signs and symptoms of Calcarea Carb are present, certainly Calcarea Carb would be the most optimal treatment. Within a few days the abdomen becomes soft and the constipation is gradually relieved. The effect of the medicine is not immediate.

Calcarea Carb is also used for the treatment of deep-seated diseases of men as well as women. It prevents the **tendency towards prolapse of the uterus**. It corrects the **menstrual dysfunctions** and excessive bleeding (menorrhagia). It not only controls the bleeding but also cures the enlarged glands. In case one cannot reach one particular diagnosis, the following three things should be used to prevent excessive bleeding during the menstrual period: Calcarea Carb, Murex, and Sabina in potency 30. These should be continued for a few months. In the beginning three times a day and then once a day, after it has started showing beneficial effects.

Calcarea Carb is an effective remedy for the treatment of **fibroids in the uterus**. Women of Calcarea constitution suffer constantly from thick **leucorrhoea**. Calcarea Carb will be very valuable for the treatment of such women who also have **tendency to abort repeatedly**. I had prescribed this remedy to one such lady who responded very well. In fact, she had already conceived before the next menstrual cycle and did not miscarry, though in the past she had lost many pregnancies. For any appropriate treatment, it is very important to exactly diagnose the cause of abortion. Ferrum Phos, Calcarea Phos, and Kali Phos are well known for the treatment of generalized weakness and **lack of blood (anaemia)**. They work very well during pregnancy and prevent abortion. The other useful remedy for the treatment of abortion is Caulophyllum. If the patient has the constitution of Calcarea Carb, then only Calcarea Carb should be administered without any hesitation and without the possible need of any other homoeopathic remedy.

Because Calcarea Carb has to be continued over a long period of time so it should be repeated at intervals instead of continuously. It should be continued for six months after the patient has apparently been cured.

A **cough which lingers on** and is associated with **blood in the sputum** is also the sign of Calcarea Carb. As in Kali Carb, the feet become cold. If the generalised weakness advances too far, such a patient will not be able to sit for long periods of time and tends to slip off the chair, and when a patient is in a moribund state and his head constantly sags down from the pillow, the proper remedy is Muriatic Acid which will work immediately. If it happens frequently, then Calcarea Carb is the better remedy. In Calcarea Carb the **lower back hurts**. The back also feels weak and it is difficult to stand up after sitting for some time.

| | |
|---|---|
| Adjuvants: | Sulphur to be used before Calcarea Carb and followed by Lycopodium.<br>Belladonna, Rhus Tox and Silicea |

| | |
|---|---|
| Antidotes: | Camphor, Ipecac, Nux Vomica, Nitric Acid |
| Potency: | 30 to CM. |

# Calcarea Fluorica
## (Fluoride of Lime)

Calcium Fluoride is a mineral element found in the form of a shiny stone all over the world. It is of immense value in the industrial world. In the human body, it is deeply related to the diseases of the teeth, bone, and elastic layer of the skin, muscles and the blood vessels. In its deficiency, the glands become stone hard while the teeth and the bones become brittle. Homoeopathic potency of Calcarea Fluor is the best remedy to dispel **the hardening of the muscles**. It is related to the function of almost every part of the body. In particular, it is very important for the proper **development of the bones**. In Calcarea Fluor patients, spurs form over the surface of the bones, and the veins become tortuous and knotty. The uterus loses its tone and tends to sag downwards. The nails become ugly. **Hard lumps form in the breasts of women**. Moreover, Calcarea Fluor should be used in this and other conditions that tend to become cancerous in nature. I have seen many patients whose swelling at the wrist (Ganglion) had become very hard. Previously I used to prescribe Ruta or similar medications, but these did not work satisfactorily. With the use of Calcarea Fluor, almost every patient benefited. Some patients develop **lumps in the folds of the knees (Baker's cyst)**. Calcarea Fluor works very well for the treatment of such lumps. As well as other indicated remedies, Calcarea Fluor should also be used in the **treatment of fibroids of the uterus**. Sometimes, Calcarea Fluor on its own may prove very effective.

Calcarea Fluor is also very useful in the **treatment of injuries to the retina of the eye**, especially if the margins have rather hardened. Stars seem to be dancing before the eyes. Spots may also develop on the cornea. Calcarea Fluor should also be remembered in the **treatment of the hardening of the blood vessels of the eyes**. Rigidity in the eardrums, ringing in the ears, discharge from the ears and the **enlargement of the adenoid glands (behind the nose)** can be treated with Baryta Carb as well as Calcarea Fluor. If the **glands have gradually become enlarged and hardened**, then Calcarea Fluor is the ideal remedy. During **nasal cold**, the discharge stinks and has a deep green colour. The bones of the cheeks and jaws become inflamed, teeth hurt and the gums swell up. The **tongue becomes**

**hard and inflamed**, the teeth become loose and hurt when eating food. The **pain in the throat** eases after swallowing hot liquids and becomes worse with cold drinks.

Calcarea Fluor is also related to the functioning of the reproductive organs in the males as well as females. Sometimes, varicose veins with a **tendency to bleed can develop in the external genitalia**. Calcarea Fluor and Baryta Carb both can be useful in the treatment of this condition.

Calcarea Fluor is useful in the **treatment of haemorrhoids** that are not only heavily swollen but also hardened. Similarly, if the **thyroid gland** is enlarged and hardened like a stone it can also be treated with Calcarea Fluor. Once I saw a patient whose haemorrhoids had become hard like a stone. I gave him Calcarea Fluor 1000. Incidentally, he had also an **enlargement of the thyroid**, which he used to keep covered under a scarf. I had no knowledge of the enlargement of his thyroid gland. After the treatment with Calcarea Fluor, the patient contracted high fever. Being a brave person he did not mind it. He understood that the high fever was due to the medicine and did not go for any other kind of treatment. Within a week, the fever subsided completely, the haemorrhoids became soft and regressed, and the goitre (enlargement of the thyroid gland) also disappeared as well. Only the skin covering the thyroid became baggy due to the decrease of the size of the thyroid underneath it. Later on, this also adjusted to its normal configuration. Similarly I treated a 90-year-old man suffering from cataract with Calcarea Fluor and Zincum Sulph in CM potency. By God's grace, his cataract cleared completely and it never recurred for the rest of his life. Apparently, surgery on the eye was contra-indicated in view of his old age. It must be remembered that Calcarea Fluor is useful in the treatment of cataract but not useful in the treatment of glaucoma. Cataract and glaucoma are different diseases with different aetiology.

In Calcarea Fluor, the patient has the tendency to be **nauseated and vomits**, and children in particular vomit undigested food. Overwhelmed with studies children can become mentally exhausted and then tend to feel nauseous and vomit. The patient may suffer from rheumatism along with diarrhoea. The **haemorrhoids are associated with pain in the back and the lower part of the abdomen**. The backache becomes worse in the early part of movement and gets better on moving around. In children, the backbone may become inflamed and the thighbone (femur) also becomes thickened and painful. There is pain in the lower back and stiffness of the neck. Nodules form over the joints of the fingers (Heberden's nodes). The **patient experiences severe pain in the knees and the legs**. The feet sweat and stink. Warts grow on the hands, arms, legs and over the back.

In Calcarea Fluor, there is patchy de-pigmentation of the skin. The skin around the operation scars shrinks. **Wounds may become infected and the edges of the wound thicken.**

Calcarea Fluor is usually a slow acting remedy. It should be used over a long period intermittently. Once the beneficial effect becomes evident, unnecessary repetition should be avoided. Sometimes it works best in high potency. Its ailments become worse in changing weather, on resting and in humid climate. Local application of heat and hot fomentation offer comfort.

| | |
|---|---|
| Potency: | Biochemic 6X or homoeopathic from 30 to CM |

# Calcarea Iodide
## (Iodide of Lime)

Calcarea Iodide is especially related to the glands. The glands swell up as in the case of many other remedies. Calcarea Iodide should never be forgotten in the **treatment of puberty goitre** in young girls. It is especially useful during the age of puberty and should be administered to such girls without any delay.

In Calcarea Iodide, **fibroids develop in the uterus**. The **internal lining of the nose and the ears become oedematous and make cyst-like swellings called polyps**. With the formation of polyps in the nose, the patient snores heavily. Calcarea Iodide 30 proves to be very useful in the treatment of this condition. It should however be used for two to three months because the glands, once enlarged, do not immediately regress to their normal size.

In Calcarea Iodide, the ulcers tend to be chronic in nature, much more so in Kali Iodide. In Kali Iodide, the ulcers become indolent.

In Calcarea Iodide, there is a **tendency for hair to fall out**. Unfortunately, there is no one standard treatment for hair loss.

It must be remembered that Sulphur is not given after Calcarea Iodide. This can be harmful. However, Sulphur Iodide given after Calcarea Iodide works very well and there is no need for giving any other remedy in the intervening period. The common routine is to give Lycopodium after Calcarea Carb, then Sulphur, and then Calcarea Carb again. However, Calcarea Iodide can be safely and directly followed by Sulphur Iodide treatment. Although Calcarea Iodide makes the patient feel somewhat better, it cannot cure the patient and that is why Sulphur Iodide should be used instead.

| | |
|---|---|
| Potency: | 30 or higher as needed |

# Calcarea Phosphorica

Calcarea Phos is a compound of calcium and phosphorus, and thus a very profoundly effective remedy. It has been commonly used in the biochemic system of medicines, although it needs to be used with extreme care. Calcarea Phos is described to be the friendliest treatment of women. Many of its symptoms happen to be the common symptoms of day-to-day diseases of women. Calcarea Phos must always be kept in mind. With the onset of puberty, young girls are subject to a variety of problems, such as **painful periods**, scanty bleeding or menstrual bleeding of variable duration. Once the periods become irregular on exposure to the cold at an early age, the problem may become a lifelong one. This can only be treated with the use of Calcarea Phos.

It is extremely difficult to diagnose the cause of menstrual irregularities on the basis of acute symptoms alone, without an in-depth study of the background of the disease. If an adult female is found to have similar irregularities, one usually forgets about her previous history i.e. puberty. However, it is necessary that the history should be dated back to early adulthood, since it is important to know when the trouble started and how it started. If the **menstrual irregularity started on exposure to the cold** during the periods, then Calcarea Phos should be used immediately. By God's grace, the patient becomes cured forever with its use. One symptom is common to Calcarea Phos and Cimicifuga: the patient feels a lot of discomfort, pain and cramping in the area of the uterus. The main difference is that in the patient of Cimicifuga, the symptoms become worse as the bleeding starts to flow more freely. In a patient of Calcarea Phos, **severe cramps and severe discomfort precede the onset of the bleeding**. Once the bleeding commences, these symptoms disappear. This symptom is the distinctive feature of Calcarea Phos.

Generally, Magnesium Phos is considered to be the best **treatment for spasms and cramps**. It is not only useful in the treatment of cramps of the uterus, but also cramps elsewhere in the body. If the spasms become better with the application of heat, then one should give Magnesium Phos. However, if the pain eases with cold, then Belladonna, Apis, Secale and Pulsatilla will be more useful. In the spasmodic pain associated with Calcarea Phos, heat offers relief.

Calcarea Phos is the best remedy for the **treatment of spasmodic pain and cramps over the sexual organs in women**. If sexual desire becomes heightened due to some diseases, not of the natural kind, then besides Calcarea Phos, Platinum Gratiola and Origanum can also be useful. Calcarea Phos is a must if the patient's **uterus starts to prolapse at the time of urination**. In Calcarea Phos, the menstrual blood consists of dark blood clots, while in Calcarea Carb and Phosphorus, the colour of the blood is red.

If the **periods begin before time**, the blood is bright red and if the periods are delayed, then the colour of the blood becomes black. Sometimes, the colour of the blood is red first and then turns dark. In Calcarea Phos, the **leucorrhoeal discharge is like the white of an egg.** Symptoms become worse in the morning. The **milk of the lactating women tastes salty** and the child refuses to suck.

A Calcarea Phos patient cries out with pain spontaneously. The chest hurts. The **cough is suffocating** in nature. The patient feels better on lying down. The voice becomes hoarse. The patient feels pain in the lower part of the left lung. On exposure to open air or cold, the patient develops rheumatism. The back and the neck become stiff. The head feels heavy. The limbs become numb. The symptoms become worse from the cold and change of weather. The patient becomes easily tired on going up the stairs. The pains start two hours after eating food. The symptoms aggravate after eating or drinking something. The symptoms subside with heat and in dry weather.

The **memory becomes affected** as a result of sudden shock. The patient likes to move away from the place so that the suffering may become less. In Calcarea Phos, the **headache** is very severe. The head feels warm and hurts deep down to the roots of the hair. The tonsils become swollen and cause difficulty in opening the mouth (trismus). Calcarea Phos is also useful in the **treatment of teething problems of children**. The teeth grow rather slowly and tend to decay. Another symptom of Calcarea Phos present in children is that they want to suck the milk all the time but they cannot retain it and vomit it out. They feel **severe pain inside the abdomen, as well as gripes**. Bleeding follows hard stools. The child develops **diarrhoea** after drinking fruit juice, the stools being greenish in colour. The

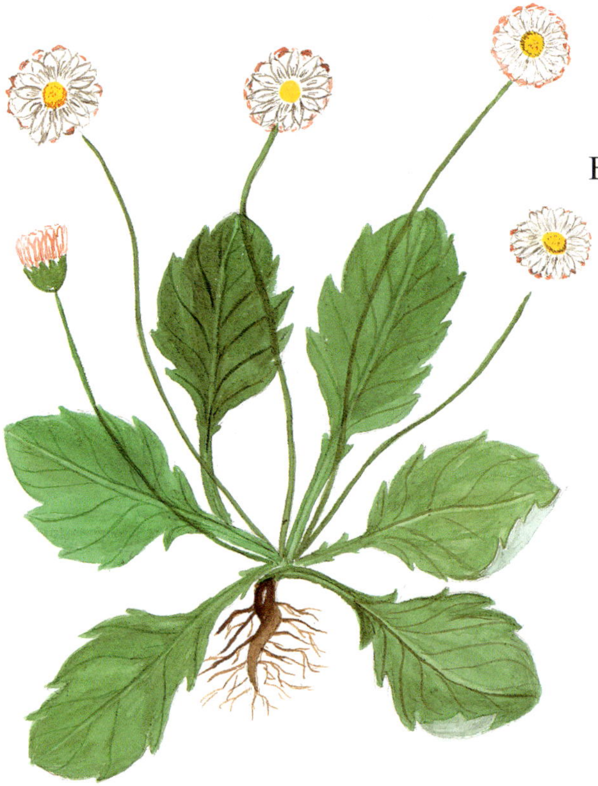

Bellis perenis

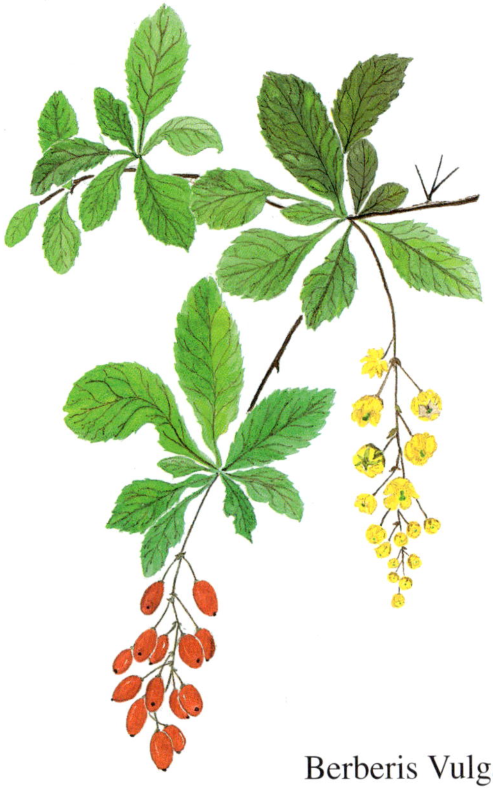

Berberis Vulgaris

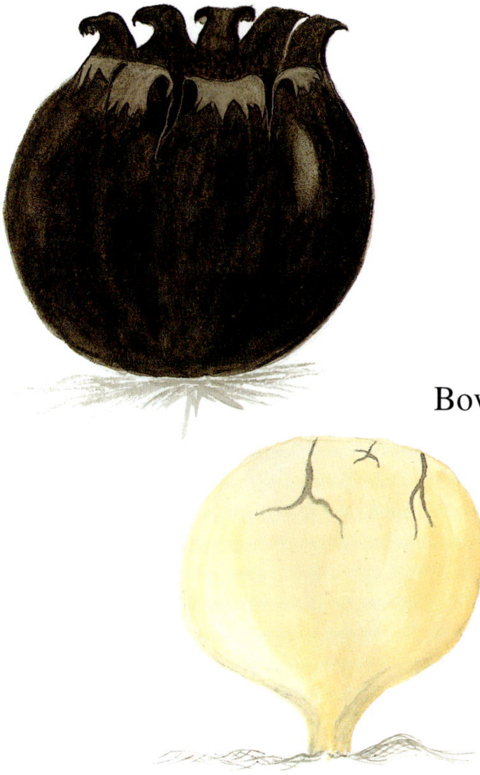

Bovista

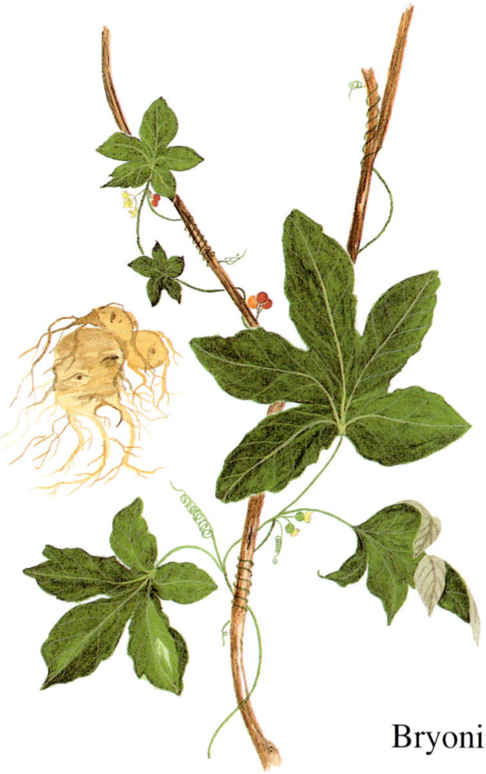

Bryonia Alba

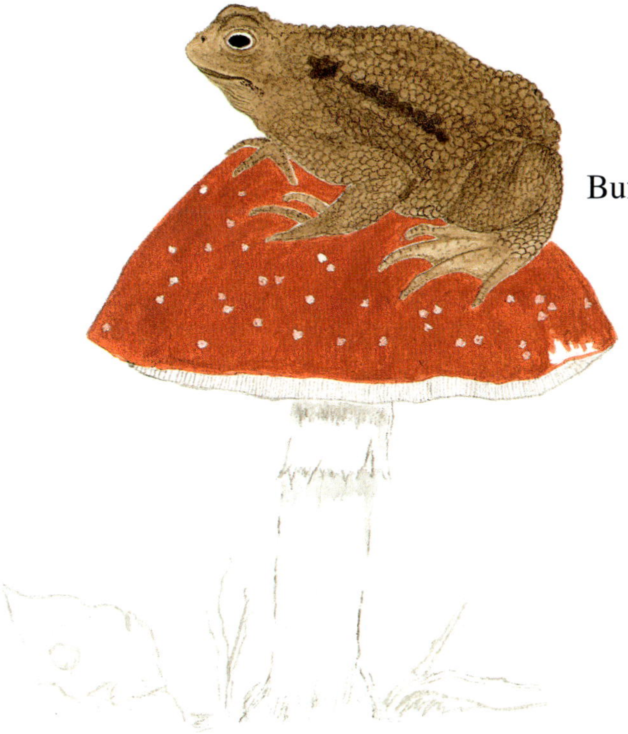

Bufo

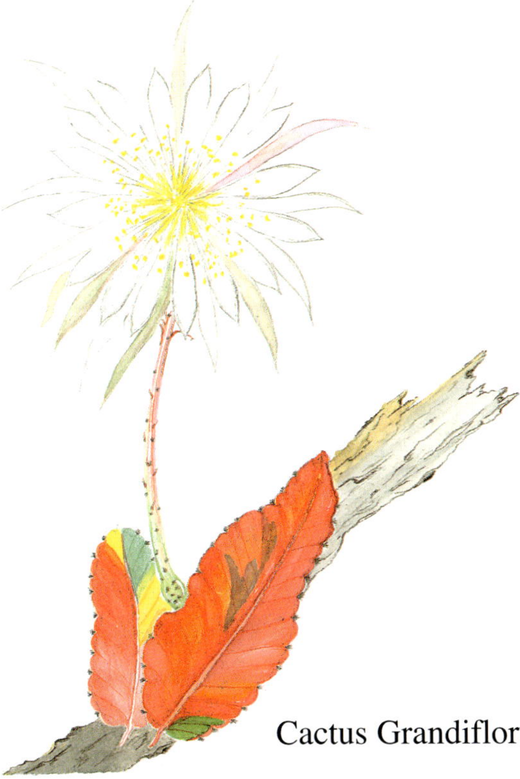

Cactus Grandiflorus

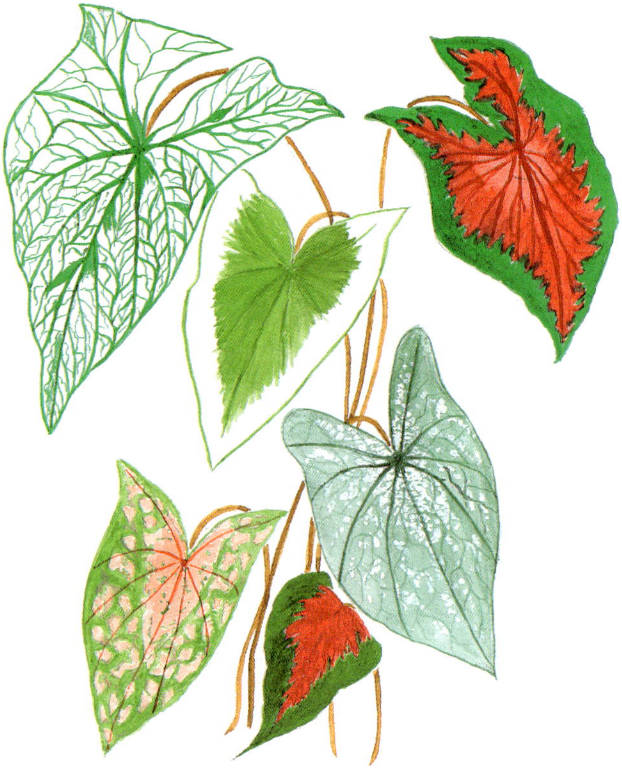

Caladiu

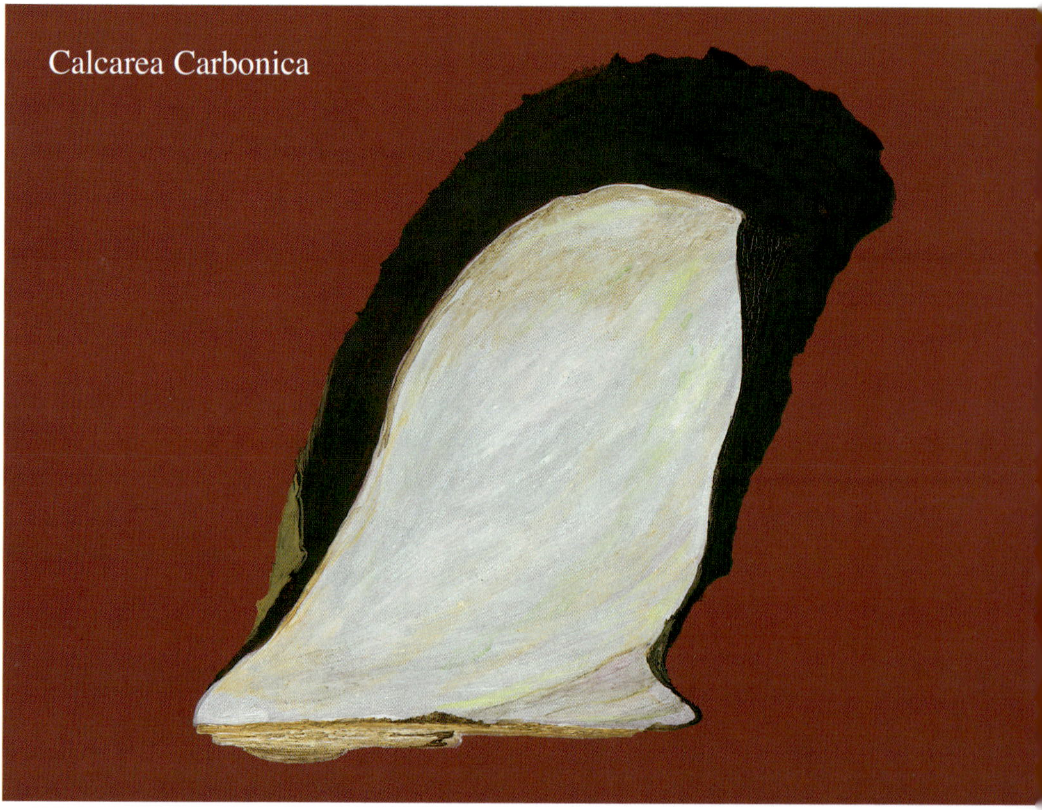

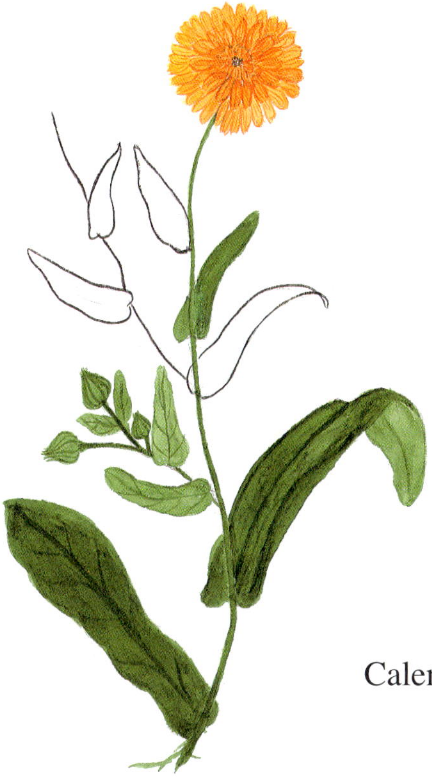

Calendula Officinalis

annabis Sativa

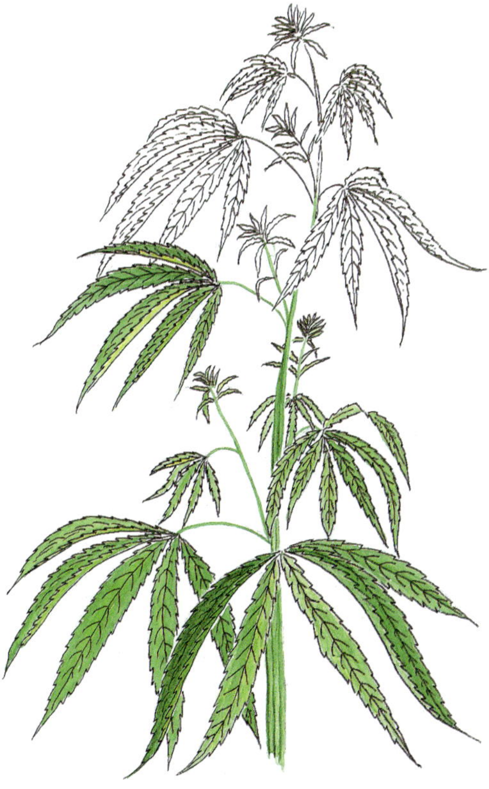

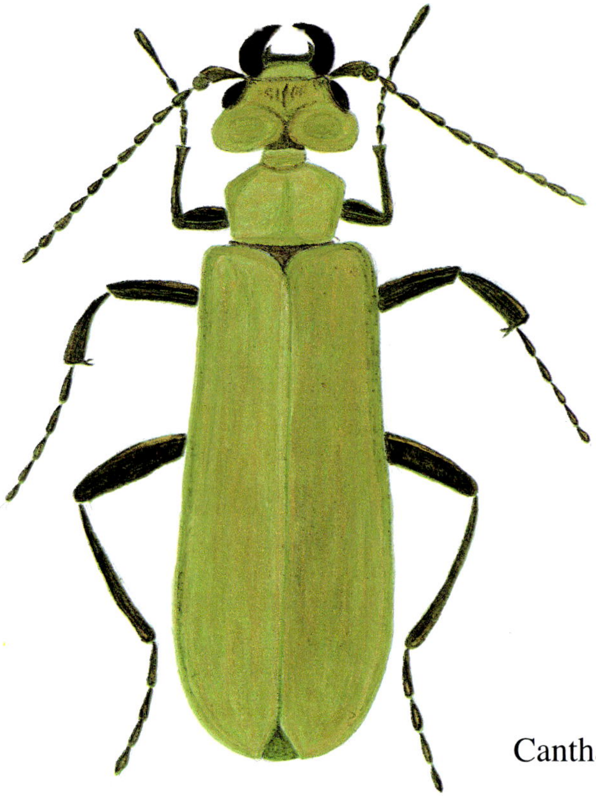

Cantharis

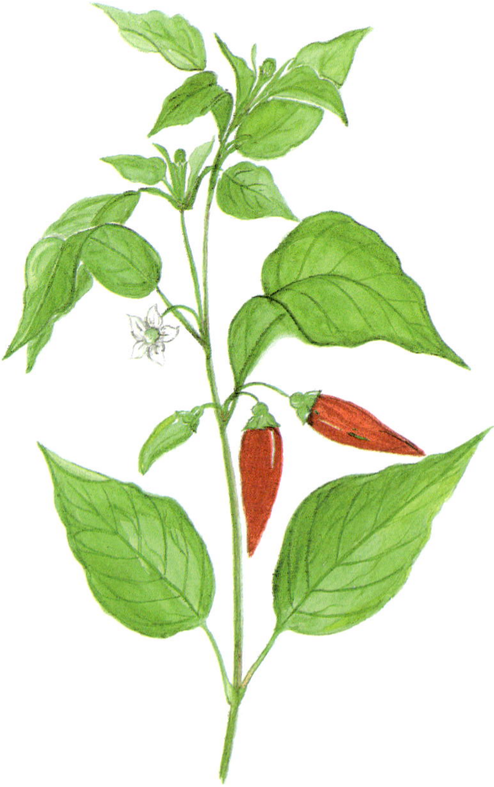

Capsicum

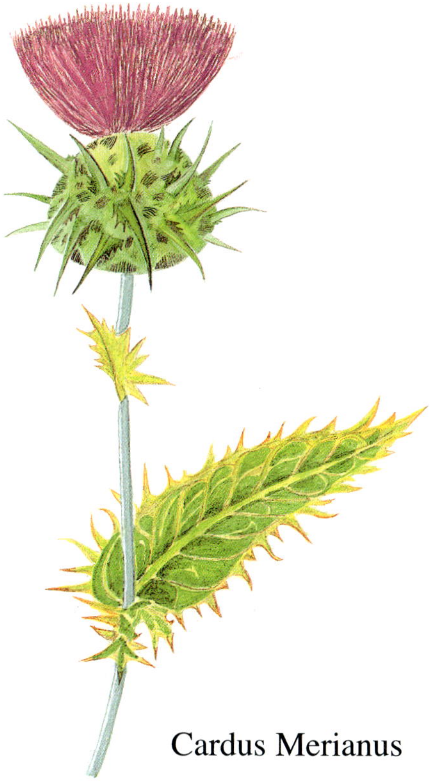

Cardus Merianus

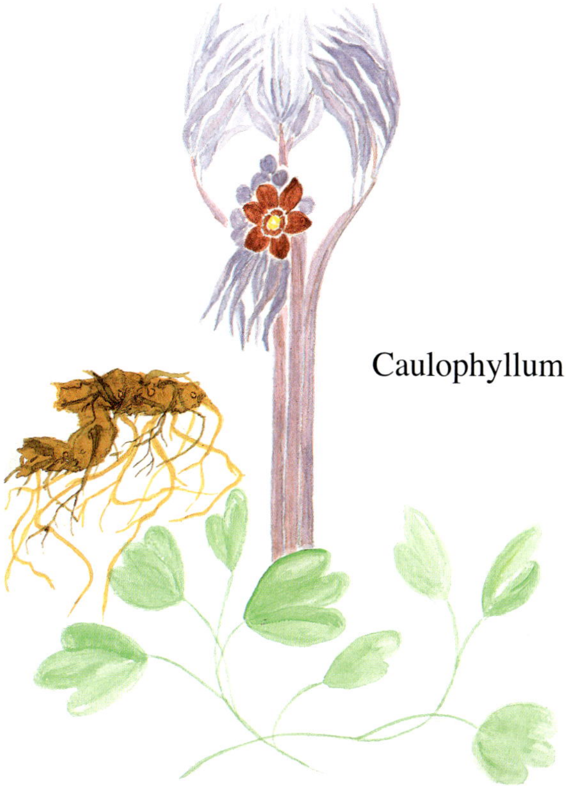

Caulophyllum

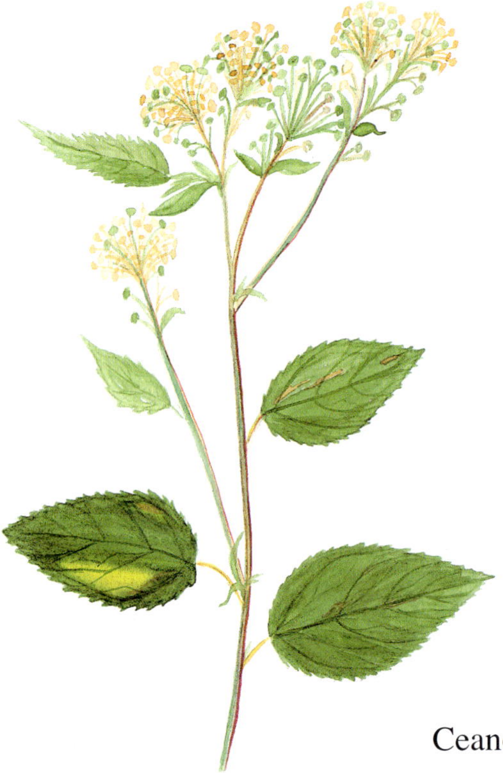

Ceanothus

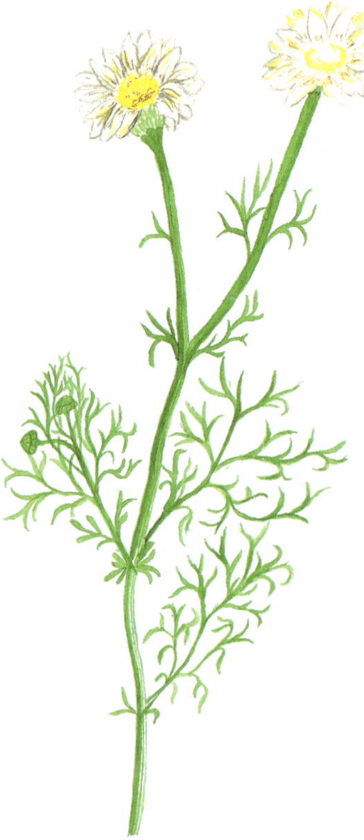

Chamomilla

patient passes enormous amounts of urine, causing weakness. There is pain over the kidney areas. The back hurts when lifting weight.

| | |
|---|---|
| Adjuvants: | Ruta, Hepar Sulph |
| Potency: | Biochemic 6X |
| | Homoeopathic from 30 to CM |

# CALCAREA SULPHURICA
# OR
# CALCAREA SULPHATE
## (Sulphate of Lime - Plaster of Paris)

The element of Sulphur is a common factor of Calcarea Sulph and Carbonium Sulph and so the symptoms of Sulphur are present in both. But the presence of carbon in one and Calcarea in the other make them distinct homoeopathic remedies of different constitutions. A special characteristic of Calcarea Sulph is the tendency to form deep **abscesses**. In this way, it resembles Sulphur as well as Calcarea Carb, and to some extent Pyrogenium. Pyrogenium is of use when the infection in the abscesses has already poisoned the blood (toxaemia). Putrefaction is also found in the deep abscesses associated with Silicea, but it usually does not affect the blood. If it happens at all, it is of very severe magnitude. The widespread pyaemic abscesses in the body resulting from toxaemia / septicaemia respond very well to Calcarea Sulph in addition to Pyrogenium. Similarly, it is deeply related to chronic sores that have the tendency to transform into **cancer,** and also controls sores to some extent. It is also useful in the treatment of the ulcers and fistulae developing when the cancers surface on the skin.

Calcarea Sulph is described as the best remedy for **epilepsy**. In recent times, the incidence of epilepsy has significantly increased and there are many reasons for this. One reason is injury to the head of the baby due to certain instruments used at the time of delivery, affecting the brain of the child. Epilepsy can also be the result of the ill effects of certain allopathic medicines. In such children, in addition to the standard prescriptions, one should look for the appropriate constitutional remedy in order to cure the epilepsy. Calcarea Sulph is said to be the one that can completely cure epilepsy. Dr. Kent, who was previously an eminent allopathic physician as well as a surgeon and understood the physiology of the human body, is of the opinion that Calcarea Sulph can totally uproot the epilepsy. Sometimes, the epilepsy is due to a tumour in the brain or it can be due to the effect of a physical injury to the brain. Sometimes it is due to the abnormal development of the skull, evident on observing the patient. In such a patient who has a permanent developmental defect of the skull, the cure for the epilepsy is apparently impossible. The statement of Dr. Kent does not hold well about the treatment of this kind of epilepsy with Calcarea Sulph. However, we can definitely say that Calcarea Sulph has significantly benefited many epileptic patients.

It is possible to treat the epilepsy which gas developed secondary to some serious illnesses of infancy, cholera and dysentery being the most salient. Whenever the diarrhoea due to gastro-enteritis or a severe kind of dysentery is treated forcibly with some allopathic medicine, there is always the danger that the child may subsequently develop **epilepsy**. I often treat such patients with Cuprum. In addition, I have also given them Artemisia in Mother Tincture form. Both of these do temporarily benefit, but I have not observed complete cure. These remedies have to be administered on a permanent basis. I have tried them in very high potency and found that the intervals between the epileptic fits prolonged, but complete cure was not obtained. It means that we should try to find out other remedies for the complete cure of epilepsy. According to Dr. Kent, Calcarea Sulph has this capability.

I have observed complete cure of epilepsy only in the condition of recurrence of that particular illness, the suppression of which had resulted in the development of epilepsy in the first place. When that particular illness relapses, it can be treated with other kinds of complementary remedies, such as Arsenic for the treatment of fever, and Mag Phos for the treatment of **abdominal pain** and colic. However, antibiotics and strong medications that suppress the illness must be avoided.

Regarding the treatment of **epilepsy,** one should study the prodormal signs (Aura), as already mentioned in reference to Calcarea Ars. In some of these patients, blood is noted to rush towards the head. Generally it is considered to treat with Belladonna however, is not proper. Belladonna only helps partially, for a short time. In some other homoeopathic medicines also, there is a tendency of blood rushing towards the brain such as in Hydrocyanic Acid. Hydrocyanic Acid causes severe spasm of the air passages, resulting in a profound congestion of the face. In the presence of these symptoms, Hydrocyanic Acid may also be one of the important remedies for epilepsy. Hydrophobinum is also related to this kind of illness. The patient is scared of flashing objects. **If there is fear of developing epilepsy on the sight of a flashing object**, Hydrophobinum would be found very useful. This may be given in combination with Hydrocyanic Acid. These are compatible and in fact are supplemental to each other for the treatment of this kind of epilepsy.

When an epileptic cannot be treated by homoeopathic remedies he should definitely be transferred to the care of allopathic physicians. A number of strong allopathic medicines have been discovered to control epileptic fits. They keep the patient drowsy to a great extent, but relieve him of the pain of the epileptic fits. In addition to allopathy, the traditional Chinese system of medicine may also be tried.

Calcarea Sulph is very useful in the treatment of **muscular pains and strains**. Whenever someone carries a heavy load beyond his capacity his back gets hurt. Calcarea Sulph, besides other remedies, may prove useful. Its action is not limited to the muscles of the back, but extends to the muscles of the entire body. It is also very beneficial in the treatment of **severe muscular strains of the limbs** due to excessive heavy lifting.

If other symptoms of Calcarea Sulph are present, whenever there is severe **flushing of the face** causing **convulsion,** not only on the face but other parts of the body as well such as the chest, arms, legs or head and there is a feeling of tightness, Calcarea Sulph can prove very effective. Calcarea Sulph is also useful for the treatment of **bone pains**, **inflammation of the glands** and generalised muscle fasciculation (twitching), especially the muscles of the face. **Calcarea Sulph, Agaricus and Kali Phos are useful in the treatment of muscle twitching under stress in feeble-minded patients**. The ailment of the patient aggravates on standing up, being more common in the women who stand for extended periods of time while cooking.

The Calcarea Sulph patient feels comfort on starting to walk, but after walking for some distance, as the circulation of the blood improves and the legs feel warm, his symptoms become worse again.

Due to his constant state of apprehension, the Calcarea Sulph patient wakes up early in the morning. This symptom along with other symptoms of Calcarea Sulph makes the diagnosis certain. Calcarea Sulph may be effective in the treatment of feeling of tiredness, vertigo or symptoms like epilepsy, resulting from mental exertion

This is also useful in the treatment of **diplopia** (double vision) and hypersensitivity to light. It is also useful in the elderly when they hear **various kinds of noises** in their ears.

In Calcarea Sulph, there is persistent nasal catarrh, which virtually settles in permanently and then destroys the inner lining of the nose. This makes the life of these patients forever miserable. Calcarea Sulph is the ideal and sure-shot remedy for this kind of nasal catarrh when associated with the other symptoms of Calcarea Sulph.

Calcarea Sulph is also useful in the treatment of **paralysis of the tongue where** the muscles of the tongue become rigid and tense. Sudden muscular cramps of the tongue and the associated sensation of suffocation is also present. This symptom is also found in Hepar Sulph. The feeling of tightness of the air passages (suffocation) and nasal catarrh is followed by constant irritation in the throat due to which even a small amount of air entering the throat or just mere speaking can precipitate a choking sensation.

The diagnosis being correct, Calcarea Sulph is also useful in the treatment of **chronic inflammation of the kidneys**. In Calcarea Sulph, the person feels warm all over and does not like to cover his body. Even the warmth of bedding may be intolerable to him.

Befitting the constitution of a particular person, Calcarea Sulph would benefit in treating **asthma and ailments of the ear** also. Similarly, it will be beneficial in curing **malaria**. In this respect, it has been learned that during the onset of fever, the chills start from the feet, but this condition has also been described in reference to other homoeopathic remedies. Thus, this particular symptom cannot be diagnostic of Calcarea Sulph.

Another feature of Calcarea Sulph is the presence of **thick, yellowish secretions from the eyes**. The **eyesight becomes foggy** and most things are only partially visible. The discharge of the ear is blood-mixed and the nasal discharge is of a yellowish colour. The throat hurts. Sputum from the throat is yellowish in colour. Similarly, the diarrhoeal stools are sticky like thick pus and may often be mixed with blood.

**Itching of the body** is not unusual in Calcarea Sulph. The **sores** discharging pus do not heal easily. Yellow scabs form over them. Pimples develop at the roots of the hair, which itch and bleed easily. In a Calcarea Sulph **child, his dry eczema** also shows similar scabs. The patients of the nature of Calcarea Sulph suffer from frequent disturbance of sleep due to strange kinds of dreams. If a few doses of Calcarea Sulph are administered, it will rid them of their strange dreams and restore their deep comfortable sleep.

| | |
|---|---|
| Potency: | 30 to CM |

# CALENDULA OFFICINALIS
## (Marigold)

Calendula lotion is used locally for the **treatment of skin sores**, but it has also been found very useful in the **healing of wounds** when taken internally in homoeopathic form. Non-healing, indolent ulcers start to heal with the help of Calendula 200. Taken internally it dries up the chronic ulcers, if its local application has not already benefited. There is a basic difference between the working of Calendula from Hepar Sulph and Silicea. Calendula builds up the inner strength of the body to repair the damage done to the tissues due to wear and tear. Hepar Sulph and Silicea fight against the infection. Calendula is very useful in the treatment of surgical wounds that do not heal normally, provided the radiation treatment has not destroyed the cells surrounding the surgical wound. Pure honey is also beneficial as a local treatment of sores and ulcers. In fact, honey has been found to be more effective than Calendula in many instances.

For the treatment of **bed sores** (Decubiti), normally Arnica and Hypericum are used. If both of them fail, Calendula in potency 200 will certainly benefit to some extent. Complete cure is also possible. Calendula is also useful in stopping bleeding after the extraction of teeth. The symptoms of Calendula intensify in cloudy wet weather.

| | |
|---|---|
| Adjuvant: | Hepar Sulph |
| Antidote: | Chelidonium |
| Potency: | Q to 200 |

# CAMPHORA
## (Camphor)

The most salient feature of Camphor is that the skin of its patient becomes very cold during the illness, though the patient internally feels very warm. He also feels very weak and debilitated. **Spasmodic conditions** are also prominent. Camphor will be found beneficial in the treatment of any sickness in which the body is very cold and there are cramps. It is also very effective in the treatment of **cholera,** especially where there is a frequency of loose stools but no pain, or sometimes no diarrhoea either. It quickly weakens the body so that the entire body feels cold. In such a condition, Camphor in a low potency is found to be very useful. If the cholera is associated with cramping of the stomach, hands and feet, Cuprum would be more optimal. However, **if the limbs feel ice-cold along with cramps** and cold sweats, Camphor would be the ideal treatment. In the cholera associated with Camphor, nausea is common. The Camphor patient feels frightened and scared, resembling Aconite, except that in Aconite there is no feeling of being cold. The feeling of extreme cold is the distinctive feature of Camphor. When, like Aconite, the sickness commences suddenly and is accompanied with fear and convulsions but the body feels very cold Camphor, instead of Aconite, would be more appropriate. Aconite would certainly be more useful if the onset of the illness is sudden and severe with the body feeling hot.

In a way, Camphor is related to Cantharis but also works as an antidote to it. In Cantharis, the linings of the kidney tubules become inflamed and there is a feeling of **burning along the urethra** with the urine passing in the form of drops. These symptoms also occur in Camphor to some extent. Sometimes, Cantharis poisoning can damage the kidney permanently and may also produce neurologic/psychiatric symptoms. In this particular situation, Camphor annuls the bad effects of Cantharis. Cantharis is not only a temporary remedy but can also neutralize the aftereffects of many other diseases permanently.

The Camphor patient becomes mentally weak. His **memory fades** and he is afraid of being left alone. He feels **dizzy** and may faint. He remains lying down quietly with his eyes closed as if he is sleeping but in fact he is not. He seems to be in another world. He may exhibit the signs of insanity and violent anger. This particular symptom is also present in Cantharis and Hyoscyamus. The inflammatory process shifts towards the brain with the patient showing signs of madness and aggression.

When the fever is secondary to the infection of the **uterus**, Camphor is also beneficial besides Pyrogenium and Sulphur. If the body is cold, the treatment should be started with Camphor. Sometimes, the fever is suppressed by some kind of treatment and the body becomes cold. At that time, Camphor is more effective than Sulphur. Once the body has warmed up and feels feverish, Sulphur and Pyrogenium should be administered together.

In Camphor, the body is extremely cold yet the patient sweats profusely. However, he does not want to be covered with anything. In fact, due to the feeling of internal heat, he likes to cast away the covering clothes. The symptom of dislike for covering clothes is also found in Secale Cor. The difference is that the Secale patient is warm and also feels warm, while a patient of Camphor, in spite of being very cold, does not like to be covered with a cloth. The symptoms of Camphor resemble those of Camomila and Aconite. The Camomila patient is of a furious nature and remains dissatisfied. He borrows things from other people but then throws them away. If such a patient does not have all the typical symptoms of Camomila, he may be treated satisfactorily with Camphor. A Camphor patient experiences the feeling of heat and cold alternatively. The body may feel warm while in the midst of the cold state of the body. The condition of alternating heat and cold changes frequently, showing that the fever is submerging deep down into the body. When the fever penetrates the backbone or transfers itself towards the brain, the body becomes cold. Nonetheless, the body keeps on defending itself against the sickness and tries to expel it. In this alternating feeling of cold and hot, Camphor is very beneficial.

In **menopause, elderly ladies** suffer many diverse symptoms like hot flushes on the face. Beside other remedies, Camphor should also be kept in mind. Ladies who obtain relief from the use of Camphor feel very cold when uncovered but sweat profusely when they have their clothes on.

The **headache** of a patient of Camphor does not involve the entire head. It may just be on the back of the head or on the forehead. The headache at the back of the head and the lower part of the neck, associated with a throbbing sensation, can possibly be treated with Camphor. Camphor is very well known for the treatment of **convulsions leading to the lockjaw**. Many a time, women go through these kinds of symptoms as a result of intense heat or marked internal weakness. One does not have to forcefully open the patient's mouth to adminster any medicine. Low potency Camphor happens to be very effective by its mere application to the lips. A characteristic feature of Camphor is that in the state of convulsion and associated lockjaw, the lips and tongue become blue.

The patient of Camphor feels intense thirst that is unquenchable. The patient wants to drink extremely cold water. While experiencing gas in the abdomen, there is a tendency towards **nausea and vomiting**. After vomiting, the stomach feels cool and calmed down. In the absence of nausea and vomiting, the body becomes very cold. Every kind of food tastes bitter.

In Camphor, the **tendency towards vomiting** is more common than the frequency of stools. The **stools** are frequent but scanty and are associated with marked weakness of the body and cramps. For repeated loose motions, vomiting and **cramping on the calves**, Veratrum Album is the top most remedy. The body feeling cold occurs in both Camphor as well as Veratrum Album, but in Veratrum Album cold sweats are visible only on the forehead. In Veratrum Album, there are two extremes of symptoms. Either there is severe chronic **constipation** or **frequent diarrhoea**. When other usual remedies prove ineffective, the chronic obstinate type of constipation would be relieved after a few doses of Veratrum Album.

When **the muscles of the urinary bladder become weak** and one needs to **strain the abdominal muscles to pass urine**, Camphor is a very useful remedy in this condition. There is retention of the urine, even if the bladder is full. There is a feeling of burning and cramping. Camphor is very obviously useful for the treatment of this paralytic condition of the bladder. Camphor also **affects sexual organs**. One may become permanently impotent due to the excessive use of Camphor. Sometimes the reaction is quite the opposite, i.e. an over-indulgence in sex which is certainly not normal. Whenever such contrasting symptoms are noticed, Camphor should be kept in mind so that it may be used as needed.

In Camphor, there is a tendency towards repeated **colds and cough with sputum (expectoration),** in this way it is equally matched to Antimonium Crude and Ammonium Carb. Both these remedies help in relieving the constant tendency of contracting such illnesses. The patient catches **cold** immediately on the slightest change of weather. The nose feels cold and starts running. The thick sputum (expectoration) tends to be stuck in the air passages resulting in a feeling of suffocation and difficulty in breathing. The deep inspiration (breathing in) provokes coughing and the heart starts beating fast.

Another peculiar symptom of Camphor is that the pain feels somewhat relieved by concentrating on the site of pain. The Camphor patient is sensitive to cold and touch; both aggravate symptoms. After a major surgical operation when the body becomes very cold and the blood pressure falls profoundly, besides Carbo Veg a few doses of Camphor will offer prompt relief.

In the state of being unconscious, the Camphor patient exhibits dilatation of the pupils of the eyes, which become fixed in one position. Everything looks so bright and flashy to him. He **envisions sparkling dots of light**. The symptoms intensify in the sunlight. The face is pale, drawn and lifeless. Cold sweating, typical of advanced cancers, is also present.

On exposure to cold, the patient develops **diarrhoea**, the stools being darkish in colour causing dehydration and profound weakness. The tongue and the inside of the mouth feel cold. The thirst is of the unrelenting type.

| | |
|---|---|
| Adjuvant: | Cantharis |
| Antidotes: | Phosphorus, Opium |
| Potency: | up to 30 |

# Cannabis Indica

Cannabis Indica is the other name for the hashish grown in the Indian subcontinent. It grows in the valleys of the Himalayas and the lofty grounds of Tibet. For long, it has been used as an intoxicating agent. The users of Cannabis Indica live in the world of their own, as if they are in the heavens. Time virtually comes to a standstill for them and recent events look ancient to them. They feel as if they are in the state of eternity. The symptoms of Cannabis Indica in homoeopathy are described as the patient floating in the atmosphere. The time does not pass or move. In a normal person, this state of inertia would make him feel seriously oppressed. The patient of Cannabis Indica does very little but thinks he has worked for many hours. His subjective feelings and emotions are overwhelming. He feels physically agitated all over, resulting in the shaking of the hands and feet. He feels extremely weak. The brain does not get enough blood. Instead, the face is flushed and the eyes staring. This condition is known as **Catalepsy**. Cannabis is very useful in the treatment of Catalepsy. The symptoms of Cannabis very much resemble those of Opium, which is the best treatment for Catalepsy. In Cannabis, the **sensitivity of the skin decreases**. The patient is lured by his own fantasies and imagination. On the contrary, in Hyoscyamus the delusions are frightful and the patient does not enjoy these scenes.

Cannabis addicts find their body divided into two parts. One is their personal self and the other is high up somewhere in the sky. This is why Cannabis addicts are considered as well connected saints.

A Cannabis patient laughs at serious matters also. He cannot control his laughter or crying. He may simply keep on laughing or crying. This indicates that his sickness is well established. The coexistence of laughing and crying like the sun and the shade, associated with a state of euphoria instead of madness, is the symptom of Cannabis Indica. Once the state of intoxication is over, the symptoms are different. Due to the intoxicating effect of Cannabis and damage to the brain, the patient is very scared of death.

A Cannabis patient has a constant fear of becoming insane. He is afraid of the dark. He keeps on making useless arguments. His thinking is irrational. Normally Cannabis addicts do not even complete their sentences. Cannabis in homoeopathic form will be found useful in treating those people who exhibit these symptoms, yet are short of being intoxicated.

The homoeopaths have done the proving and have come to the conclusion that the mind of a Cannabis patient is bombarded with thoughts, and owing to his inability to express them, his speech is rather disjointed. His thoughts are rather stirred-up. His mind is occupied with multiple irrelevant thoughts. He begins to talk normal and then suddenly becomes lost because of a new thought popping up. He becomes excited and starts talking about a new idea. He becomes lost in an imaginary world of his own. He enjoys music. Sometimes he becomes overwhelmed with his emotion and excitement. The Cannabis patient experiences a **throbbing kind of headache associated with pounding of the heart**. There is heaviness at the nape of the neck and throbbing at the temples.

It is an established fact that the thoughts of one person may be transferred to another person's mind (telepathy). Some thoughts from a remote mind may be detected through the so-called sixth sense. Many well known scientists also have testified that there is a deep down capability of such detection in the human body. If a person exhibits this kind of symptom due to any mental disorder, Cannabis should be utilised.

A Cannabis patient **grinds his teeth during sleep**. He **stammers while talking**. He is not hesitant to drink water but does not like to wash his hands, feet or take a shower with water. His stomach is full of gas which makes the belly tense.

A Cannabis patient **passes urine frequently.** In Opium, urination is less frequent and the other body secretions also reduce in quantity. In Cannabis, the ailments of the kidney are not unusual. The patient passes urine frequently but has hesitancy in the beginning and at the end of the act of urination. There is burning and mild scalding along the urethra. This also happens in Cannabis Sativa more than in Cannabis Indica. Thus, it is also used in the treatment of Gonorrhoea. Some patients of Gonorrhoea may be cured with one dose of CM Cannabis Sativa. It brings the suppressed Gonorrhoea to the surface and then cures it. Merc Cor CM is also described to be useful in its treatment.

In Cannabis Indica, there is **suppression of menstruation and tendency towards abortion**. The sexual urge is enhanced. The symptoms pertaining to the heart aggravate at night. There is nightlong sensation of pressure on the chest and suffocation, relieved during the day on walking around. With the onset of night, the symptoms return.

Some people develop **humpback** due to the weakness of the muscles of the back. Cannabis Indica administered at the beginning of the symptoms will help prevent this deformity of the back. Once the disease is well advanced, there will be no useful effect of this remedy. Cannabis Indica will be of use when the person feels pain in the legs and lower part of the body on walking. The arms and hands feel shaky and then the lower body may also be similarly affected. The legs feel rather numb and weak. Another symptom of Cannabis Indica is that the person feels sleepy yet cannot have good sleep. In Cannabis Indica, the skin feels tense and drawn, as in Opium. The symptoms of Cannabis Indica aggravate in the morning, and from lying on the right side and on smoking tobacco. Fresh air and rest offer relief. The patient feels like going to sleep but cannot.

| | |
|---|---|
| Potency: | usually 30 or very high |

# CANNABIS SATIVA

The symptoms of Cannabis Sativa very much resemble those of Cannabis Indica. In fact, many homoeopaths use one for the other, however, they also tend to annul each other.

The symptoms of Cannabis Sativa are more intense than those of Cannabis Indica. For example, the double personality in Cannabis Indica is well known. The patient feels confident that he belongs to both the worlds. On the other hand, in Cannabis Sativa, the patient has persistent doubt of his personal being. He cannot definitely place himself. He loses control over his speech and writing. While writing, he frequently changes the words. His speech is incomprehensible. There is frequent and unnecessary mixing up of words. While talking, he feels as if somebody else is talking. Psychiatrists have extensively studied this condition but cannot cure it and just prescribe tranquilizers. In homoeopathy however, the appropriate remedy can cure the patient.

A Cannabis Sativa patient feels as if drops of cold water are falling on the top or the back of his head.

The **eyes of a Cannabis Sativa patient are congested with blood**. The veins become visibly prominent in and around the eyes. The nose also bleeds. One cheek is red, while the other is pale. This also occurs in Pulsatilla. In Cannabis Sativa, there is dryness of the mouth and throat. There is a feeling of choking and difficulty in swallowing. The patient feels awfully tired.

The **kidneys get inflamed**. Urine comes in drops, associated with a burning sensation (scalding micturition). At the end of the micturition, there is a sensation of severe stitching type of pain. The severe spasm at the urethra and the meatus cause great discomfort. There is pain in the urethra, which the patient feels while walking as well.

Asthma too is a symptom of Cannabis Sativa, associated with rumbling over the chest. In fresh air, the patient feels relieved. Cannabis Sativa may very well be the remedy for symptoms of the **bladder associated with asthma**. In fact, many chest problems are the result of suppression of gonorrhoea causing asthma and its deleterious effect on the urethra. Cannabis Sativa is very useful in treating the urethritis caused by gonorrhoea associated with symptoms of asthma.

In Cannabis Sativa, the patient feels as if drops of water are pouring out of the heart. There is palpitation along with the feeling of pain. Knees hurt while going up the stairs and the legs feel heavy. Lying down, also aggravates the symptoms.

| | |
|---|---|
| Antidote: | Camphor |
| Potency: | 30 |

# CANTHARIS

Cantharis is a very poisonous fly. In the old days, seamen used to give its poison to prostitutes for its aphrodisiac action. In those days, the sea ports used to be the centre of sexual obscenity. Nowadays, the use of Cantharis is prohibited by law. The sting of this fly causes intense burning.

In homoeopathic form, its poison is utilized to relieve a **burning sensation**. Its blisters are not that big. For the treatment of large blisters, Rhus Tox is better than Cantharis. Intense burning is also a symptom of Rhus Tox. Rhus Tox 1000 given a few times will ameliorate the unusual burning pain of the entire body. In such a condition, Calendula can also be used.

In Cantharis, the patient expresses sudden total indifference to his surroundings, perversion of the mind and loss of consciousness. His mind is occupied with strange and weird thoughts. The symptoms point towards Cannabis Indica as well, but the main distinctive point is that in Cannabis Indica, the patient enjoys his perverted illusions and does not suffer. In Cantharis, the patient is in a state of frenzy due to the **cloudiness of the mind**. He does not know what he is doing. He also feels as if he is possessed by a demon and is talking under the influence of the possessing force. These kinds of symptoms also happen in Cannabis Sativa.

While under the effect of the poison, the patient loses his self-identity and feels himself under the influence of a foreign power. If this particular symptom becomes permanent, it is due to some mental problem rather than Cantharis. High potency Cantharis might relieve the sickness. The Cantharis patient is of **aggressive nature** and likes to torment others. He can become extremely angry. Cantharis in high potency can be useful in treating a sadistic type of person showing aggressive sexual behaviour.

In Cantharis, the patient has a **fear of water**. Mere reflections on the surface of water can throw him into a state of convulsion. He is intensely restless leading to extreme anger. The burning associated with Cantharis is very troublesome. He has fits of anger and ferocity and has the tendency to kill. There is an obscene type of talking by innocent young girls which resembles that of Hyoscyamus. Cantharis is also very useful in treating severe stabbing type of pains.

Along the course of the nerves, painful blisters form, more so on the face (Herpes). They may leave deep ugly scars. When on the eyes, the patient may become blind or this may result in the loss of one eye. It is very important to start the treatment promptly. Commonly, the combination of Arsenic, Ledum and Lachesis is very beneficial. In the absence of restlessness, Arnica, Lachesis and Ledum should be administered at once. If these two formulas do not work satisfactorily, Cantharis should be administered without any delay. In the case of really big blisters, Rhus Tox is found to be very useful. Compared to Rhus Tox, the restlessness of a Cantharis patient is very intense, resembling Arsenic. The colouration of the blisters of Cantharis changes fast and the surrounding skin becomes dark with signs of impending gangrene. In this situation, Cantharis must be given immediately. The skin of the Cantharis patient feels severe burning from simple touch. Cantharis is of great use for treating the hypothermia due to intense cold. Thus, it may once again perk up the fading body defences. In Cantharis, the stomach distends with gas. There is a burning sensation in the gullet (oesophagus) and the stomach, along with severe thirst.

Merc Cor is chronic of Cantharis. Merc Cor CM rapidly relieves the intense urinary symptoms. Cannabis Sativa in CM also works very well. Natrum Mur 200 or other high potency can also be useful. Cantharis is a very effective remedy for urinary symptoms associated with passing albumin in the urine. In the absence of albumin, the urine of a Cantharis patient is of a dark red colour.

There are certain special symptoms pertaining to menstruation. The periods are frequent and excessive in amount. The colour of the menstrual blood is darkish. After the delivery of a child, if the placenta is retained (in Secal as well as in Cantharis) then the infection of the uterus may lead to gangrene formation. In case, the infection has not far advanced, the uterus remains chronically inflamed associated with persistent foul discharge. The ovaries feel painful and burning. The heartbeat is weak and irregular. There is pain in the lower part of the back. The symptoms of Cantharis intensify with touch, cold water and on urination.

| | |
|---|---|
| Antidotes: | Aconite, Camphor, Pulsatilla, Cannabis Sativa |
| Potency: | 30 or very high |

# CAPSICUM
## (Cayenne Pepper)

Capsicum is prepared from red pepper. As a common notion, when a thin, lean person is found to be restless, it is said that it is his reaction to the pepper. However, the Capsicum patient is different altogether. He is fat, flabby and shows venous spiders on his face. His complexion is that of an alcoholic. The alcohol affects the small blood vessels of the face, which turn into reddish looking spider webs. The ingestion of chillies also causes enhancement of the circulation to the skin. Whether the food is hot or cold, the patient is hypersensitive to both. Hot things feel hotter and cold things seem colder than they actually are. When a person, in the habit of taking too much pepper, gives it up, his appetite becomes suppressed because his digestive glands and the lining of the stomach have been tuned to work under the stimulating effect of the chillies. When he resorts to taking pepper again, his glands become active and produce acid for digestion, which in turn stimulates the appetite.

Even though hot pepper causes burning and gives the feeling of warmth, nevertheless the Capsicum patient is of a cool nature and likes to live in well-heated room. A strange quality of the patient is that he does not like to live outside his home for long. He feels homesick even if he is not in the habit of taking too much hot pepper. A mere administration of two doses of Capsicum may somewhat diminish his anxiety to return home.

A Capsicum patient is stubborn in nature. It has been seen that in areas where a lot of hot pepper is consumed, the people there are usually of a stubborn nature, but not everyone who eats pepper is essentially of such a nature. An **angry nature with irritability and dissatisfaction** resembles Chamomilla. One cheek is red and the other is pale. This is commonly seen in diseases of the children. The scalp sweats. The patient thinks of committing suicide but does not dare. He is rather scared. He likes to live alone. The head or some other part of the body feels magnified. It can also happen in Sabadilla. In Capsicum, there is a feeling of throbbing. His **severe headache** becomes worse while resting, while movement makes it subside.

The **bone behind the ear becomes red and swollen** (mastoiditis) after a sore throat. This then becomes chronic. Phytolacca and Conium are also useful in treating this condition.

In cold, due to Capsicum, the face of the patient is flushed but cold. The tip of the nose is red. There is feeling of burning and irritation inside the nose. The nose may even be blocked. The Cough is associated with a foul smell and there is pain inside the throat. **Small blisters form on the tongue**, which are painful to touch and cause difficulty in swallowing.

In a patient of Capsicum, **premature wrinkling** of the skin is usual. The skin loses its elasticity and thick lines become prominent. Capsicum is useful in treating flabby muscles associated with defective circulation.

Capsicum may be used in the treatment of **measles** when the face is markedly congested and no other treatment works. Another special characteristic of Capsicum is that the **tonsils swell** but they are soft and can be reduced in size by pressure, like a sponge.

In Capsicum, **burning in the stomach** after food is very pronounced. **Dysentery** and diarrhoea are associated with a feeling of warmth inside the belly. The burning sensation (tenesmus) continues after defecation. There is an intense desire to drink cold water. Haemorrhoids burn and are swollen and red.

Persistent **hoarseness of voice** is also a symptom of Capsicum. If other symptoms of Capsicum are present, this remedy will prove effective. For the hoarseness of voice, Phosphorus, Causticum, Sulphur, Lycopodium, Coca, Psorinum and Borax are used.

The irritation of the larynx (voice box) and trachea provokes **dry cough,** along with a hissing sound in the chest and pressure on the bladder on coughing. There is chest pain on breathing and pain on the left lower ribs in the heart area. Other symptoms of Capsicum are a dislike for the open air, relief of symptoms with heat and taking food, aching over different parts of the body, random **twitching** of the facial muscles, and prominence of the bones at the temple associated with inflammation.

Capsicum is useful for the treatment of elderly people who have been involved in intellectual work throughout their lives but in later years of life, due to changing circumstances could not afford an easier lifestyle.

| | |
|---|---|
| Antidotes: | Cina, Caladium |
| Potency: | 30 to 200 |

# Carbo Animalis

Carbo Animalis is very similar to Carbo Veg. Carbo Veg is prepared from the coal of vegetable matter, while Carbo Animalis is prepared from the animal ashes. Although they are chemically very closely related, yet in certain symptoms there is a clear distinction between them.

The ailments related to the symptoms of Carbo Animalis have a tendency to change to cancer. It is particularly useful for the diseases of old age. Typically, the patient is anaemic, his face is sallow, the limbs become weak, and the body defences start to decline. As in Carbo Veg, the glands become hardened, with the tendency towards becoming cancerous. Like Aesculus, Carbo Animalis is useful in the treatment of clotting of the blood inside the veins, and the formation of spider webs on the skin.

The Carbo Animalis patient is usually sad and depressed and likes to be alone. Mostly, he is quiet. At night, he is restless and frightened. The blood flows towards the head. The mind is confused. The eyesight is dim and the eyes feel heavy. There is pain at the nape of the neck. Lips and cheeks are bluish. The nose swells and bluish lumps develop on its surface. Hearing declines and it is difficult to recognize the direction of the source of sounds. There is dry nasal cold with loss of sense of smell. Copper coloured pimples and acne develop on the face. The head and the face feel warm. Warts appear on the face and on the hands of old people. The patient has scary dreams.

The **stomach of a Carbo Animalis patient feels weak and empty**. After taking food, he feels weak and tired. Heavy lifting or hard labour physically exhausts him. The hips and wrists hurt.

The conventional doctors suggest surgical removal of the uterus as a **treatment of cancer of the cervix**. This does not necessarily succeed, however early administration of Carbo Animalis will cure the condition. It is also useful for the treatment of generalized inflammations of the uterus and associated pains. The erosion at the cervix of uterus is associated with **leucorrhoea** of burning nature. In Carbo Veg too, there is a similar burning sensation internally.

Outwardly, the patient feels calm and cool. The prompt usage of Carbo Animalis for the treatment of the burning type of leucorrhoea can pre-empt the development of cancer.

Carbo Animalis is very useful for the **treatment of nausea in pregnancy** which is worse at night.

Carbo Animalis must not be forgotten when a woman feels **weakness during lactation** and suffers from mental exhaustion. This is a good remedy for cancer of the uterus as well as cervical cancer.

The special characteristic of Carbo Animalis is the swelling of the lymph glands along with a bluish colouration of lips and cheeks.

In Carbo Animalis, **women have more frequent, heavy and more prolonged bleeding (menorrhagia)**. The menstruating woman becomes very weak. As in Sepia, a saddle-shaped darkish area develops on the nose extending to the cheeks. In the absence of its own specific symptoms, Sepia will not relieve this. A Sepia lady is usually of a slim build, feels aloof amongst the near relatives and **loses affection** especially towards her husband and children. In fact, she feels indifferent towards them. If such a patient also has a typical mark on the nose, Sepia should be administered. If ineffective, Carbo Animalis must be tried. In my experience, Carbo Animalis is very **effective in ailments developing after childbirth**. It also cures the mark on the nose. It is useful in treating the nausea of pregnancy. While associated with other symptoms of Carbo Animalis, it is very beneficial in treating the induration of mammary glands and the pain thereof.

It is also useful in the **treatment of deafness**. Often, both ears become deaf and voices cannot be recognised. The direction of the sound is also difficult to ascertain. Amongst the remedies for deafness is Chinopodium. If the deafness is due to the degeneration of the nerves, or sequestered secretions inside the ear, Chinopodium 30 or 200 should be used for two to three months. Sometimes, such a patient suddenly feels better. Before the recovery of his hearing, he feels frequent gusting of air into the ears.

Carbo Animalis is not the treatment of locked up discharge in the ear but it is the treatment for nerve deafness affecting both ears. Chinopodium often affects one ear.

Carbo Animalis is a good medicine for the **treatment of acne** and swelling of hands and feet due to cold. It also prevents against the tendency of the formation of warts on hands and face. Sometimes, due to structural mal-development, the bones start thickening and have a tendency to transform into cancer (Paget's disease). If any abnormal change is noticed like this, Carbo Animalis should be promptly given. The ankles of Carbo Animalis patients are weak and turn in easily and repeatedly. To prevent this tendency of spraining of the ankle, Carbo Animalis 30 should be given to strengthen them, but Bellis should not be forgotten in such a condition.

The **hands become numb, the wrists and the calves hurt** along with cramps during walking. The small joints of the body become stiff. The **back feels taut** and hurts.

In Carbo Animalis patients, the lungs develop lesions and the chest feels cold. There is **greenish sputum along with cough**. The patient's sweat is malodorous during the night. The symptoms aggravate in cold air, while heat relieves the symptoms.

| | |
|---|---|
| Adjuvants: | Helonias, Calcarea Phos |
| Antidotes: | Arsenic, Nux Vomica |
| Potency: | Usually 30. For the treatment of cancer, potencies of 200 to CM may be used. |

# CARBO VEGETABILIS

The vegetable carbon i.e. coal prepared from wood, is called Carbo Veg. Dr. Hahnemann experimented with this on himself and noticed its long-lasting effects and therefore used it in the treatment of deep, chronic illnesses. In allopathy, Carbo Veg tablets are used to combat gas in the abdomen. To some extent, they absorb some gas, but have no effect on the acid production by the stomach. In homoeopathy too, Carbo Veg is used for **excessive gas in the stomach**. In addition, it controls production of gas by suppressing the causative mechanism.

Carbo Veg is **one of the most potent life-saving treatments**. When a serious sickness advances and brings the patient on the verge of death, Carbo Veg plays a very important role in reviving the dying patient. It is extremely difficult to encompass the basic mechanism of its extraordinary functions, but it has been repeatedly found to be very effective in bringing a dying person back from the verge of death. It restores the body temperature. In view of this, I thought that Carbo Veg would certainly raise a lowered blood pressure. On use, I found that **it definitely elevates the blood pressure**. I also noted that it does not elevate the blood pressure blindly. There is certainly no danger that Carbo Veg would unnecessarily raise the blood pressure to an abnormal level, it simply normalizes the blood pressure after it has seriously dropped. Normally, the blood pressure drops profoundly when the patient is at the point of death. A single dose of Carbo Veg starts warming up the body. Once I happened to see a patient who had suffered a very severe heart attack. He was virtually dead when I saw him. His forehead was covered with profuse cold sweat and the breathing was hardly noticeable. I dropped two or three drops of Carbo Veg into his mouth. Within a very short time, he started breathing normally. The cold sweats disappeared from the forehead, and his body started to warm up gradually. I then gave him the specific remedies to strengthen his heart which, with the help of Carbo Veg, became very effective. I have used Carbo Veg in many other patients and have always found it very effective. It should be in the first-aid kit for saving lives.

Carbo Veg is also deeply related to **asthma**, especially when the patient's temperature has dropped, there is profuse cold sweating and the patient is so weak that he cannot expel the secretions from his

chest. This kind of patient may be of two types: one exhibiting the symptoms of Ammonium Tart whose initial symptoms have been of Ipecac. The symptoms of Antimonium Crude are the worst type of symptoms of Ipecac. The stomach becomes inflammed, resulting in the tongue being covered with a dirty white coating. When the condition of this patient further aggravates, and he is unable to expel the sputum from his chest due to severe weakness, Antimonium Tart may well stabilise the condition of the patient and bring him back from this dangerous situation. However, Antimonium Tart is not curative for asthma. Carbo Veg resembles Antimonium Tart. Once I saw a patient who was seriously sick with asthma. When I gave him Carbo Veg and his body gained strength. He coughed out the expectoration and his sturtrous breathing became normal. When given the appropriate asthma treatment, he recovered completely. It proves once again that Carbo Veg is a vital homoeopathic remedy when the patient is in moribund state. Typically, the asthmatic patient sweats profusely, is cold and has air hunger. For this purpose, fanning on the face helps. On the contrary, the Arsenic patient does not sweat, and his chest does not rattle with accumulated secretions.
Carbo Veg is very useful in treating the **failing heart muscle**. It is the best tonic for the muscles. When **the pressure of gas from the stomach** is directed upwards, Carbo Veg is very beneficial. The accumulation of gas in the stomach is mentioned in reference to many homoeopathic medicines. This alone will not help to arrive at the correct diagnosis. One has to try different medicines. There is no equal to the long, vigilant experience of the treating physician. With repeated use, the remedies start manifesting their symptoms which may not have been detected with formal proving. Gas in the stomach is also mentioned in relation to Arsenic Iodide. In fact, it is the treatment for the peptic ulcer of the stomach and its deleterious effects. In Carbo Veg, the gas is in the upper part of the abdomen and smells foul. The stools in Carbo Veg diarrhoea also smell foul and the patient feels extremely weak. As such, its symptoms resemble those of Baptisia. Baptisia however, works more profoundly in such a condition as well as for the treatment of foul-smelling diarrhoeal stools of typhoid. Carbo Veg is of no use in typhoid diarrhoea.

The symptoms of Carbo Veg also include **numbness of hands and feet**. **Legs feel numb too**, especially the calf muscles. In medical terminology, the calf muscles are called the second heart, because they pump back the venous blood towards the heart. One may feel light-headed on sudden standing up, showing that the calves have not pumped the blood back up sufficiently. Carbo Veg is very useful to treat this condition, because it not only elevates the blood pressure but also invigorates the calf muscles. This is how it helps to revive a dying patient.

Another important characteristic of Carbo Veg is that it prepares the body to properly react to Kali Carb. Many of the symptoms of Kali Carb resemble those of Carbo Veg, but Carbo Veg is a relatively mild remedy while Kali Carb produces a strong body reaction. Most Kali Carb diseases are chronic in nature. The direct initial use of Kali Carb may produce a serious reaction. Therefore, Carbo Veg should be given first before administering Kali Carb, especially for the treatment of joint pains in hands, feet and wrists.

When I first started homoeopathy, I used Carbo Veg. My experience showed that Carbo Veg itself has some beneficial effects on the pains and aches, especially **backache and muscular pains**. However, if **blood pressure is high** and the face is flushed with blood, Belladonna and Aconite are more effective than Carbo Veg. In addition to Aconite and Belladonna, Carbo Veg and Kali Carb may also be used after Rhus Tox. After these, Calcarea Carb would further prolong the effect of Aconite, Belladonna and Rhus Tox. All these homoeopathic remedies contain the element of Carbon, which is deeply related to the muscles.

In a Carbo Veg patient, the acidity in the stomach is not due to excess of hydrochloric acid but rather due to the lack of it. When the normal acidity of the stomach (hydrochloric acid) is not sufficient, food starts decaying and produces foul acidic substances, resulting in severe compromise of the process of digestion. In simple terms, it may be said that the stomach has two ends that are capable of remaining open or closed. The upper end of the stomach is the cardic end, and the lower end is known as the pyloric end. The foul acidic matter puts both ends into a state of contraction and the blocked-up food containing foul acidic contents produces gas, distending the stomach. Under pressure, the upper end may open letting the foul-smelling gases, as well as the acidic contents of the stomach, regurgitate. This produces burning and foul eructation or belching. The pyloric end opens only under very high pressure. Normally, digestion of the food in the stomach takes about three hours. After this, the stomach contents are let to pass into the intestines and the foul gas also enters the gut. These foul contents work as a good medium for the growth of germs and worms which cause further putrefaction. Carbo Veg is used in controlling this vicious symptom complex and after use for some period, it normalises the digestive system.

When given in appropriate potencies, Carbo Veg as well as Carbo Animalis, helps to kill germs and worms in the intestines. However, some kinds of bacteria and worms settle permanently inside the stomach and intestines and are difficult to completely eradicate.

In my experience, the most effective medicines to kill **worms in the intestines** are Santoninum, Cina and Teucrium. I have also used Sabadilla for the same purpose, even though most of homoeopathic books only describe Sabadilla in reference to sneezing and irritation of the nose due to allergies. I believe that the allergy of the nose and itching can be secondary to the presence of worms in the intestines. The irritation they produce inside the stomach and the intestines also gets referred to the nose and the face. In Boericke, Sabadilla has been mentioned for the treatment of worms, although Boericke does not specifically describe its use for worms under Sabadilla. Carbo Animalis is probably the most effective remedy for **hookworm** infestation of the abdomen. Besides these, there are many more homoeopathic remedies for the treatment of worms. A detailed repertory should be consulted as needed.

In Carbo Veg, there is a tendency towards **hoarseness of the throat** in the evening. **Hands and feet become numb**. There is physical as well as mental lethargy. In fact, the entire life process becomes sluggish. There is a feeling of burning inside, while the patient feels cold outwardly. The patient takes no interest in any kind of news, be it of sorrow, happiness or something startling, as if he does not care. It seems as if he is not tuned to think any more.

In Carbo Veg, the **headache** is usually towards the back of the head. It starts with the onset of cold and then makes the entire head throb as if being hammered. This also happens in Natrum Mur. The **hair tends to fall**. Cold sweats appear on the forehead. Its patient gets frightened at night and thinks of demons and the devil. The **ears discharge foul smelling material** indicating the presence of deep infection and fever. In Carbo Veg, the **chronic cold** can afflict any part of the body making the patient permanently sick. If the chronic cold of a Carbo Veg patient is suppressed by some other treatment, it may result in serious consequences later. Hence, the chronic cold should better be treated with Carbo Veg.

Carbo Veg will also clear the picture of suppressed diseases. Carbo Veg will best treat sores in the mouth and white blotches, inflammation of the gums and loosening of the teeth, if its other symptoms are also present.

It is also very useful for the treatment of **ulcers in the stomach,** which result in foul smelling diarrhoea and swelling of the liver. The limbs become flabby and the legs and feet gradually start withering away. The feet may suffer in many different ways. Carbo Veg is also useful in the treatment of **varicose veins**.

Carbo Veg is also very useful in the treatment of the early stages of **whooping cough and rattling chest**. The cough of a Carbo Veg patient resembles that of Lachesis. Asthma comes on suddenly at night.

Carbo Veg should be the treatment of choice for a prolapsed uterus associated with foul smelling, darkish vaginal discharge. Carbo Veg is also very useful in the treatment of lactating mothers when the milk is not enough; they are very weak and suffer from remittent fever. Carbo Veg patients usually see fire, stealing and accidents in their dreams.

| | |
|---|---|
| Adjuvants: | Kali Carb, Drosera |
| Antidotes: | Camphor, Ambra Grisea, Arsenic |
| Potency: | 30 to 200 |

# CARBOLIC ACID

At one time Carbolic acid soap was used in hospitals and dispensaries as an antiseptic. It has a very pungent smell. Usage in homoeopathy is quite different. Carbolic Acid in Homoeopathic form is the best treatment for severe allergic reaction to a **sting by a bee or a wasp**. A dose or two can offer complete cure.

Carbolic Acid acts on the **sensory perceptions of the body**. Its patient has an unusually sharp sense of smell. The normally imperceptible smell may easily be noticed by the patient of Carbolic Acid.

In Carbolic Acid, the pain is severe and sudden in nature. It comes on suddenly and disappears just as fast. Some parts of the body may be numb. Some parts feel as if tied in a rubber band. Carbolic Acid has been found very useful in the treatment of mouth ulcers.

There is **neuralgic type of pain in and around the eye**. Carbolic Acid would prove very useful in treating such a pain that has settled inside the eye.

One symptom of Carbolic Acid is that there is complete loss of appetite. The **abdomen becomes distended with gas**. Excessive amount of distension of the abdomen in a localised area is typical of Carbolic Acid because Carbolic Acid causes spasmodic constriction of the intestines at different places. The gas gets loculated between the so formed constriction rings. Carbolic Acid should be well-remembered for treating such sicknesses.

The Carbolic Acid patient has a bad taste in the mouth. There is no sense of thirst, and a loss of appetite. Sometimes, he experiences severe constipation and at other times, severe diarrhoea. The stools smell very offensive. In the case of constipation, even the breath smells foul. What this shows is that the foul gases cannot be expelled naturally. Instead, they become absorbed through the walls of the intestines and reach the lungs via the blood, resulting in bad breath.

Carbolic Acid is very important for treating **albumin** in the urine. Some patients excrete so much albumin in the urine that it becomes dark like black ink. Terebinthina too, is very useful in treating this condition. The Carbolic Acid patient frequently gets up at night to pass urine, which may very well be due to **enlargement of the prostate gland**. Carbolic Acid is very useful in the **treatment of infections of kidneys,** as well as prostate gland. Carbolic Acid must be kept in mind for any increase in the frequency of passing urine at night. Some physicians advise Carbolic Acid to be used in potency 1X; I however do not have any personal experience of that.

Carbolic Acid may be very useful in the **treatment of severe backache, especially when it is radiating down to both the buttocks**. This is its typical characteristic.

Carbolic Acid may be the curative treatment for **leucorrhoea developing before puberty.** Typically, the periods and leucorrhoeal discharge smell foul.

Carbolic Acid would cure cramps in the feet and legs, as well as generalized bone pains, if the patient has the general disposition of Carbolic Acid. The skin signs of Carbolic Acid are the development of blisters with itching, burning and pain.

| | |
|---|---|
| Antidotes: | Vinegar, Chalk, Iodum |
| Potency: | 30 |

# Carboneum Sulphuratum

## (Alcohol Sulphuris – Bisulfide of Carbon)

Carboneum Sulph contains the elements of Sulphur and Carbon, therefore it profoundly affects the functioning of the human body. Its range of action is very wide and it is useful in the treatment of deep-seated illnesses.

The patient of Carboneum Sulph, like that of Carbo Veg, enjoys open fresh air. Though his body may be cold, he would still like to keep the windows open for the want of oxygen. Carboneum Sulph contains Sulphur, which has a completely opposite effect. Its patient likes to keep the windows open, but cannot tolerate drafts of air. As in many other Homoeopathic remedies, the patient feels heaviness on the chest while going up the stairs and feels very weak. The discomfort of the chest behind the sternum may very well be due to angina, therefore it should not be neglected; instead it should be clinically evaluated and investigated. The pressure of the chest is not always necessarily due to a heart problem. It may well be due to disorders of the nervous system, lungs or stomach. Thus, the pressure of the chest is not a diagnostic sign in itself.

The symptoms of a Carboneum Sulph patient **aggravate on taking a bath** that is due to the element of Sulphur in it in which there is a dislike for taking a bath. It should however be remembered, that a patient of pure Sulphur is simply scared of bathing, but his symptoms are not aggravated on taking a bath, while the symptoms of a Carboneum Sulph patient actually aggravate on taking a bath.

Some Homoeopathic physicians have opined that Carboneum Sulph is the best treatment for a severe type of **Lupus** of the face, it can, in fact, cure the condition. I am of the opinion that it should be further tested. I have myself done a lot of study on this matter, but have not found any specific correlation of Carboneum Sulph to Lupus to distinguish this from other remedies.

Carboneum Sulph has been found to prevent the spread of **cancer** also. Carbon and Sulphur together have a profound effect on the human body. The remedy, which could cure a serious illness like Lupus, must obviously be strong and profoundly effective. Every kind of cancer needs to be treated by one particular medicine. However, some medicines are such that they can stop the spread of all cancers for a year or two. In that period, an appropriate remedy may be found. Carboneum Sulph, Arsenic Iodide and Graphite are the three top remedies of this nature. For **cancer of the skin**, Pyrogenium and Psorinum are also useful. Their patients have an individual and specific constitution of their own. When the know-how about a patient is limited, the treatment should be started with Arsenic Iodide, which is also very useful in the treatment of **cancer of intestines**.

Carboneum Sulph is also related to **joint pains**, especially when they are chronic in nature. Carboneum Sulph will gradually offer cure. In Carboneum Sulph, there are **cramps in the arms and the legs**, along with repeated episodes of long-lasting, undulating pain. The **arms and hands become numb** and the nerves become inflamed.

The elements of Carbon and Sulphur in the Carboneum Sulph have completely opposite symptoms. Sulphur is hot, while carbon is of a cold nature. In Carbon, the patient feels cold and is cold, though internally he may have a burning sensation in some places. In Sulphur there is a feeling of constant heat, which becomes part of one's life. The hands, feet and scalp burn, as in Pulsatilla. However, in Pulsatilla, there is no thirst while a patient of Sulphur feels very thirsty.

A patient of Carboneum Sulph cannot tolerate cold. He falls ill as soon as his feet become cold. The feet of a Carboneum Sulph type of patient must always be kept warm.

Some of the symptoms of Carboneum Sulph resemble those of Arnica. In Arnica, the patient feels badly beaten all over, irrespective of being physically injured or not. The Carboneum Sulph pain is also of similar nature. Carboneum Sulph is very important in the treatment of **psychological symptoms.** Such a patient is aggressive, intolerant, has intense anger, is unable to distinguish between right and wrong, and has a tendency towards committing suicide. The **scalp is dry, with dandruff and the hair tends to fall**. Carboneum Sulph is also very useful in the treatment of **diseases of the eyelids**, especially when the patient is of the appropriate constitution.

In Carboneum Sulph, the headache is mostly on the left side, but may also be on the right. Commonly, it is only one-sided.

**Weak eyesight** and inability to distinguish between colours is also a symptom of Carboneum Sulph. In a patient of Carboneum Sulph, **the discharge from the ears** is foul smelling and mixed with blood. The **hearing decreases**, along with **ringing in the ears (tinnitus)**. Due to the **involvement of ears**, the person feels dizzy. The **tongue becomes insensitive**. Along with **itching, small ulcers** form which then spread. Pimples appear on the face. A special feature of Carboneum Sulph is the insensitivity of the lining of the skin and the inner linings (mucus membranes). The skin also becomes insensitive. The numbness of the inside of the mouth and especially of the tongue is very pronounced. The nerve fibres under the skin and the mucus membranes become afflicted, causing insensitivity of the surfaces. The teeth become very sensitive to cold once their nerve endings become exposed.

On exposure to cold air, the symptoms pertaining to the teeth and the face become aggravated, and there is **increased sensitivity**, not only at the nerve endings of the teeth, but on the entire face. The generalised, firm **enlargement of the glands** also is found in Carboneum Sulph.

Carboneum Sulph is useful in the treatment of many **sexual weaknesses of men** as well as women. The ovaries shrink in size, which in fact is a precursor of cancer. In this condition, Carboneum Sulph should better be instituted in relatively high potency like 200.

Carboneum Sulph will cure the **stiffness of the toes and the ankles** if the patient is of Carboneum Sulph constitution.

| | |
|---|---|
| Potency | 30 to 200, 1000 or CM as needed |

# Carcinosin
## (Cancerous Tissue)

Homoeopathic doctors have devised different remedies from cancerous materials, the salient one being Carcinosin. It is produced from the cancer of the lungs. Dr. Brunt experimented on this first and then Dr. Clarke performed further tests on it.

Carcinosin is very useful in treatment of the **cancer of the breast**. Carcinosin is also beneficial for the treatment of **varicose veins** on the legs. By using Carcinosin on a patient with **cancer of the intestines**, the **threadworms** and other germs thriving on the extracts of the intestine are expelled in the stools. In a potential patient of a cancerous family, the administration of Carcinosin will manifest externally, the suppressed tendency of developing a cancer in the form of enlargement of the glands on the neck or the tonsils, which become very painful. This is a typical sign, though not described in books. I have found this in my own homoeopathic experience. This potentiality of developing cancer is not limited to any country, region or climate, but applies uniformly to the entire world. People who show such reaction would benefit significantly against the development of cancer. However, also according to Dr. Kent, Carcinosin decreases **the severity of pain, stinging and burning due to cancer**. A patient may live for years without much discomfort. According to Dr. Kent, it does not cure the cancer, but slows down its growth and spread to a significant extent. I have often found the opinions of Dr. Kent to be true. Maybe his comments on Carcinosin are also correct. I have used it in the treatment of some cancer patients with success. For years, they did not show any signs of recurrence. Thus, for the majority of cancer patients, Dr. Kent is right.

Besides Carcinosin, two other medicines have been prepared from bacteria growing on the cancerous tissues. Unfortunately, they have not been found to be very effective in the treatment of cancer. Micro Coccine has been prepared from Micro Coccus. Dr. Winter has found it useful to control the hypersensitivity of cancer. The other remedy is Oslo Coccine. This has not been found useful in the treatment of cancer, but has been found very useful in treating influenza. Dr.

Foubister has written in an article that the administration of Carcinosin does not show up all symptoms of cancer as proving; it only produces changes in the susceptible areas of the body. Maybe, the reactive enlargement of the lymphatic glands might be due to the presence of cancerous elements. More testing and research is required for this. Dr. Foubister has described how, that after using Carcinosin, the body starts reacting in the form of elevation of the body temperature.

According to Dr. Foubister, for people who are susceptible to the development of cancer, the following remedies could be used such as, Tuberculinum, Medorrhinum, Natrum Mur and Sepia. The detailed account of these remedies is found in the relative chapters of this book. Alumina, Arsenic Album, Arsenic Iodide, Pulsatilla, Staphysagria, Phosphorus and Calcaria Phos are also very useful and must be kept in mind regarding the treatment of cancer. Sepia and Staphysagria are deeply related to illnesses secondary to emotional suppression. Cancer may be one of them. Phosphorus and Calcaria Phos are deeply related to the **cancer of the bone** and they are related to the **lungs** as well. Lycopodium is related to the cancer of the gall bladder and the pancreas. The usefulness of Lycopodium is in diluting the bile of the liver. Silicea has been found to be very useful in treatment of **cancer of the prostate**. Besides this, Silicea CM has been extremely useful in the treatment of AIDS. AIDS, like cancer, is considered to be untreatable. In many countries, under my guidance, Silicea CM has been tried on AIDS patients. Many of them have responded surprisingly well. The medicines related to cancer treatment need further research. The cancer patient should be thoroughly evaluated clinically, before starting the homoeopathic treatment. Reassessment must be done after the treatment has been given and the resultant changes noted. Facilities at modern clinical laboratories should be utilised.

All the homoeopathic remedies for cancer should be carefully studied and their specific symptoms remembered. In this way, everyone will be able to benefit, along with humanity at large. The condition is that all successful experiments should be made publicly known to others for the benefit of the world. The alternating use of Carcinosin and Radium Bromide in potency CM can minimize the dangerous effects of radiation.

| | |
|---|---|
| Adjuvant: | In view of the nature and severity of cancer, besides Radium Bromide, one or more of the above mentioned remedies can be used. To prevent the cancers of the bone and lungs, and their spread, Phosphorus and Bryonia are very essential. They should be given in potency 30 and if potency 30 does not work any more, the potency should be increased to 200. |
| Potency: | 200 to CM |
| PS: | Should be given once in two weeks. If the surgery has been performed in view of the severity of the cancer, it may be given in potency CM daily for a few days. Restlessness after surgery can respond to Arsenic CM. Only one dose should be given and should not be repeated unless the restlessness becomes severe again. In that condition, it must be repeated. |

# Carduus Marianus

Carduus Marianus is very **important for the treatment of liver diseases** and I have often used it regularly on patients with liver problems. Even on prolonged use, it has not produced any untoward side effect. Its main action is on the liver and the **circulatory system**.

Commonly, it is considered as the remedy for liver problems. It also has many other features like the **tendency to nose bleed** along with the feeling of cool breeze over the head. The eyes feel great outward pressure and **the eyeball protrudes out**. This particular sign is also noticed in Belladonna. In Carduus Marianus, the bleeding from the nose is preceded by **irritation inside the nose.**

In Carduus Marianus, there are **symptoms pertaining to the stomach also**. This is due to the fact that whenever there is a problem with the liver, the stomach is also affected. The taste inside the mouth is bitter and unpleasant. The tongue shows a dirty coating. There is loss of appetite. There is typical bad odour from the mouth, secondary to the **stomach dysfunction**. A stomachache, moving from the left to the right, is also a sign of Carduus Marianus. It shows that the liver disorder has disrupted the stomach function also. By this time, the patient vomits dark blood. There is pain on the chest and over the right-sided ribs, which becomes worse on movement. The pain over the chest may radiate to the shoulders, the back and the upper abdomen.

When the patient is lying on the left side, he feels pain on the right side, as if somebody is dragging him downwards. This symptom is noted in other remedies as well.

Carduus Marianus has been found to be very useful in the **treatment of stones in the gall bladder**. The lining over the gall bladder becomes swollen and painful. There is a **piercing sensation over the spleen**. The skin over the left side of the body becomes hypersensitive and sore. There is **severe chronic constipation**. Stools are clay coloured. Bleeding piles develop and urine is deep-coloured.

Due to the diseases of the liver, there is a **cough** affecting the lower part of the right lung. There is pain over the scapula like the patients of Chelidonium and Aesculus. There is pain over the right buttock and the hip joint, which radiates down the leg. **Muscular spasms** also occur. Carduus Marianus is very useful in the treatment of hip pain which gets worse on movement. In a patient of Carduus Marianus, there is a tendency to develop **varicose veins**. In all such remedies associated with bleeding of dark coloured blood, there is a tendency to develop spider webs of blue colour. Feet become swollen (oedematous). Cramping of the feet and the calves make walking difficult. Cramps of the legs which develop on walking fast, are best treated by the combination of Bryonia and Arnica. When the disease has reached an advanced stage, the patients of Carduus Marianus may not even walk a few steps. The feet become weak. Carduus Marianus is also useful in the treatment of influenza affecting the liver.

| | |
|---|---|
| Potency: | Q to 30, but mostly used in the form of Mother Tincture. |

# Caulophyllum

Caulophyllum is a very effective treatment for the **gout affecting the small joints of the hands and feet**. It is also useful for the treatment of fleeting joint pains of the hands and the feet due to reasons other than gout. Affected areas have a tendency to go into spasms.

I have found Caulophyllum very effective in the treatment of certain forms of, which has not been previously mentioned in books. This pain radiates from the back into both the legs or just one leg. The back pains in the patients of Caulophyllum nature resemble the pain during pregnancy. On that basis, I have tried it in the treatment of sciatica. Sciatica is the pain along the course of the nerve which is called the sciatic nerve.

Caulophyllum is a very useful and important **remedy during pregnancy**. It invigorates the uterus. I have often used it to treat a threatened abortion/miscarriage, and by the grace of Allah, found it very useful to avert this condition.

If the labour pains radiate towards the inside of the thighs or over the course of the sciatic nerve instead of being directed towards the uterus, and there is **spasm at the neck of the uterus**, Caulophyllum is the best remedy to alleviate this situation. Secale Cornutum is also very useful to treat the spasm at the cervix uteri. However, the tightness is much more severe in the case of Secale than Caulophyllum. Besides, there are other symptoms of Secale which distinguish it from Caulophyllum. However, Caulophyllum will be useful to treat severe tightness at the neck of the uterus caused by the misuse of Secale. Many homoeopaths advise regular use of Caulophyllum in the last month of pregnancy in 30 potency. This facilitates childbirth and the convalescence after becomes smooth and uneventful.

Sometimes **the foetus is not positioned properly** in the uterus and delivery becomes impossible without surgery. Even Pulsatilla may not be able to rectify the position. In this condition, the administration of Caulophyllum 200 along with Arnica 200 may normalise the position of the foetus in the uterus. If the position of the child inside the uterus does not correct itself with the administration of Arnica and

Caulophyllum, given two to three times a week for two weeks, then the obvious treatment would be surgery. The timing for the surgery will of course be decided by the surgeon. Sometimes surgery may be required even before the pregnancy has reached full term.

Caulophyllum is the best remedy for treating **brown spots (freckles) on the faces of women** and may be useful in men also. Spots may completely vanish from the face and disappear forever. Caulophyllum may be useful in treating the dark facial discolouration which will be recognizable along with its general features. The best remedy of course is still Arsenic Sulfuratum while to the patients of Secale Cor nature, Secale Cor would be the most ideal treatment to normalize their facial complexion. The effect of Caulophyllum is neutralized by the use of Coffee; therefore during the administration of Caulophyllum, Coffee should be avoided.

| | |
|---|---|
| Adjuvants: | Arnica |
| Potency: | 30 to 200 |

# CAUSTICUM

Causticum is a profoundly effective Homoeopathic remedy which has been found very useful in the treatment of many day-to-day illnesses. It is normally used as the instant **treatment of muscular paralysis, especially facial palsy**, though it is also useful in many other illnesses. The Causticum symptoms progress gradually. The paralysis that follows exposure to cold is usually considered as having occurred suddenly. In fact, the patient has been exposed a few days earlier and then suffers from gradual progressive restlessness, weakness and tiredness before exhibiting the symptoms of paralysis. **Paralysis of a sudden kind** is seen in Aconite. In the case of Causticum, the exposure to cold occurs two to three days, or at least twenty-four hours before the onset of signs.

**Stammering** due to partial paralysis of the muscles of the tongue, but not due to fear, is best treated with Causticum. However, once a child starts stammering, an element of fear also prevails. In such a situation, the combination of Stramonium and Causticum will offer much faster relief from paralysis.

In the illnesses of Causticum, the nerves become afflicted resulting in permanent changes in the muscles. The glands become hard. If the paralysis prolongs, the limbs become stiff and contracted. Causticum is the ideal treatment if other symptoms of Causticum are also present.

**Hysteria** is another condition in which successive fits gradually become more and more severe leading to convulsions. The patient of the nature of Causticum is over-sensitive and can neither tolerate noise nor light touch. Cold and the heat both do not suit him. Usually the spasm affects individual muscles. **Joint pains** associated with Causticum are relieved by the application of heat, except in the case of the fingers where cold offers greater relief than heat. Similarly, the **cough** associated with Causticum also responds better to intake of cold water. The patient of a Causticum nature suffers more in the hot climate or with heat, except in the areas of the throat and the hand. Causticum by nature causes restlessness.

Causticum is also related to **epilepsy**. However, epilepsy resulting from a deformity of the skull or a severe accident is not amenable to any kind of medicine. For this, surgery is the only treatment. In America, a neurosurgeon was awarded a Nobel Prize for the successful surgical treatment of thirty-four epileptic patients.

In Causticum, if the **symptoms relating to the skin are suppressed** by any means, then **mental illnesses** ensue.

The **headache that may potentially result in a stroke** can be treated with Causticum. Some kinds of severe headache may render the patient **temporarily blind.** If in such a patient, the vision returns and there are no paralytic signs, Gelsemium would be found more effective than Causticum. In case of paralytic symptoms, Causticum would be the most ideal remedy

The slowly **progressive drooping of the eyelids** (ptosis) also requires Causticum. This condition develops and progresses slowly and so will be the road to recovery. The treatment with Causticum should be continued with perseverance. At times, the alternation of Sulphur and Causticum will also be found to be useful.

Sometimes, the patient sees spots. Green spots specify Causticum. In Causticum, there is a tendency to develop **warts**. Thuja and Medorrhinum are both useful in the treatment of fine, soft warts but when the warts are large and in abundance, Causticum and Nitricum Acid are more useful. Warts related to Causticum appear on the face and the nose, especially a big warty area over the nose establishes its diagnosis.

Another symptom of Causticum is the development of paralytic symptoms in the throat. The **voice is hoarse** in the morning. The symptoms gradually develop and can progress to difficulty in swallowing. The patient is afraid of choking himself by entry of food into the air passage. This symptom may be associated with many other Homoeopathic remedies. But a successful outcome rests on the constitutional remedy.

The Causticum patient is not usually superstitious. Sometimes he may lose his appetite altogether at the sight of food.

Sometimes, women develop **urinary retention/stoppage at the time of childbirth** due to anxiety, pressure or inflammation of the kidneys.

Causticum becomes indispensable to combat this urgent situation. In fact, it becomes a life saving measure in some cases. I have found in my practice, that some women do not pass urine for twenty-four hours after giving birth. On administering Causticum, they first passed blood-mixed urine, showing that the kidneys were only inflamed and not totally shut down. The blood in the urine started clearing and urination became free and normal. After this, they were given a course of Pareira Brava Q, which acts as diuretic and washes the kidneys naturally clean. In other situations when **urinary stoppage** occurs, Causticum has a different role. For example, the patient cannot pass urine while sitting. When the patient stands up, the pressure expels the urine involuntarily and unknowingly. Causticum has been found significantly useful in treating this condition.

In Causticum, sometimes there is paralysis of the lower part of the large gut (rectum) and the patient suffers from faecal incontinence. The stools become hard in the rectum in the form of stones. The patient happens to pass those hardened stools while walking, unknowingly. Such patients are rare but in my experience, and I have seen two or three, all of who were old people.

The patient of Causticum exhibits a reddish glare on the tongue. Women experience pain and spasms in the lower abdomen before their periods, which cease once menstruation begins. When bleeding stops, the spasms recur. The spasms get better when menstruation resumes.

When **periods stop as a reaction to some shock**, fear or at the death of a dear one, Causticum may be useful to abate this condition. Similarly, **nursing mothers may stop producing milk** due to sudden shock or severe grief. Causticum will restore their lactation.

The **paralysis of the throat** in a Causticum patient is not only related to the muscles of swallowing but also affects the voice box.

The three Homoeopathic remedies Phosphorus, Bryonia and Causticum are very similar. In short-lived illnesses, they can be given together without any danger. In fact, the combination works at a greater advantage. This combination should not be used in a potency higher than 30. If this combination does not prove to be effective, then one of these remedies whose symptoms match with the patient the most, may work on its own.

| | |
|---|---|
| Adjuvants: | Carbo Veg, Petrosel |
| Antidotes: | Colocynth, Dulcamara, Guaiacum, Nux Vomica |
| Potency: | 30 to CM |

# CEANOTHUS

Ceanothus is a tea-like shrub growing wild in the state of New Jersey, USA. It is used in the treatment of **symptoms related to the spleen**. The spleen is commonly afflicted by malaria. Such patient suffers from deficiency of Haemoglobin (red blood content) - **anaemia**. Its symptoms are in general, more prominent on the left side. The side feels heavy and swollen. If only the liver is enlarged, the upper part of the belly feels hard on the right side; but if both spleen and the liver are enlarged, both sides feel hard. To my knowledge, there is no better treatment for splenic disorders than Ceanothus. When the spleen is hardened, the blood vessels also harden. This results in high pressure in the veins of the spleen and liver (chronic portal hypertension); Ceanothus lowers this pressure. The commonly described **high blood pressure** (hypertension) is usually related to the heart and the kidneys. However Ceanothus should be used in portal hypertension due to the liver and spleen derangement.

Very often, anaemic women suffer from **continuous vaginal bleeding**, which is like thin, diluted blood. Ceanothus is very useful for combating this situation too.

The patient of liver and spleen often suffers either from constipation or diarrhoea. The Ceanothus patient usually has **diarrhoea**. Urination is frequent, the urine being frothy and greenish in colour. It contains both **bile pigment and sugar**. In this regard, another medicine, Tinospora Cordifolia is worth mentioning. This is an ayurvedic medicine specially used for spleen problems and has be found to be quite useful.

The symptoms of Ceanothus aggravate on movement and from lying on the left side.

| | |
|---|---|
| Potency: | Mother Tincture or 1X |

# CHAMOMILLA

Chamomilla is prepared from a bushy plant growing wild amongst the crops of wheat and corn. It has been used to treat various diseases. In particular, it is useful to tone up the uterus weakened after childbirth. Many people use its leaves as tea. In homoeopathy, the fresh plant, along with its flowers is ground and mixed in alcohol. This is ideal to treat **hypersensitive and irritable children** who happen to be very stubborn and who lose their temper easily. They become furious over trivial matters and are very difficult to handle when sick. Nothing calms them down. They will ask for something and once their demand has been met, they throw away the object. They will demand to be taken to some place, and having reached there, they will question as to why they were brought there. They are very rude during an outrage. One of the reasons for this is, that the Chamomilla patient happens to be more sensitive to suffering than normal people. His ailments are related to nerves and emotions. Chamomilla is ideal to treat people of an extremely sensitive nature. Outwardly, they may be very ill mannered, but deep down they are **very sensitive**. Usually they are silent, yet can explode over a trivial matter and become very tense. On the face of it, they are quiet and lazy. Chamomilla, given in high potency, provides prompt relief to such a patient. While his emotions come under control, the other medicines get a chance to work.

It must be remembered that Chamomilla patients with extreme mental anguish will not respond to other remedies unless the mental state improves as all of the body's energy is focussed in one direction.

A patient may apparently be of the Chamomilla nature, but may not exhibit its complete set of symptoms and thus may not benefit from Chamomilla. It is not always necessary that the working nature of a remedy and the constitution of the patient be a complete match. The physiology of the human body is very elaborate and intricate, therefore one particular remedy may need to be followed by many more.

Chamomilla is ideal for the treatment of hypersensitive patients exhibiting mental anguish causing **jerking and twitching (tonic contractions) of the muscles**. The patient feels as if caught in a vice.

The entire neuromuscular system is in disarray. Chamomilla is somewhat similar to Coffea, Nux Vomica and Opium. The patients of Coffea and Nux Vomica are also of very sensitive nature. The patient of Opium is apparently listless, carefree and stuprose, but deep down he is very sensitive. The Opium poisoning makes the patient very irritable and restless. When given in a larger quantity, the first reaction caused is unconsciousness, then **mental anguish** and irritability followed by state of withdrawl. In addition, some symptoms resemble those of Chamomilla. On that basis, some Opium patients are of a furious nature, they like to be left alone and are silent. Anything can provoke them and make them very irritable.

Chamomilla offers immediate relief in children who develop **convulsions** due to any ailment and fever (their nature being that of Chamomilla). Chamomilla is very useful in the treatment of **dysentery of children**, when the stools are sticky and of green colour, as if grass has been mashed into them. Ipecac is also a very good remedy in this situation. The stools are of a similar kind but the constitution is quite different.

In Chamomilla, heat brings relief to most pains, except for the neuralgic pain of teeth, face and the jaw, which respond favourably to cold. Nerve endings of a patient, when covered, will get relief by warmth but when the nerve endings become exposed, heat aggravates the symptoms. These details are not mentioned in most books. The treating physicians must carefully study all the symptoms so that no confusion is left and the proper remedy may be identified.

The **toothache** of a Chamomilla patient starts at night and disappears in the morning. Usually it is more intense in the first part of the night. After midnight, the pain starts dissipating. The toothache of an Arsenic patient lingers on throughout the night. In Chamomilla, there is **swelling of the gums** along with the formation of blisters and the gums start receding from the teeth. People who do not clean their teeth properly also begin to suffer from these kinds of symptoms.

As a matter of fact, Chamomilla patients are narrow-minded and they are somewhat mean. They do not care for others and have no sympathy for them. They are very sensitive for their own sake. They are self-centred and self-interested. To lose one's temper with others is part of the same constitution.

The Chamomilla symptoms worsen at about 9 a.m., like Natrum Mur and sometimes at 9 p.m. also. The patient hears **noises in the ears** like firecrackers going off. The ear is very sensitive to wind draft, aggravating the symptoms. Otherwise, the patient likes open air but keeps the ears covered. People who use a scarf either feel very cold or dislike the air, but the patient of Chamomilla is different, he merely protects the ears but not the face.

Chamomilla is the best remedy for an angry type of person who **has a sore throat**, associated with spasms and inflammation. The Chamomilla patient feels awfully thirsty. **Sleeplessness** due to Coffee, in general responds very well to Nux Vomica but to dispel all the side effects of Coffee, Chamomilla is more effective. Similarly, the ill effects of Chamomilla can be neutralised by Coffee.

Chamomilla is mentioned to be a good treatment when a person develops gas smelling like rotten eggs and belches out the same odour.

In allopathy, doctors use morphine as analgesic, especially during a heart attack. Morphine may cause severe **vomiting** which can be usefully treated by Chamomilla. In Chamomilla, the **abdominal pain** bends the patient over, as in Colocynth. The pain is unbearable, located at the umbilicus and the liver area. After a furious fit, the patient develops a colicky pain in the abdomen. The belching is malodorous. The patient dislikes anything hot. The tongue is yellowish and the taste is bitter. Vomiting also tastes bitter. The abdomen feels very heavy. All these are the symptoms of Chamomilla.

Some women pass blood clots during their **menstrual period**. It looks as if the inner lining of the uterus is being shredded and peeled off. This particular condition is closely related to Chamomilla.

A Chamomilla patient will develop **convulsions during pregnancy** and at the time of childbirth. Chamomilla should also be remembered for the treatment of **excessive bleeding after childbirth**. Often, this alone may control the post-partum haemorrhage. Some lactating women may develop cramps of some part of the body. In particular, if this spasm is that of the legs or the neck, a dose or two of Chamomilla will provide relief. In fact, Chamomilla will prove to be beneficial for the nursing child also. A suckling baby can get the medicine through its mother's milk but this is not always the case. If possible, he should be treated separately. If the symptoms of the child are similar to the constitution of his mother, then treating the mother only may suffice.

Chamomilla is also useful for the treatment of **cough**, especially coughing during sleep or on getting furious. Chamomilla also invigorates the resistance during an epidemic of **whooping cough**. Chamomilla will be more effective if the child is of irritable nature, but it can be useful in the simple seasonal type of cough too.

Chamomilla is most essential to treat the persistent peevishness and restlessness associated with diarrhoea during **teething**. If the child is in the habit of **crying and screaming** at night due to dreadful dreams, he should be treated with Chamomilla.

Chamomilla is one of the topmost remedies for the treatment of **earache**. In fact in this condition, one of the three following remedies is routinely used. If the child cries and feels helpless, he should be treated with Pulsatilla. If he cries with anger, then Chamomilla should be administered. When none of these two symptoms are present, Alium Cepa will often work.

| | |
|---|---|
| Antidotes: | Nux Vomica, Coffea |
| Adjuvants: | Belladonna, Mag Carb |
| Potency: | 30, 1000 or sometimes CM |

# CHELIDONIUM

Chelidonium is very useful in **most liver disorders**. In addition, it is deeply related to coughs also. Its cough originates from the right lung. For the treatment of **repeated coughing due to the irritation of the throat** that does not respond to any other medication, Chelidonium will be found to be extraordinarily useful. Once, there was a patient who suffered from a cough for many years. I prescribed Chelidonium to him, combined with Rumex. By Allah's grace, he became well very soon. Rumex too, is very useful for the treatment of chronic cough, especially of the dry nature.

The Chelidonium **cough** is typically associated with persistent irritation of the throat, burning and unease. Due to this, the patient becomes restless and gets tired of this condition. Chelidonium is extremely useful and effective in this condition. It decreases the severity and frequency of the cough, making it mild and harmless. This naturally relieves the irritability and anger of the patient, and with other remedies, the cough would gradually be cured, though not immediately.

The Chelidonium cough is associated with a small amount of sticky phlegm that is difficult to expel. Even if expectorated, the throat is still not cleared. Irritation soon resumes. In such a situation, Coccus should also be added to Chelidonium.

Chelidonium is very effective in the treatment of **jaundice,** as well as **pneumonia** and **pleurisy,** in which there is inflammation of the outer lining of the lungs in the lower part (basal pleurisy).

The urine of a Chelidonium patient is yellow with a pungent smell. When **constipated**, the stools are in the form of small rounded balls, like goat's droppings. If **diarrhoea** sets in, the colour of the faeces is brownish clay. Constipation and diarrhoea alternate with each other. The **abdominal pain** radiates to the back. After taking food, the symptoms of the stomach ameliorate. The patient likes hot food and hot fluids, especially hot milk.

Chelidonium is also useful in the treatment of **gall bladder stones**. This pain radiates towards the back while the pain in a patient of

Berberis Vulgaris radiates in all directions. Chelidonium resembles Bryonia as well. Its symptoms are generally on the right side and worsen on movement, but the difference is that the patient likes to sleep on the side of the symptoms, while in Chelidonium, if the patient sleeps on the affected side his symptoms get worse. In Chelidonium, heat intensifies **headache**. In hot countries, this may be used for the treatment of headache due to heat exposure.

In Chelidonium, the headache is associated with **drowsiness and vertigo**. The head feels heavy and numb. There is a tendency of falling forward. The **headache** radiates up to the back of the right ear towards the shoulder. There is pain over the right shoulder and the right side of the chest. The **cough** is associated with small amounts of phlegm. The palms and wrists hurt, while the tips of the fingers are ice-cold.

Sclera of the eye (i.e. the white of the eye) becomes yellowish. On looking up, the eyes hurt and the tears flow constantly. The **neuralgic pains become localised above the right eye**. The complexion of the patient is yellowish which is much more evident on the cheeks and over the nose. The skin is dry and yellowish. The tongue is also yellowish and flabby. Due to the associated **liver disorder, there is a tendency to vomit**. The kidneys feel irritated and inflamed and there is debris in the urine. When touched, the body hurts. There is pain at the hips and the thighs. As in many other remedies, an unbearable pain in the heels is also a symptom of Chelidonium.

| | |
|---|---|
| Adjuvants: | Lycopodium, Bryonia |
| Antidotes: | Chamomilla |
| Potency: | 30 to 1000 |

# CHENOPODIUM
## (Jeros Oak)

Chenopodium is prepared from oak trees grown in Jerusalem. It is a fairly broad-spectrum remedy. It is related to the nerves and paralysis related to them. According to most physicians, there is no curative treatment for the **deafness resulting from the paralysis of the auditory nerve**. Once the nerves are dead there is no hope of reviving them, but recent research has shown that when a nerve has been damaged, the ends of the adjoining nerves spread out to compensate for the loss. In particular, modern scientific research has proved that when the nerves inside the eye degenerate, new ones start developing. Sometimes when an eye has been lost, nerve fibres develop from the healthy eye to connect with the dying and dead nerve fibres of the affected eye. More experiments are being done. No doubt, the dead nerves do not vitalise, but other nerves spread out to substitute them. If the nerve endings are not completely dead, Chenopodium may revive the dying nerve fibres.

Most Chenopodium patients can hear only some sounds. For example, they may not be able to appreciate the voice of men but can appreciate the voices of women and children. Because they cannot hear so-called low-pitched (heavy) sounds, they can perceive ones that are high-pitched. Many such patients who had limited hearing got significantly better with the use of Chenopodium. Sometimes, the patient feels **vertigo due to the ear problem**. The **hearing decreases** and there are noises in the ears. In this situation, Chenopodium will restore the hearing. Chenopodium will restore the functions of the auditory as well as vestibular nerves. If the voice is suddenly lost, Chenopodium benefits this condition too.

Chenopodium is also useful in the **treatment of right-sided paralysis of the body** (hemiplegia). It is also useful in the treatment of shoulder pain. Lycopodium is also useful in the treatment of right shoulder pain, but in Chenopodium the pain is on both sides. In Chenopodium, as in Opium, there is a tendency of developing apoplexy that is more pronounced in the case of Opium, but the Chenopodium apoplexy can also resemble that of Opium. Suddenly, the face of such a patient becomes red and congested. The Chenopodium patient also suffers from sudden vertigo. The inborn tendency to develop vertigo is also a symptom of Chenopodium. This condition is called Meniere's disease. In this disease, there is repeated vertigo associated with severe vomiting. Chenopodium is also effective in treating lethargy, insensitivity, unconsciousness, partial paralysis of the nerves, and in the enlargement of the tonsils and neck glands.

The Chenopodium patient suffers from **severe pain in the backbone** that spreads out over the shoulders and chest. **Urination** is very frequent, the urine being yellowish in colour and frothy. There is an associated tingling sensation at the urethra. Yellowish material deposits on the walls of the container. This sign is also present in Chelidonium.

Some doctors have prescribed Chenopodium for the treatment of roundworms and hookworm infestation. When Chenopodium oil is given in repeated small doses, after some time the patient becomes free of these worms. I however, have not practised using Chenopodium for this purpose.

| | |
|---|---|
| Potency: | Chenopodium is usually used in potency 3 but I have found it very useful in potency 30. For worms, Chenopodium oil is given 10 drops every two to three hours. |

# Chininum Ars
## (Arsenite of Quinine)

Chininum Ars is the treatment for the disorders of blood formation (haemopoetic system), resulting from chronic illnesses, associated with hypo function of the liver and dysfunction of the bone marrow. Due to the lack of blood (anaemia), the face is somewhat swollen and pale. Wrinkles appear on the face reflecting senility. The patient feels weak and listless. Chininum Ars is the examplary treatment for such patients. However, one cannot benefit without understanding the basic constitution of Chininum Ars.

Chininum Ars is a compound of China and Arsenic. It is prepared from the bark of Cinchona, which used to be the source of quinine (considered to be the best medicine for **malaria**). Later on, more medicines were discovered for the treatment of malaria, though quinine has its own unique status.

Chininum Ars is very useful in **combating the residual ill effects of malaria**. The liver and spleen enlarge; the skin is dry, lacking normal lustre. The skin looks yellow all over. The person frequently gets out of breath and loses his appetite. Such patients do not recover immediately with Chininum Ars, therefore, it should be used over a long period and then it works wonders.

Cold air aggravates the symptoms of Chininum Ars. There is a constant **feeling of slight cold** in the body. There is chronic **diarrhoea** in which stools are watery and putrid. Various parts of the body are swollen. The patient does not want to move. Instead, he likes to lie down still. In Chininum Ars, there is **throbbing in the muscles** which can be felt to the fingertips. The pulse is weak, thready and slow.

In Chininum Ars, like Lachesis, the symptoms aggravate after sleep. The body feels restless, more so by the evening. Many patients have a guilty conscious and firmly believe that they cannot be forgiven. The Chininum Ars patient feels guilty over trifle misgivings and becomes **suspicious-minded (a victim of fear and superstition)**. Sometimes such patients may experience odd visual hallucinations.

During fever, a Chininum Ars patient suddenly jumps out of bed with fear. He remains restless, gradually loses hope and becomes sick of life. Noise is unbearable and the memory becomes weak. Such patients, who have lived luxurious and vulgar lives, are more likely to develop the symptoms of Chininum Ars.

In Chininum Ars, due to the weakness of the nerves and lack of blood, the patient feels **jerking during sleep**. This symptom has been mentioned in reference to many other remedies but is a symptom of Chininum Ars as well. Sometimes, the patient wakes up due to the feeling of pain that spreads through the body like a flash of lightning. In Chininum Ars, the symptoms resulting from low blood pressure are the same as those in Arnica and Belladonna associated with high blood pressure. The arms, legs, hands and feet become cold, but then the blood pressure rises. This is a specific symptom of Chininum Ars.

In Chininum Ars, weakness is more pronounced on the right side, such as the right side of the neck and the **right arm**. When the weakness advances, one may have **convulsions.** At night there is headache. Nasal cold also causes headache. In general, when the cold is suppressed, the headache gets worse. There is a **feeling of being hammered over the head** that is usually due to the lack of blood. This symptom is also salient in Natrum Mur (because Natrum Mur also is one of the best treatments for anaemia). In this, the blood becomes more dilute. In Chininum Ars, the lack of red blood cells cause anaemia, so the swelling noticed in Chininum Ars is soft and pitting in nature. The muscles of the scalp also hurt. The symptoms aggravate in the cold.

In Chininum Ars, there are **symptoms related to the eyes** as well. Light irritates the eye and produces warm tears. This symptom is also found in Natrum Mur. As far as the eyes are concerned in Chininum Ars, ulcers are found in not only one but in both eyes. The tendency towards developing **ulcers and eczema simultaneously** is also present in Chininum Ars, as in Arnica. In Arnica, if there is irritation in one eye it will eventually cause irritation in the other eye as well. Both eyes hurt at the same time. This happens in Chininum Ars also but the patient sees **flashing stars and flames**, which are more marked in the left eye than the right. Tears form in the left eye. There is a feeling of pain. There is **noise in the ears** and voices are heard.

The hearing either becomes unusually sharp or the patient starts becoming deaf. These contradicting symptoms are specific to Chininum Ars.

The nose discharges **blood-mixed fluid or offensive smelling pus**. The nose starts decaying from the inside. There is peeling of the lips and the tip of the nose. The face is pale, earth coloured and swollen like yeast. A strange kind of glare appears on the face, typical of anaemia. The inner linings of the mouth cavity may bleed. Streaks appear on the tongue. The colour of the tongue may be black, brown, white or yellow. The **gums become swollen** and they start receding from the teeth. There is distaste in the mouth; even the best food tastes awful. There is unrelenting thirst, toothache at night and grinding of the teeth which disturbs the sleep. The throat is dry and sometimes there is a stinking smell from the throat. This is a grave sign because it shows that the **sores inside the mouth are far too serious and have become necrotic.** If all the symptoms of Chininum Ars are not evident in this kind of patient, Arsenic in high potency should be administered without delay. One symptom of Chininum Ars is that the person feels discomfort on swallowing a drop of water or a morsel of food, even if the throat is not evidently diseased. There is a need for constant hawking to clear the throat.

Sometimes in Chininum Ars, the appetite is completely extinct and one has a bad taste in the mouth, while at other times, there is an intense never-ending appetite to eat. As soon as food is taken, the abdomen becomes full. There is a feeling of **burning and acidity** and soon after taking food, the patient feels hungry again. He cannot digest fish and eggs but definitely is not allergic to them. In case of **allergy to eggs**, just one dose of Calcaria Carb in high potency may do the job. It normally works, though not always.

In Chininum Ars, **nausea does not let the patient sleep**. As soon as the nausea is treated, the person goes to sleep but soon afterwards, he **vomits**, meaning that the nausea was only temporarily suppressed yet its real cause persisted.

All the abdominal ailments produced after malaria are found in Chininum Ars. **The liver and the spleen are enlarged** but the rest of the abdomen is shrunken and drawn in. The stools are dry and lumpy due to constipation. In Arsenic patients, some fruits cause diarrhoea.

In Chininum Ars, **haemorrhoids or piles** are also found, which are markedly swollen and bluish. They also itch. In the urine, the patient passes albumin and sugar. Chininum Ars is useful in the treatment of sexual weakness of men as well as women. Women suffer from an **abrasive type of leucorrhoea** and the discharge is mixed with blood. The **menses are copious in amount**, free, offensive smelling and black or yellowish in colour. They may continue for a long time and then suddenly stop altogether. If the peculiar symptoms of Chininum Ars are also present, then this remedy, by Allah's grace, cures all the symptoms.

In Chininum Ars, there is a feeling of **spasm and paring in the windpipe, along with the sensation of suffocation**. Deep breathing is difficult because it causes irritation inside the air passage. Symptoms of **Asthmatic cough** can also be present.

There is pain at the area of the heart, with feelings of tightness and suffocation, convulsion, swelling, weakness and palpitations. The hands and feet become cold. There is severe **cramping of muscles in the calves**. There are rheumatic pains in the body and pain in the knees and legs. The patient sleeps peacefully only in the latter part of the night.

It must be kept in mind that all the above symptoms, which are due to the lack of blood, will be treated by Chininum Ars. If these symptoms are present, and the person is not anaemic, the above remedy might work, but only sparingly.

| | |
|---|---|
| Potency: | from 30 to 1000 |

# CHOLESTERINUM

This remedy is prepared from bile. It is very useful in the **treatment of liver and gall bladder diseases**. It is the best treatment for gall bladder pain (billiary colic). In my experience, I have found it very useful in the treatment of the diseases of the liver, gall bladder, spleen and pancreas. It is also very useful in the treatment of the **cancer of the liver**. It prevents deposition of fat in the body. It is also useful in lowering **blood cholesterol** level. In America, patients have tried many modern medicines to lower cholesterol which did not work, but with the use of Cholesterinum, they noticed significant effect.

Cholesterinum is also useful in preventing **inflammation of the gall bladder and pancreas** and **prevention of stone formation**. If given at the initial stage, the patient will be saved from many possible complications. If the stones have already formed, use of Cholesterinum will soften and dissolve them. Within a short time, the stones disappear.

Cholesterinum is also very useful in treatment of **jaundice** and an **enlarged spleen**. Cholesterinum patients usually exhibit restlessness and general unease. There is loss of sleep, though not to the extent as in Arsenic and there is no irritability of Chamomilla. It is also useful for the treatment of suffocation.

Morphia annuls the effect of Cholesterinum.

| | |
|---|---|
| Potency: | 30 |

# Cicuta Virosa
## (Water Hemlock)

Cicuta Virosa is one of the best treatments of convulsions. **Convulsions and convulsive fits** are its typical sign. When there is increased mental anguish, hypersensitivity and intolerance, where even the slightest pressure causes tingling of the muscles, then some patients may go into a convulsion which starts from the centre of the body and spreads towards the periphery. In Cicuta Virosa, this symptom is just the opposite of other remedies, where the state of convulsion generally starts in the periphery of the body, i.e. the fingers or soles of the feet, and then spreads towards the upper part of the body. But in Cicuta Virosa, if there is severe cramp and colic at the stomach, then it spreads into the other organs. There is tightness of the neck and a spasmodic convulsion which then shifts to the lower part of the body. The spread of the spasmodic condition, starting in the centre and spreading to the periphery, is the special feature of Cicuta Virosa.

In Cicuta Virosa, the convulsion generally starts at the stomach or heart, in the form of tingling. The patient is more sensitive than usual in reacting to an **injury to sensitive areas** or when a thorn pierces the body. If this leads to convulsions, then Cicuta Virosa is a useful remedy. Arnica and Ledum are also very effective remedies. Besides these, Hypericum, Staphysagria and Ruta are also useful in the treatment of injuries to the nerves and the resulting signs and symptoms.

Some symptoms of Cicuta Virosa resemble Catalepsy. In this condition, the mind becomes stunned temporarily. The **patient forgets** who he is and where he is. There is a wave of confusion starting in the head, resulting in the patient becoming completely unaware of his surroundings. Cicuta Virosa is very important in the treatment of this condition.

The difference between apoplexy and catalepsy is that in apoplexy, the brain becomes functionless as a result of clotting of the blood and the patient becomes paralysed and motionless. In catalepsy, the patient is apparently lethargic but when questioned, he can answer properly. After that, he does not remember what has happened. He confuses the present with the past. He is surprised at the sight of an old friend, wondering if he has seen him somewhere before.

Cicuta Virosa is very useful in treating the severe **muscular spasm on the back of the head and the neck**, resulting in the turning of the neck backward (opisthotonus). In Cicuta Virosa, the spasm is towards the back of the neck and the person becomes rigid backwards. In addition to this, Cicuta Virosa is very useful in the treatment of **rigidity due to meningitis**. In epilepsy, if the person falls backwards, Cicuta Virosa will be of use. In other words, the conditions resembling epilepsy and the ones resulting in head injury should be carefully studied regarding their special symptoms. It must be remembered that its convulsions spread from the centre towards the periphery.

Some of the mental symptoms of Cicuta Virosa resemble those of Natrum Mur. In old age, the arteries become narrow due to arteriosclerosis and blood flow to the brain is reduced. When such patients also develop stomach upset, they will suffer from amnesia (brainfag). Nux Vomica is useful for its treatment. The ailments of Cicuta Virosa are related to the **nerves**. When there is a severe spasm at the stomach, Cicuta Virosa will be useful, otherwise it will not be. One peculiar mental symptom of Cicuta Virosa is that a patient with an advanced disease cannot distinguish between the tastes of different items. The **taste buds** are afflicted; they become **insensitive**. The patient cannot distinguish between uncooked and cooked food. He will eagerly ingest both. Some children like to eat coal, clay, lime and paper. This is due to a lack of calcium. It has nothing to do with the nervous system.

The patient of Cicuta Virosa behaves in a childish way. He jumps over the bed, talks strangely, dances, sings and screams like a child. His thoughts are foolish. If he has a fit of **epilepsy** due to sudden fear, Aconite 1000 given promptly can be beneficial. However, it does not cure it. Cicuta Virosa is the ideal permanent curative medicine for the treatment of such convulsions or epileptic fits resulting from fear. When the intensity of the fit subsides, these patients become deeply downcast. This is an additional symptom peculiar to Cicuta Virosa.

Cicuta Virosa is good in the treatment of **residual ill effects of old injuries**, especially those from head injuries resulting in paralysis. Generally, Natrum Sulph and Arnica are quite useful, and after that is Opium and Plumbum. However, if **convulsions or epilepsy develop after these injuries**, Cicuta Virosa can treat these conditions. This is also the treatment of a **squint** resulting from the head injuries. However, before this, Arnica and Natrum Sulph should also be used. If due to fear, the eyes move upwards, the pupils dilate and a squint appears, then there is no better treatment for this condition than Cicuta Virosa.

The skin symptoms of Cicuta Virosa are related to the nerves, such as, a feeling of **irritation** after shaving. The movement of the razor on the skin causes tension in the underlying nerves and the roots of the hair become hypersensitive. The nerve symptoms usually direct themselves to the overlying skin. At this stage, the treatment becomes difficult. However, if the characteristic symptoms of Cicuta Virosa are present, this particular remedy would work. Small pea-size bumps also develop over the hands and the face. The associated **eczema** does not itch. Thick lemon coloured scabs develop over the bumps.

When a **fish bone gets stuck in the throat**, Silicia offers prompt relief. However if there is subsequent tightness and restlessness in the throat, Cicuta Virosa will offer relief.

In Cicuta Virosa, the entire body shakes. The arms and legs feel weak; **sudden jerky movements** are followed by a severe weakness of the legs, which feel unstable and cannot support the body weight. The patient feels **dizzy** and sweats on the head during sleep. A typical eye symptom relating to Cicuta Virosa is that the person feels the words are disappearing while reading. Things look as if they are moving closer and farther alternatively. Hearing decreases. Swallowing is difficult. The throat is dry. There is tightness in the upper food passage (oesophagus or gullet). Thirst is intense. There is burning, hiccupping, presence of gas and **distension of the abdomen**. These are all symptoms of Cicuta Virosa. There is **morning diarrhoea** and the desire to keep on passing urine. The chest feels tight with a feeling of suffocation. There is difficulty in breathing and the breathing organs, like the larynx and trachea, feel tight and constricted. There is a feeling of warmth inside the chest.

In women, during their **periods**, there is severe pain at the uterus and the coccyx. At the time of childbirth and afterwards convulsions occur.

In Cicuta Virosa, the symptoms get worse with touch, gusts of cold air, injury and tobacco smoke. Heat relieves the symptoms.

| | |
|---|---|
| Antidotes: | Opium, Arnica |
| Potency: | 6 to 200 |

# CINA

Cina is very famous for the treatment of **worm infestation** in children. Its peculiar nature is that of ill temper. Its patients (children) get outraged over trivial matters. Nothing can please them. They are very sensitive. Their hypersensitivity is not only of their nature but it also **affects their skin**. The patient does not let anybody come near him or touch him. Even a light touch with the hand is unbearable. He hesitates to face a stranger. Like the patient of Chamomilla, the patient makes strange demands, and when the demand is met, he throws away the object. Being stared at by somebody upsets him.

The Cina patients **grind their teeth** during the night, which is interrupted by frequent jolting and waking up. Fear scares them and wakes them up. In their frightful dreams, they see dogs, demons and ghosts. They scream during sleep and wake up trembling. The children like to sleep on their hands and knees.

The Cina patient has a peculiar glossy gleam in the eye. He experiences an array of colours, especially yellow. The pupils are dilated. The patient experiences blackouts. There is constant irritation inside the nose, which needs to be **constantly rubbed**. The irritation is never ending. The margins of the nostrils shrink inside. Around the mouth and the lips, yellowish or bluish round spots develop.

**Convulsions** are a special characteristic of Cina. The limbs feel tight and jerky. As in Cicuta, the neck of the person arches backwards (Opisthotonus). The fingers turn in. There is a feeling of chilliness and quivering all over the body. When such a patient is patted on his back, he develops headache.

The symptoms of Cina aggravate after taking food. The patient feels very hungry. The child throws up clotted milk. The nature of Cina resembles somewhat with that of Aethusa. Besides the mind, heat affects the stomach and intestines; but the symptoms are expressed a little differently than in Aethusa. In Aethusa, the child vomits milk as soon as he drinks it and is mostly constipated but in Cina, diarrhoea or dysentery is more common. The stools are mixed with a whitish sticky material (mucus). When the infection has become well established, the diarrhoeal stools become green in colour.

In a Cina patient, the sensation of touch and taste are either enhanced or reduced significantly. In other words, they are out of balance. Often, the patient eats one thing and perceives the taste of something else. Ingestion of food, milk or water causes a rumbling noise in the throat. This symptom is also found in Cuprum and Arsenic. Cuprum is also useful for the treatment of worm infestation.

The stools of a patient of Cina are foul-smelling and propulsive, like Podophylum. A peculiar symptom of Cina is that when the child lies prone on his stomach, his diarrhoea stops showing that pressure over the abdomen offers relief. Cina should not be forgotten in the treatment of **epilepsy developing after a malarial attack**.

In Cina, there is violent coughing in the morning, and one may develop spasms of the throat due to incessant coughing. There is pain in the chest. The attacks of whooping cough also occur. In women, during pregnancy, sudden unexpected news of happiness or grief can precipitate headache or pain in the abdomen which can linger on for quite some time. Cina can be administered to control this kind of suffering. The symptoms of Cina aggravate after food at night and in hot weather.

| | |
|---|---|
| Antidotes: | Camphor, Capsicum |
| Potency: | 30 to 200 |

# CINCHONA OFFICINALIS
## (China)

China is prepared from the Cinchona tree. The well-known anti-malarial medicine quinine is prepared from the bark of the same tree. In homoeopathy, this is called Cinchona but it is more commonly known as China. An effective and useful medicine, it is extremely beneficial to **annul the bad aftereffects of malaria**. It is used in the majority of malaria cases. Cinchona overcomes the symptoms of malarial fever, which it suppresses. In most malarial patients, the symptoms continue to exist in a suppressed form. These after effects and suppressed symptoms of malaria are amenable to treatment with homoeopathic China. Sometimes, it can be useful in the treatment of malaria fever as such. Normally in the cold weather, one does not feel too thirsty. But when intense thirst is felt in cold weather and fever becomes high, the patient feels thirsty again. In this particular symptom, probably the best treatment would be China.

It has been repeatedly said that in the case of malaria, no medicine should be given when the fever is coming on. The best time to administer medicine is when the fever is subsiding or has subsided or there is an onset of a new attack of fever. After the malarial attack, the malarial parasites settle in the liver. Thus the ideal time to administer medicine is when the malarial parasites are on their way to settle in the liver. Most of them will be destroyed with treatment but if some happen to survive, they will definitely become weakened. Similarly, the treatment should be repeated after the next episode of fever. The statement I have made seems philosophical, but it is a hard fact that I have personally observed time and time again, and many other homoeopaths will agree with me.

China is also very useful in curing the **weakness and other side effects of malarial fever**. Its patient is very sensitive to touch. Movement aggravates his condition. Cold air is unbearable. All the nerves happen to become very excitable. Mental fatigue and physical weakness are typical signs of China. The patient becomes extremely irritable, careless, depressed and bad-tempered. He cannot concentrate. While talking to others, the conversation is often interrupted. The associated severe **headache** that spreads down the neck feels better by applying pressure and in a warm room. There is a feeling of throbbing over the forehead. The patient does not tolerate light pressure, yet at the same time he feels relief by deep pressure. Touch, a draft of air and a thump of anything aggravate the headache. Darkish blue rings form around the eyes. Due to the affliction of the liver, the eyes become yellow and feel heavy. Vision becomes dim, and temporary blindness may also ensue.

**Digestion is slowed down**. Fruit and sour food hurt the stomach. Food is not digested properly. The abdomen distends. China would be ideal to treat the inflammation of liver and spleen with jaundice and pain at the gall bladder area, if the patient's constitution matches that of China. In this condition, China 30 should be used continuously over a long period.

The China patient **has a tendency to bleed.** There is **bleeding from the throat, nose and uterus**, which is also associated with cramps. Periods start before their due time. **Leucorrhoeal** discharge is mixed with blood. China would be an important remedy during childbirth when labour pains stop due to bleeding and convulsions start, if the other symptoms of the patient are also of the nature of China. Post-partum bleeding continues for a longer period and smells foul.

The arms and legs of a China patient hurt as if sprained and jolted. The tonic **contractions of the muscles, like epilepsy,** and the paralytic weakness of the affected part is also a symptom of China. There is a rush of blood towards the head, **ringing in the ears** and blackout in the eyes. In the state of commotion, the patient becomes unconscious. The patient feels restless and sleepless due to weakness after losing blood. In women, after bleeding and due to nursing the child, anaemia develops. They sweat at night. The skin feels cold. One hand feels cold and the other warm. The hands and feet of China feel weak and shaky. The gums swell and the **teeth become loose, resulting in a severe pain on chewing**, as if the teeth have become too long. Taste is bitter. Food also feels bitter or extremely salty in taste. Thereby, the patient hates food. Milk upsets the stomach. The associated chronic form of **diarrhoea** is aggravated at night. Unlike China, the diarrhoea of Petroleum starts during the day and stops before the night sets in.

In China, the abdomen becomes distended but the flatus does not smell. This particular symptom is saliently described in homoeopathic books.

| | |
|---|---|
| Adjuvants: | Ferrum Phos, Calcaria Phos |
| Antidotes: | Arnica, Arsenic, Nux Vomica, Ipecac |
| Potency: | Generally 30; otherwise 200 or 1000 |

# Cistus Canadensis
## (Rock Rose)

Cistus is prepared from a flowering plant which grows wild in snowy areas. The nature of this medicine is very cold. Every kind of ailment related to it carries the feeling of chill and cold.

Cistus is a profoundly effective antisporic medicine, meaning that it is basically related to skin diseases. Whether these diseases involve glands or mucous membranes, they are still called as Psoric. Cistus is one of those medicines used for the treatment of psoric ailments. Thus, it is very important in the treatment of gravely dangerous diseases. Lupus and cancer too are not beyond its jurisdiction. Compared to Calcaria, it is somewhat mild but in some diseases, it actually works better than it and also over the diseases of the glands. It is also useful in the treatment of intestinal diseases. In **intractable diarrhoea** which does not respond to any other medicine, especially when associated with inflammation of the glands, one should not forget Cistus. Similarly, the **chronic cold** in a patient who has the disposition of Cistus will not be treatable with any other kind of remedy. Such patients are, in general, flabby and pale in colour. They easily become short of breath, especially on climbing heights.

Peculiarly, Cistus is very effective in treating **headache during fasting**. Lycopodium, Bryonia, Nux Vomica and Gelsemium also may be useful in treating the headache resulting from prolonged fasting or starvation.

In Cistus, often the irritation is not manifest externally but remains suppressed in the deeper layer of the skin. Therefore the skin feels uneasy with a sensation of crawling like the movement of ants over it. The patient may feel a sinking of the heart and as a reaction, he constantly pounds the area over his heart with his hands. Prolonged itching over the skin makes the disease manifest externally. Blisters form that bleed when scratched. The use of Cistus will offer relief to the patient. However Cistus should be repeated often, with intervals, to cure itching of long standing. It is indeed a very strong and effective medicine. The experienced capable physicians have claimed that this alone can cure **Lupus of the face**, which is considered almost incurable. Cistus is well known in the treatment of **cancer of the lower lip**.

The symptoms of Cistus related to the **teeth and gums** resemble those of Sulphur, except that in Sulphur there is intense burning and stinging sensation, and the teeth tend to rot. In Cistus, the jaw muscles become weak resulting in relative loosening of the teeth, but there is no burning sensation. The cold in the patient of Cistus also is devoid of any burning sensation. The nose, in fact, feels cold inside. The feeling of cold actually brings on the symptoms of the common **cold**. The timely use of Cistus will stop the cold developing. Once the cold has settled and there is an accumulation of discharge in the nose (which causes burning when scratched) Cistus should be used. In the case of Arsenic, the burning sensation continues even in the presence of discharge. In the case of Cistus, when the discharge is let out, the patient feels relief. There is a cold sensation in the mouth and throat. The dry cold air provokes pain. The **throat/pharynx becomes inflamed** and then proceeds to pus formation. Secondary to the inflammation of the throat and pus formation, the **person's head turns to one side** (due to spasm of the overlying muscles of the neck). The patient feels cold in different parts of the body. There is a feeling of cold in the stomach and the abdomen before and after taking food. The patient likes to eat cheese. The **stools are thin, watery and propulsive,** and more frequent in the morning. The patients, especially women, love to eat spicy food. In Cistus, the skin of the hands becomes hard, dry and thick and **itches** a lot. The patient cannot sleep due to restlessness.

Cistus is also useful in the treatment of the **diseases of the breast in women** (mammary glands). Though there is no one specific sign, probably the presence of other symptoms would settle the diagnosis. Enlargement of the mammary glands can sometimes transform into cancer. Cistus could be one of the possible remedies. The presence of a chain of swollen, enlarged glands in the neck is a typical sign of Cistus. Absence of the involvement of the glands inside the throat and outside on the neck rules out the diagnosis of Cistus.

Cistus may be of use in the treatment of intractable **itching of the ear**, which develops sores as a result of scratching, and then pus formation. The **cough** of Cistus is also, associated with itching and irritability. The disease process being seated in the deep tissues will not benefit from superficial scratching unless the disease manifests itself externally on the surface of the skin. According to allopathic science, diseases deep inside the body and the ones on the surface of the skin are different. But according to the homoeopathic view, both are the manifestation of one basic weakness, affecting the inner linings, the glands, as well as the external surface of the skin.

Cistus is very important for the treatment of **nail problems**. Many diseases, when well established, affect the nails. Streaks form over the nails, which become thick and deformed. Cistus is a prominent remedy for treating the skin condition due to chronic diseases. There are some other medicines also which can be used for the treatment of the nails. In Cistus, any kind of deformity of the nails can be expected. Other symptoms of Cistus being present, this would be the most ideal and the best remedy to treat the skin condition. The symptoms of Cistus aggravate on touch, movement, draft of cold air, at night and by mental work. The symptoms ameliorate after taking food or bringing out sputum.

| | |
|---|---|
| Adjuvants: | Conium, Carbo Veg, Calcaria and Argentum Nitricum |
| Antidotes: | Rhus Tox, Cepia |
| Potency: | Commonly 30 but high potency may be used as needed |

# CLEMATIS ERECTA
## (Virgin's Bower)

Clematis is a profoundly effective remedy related to all **skin diseases**. As a result of ingesting Clematis poison, various kinds of skin diseases will result, like eczema, itching and formation of blisters and pimples. Regarding its effects on the skin, it resembles Rhus Tox, but is much more powerful. It is effective against the tendency to develop cancer, especially the **skin cancer** called **Epithelioma**. In Clematis, the skin symptoms become worse on exposure to cold water, cold weather or cold air, except the problem inside the mouth. The pain in the gums is relieved by application of cold water, whereas heat aggravates it.

The **blisters** of Clematis tend to make yellowish pus. Conditions like ringworm and different kinds of **eczema** are also well within the range of action of Clematis. Red pimples form over the skin, which burn intensely. These pimples form mostly over the head, hands and face. With the exception of eczema, there is a feeling of something creeping over the skin. Scratching offers temporary relief. There is pain over the temples and dispersion of thoughts. Open air offers relief.

Clematis is used in many **diseases of men** relating to the reproductive system, especially the inflammation of the right spermatic cord and inflammatory swelling of the right testis (orchitis). It only acts on the right side. The associated urinary symptoms may be sensitivity along the urethra and frequency of scanty urination followed by scalding at the end. The flow of urine is rather interrupted and sometimes may be in the form of drops, and the dribbling may continue for a minute or two after the act of urination. It is also effective in treating the inflammation of the bladder on the right side.

**The overall symptoms of Clematis are the same as that of suppressed Gonorrhoea.**

The **toothache** of Clematis gets worse at night and with the smell of tobacco, especially when the bed is warm.

In Clematis, the **eyes burn severely** and feel warm as if on fire. A draft of wind is unbearable. Eyes water and swell, especially the left eye. The patient feels difficulty in opening the eyes.

A peculiar symptom in Clematis is that the patient feels generally weak after taking food. The arteries throb and pulsate. The patient feels full as soon as he takes food. There is a strong, piercing type of **pain from the chest down to the abdomen**, getting worse on breathing in.

The characteristic point about Clematis is that its **symptoms aggravate in proportion to the size of the moon**. The symptoms also become worse after taking a shower.

One thing to be remembered about Clematis is that when it is administered to the patients, their mouth feels very dry and they feel thirsty. The resulting thirst will not be quenched by taking water. The patients should be warned about this symptom.

| | |
|---|---|
| Antidotes: | Bryonia, Camphor |
| Potency: | 30 to 200 |

# COCCULUS
## (Indian Cockle)

Cocculus is famous for the treatment of **vertigo**. Vertigo results from an imbalance of fluid in the deeper part of the ear (inner ear) or due to the weakness of the vestibular nerve which carries the sensation of balance from the ear to the brain. The resultant delay in nerve conduction results in dizziness and the person cannot maintain balance. When the patient turns his head one way or the other, the message about the movement does not reach the brain promptly.

Due to the **weakness of the nervous system**, the physical efficiency and the efficiency of the brain is disturbed. The patient feels tired and weak. Later, this weakness may turn into full-fledged paralysis. The victims of this condition are usually people who become mentally exhausted after taking care of their near and dear ones for a long time. They virtually remain awake day and night and are in constant state of fear and anxiety. The resultant physical and mental exhaustion will be cured by Cocculus.

This exhaustion usually does not affect midwives and nurses because they take care of the patient as a part of their professional duty. They do not have any direct personal relationship with the patient. Generally, their physical fatigue does not convert into nervous tension.

In the Cocculus patient, the body starts feeling weak as a result of mental pressure, supplemented with physical exertion or physical exertion with mental anxiety. The patient does not sleep well. He is always in a state of anxiety and apprehension, which results in headache. There is a tendency to develop **vertigo, nausea and vomiting**. The symptoms get worse with movement. It further gets worse by stumbling during walking. The symptoms are aggravated during travel. One must always keep Cocculus as the initial treatment for **imbalance resulting from sudden motion**.

The skin of a chronic Cocculus patient shivers. The **hands tremble when picking up an object**. There is loss of coordination in the movement of the limbs resulting in imbalance. The patients cannot make a quick turn. They have to turn slowly to avoid severe dizziness.

Some symptoms of Cocculus resemble those of Belladonna. In Belladonna, the **dizziness** gets worse with sudden motion but this is due to the variation in the pressure of the blood towards the brain. In both Cocculus and Belladonna, a slight noise and sudden jerk become unbearable. In both, the patient suffers from sleeplessness and mental anguish. Unlike Belladonna, the face of a Cocculus patient is of normal complexion and there is no unusual flow of blood towards the face. In Cocculus the muscles become stiff and taut. To contract or stretch the limbs causes severe pain.

In Cocculus, the patient feels severe **colicky abdominal pain**. There is **griping and cramping over the stomach**. Sometimes, the pain makes breathing uncomfortable. Some women may actually become unconscious due to severe pain. The patient dislikes food and their appetite disappears.

In Cocculus, there is a delay in message relay from one point to another. There is also a feeling of time passing rapidly. The **legs become paralysed** and numb or insensitive. The background of this paralysis is a long period of worrisome night vigil, problems and apprehension.

Due to **mental anguish** and nervous exhaustion, the Cocculus patient answers questions very slowly. He is lost in his own thoughts. He often gets severely depressed. The head feels heavy. In addition Cocculus is useful in the treatment of **headache** secondary to heat exposure, like Belladonna and Glonoine.

In Cocculus, the **eyesight becomes foggy,** but this does not last long. Due to nervous weakness, it becomes blurred temporarily. Mental fatigue is also temporary. The **inability to open the eyes, especially during night, due to severe pain in the eyes, swollen eyelids or constriction of the pupils,** are also the symptoms of Cocculus.

In Cocculus, there is a metallic taste in the mouth, which is somewhat acidic. There is a feeling of **acidity in the stomach** along with the tendency of **nausea and vomiting**. In Cocculus, there are some symptoms similar to malaria but the aches are only in the legs rather than the whole body. The **fever** associated with nausea and **vertigo** will respond to Cocculus.

In Cocculus the patient cannot bear the smell of food, which in fact causes nausea. This symptom is also present in the case of Colchicum. Whenever a **gland is inflamed and enlarged**, the treatment could be Kreosotum or some other homoeopathic remedies, but in Cocculus the swelling and inflammation is secondary to paralysis. Similarly, due to the **paralysis of the intestines and the muscles of the abdomen, the patient gets constipated** and finds it very difficult to expel the stools.

In women, the **periods are either too frequent or much delayed** and continue for much longer. These symptoms are present in other remedies also. For a proper diagnosis, the specific symptoms of Cocculus must be kept in mind. If so found, Cocculus will be the ideal treatment. The specific symptoms of Cocculus are generalized weakness, partial paralysis, movement aggravating the symptoms, and delayed conduction of sensation along the nerves. **Copious watery discharge** in between the periods is specific to Cocculus. It gradually makes the patient very weak, so much so that she talks with great difficulty. The right and left hands become cold and hot alternately and can become numb also. Similarly, the patient may have cold sweats alternately. A Cocculus patient cannot tolerate gusty wind or the wind draft. He is oversensitive to both cold as well as hot air. The symptoms aggravate in the open, sun and warm bedding, as well as at nighttime. Generally Cocculus is used in potency 30 but when there is paralysis of the lower half of the body, it needs to be given in potency CM, to be repeated after a long period. This kind of paralysis is treatable with Cocculus and only Cocculus; otherwise the patient remains untreated for life.

| | |
|---|---|
| Antidotes: | Coffea, Nux Vomica |
| Potency: | Usually 30, but in case of the specific paralysis, up to CM. |

# Coccus Cacti
## (Cochineal)

Coccus Cacti is commonly used in the treatment of day-to-day superficial and short-lived ailments. Yet, it is a profoundly active medicine with the capability of curing chronic illnesses within its jurisdiction. So it should not only be taken as a simple, temporary type of remedy.

In Coccus, all the discharges are sticky long and threadlike. The threadlike pus resembles wool or a woven rope. The presence of similar type of expectoration in **whooping cough** is suggestive of Coccus Cacti. In this way, Coccus is like Kali Bichrome which it resembles in the sense that its expectoration is also sticky and thready, and it is also useful in whooping cough.

Coccus patients remain sick during the winter season and do not get better until the onset of summer. They cannot get rid of cold and catarrh. If the nasal discharge is threadlike, then Coccus should be utilized without hesitation. In fact, it works promptly, effectively and for a long time. **The cough and the cold** become worse in a warm room, while the cold and cold water relieve them however the symptoms recur soon. This contradicting behaviour of the remedy should always be remembered. Body heat resulting from exercise proves harmful. Exposure to cold establishes the ailments deeply, while inner heat also aggravates the symptoms. Sometimes, external heat may also make the symptoms worse.

The difficulty in breathing experienced while making an ascent is due to the accumulation of sputum in the chest. It is not related to the weakness of the heart. Once the patient vomits out the expectoration, the chest feels light and going up heights will not be difficult anymore.

In Coccus, the cough arises out of the need to expel the expectoration (which causes spasm in the throat). The distinguishing sign of Coccus is the sensitivity of skin and inner linings, resembling the plant 'Touch-me-not', which withdraws on touch. Sensitivity of the throat is a special symptom of the Coccus ailment. In Coccus, there is sometimes difficulty in swallowing also.

In Coccus the urinary symptoms such as the urgent need to urinate, passing small brick red particles and gravel in the urine, and the presence of uric acid causing a stabbing type of pain from the kidney down to the bladder (renal colic), are of great importance. Sometimes the urination may suddenly stop altogether.

Regarding the symptoms in women, menstrual blood is thick, dark and contains large blood clots. This may be associated with an inability to pass urine (i.e. retention of urine). The periods become interrupted, resuming only at night.

After the running nose stops, the yellowish sticky secretions stick inside the nose. After blowing the nose, the inner lining feels as if it is burning. The patient feels extremely thirsty. Mental depression, solitude and silence or excessive talking, are also the symptoms of Coccus (like Lachesis). In Coccus, the catarrh can also affect the stomach, intestines and inner linings.

| | |
|---|---|
| Potency: | usually 30 |

# COFFEA CRUDA
## (Unroasted Coffee)

Coffee is used as a favourite drink in most countries of the world, especially in the western world. Coffee dispels sleep. It stimulates the nervous system, and enhances the flow of ideas and mental alertness. The **person cannot go to sleep** even if he so desires and tries.

The homoeopathic Coffea Cruda is prepared from the unroasted Coffee bean. If sleeplessness is due to excessive talking or mental commotion, a dose or two of Coffea bring about peaceful sleep. The person is whisked into sleep without any preliminary slumber. Nux Vomica also has a similar feature of bringing about sleep rapidly. One symptom of Nux Vomica and Belladonna shared by Coffea is that the noise agitates the person and loud voices perturb him. However in Coffea, the noise provokes pain up to the periphery of the limbs. Also, noise rekindles the previous pains of the leg or the knee. In fact, the re-appearance of old pains due to the noise is a typical feature of Coffea.

The symptoms of Coffea are brought about by sudden joy rather than to grief. In other words, sudden, happy news causes mental commotion. A loss of sleep due to profound grief needs to be treated with different kinds of remedies.

The Coffea patient reacts badly to intake of alcohol. In the countries where drinking is extremely common, a Coffea patient would refrain from drinking alcohol for fear of serious reaction, and alcoholics often use coffee to dispel the effects of alcohol.

In a patient of Coffea, the **hypersensitivity of the skin** is extreme, and is in the form of a strange kind of tingling and discomfort. Regarding the extreme sensitivity of the skin, Zincum Metallicum is the next in order.

A Coffea patient has strong intolerance towards the sound of footsteps. Itchy rashes appear on the skin. These are red in colour. They appear and then disappear equally fast. The underlying mental anguish causing these eruptions does not last long. The skin conditions secondary to the disorder of the stomach and blood, do however, last a long time.

Coffea by nature is a rapidly effective form of treatment. It **works promptly to induce sleep when the sleeplessness is due to severe mental commotion or mental exhaustion**. Similarly, it benefits other ailments pretty rapidly also. Some of the patients of Coffea develop **hysteria**. Under the heavy emotional overlay, they lose consciousness. Their **jaws close together tightly**. Severe headache and **neuralgic pains** (trigeminal neuralgia) on the face and a tendency towards diarrhoea are also amongst the symptoms of Coffea.

Coffea patients are extremely intelligent. They react immediately when addressed. Their senses become sharp as does their **sense of hearing**. They can perceive distant sounds and voices inaudible to others. When they retire to sleep, they cannot do so. Instead, they hear the distant barking of the dogs or sounds produced by other animals. These unusual sounds intensify some of their preexisting symptoms. Interestingly enough, these patients happen to recall their good old days, including the poetry they have read in the past. Their mental capability is enhanced immensely. Their thinking is not merely superficial but their thoughts are very deep and broad. The commotion provokes their subconscious mind bringing back old memories and perception of distant sounds. They can also recall good old tastes and fragrances. All these are the happier and enjoyable components of their overall symptoms.

A Coffea patient is also very sensitive to cold. The pain inside the mouth however, benefits from ice cold water (the usual neuralgic pain does not follow any particular rule). The **toothache** of a Coffea patient definitely responds to cold application.

The face of a Coffea patient is usually not congested or flushed but in some situations the blood may rush towards the head. The face and the head then become warm, but the patient remains fairly conscious and alert. Unlike Belladonna, he is not drowsy.

Another typical sign of Coffea is that the patient feels as if something is cracking open on the back of his head.

Nux Vomica is the most effective treatment to annul the effects of Coffea. Among the Coffea symptoms in women, there is **intense genital itching**. The heartbeat is very fast, and may become irregular on hearing sudden happy or sad news. The blood pressure rises, while the urinary output decreases.

| | |
|---|---|
| Adjuvant: | Aconite |
| Antidote: | Nux Vomica |
| Potency: | 30 |

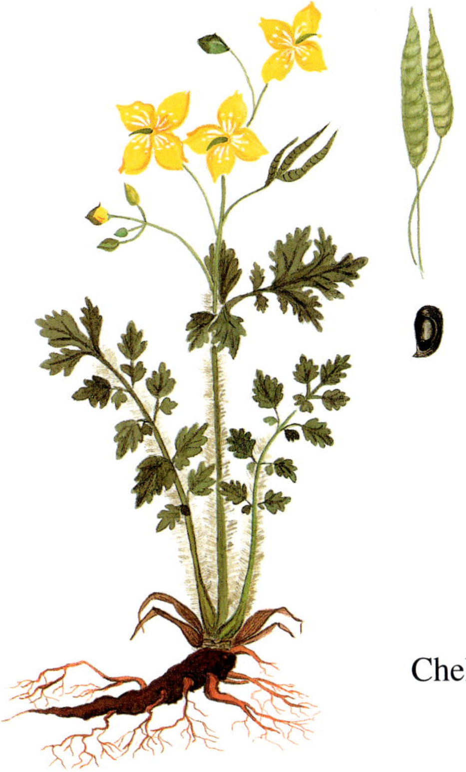

Chelidonium Majus

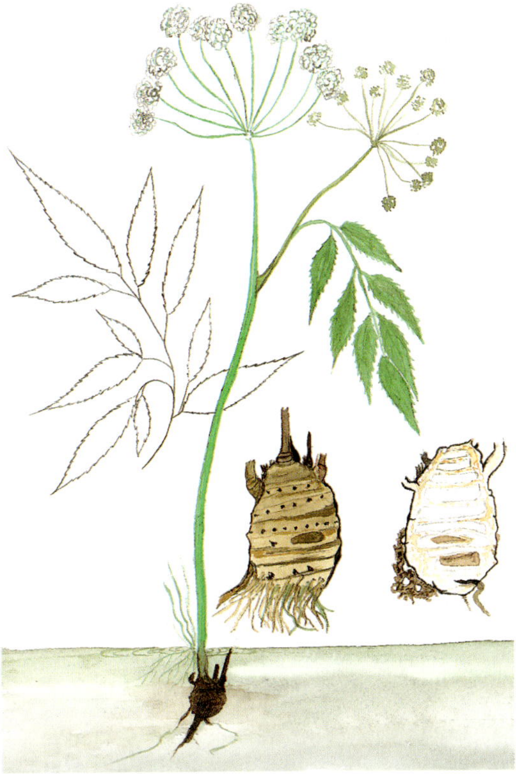

icuta Virosa

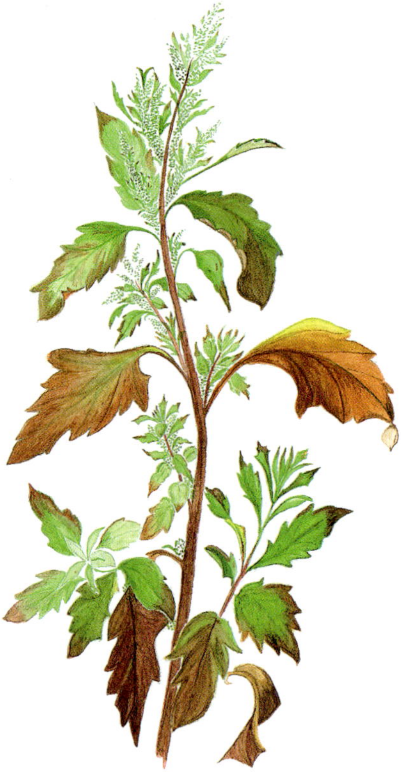

Cina

Cinchona Officinalis (China)

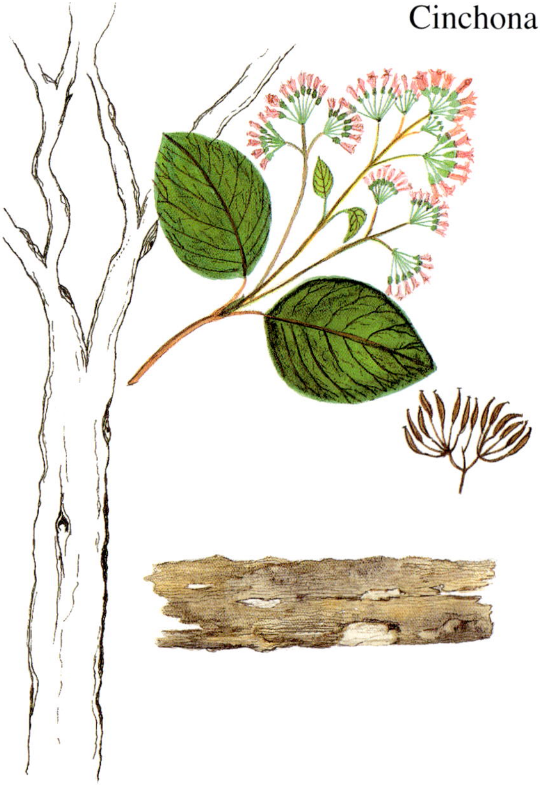

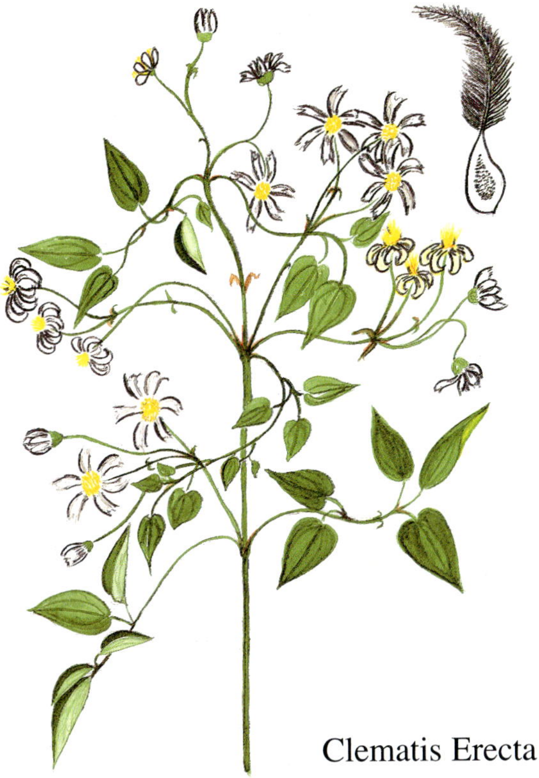

Clematis Erecta

occus Cacti

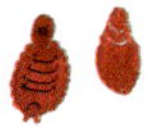

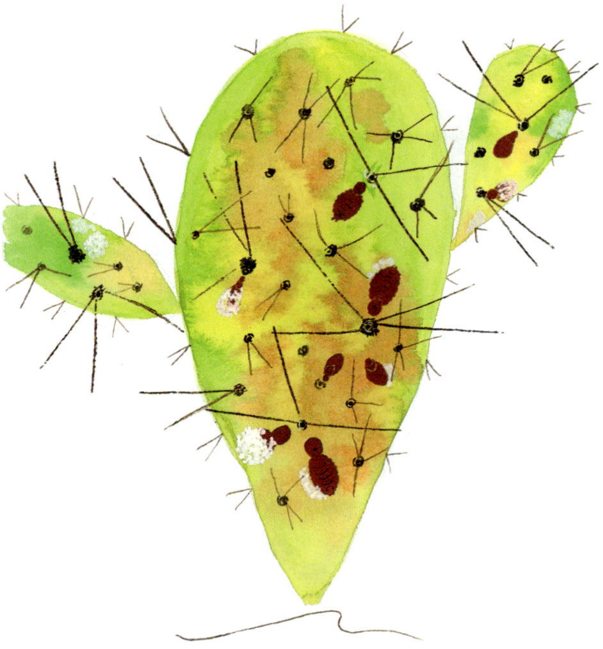

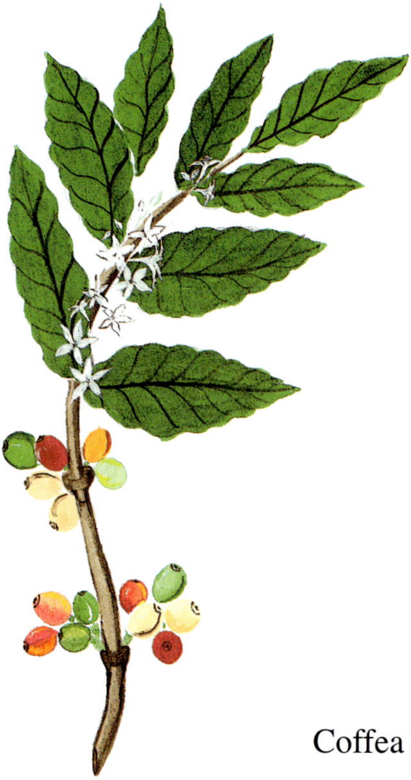

Coffea Cruda

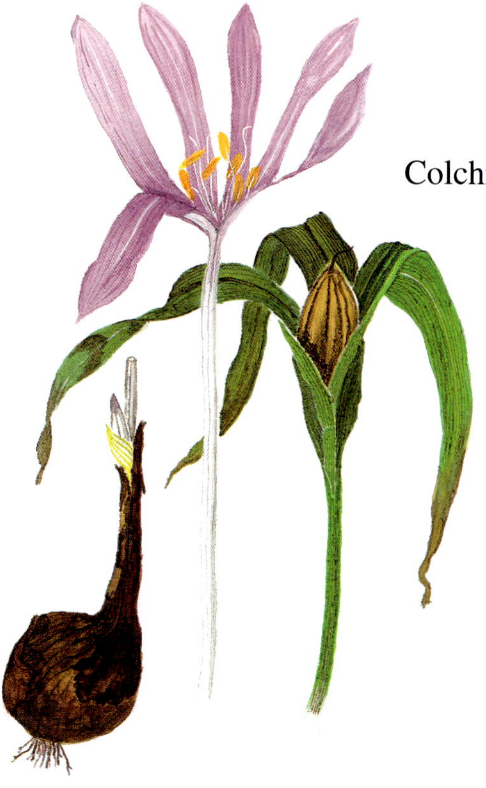

Colchicum

Colocynthis

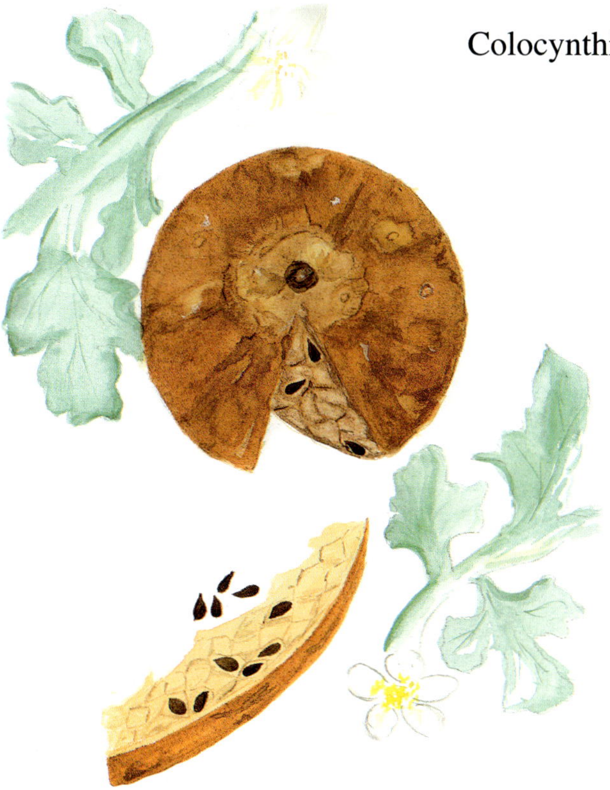

Conium Maculatum

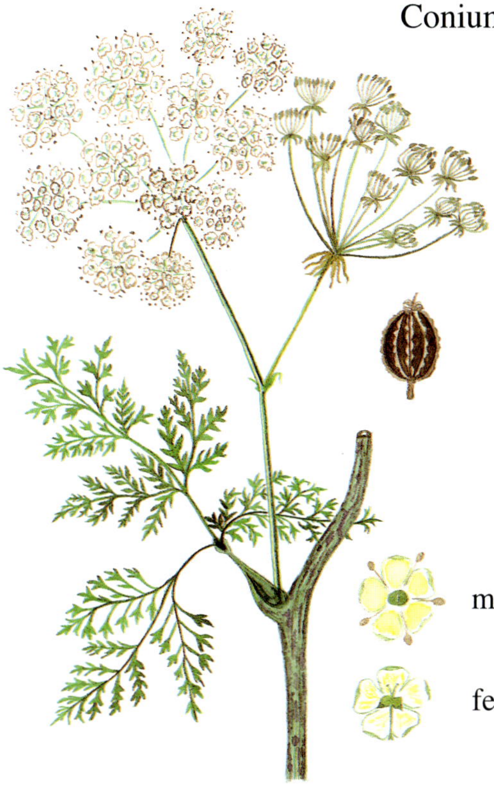

Crotalus Horridus

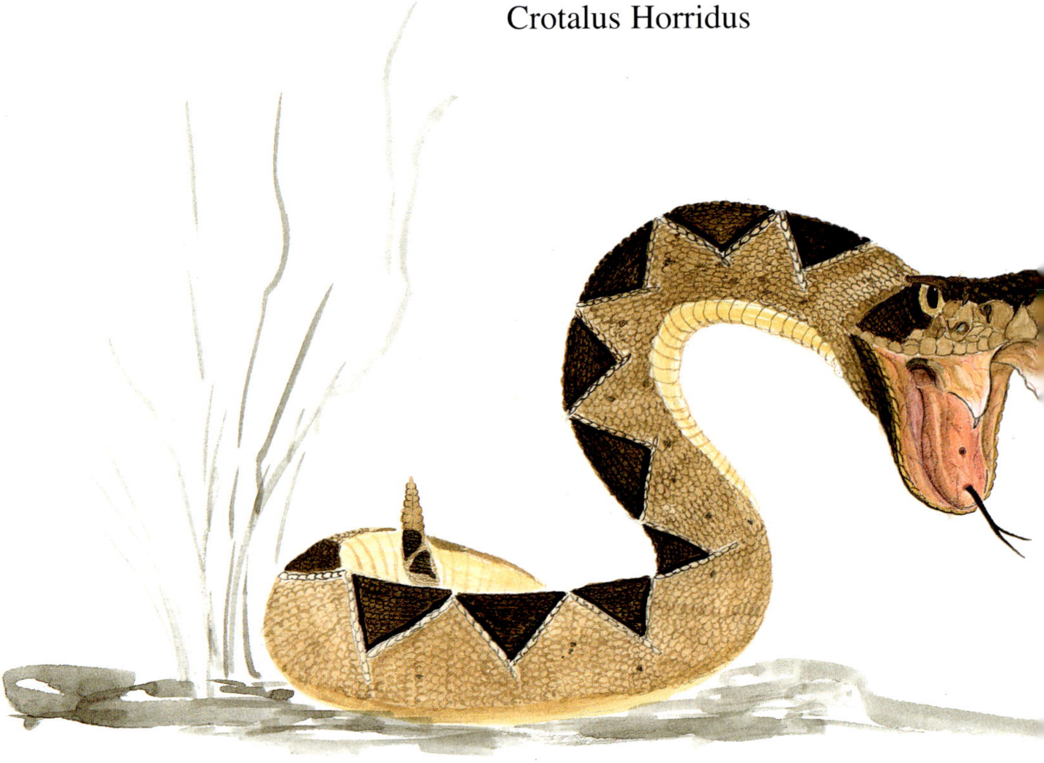

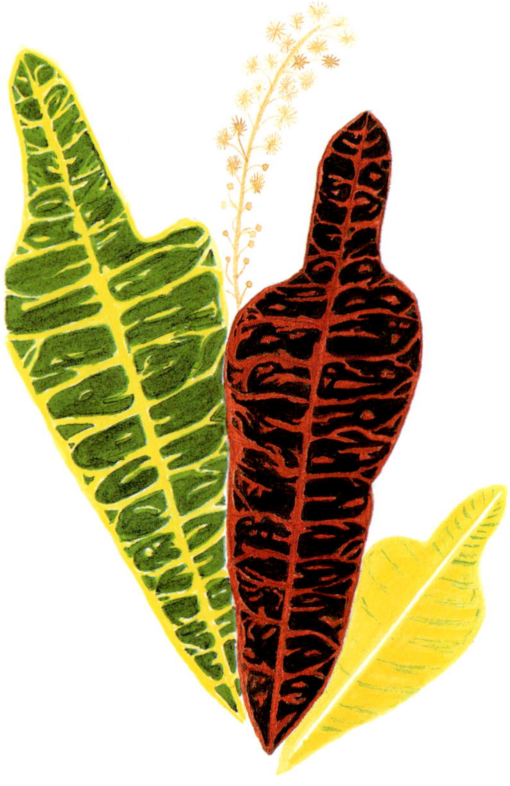

Croton Tiglit

yclamen Europaeum

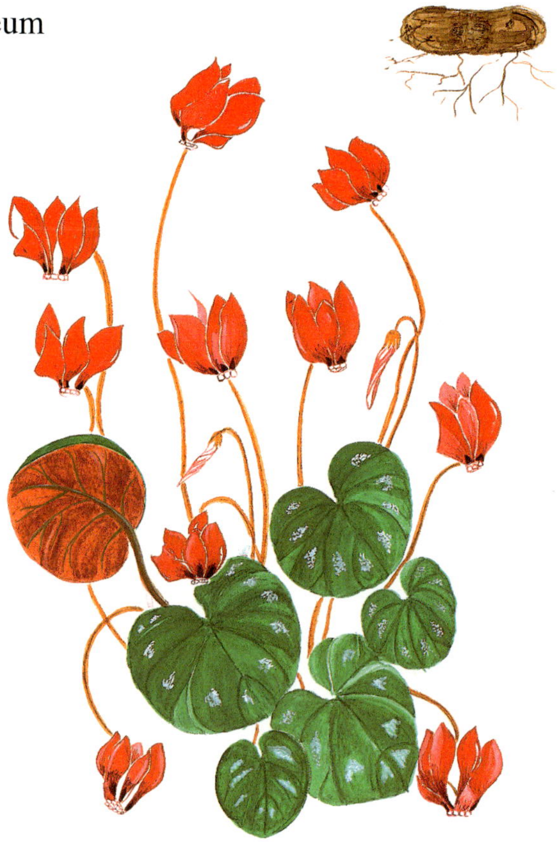

Digitalis

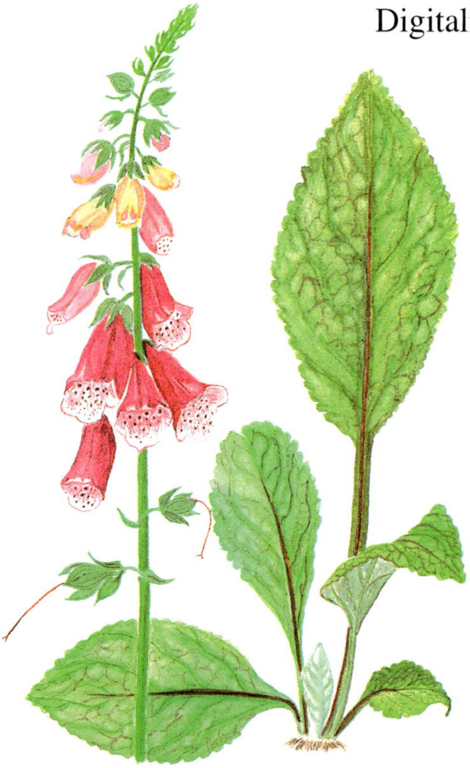

Dioscorea Villosa

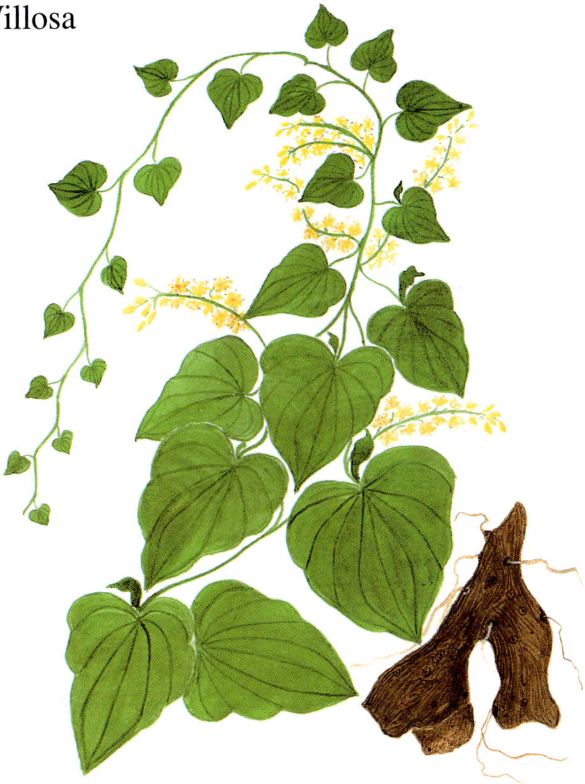

Drosera Rotundifolia

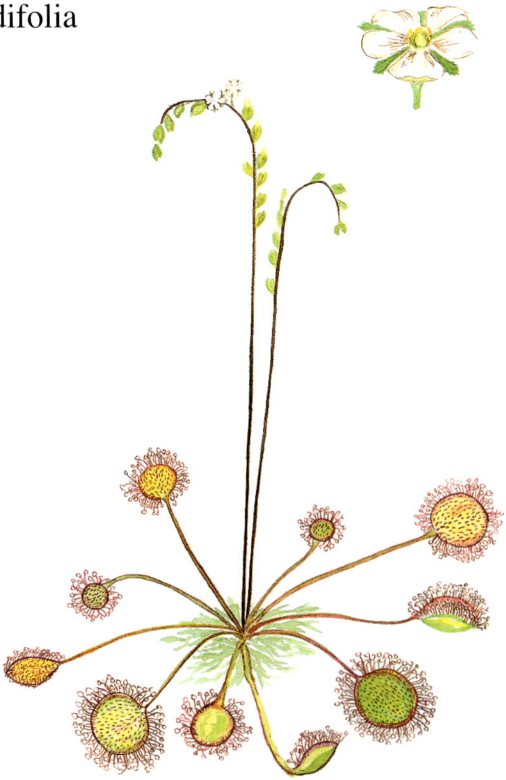

# Colchicum
## (Meadow Saffron)

This medicine is prepared from the flowers of wildly growing saffron (in the midst of green meadows). Its most salient effects are on a severe kind of gout associated with fleeting joint pains, a strong sensation of nausea from the smell of food and severe **abdominal cramps**. The patient suffers from severe offensive diarrhoea. All the symptoms intensify on the stoppage of excretions from the body. The symptoms worsen in the cold and damp weather, especially if the urinary output decreases due to kidney dysfunction or when sweating stops due to some external causes. The symptoms also aggravate in very dry, hot weather. The symptoms of gout may appear inside the eyes and on the teeth, more so when the deposits of gouty material settle on the gums.

This in general is the introduction of Colchicum. Now we will describe its symptoms related to the individual organs of the body as follows:

**The face**: The face becomes swollen, the skin feels tingly. The cheeks become red and sweaty. The temperament is of anger, like Chamomilla.

**The stomach:** Regarding the disorder of the stomach, the tongue burns and the teeth ache. The mouth is dry with the feeling of intense thirst. The smell of food, especially that of fish being cooked can cause severe nausea, so much so that the patient becomes unconscious. The stomach either feels very hot or extremely cold.

**The abdomen:** The abdomen becomes distended with wind due to severe intestinal cramping. The extreme type of distension in the abdomen is found in cattle like cows, buffalo, sheep and horses (after they have been fed fodder containing Hydrocyanic Acid). When a similarly severe distension is found in human bodies, a few pellets of Colchicum in homoeopathic from will actually work like magic. The effect is so apparent and certain that even the staunch opponent of homoeopathy cannot deny it. The kind of severe abdominal distension mentioned above compels the farmer to call for a veterinary surgeon to pierce the abdomen of the animal with a knife to let out the air, but most often the animal is always at the point of death. It has to be immediately slaughtered before it dies. Unfortunately, the scientists of today still cannot understand the effectiveness of this remedy in potency 200 or 100 which practically does not contain any material substance of the medicine, but produces an undeniably certain effect.

**The back:** There is pain in the lower part of the back radiating down to both the hips. The pain feels better on resting or on applying local pressure.

**The skin:** Rosy red spots form over the skin and there is tendency towards urticaria. In addition to severe abdominal distension and cramping, the patient passes jelly-like discharge with the stools and this is associated with tenesmus. Such patients commonly suffer from dysentery in the autumn season. The stools contain large pieces of the broken down inner lining of the intestines in the form of small pieces of tape.

There is paralysis of the function of the large gut, which is of temporary nature. This results in the inability to excrete in spite of feeling the urge. As the patient strains himself without success, other physical means need be adopted to relieve the constipation.

Rheumatic pains develop in the hands, feet, arms and the legs affecting mostly the joints. The rheumatic pains are fleeting in nature and become worse at night. The typical gout involves the big toe and the surrounding soft tissue. The overlying skin becomes wet, markedly swollen, shiny and hypersensitive to touch, even the touch of cloth over it. Such patients cut their shoes around the big toe to keep it exposed so that the pain does not aggravate too much while walking.

**The urine:** When the urine becomes scanty and is of deep brown colour mixed with blood, the joint pains become greatly aggravated.

**The heart:** If the diarrhoea is attempted to be suppressed with strong allopathic medicines, the heart may be afflicted and difficulty in breathing will ensue.

Potency: 30 or 200 but some homoeopaths use it in potency 3.

# COLOCYNTHIS

Colocynthis is very useful in the treatment of suddenly developing ailments such as **severe abdominal pain**. The abdominal pain is relentless. It doubles the patient up bending forward. The pressure due to forward bending, offers relief by pressing on the affected area. The local application of pressure and heat offers relief. Similar symptoms appear in the case of Magnesia Phos. So in an emergency situation, I advocate the use of a combination of Colocynthis and Magnesia Phos, and by the grace of God, a rapid relief will be obtained.

Colocynthis is basically the remedy for diseases of the **nervous system**. Whenever there is pain over the limbs, the adjacent muscles contract, causing the sensation of being caught in a vice. Abdominal pain is associated with cramping of the intestines. Colocynthis is related to the small nerve fibres, therefore the cramping of the intestines, the pain at the back and the arms usually remain localised, thus sparing the rest of the body. Contrary to this, the sciatica pain radiates from the back down the legs and the pain of the arm is referred to the entire extremity.

Colocynthis **pains** come in the form of an attack. Every second attack is stronger than the first one. The pain keeps slowly and steadily increasing in severity. The administration of Colocynthis offers prompt relief. Some men develop severe pains and aches due to financial loss in business or severe shock. Some women feel a boring type of pain over the ovaries, the severity of which doubles them up. The ovaries develop small tumours inside them.

While opening the bowels, the associated urination causes burning along the urethra and sometimes there is a discharge of material like the white of the egg, which smells offensive and is associated with itching. Sometimes, the patient passes small crystals in the urine, which settle on the walls of the lavatory. Sometimes, there are severe cramps in the whole of the abdomen at the time of passing urine. The susceptible patient of Colocynthis is of delicate constitution and physical appearance.

The **headache** associated with Colocynthis is very severe. Eye movement makes it worse. There is pain over the facial nerves, which feels better on the application of local pressure and heat. The use of Colocynthis offers unusually fast and effective relief. The Colocynthis pains are of undulating pattern. Every second wave of pain is stronger than the previous one, so much so that the patient screams with it and develops **hysterical fits**. A few pellets of Colocynthis in homoeopathic form offer immediate relief. The beauty of homoeopathic treatment is that it offers immediate relief in many day-to-day ailments. With the administration of Colocynthis, the pain disappears as fast as it had appeared. Colocynthis can be used for these kinds of pains, irrespective of where they are over the body. Its effect is prompt and as soon as the patient feels relief from pain, he goes to sleep.

| | |
|---|---|
| Antidotes: | Nux Vomica, Tobaccum |
| Potency: | Usually 30, but sometimes up to CM. |

# Conium Maculatum
## (Poison Hemlock)

The deadly poison Conium is derived from a plant, which in Urdu is called 'Shackran' and in Latin and English is called Hemlock. This plant grows abundantly in most regions of the world. The word Conium is derived from the Greek work Konas, which literally means "to cause dizziness". The poison produces severe vertigo. In the tenth century, this poison was also used in the treatment of diseases of lymph glands, epilepsy and whooping cough but due to its severe deleterious effects, its usage was gradually reduced and then abandoned. In the Roman and Greek empires, it was used as a legal means to cause death of the criminals subjected to capital punishment. This is the same poison that was presented to Socrates. It paralyses the entire body starting from the feet upwards. Before death, the symptoms are severe dizziness, convulsions and then progressive unconsciousness.

In homoeopathic form, Conium is used for the treatment of all the symptoms described above. Some other homoeopathic remedies, like Belladonna, Gelsemium and Cocculus are also known to be used in the treatment of vertigo, but the difference of Conium from the others is that the patient feels severe type of dizziness while lying down. The bed seems to be spinning and the slightest movement of the eye increases dizziness. Young widows or impulsive type of young women who cannot get married may start suffering from different symptom complexes including typical symptoms of dizziness due to the suppression of their emotions. If the symptom of severe dizziness is also present, Conium will relieve their other symptoms also.

Conium is also useful in the treatment of **weak eyesight**. Conium is very important in the treatment of **hardened lymph glands**, which it softens. As long as the glands do not transform into cancer, these are not painful. Without doubt, Conium is very important in the treatment of **cancer of the stomach**. The trouble is that in the early stages, the cancer of the stomach is painless. If the treatment is started late, which usually is the case, then Conium will offer only temporary relief. It makes life somewhat comfortable but it cannot totally eliminate the deep-seated roots of the cancer. Sometimes, the relief is very obvious as if the cancer has disappeared. In fact, the cancer is not cured, but is simply suppressed temporarily under the effect of Conium. It is said that the cancer reappears in three to four years, and then takes up a fatal course. The cancer should preferably not be diagnosed on the basis of gastric symptoms only. However, if somebody has the general signs and symptoms of Conium, especially vertigo, then it should be used without any delay. By doing this, the patient may be spared from cancer.

In Conium, the symptoms become worse with the cold. The glands, once enlarged, do not regress to their original size. Sometimes, the patient experiences a stabbing type of pain in the abdomen. **Blisters develop around ulcers**. The **glands swell on both sides of the neck,** descending down the sides of the body. They become hard with the progression of the disease. Even if the glands are cured, they will not revert to their previous normal size. The auxiliary glands also get swollen and tend to ulcerate. Multiple **small nodular lumps** develop in the mammary glands of women. One symptom of Baryta Carb i.e. formation of **small fatty lumps** under the skin is similar to Conium. The fatty lumps become ugly and if they do not respond to Baryta Carb, other remedies should be used, and Conium is definitely one of them.

The cancerous nodules which fungate on the surface of the skin can best be treated with a paste made out of honey. Scientific research on honey supports this observation. The new scientific research on honey is also supportive of the Quranic injunction about the extraordinary curative effect of honey.

Trembling of the body, convulsions, weakness and vertigo present the general picture of a Conium patient. The bladder becomes weak, the liver enlarges and the glands swell. A difficulty in urination and the inability to evacuate the bladder completely may very well be the sign of an enlarged prostrate gland. In this condition no delay should be permitted in initiating the use of Conium because, if the patient is constitutionally Conium, the delayed treatment may lead to cancer of the prostate. In my opinion, the best treatment of cancer of the prostate is Silicea CM. It should be given once in a fortnight, and by the grace of God, a few doses can cure the person. However, Silicea would only be useful if the general picture of the patient is that of Pulsatilla or Silicea. Regarding the nervous system, the symptoms of

Conium are a **weakness of memory** and general intellectual weakness. The patient cannot think deeply. This weakness can lead to the development of arteriosclerosis.

A Conium patient is generally very bad-tempered and irritable. He gets agitated over very trivial matters. He is restless and expresses his boredom.

A Conium patient cannot tolerate alcohol and other narcotics, which can produce quivering and mental as well as physical weakness. He also feels severe headache.

Many of the symptoms of Conium resemble those of Cocculus. In both, the patient feels dizziness, but the difference between the two is that in Conium, the dizziness is felt when the person is lying down (his bed spins around him) while in Cocculus the dizziness is noticed on standing up or on walking.

In a Conium patient, the **residual effects of severe grief** manifest in the form of intellectual weakness or loss of memory.

Wherever the symptoms and signs of Conium become apparent, the overlying skin also feels numb. The skin becomes yellowish, vesicular bumps appear, discharging malodorous exudates. In addition to actual sleep, the person starts sweating on just closing his eyes. **Drooping of the upper eyelid** is a specific symptom to Conium.

When the eyes become inflamed, they become very sensitive to light and the patient feels confounded, but in Conium even if there is no **swelling or inflammation of the eye**, the sensitivity to light is still increased and the eyes water. This is specific to Conium.

In Conium, there is a tendency towards the **formation of ulcers and chronic sores**, so much so that the ulcers of the cornea can be completely cured with Conium. The paralysis caused by Conium progresses slowly. When given on time, it prevents further spread of the disease, providing rapid cure. Once the paralysis is established, it takes a long time to get better.

Sometimes, there is paralysis of the circular fibres in the wall of the gullet, causing difficulty in swallowing. Conium is certainly one of many other remedies to be used in this condition.

Sometimes, the women experience a **sensation of heaviness and sagging of the uterus**. The paralytic state of the uterus due to grief after the death of the husband or after separation, which is slowly progressive and associated with numbness of the skin **and numbness of the hands and feet** and dizziness, then Conium must be administered. If there is an **associated inflammation of the cervix** (neck of the uterus) also, Conium will be found very effective. Even if the patient is not of the constitution of Conium, the administration of Conium will do no harm when given along with the other appropriate remedies.

Conium is also useful in the treatment of **venereal diseases** of both men and women. Conium should be the first to be utilised when the bleeding in the initial part of the menstruation is less and it is associated with cramping of the uterus. In a patient of Conium, there is a tendency towards the formation of glandular swellings and lumps in the breast and over the entire body. These nodules gradually keep on forming without any apparent sign of cancer.

| | |
|---|---|
| Potency: | Usually 30, but in deep established diseases, where there is a danger of cancer formation, it is given in CM potency and it is found to be very effective. |

# Crotalus Horridus
## (Rattle Snake)

This remedy is prepared from the venom of a very poisonous and dangerous type of snake commonly called the rattlesnake. The snake keeps on constantly rubbing its body producing a rattle-like sound. This snake is found in almost all the countries of the world, especially in the deserts and rocky areas that abound in salt in the soil. The snake likes to live in moist areas where it stays asleep. When stepped on by somebody or by its prey, it attacks suddenly. Its poison is very quick in action. The face of the patient becomes extremely fearful and dreadful, and he dies within no time at all. Mostly, there is no time for treatment to be administered. The farmers in the province of Sindh in Pakistan are quoted to say that when this snake bites, it seems to tell its victim to fall away from him so as not to crush him, since death is so instantaneous.

The effects of the snakebite are generally very long lasting and show up in the spring season. The snakes, which normally hibernate in the cold weather, become active in this season. After hibernation, when they become active, their poison is very deadly. In case the person bitten by a snake happens to survive, due to a relatively small dose of the poison, his symptoms reactivate in that particular season again and this happens repeatedly every year. In the spring season, snakebite wounds start hurting and the ailments related to the snakebite are aggravated. The spring season is known for **allergies** of many kinds, which respond to the treatment with Lachesis prepared from the snake venom. It does not do equally well on everybody rather, other remedies also need to be given. Apart from Crotalus, Alumina and Sabadilla can be useful but Lachesis is the most effective.

The main effect of Crotalus is on the liver. By the grace of Allah it will rapidly control progressive **jaundice**. The patient of Crotalus is extremely nervous and tremulous. The tongue also quivers when pulled out of the mouth. The patient feels tired on simple movement. Paralysis develops. The **blood becomes dark** in colour and exudes from everywhere, especially the junctional areas, where the outer skin and the inner lining meet. **Sudden severe illnesses like paralysis and spontaneous bleeding** from any part of the body should remind one of the snakebite. The exuding blood is liquid and of dark colour. Within the circulatory system, the blood coagulates like the curdling of milk. The blood that exudes is like dirty water mixed with blood. In the case of some other snakebites, the venom, rather than clotting the blood, makes it thin. This kind of venom affects specifically the nervous system.

Crotalus is very useful in the treatment of **strange mental conditions** like delirium, **mumbling** and shortness of temper. When somebody wants to talk to the patient, he will immediately interrupt, shut him up and then start talking himself. He cannot tolerate anybody else talking in his presence. In order to continue the conversation, he will devise some story, but will definitely cut everybody else's conversation. Excessive talking is also noticed in a patient of Lachesis whose conversation is irregular and confusing. A patient of Crotalus also talks very fast and keeps on making stories, but he is not mentally aggressive. Rather, he is slow and tends to be sleepy. He is fearful of death, tends to cry and experiences cold sweats. The **headache** and **dizziness** alternate. When resting, he suffers from headache, and when moving he feels dizzy. **Sleep aggravates** the symptoms, especially the headache which becomes very severe. Sometimes, the patient wakes up due to a headache that he did not have before he went to bed. Raising the head up also aggravates the suffering. Waves of severe headache undulate from the back to the front of the head, resulting in severe weakness.

Whenever the patient of snakebite suffers from some special illness, dark offensive blood exudes from the previous snakebite wounds, especially in the spring season. In the presence of diabetes, large dangerous kind of **abscesses** (carbuncles) form on the neck and the back, which spread rapidly and deep into the tissues. There is associated marked swelling around them. Crotalus would be very useful for the treatment of both these conditions. In such carbuncles Arsenic and Anthracinum are also effective. When women develop **typhoid during pregnancy** resulting in abortion, Crotalus will prevent against the subsequent possible complications.

In Crotalus, sometimes, the patient either sleeps too much or does not sleep at all and both these conditions alternate with each other. When drowsy, it is difficult for him to get up. Once he is awake, it is difficult for him to go back to sleep.

One thing is common in Crotalus and other snake venoms that the patient becomes **suspicious minded**. He does not trust anybody and thinks that somebody will poison him. The patient has a strong desire to drink alcohol. The best **treatment to break the habit of drinking alcohol** is Sulphuric Acid i.e., one drop of Sulphuric Acid dissolved in a glass of water, given three times a day. Crotalus is ideal remedy for a grossly obese alcoholic who has a craving for spicy food.

The eyes of a Crotalus patient are yellowish, with the appearance of **dark rings around the eyes**. The eyes have burning pain as if somebody has pierced them with a knife. There is a tendency to bleed inside the eye. The **vision becomes hazy**. Sometimes, due to extreme weakness, the eyesight may be totally lost. **Light is unbearable** (photophobia).

There is **bleeding from the ears**. The right ear becomes deaf due to the **affliction of the nerves of the ears**. The dysfunction of the ears causes vertigo. There is mild earache, throbbing sensation and hypersensitivity to loud noise. In Crotalus, **the nasal discharge** is mixed with blood. There can be a nosebleed (Epistaxis), the blood being dark and clotted in the form of woven thread. The lips swell and become numb, the face also becomes pale and swollen. The dryness of the tongue and the throat makes speaking and swallowing difficult. The tongue is red, dry and swollen. When such a patient develops **cancer of the tongue**, the condition would warrant the use of Crotalus.

A Crotalus patient cannot tolerate any kind of clothing around the stomach area. His stomach cannot hold anything and it throws up its contents. The material thrown up contains bile. The **vomiting** may be of pure blood. The stomach feels empty. Either the patient is **constipated** or has **diarrhoea**. The diarrhoeal stools are dark in colour, rather thin, but smell offensive and are mixed with blood. The urine is red or yellowish in colour. The kidneys become inflamed. There is a pain in the liver area. The heart feels weak but beats fast. The pulse is generally very rapid or becomes very weak.

**Joint pains** are also a symptom of Crotalus. The glands become swollen. The hands and feet also swell and there is stiffness and pain in the toes. The headache and stomach symptoms get better in the open but the cough becomes more severe. The entire body shakes, the skin becomes hypersensitive and pale in colour with the tendency towards boils. The face is pale and listless. If a girl fails to have periods and her face becomes covered with acne then Crotalus would be the ideal remedy for this condition. This will restore her periods and reduce the congestion on her face.

Crotalus is not only an acute remedy in fact it is very useful in the treatment of chronic illnesses also. When the **body becomes weak**, the hands shake and **tremors** develop in the middle-aged people, Crotalus would not only be found useful, but its use becomes unavoidable.

The symptoms of a patient of Crotalus become worse when lying on the right side. There is a feeling of intense cold in the stomach and in the abdomen, as if ice has been placed over them. This sensation can be an early sign of **cancer** of the intestines or stomach. Timely use of Crotalus will obviate the formation of cancer. Such symptoms must well be kept in mind to avoid unnecessary complications.

Crotalus is also used for the treatment of wind in the stomach and **stomach ulcers**. Crotalus can cure the excessive bleeding originating from the **cancer of the uterus**. The eyes of such a patient become pale as if she has developed jaundice. This is a typical sign of Crotalus. The **weakness of the heart** is also a sign of Crotalus. This symptom is found in almost all the cases of poisoning due to snakebites. In particular, there is a feeling of the trembling of the heart during the menstrual period. The hands also shake and become swollen. The legs become numb and there is a possibility of developing left-sided paralysis of the body (hemiplegia). The **menstrual periods last longer than usual**. Severe pain radiates down the legs. There is a feeling of **weakness of the stomach**. There is excessive bleeding and a feeling of prolapse of the uterus after the childbirth. Due to severe stiffness and pain, the patient feels great discomfort over the legs and keeps moving the legs constantly.

| | |
|---|---|
| Antidotes: | Lachesis, Camphor |
| Potency: | 30 to 200 |

# Croton Tiglium
## (Croton Oil Seed)

Croton Tiglium is a very well known purgative. Its patient develops sudden diarrhoea associated with griping and a continuous urge to pass stools. As a result, the patient becomes very weak. The skin symptoms of Croton resemble those of Rhus Tox. Blisters full of secretions form over the skin along with an itching and burning sensation. One noticeable difference between Croton and Rhus Tox is that in Rhus Tox when the eczema gets better, the healthy skin appears underneath. Next time, the **blisters** do not form at the same place. Afterwards, if the eczema returns, the previously affected part may become eczematous as well. In Croton, the blisters will form over the previously healed healthy areas leading to the development of an obstinate type of eczema.

Rhus Tox and Croton affect the intestines similarly. Croton is very useful in the treatment of **chronic dysentery and diarrhoea**. Unlike Rhus Tox and other anti-diarrhoeal remedies, the diarrhoea in a patient of Croton is sudden and propulsive. When children develop diarrhoea soon after taking milk, Croton would be the most probable remedy. The **nausea** in Croton is like that of Ipecacuanha. In Ipecacuanah, however, there is only nausea but no vomiting. In the case of Croton, there is nausea and diarrhoea but no vomiting.

In Croton, the **stomach distends with wind** and there is rumbling noise in the intestines. It feels as if the intestines are full of fluid. The stomach feels empty and hungry. In Croton, the skin and the abdominal symptoms alternate with each other.

A variety of eye symptoms are also found in Croton. The **eyes become red and sore**. Pimples and blisters form over the swollen eyelids. These symptoms are also noticed in other homoeopathic remedies but when there is inflammation of the intestines (Enteritis), the most likely remedy is Croton. In Croton, the eyes sink back due to dehydration. In Paris Quadrifolia this very symptom may be related to a wider range of ailments, so much so that the women can feel as if threads are being pulled out of their breasts causing severe pain, which makes sleeping difficult at night. Croton and Paris differ with each other. In the former, there is diarrhoea while in the latter there is no diarrhoea. In Croton, there is a feeling of pull with a rope under the umbilicus. This kind of sensation is also noticed in Plumbum.

Regarding **eczema** in children, especially the kind involving the scalp, Croton and Sepia work very much alike. But the typical symptoms of Croton would differentiate the picture from that of Sepia.

There is a variety of homoeopathic remedies related to the **eczema over the genital organs**. Croton is on the top of the list. Rhus Tox, Anagallis and Graphites are also famous in the treatment of this kind of eczema. The blisters in Croton are smaller than those of Rhus Tox. Similarly the fluid content of the blisters is also less in Croton. Croton and Rhus Tox work as antidote to each other. In Rhus Tox there is no diarrhoea.

The panacea for the treatment of the severe kind of diarrhoea resulting from Croton is Podophyllum. In Podophyllum too, the **stools** squirt out forcefully. The itching associated with Croton is best treated with Rhus Tox.

Anagallis is well renowned for the treatment of **itching of the palms**. The **itching and eczema** of Rhus Tox is usually on the **back of the hand**. Anagallis is the treatment for a similar condition of the palms of the hands. Burning is milder in the case of Anagallis compared to Rhus Tox. The reappearance of the eczema of Anagallis over the previously affected area resembles the similar tendency in Croton.

The ailments of Croton get worse in hot weather. The patient is restless, confused and sallow. There is a feeling of severe pressure and pain on the forehead. There is a feeling of **heaviness in the head and vertigo**. The cough may also provoke an attack of Asthma. The patient starts **coughing** as soon as he puts his head on the pillow. The patient cannot lie down and finds it impossible to take a deep breath.

Croton should not be forgotten in treating **discharging** ears with severe itching. A feeling of burning in the food pipe (oesophagus) is also a specific sign of Croton. The stomach feels weak.

In Croton, **the urine is frothy and of orange colour at night**. When settled, sticky particles rise to the surface. During the daytime, the urine is yellowish in colour and contains white particles.

In Croton, the symptoms aggravate on eating, touching the affected area and at night.

| | |
|---|---|
| Antidotes: | .Antimonium Tart, Rhus Tox, Podophyllum |
| Potency: | 30 to 200 or up to 1000 |

# CUPRUM METALLICUM
## (Copper Metal)

Copper is a metal of reddish brown colour, which is utilized to make various instruments, weapons and electric wires. It is soft in consistency, so it is mixed with other metals to make different alloys. These alloys have proved useful due to their differences, particularly in industry. The people working with Copper gradually start developing the symptoms of Copper poisoning, such as severe abdominal colic, cholera, cough and convulsions. The homoeopathic remedy prepared from the Copper powder is called Cuprum.

**Convulsions** are the most prominent characteristic of Cuprum and one cannot think of Cuprum without them. The convulsions are very severe and unbearable; the patient in agony wishes to die. Severe convulsions and tightness are uniformly present in any ailment of Cuprum and this condition affects all the muscles of the body. Cuprum will prove very useful in the treatment of **epilepsy and cholera**, especially when associated with convulsions and blue coloration of skin. During a convulsion, the hands form into a tight fist. Similarly, the feet twist downwards. The severe contractions of the hands and feet then proceed upward towards the legs and the arms and then the entire body becomes stiff and contracted.

Sometimes, the spasmodic condition affects the blood vessels going to the brain, as a result of which the patient talks absurdly, **loses his memory** and can become delirious or even unconscious. The muscles exhibit tonic contractions and convulsions. There is twitching and fasciculation of the muscles. The **jerking of the muscles** is on the side opposite to the one the patient lies on. In Cimicifuga, the twitching is on the same side as the person is lying on. The stiffness of the entire body associated with **unconsciousness** as in epilepsy is a typical sign of Cuprum. However, if a person is unconscious but the twitching is only on one part of the body or another, without generalised rigidity, the patient is not one of Cuprum.

Cuprum is also very useful in the treatment of **whooping cough and asthma**. In my opinion, Cuprum must be used to treat the convulsions associated with coughing and asthma. Cuprum offers prompt effective relief when the patient feels the spasmodic contraction of the windpipe (trachea) in warm weather, becoming better on the local application of ice or something cold. The spastic tightness at the sides and the lower part of the chest is very troublesome. The patient feels as if he is going to die. There is a stabbing type of pain starting from the chest going towards the back. In fact, this results from the convulsion and Cuprum works magically to relieve it. Keeping this in mind, Cuprum is also useful in the treatment of **biliary colic** and convulsions.

When an old person happens to marry after a long period of celibacy, he may experience convulsions, which may radiate upward towards the legs and then back after sexual intercourse. Cuprum is the best treatment for this condition.

Cuprum is the ideal remedy for treating the **convulsions during menstruation**, which start from the fingers and then spread through the entire body. The body becomes rigid. If there is unconsciousness, **delirium** and the eyes become fixed directed upwards, Cuprum should be administered promptly. Cuprum is the best remedy for treating epilepsy in which the **headache** starts from the nape of the neck and then radiates towards the forehead. There is an element of frequent convulsions and jerking of the fingers, making the patient scream. There is incontinence of urine or faeces.

Cuprum works equally well for relieving the violent contractions of the muscles which bend the joints or make the joints straight (i.e. the flexor and extensor muscles). The contractions of these muscles cause severe pain, but when the muscles become completely flaccid, they cannot be put into use under command (voluntarily). An epileptic patient of Cuprum usually suffers from severe headache following convulsions.

Sometimes, a woman **loses her eyesight at the time of childbirth** due to the rupture of a blood vessel supplying the brain, which can lead to permanent blindness. However, in Cuprum, the **blindness is transitory**, because it is due to the spasmodic narrowing of the blood vessels, rather than the rupture of these vessels. Transitory blindness observed at the time of childbirth in the presence of other signs and symptoms of Cuprum will, by God's grace, be definitely benefited with Cuprum, which will also **facilitate the childbirth**.

Some conditions pertaining to the mind are very evident in the patient of Cuprum. The patient is inflexible, remains sad, and keeps on uttering words that he really does not mean. The mind feels empty. There is headache, and a noticeable reddish blue hue and inflammation. The patient feels as if hot water is being poured over his head. There is severe vertigo and the head seems to be sagging forwards. There is **severe pain at the forehead, temples and the nape**, which is aggravated on application of local pressure, and there is pallor of the face with a bluish tinge. The patient remains lost in deep thoughts. The lips are bluish and during the unconscious state, the jaws lock tightly and there is frothing at the mouth. The nose becomes heavily congested with blood. The sense of smell is lost, and there is a metallic taste in the mouth. The patient spits a lot. The tongue becomes paralysed, and the person starts stammering. The patient protrudes his tongue like a snake, contracted and narrow.

One sign of Cuprum is the **hiccuping**, which results from the spasm of the diaphragm. Drinking cold water would relieve the nausea and vomiting. **Nausea and vomiting** occur on exposure to the cold. Severe abdominal colic, frequent scanty stools associated with severe attacks of convulsions, distention of the abdomen, which hurts on light pressure or touch, and the drawing in sensation of the abdomen are all signs of Cuprum.

Cuprum is one of the three commonly used remedies for cholera. Its distinguishing features are very obvious and easily recognisable. In cholera, the colic starts in the stomach which is very severe, but the stools though diarrhoeal are interrupted and scanty rather than free. There is violent twisting of the hands and feet but the cramps of the calves are much more severe than any other kind of cramps. Along with these spasmodic signs, there is generalised bluing of the body establishing the diagnosis of Cuprum. Other two remedies used for cholera are Camphor and Veratrum Album.

Sometimes, young girls experience **severe tightness over the back and the abdomen** during their periods. If these cramps migrate to the calves, Cuprum would be the most appropriate remedy. In this condition, the patient has mild nausea and diarrhoea too. The occurrence of epileptic fit during menstruation is also a sign of Cuprum. If this condition is observed at the appearance of new moon, then Silicea would be found more useful.

| | |
|---|---|
| Adjuvant: | Calcarea Carb |
| Antidotes: | Camphor, Belladonna, Hepar Sulph, Staphysagria, |
| Potency: | From 30 to 200 |

# Cyclamen Europaeum

Cyclamen Europaeum is prepared from the root of a plant famous for the bizarre stories surrounding it.

Cyclamen is the remedy full of conflicting qualities. Its patient does not want to move at all, even though movement relieves his symptoms. The patient is afraid of going into the open although the open air relieves his symptoms, especially those of cold and cough. His desire not to move or walk around is based on the **weakness of his body**. Associated with this remedy are the symptoms of severe diarrhoea and vomiting, severe stomach upset, and a salty taste in the mouth. In women, the menstruation becomes irregular. **Periods become more frequent, copious in amount and the blood is black and clotted**. With movement, the bleeding becomes less. All these are signs of Cyclamen. Cyclamen is very important in the treatment of progressive anaemia resulting from excessive menstrual bleeding. Both sexes can have various kinds of disorders of the urinary system and of sexual weakness.

The Cyclamen patient is very restless at night. He **feels weak on walking**, although, walking relieves his aches and pains to some extent.

In a patient of Cyclamen, the **mental state fluctuates**. Out of sudden happiness, he may become delirious or then feel tired and down. His mind is empty. He does not even want to speak. He is irritable and hates to do anything.

A female Cyclamen patient feels lonely and presumes that everybody is talking ill of her. A number of young girls have the same feeling. I have tried Sulphur and Stramonium to treat such girls, but did not find any obvious beneficial effects. Perhaps, Cyclamen could have been useful.

In Cyclamen, the **headache** is very severe. It feels as if the head is going to explode. It starts in the morning. The patient sees stars before the eyes. The eyesight becomes blurred. A peculiar type of **eye squint,** in which the eyeballs turn inwards, is very amenable to treatment with Cyclamen. The eyes feel warm. There is **double vision** (diplopia). At times, the eye conditions can be secondary to the stomach upset. The pupils become dilated. Half of the field of vision

is lost (hemianopia) and spots of different colours appear before the eyes.
In Cyclamen the **right ear hurts**, feeling drawn in. Thundering noises are heard in the ears so the hearing is also affected.

In Cyclamen, there is a feeling of **burning, dryness and scraping** in the throat. The patient does not usually feel thirsty, but during a fever, especially in the evening, he feels very thirsty.

The **stomach symptoms** of Cyclamen are comparable to those of Pulsatilla. The patient hates fatty food. His stomach feels hot and burns and is much worse after drinking coffee. A typical symptom of Cyclamen is that every time the patient drinks coffee, he will have diarrhoea. The hiccuping associated with stomach upset is also a characteristic of Cyclamen. Cyclamen is similar to Gelsemium regarding the feeling of the dryness of the mouth, lack of thirst and **excessive urination**. Usually, the patient also sweats much less, however, while sick, he sweats a lot. The **quantity of the urine is much increased**. The urine is colourless like water and passed frequently.

The **phlegm** in a patient of Cyclamen is **whitish**. It means that the invasion by the bacteria has not been severe and the obvious infection has not been established. In Cyclamen, the patient experiences a **suffocating cough**.

The superficial bones hurt. There is **severe cramping of the right thumb and the index finger**, which becomes worse on writing. The **heel of the foot throbs like an abscess**. Sometimes this kind of pain may be associated with the formation of bone spurs which need needing prolonged treatment as a result of which, the excessive outgrowth of the bone may stop. Once these spurs develop to a significant size, surgery is indicated. The remedies implied to relieve this kind of heel pain are Arnica, Ledum, Ruta, Calcarea Flour, Rhus Tox, as well as Calcarea Carb.

In Cyclamen, scratching relieves the itching. The itchiness (pruritis) is relieved at the onset of menstruation.

| | |
|---|---|
| Potency | 30 to 200 |

# Digitalis

Digitalis is a renowned form of treatment used frequently in the diseases of the heart. In allopathy, it is used to control rapid heartbeat (tachychardia), as well as an irregular heartbeat (arrhythmia). It slows down the pulse rate and controls its irregularity. However, it has to be used for longer periods with increasing dosage, but its beneficial effects last only for a short period. Since it needs to be given in more and more amounts, it can accumulate in the body and cause an injurious effect. Under these circumstances, all allopathic doctors are compelled to stop this medication. As soon as it is stopped, the beating of the heart becomes extremely fast and uncontrollable again. The power of the heart muscles becomes like an ineffective flutter after which the heart starts to fail. In fact, the slowing of the heart is a temporary effect. It does not increase the strength of the muscles of the heart. It only restricts the heartbeat to a certain limit. The result is that these muscles, gradually, fail completely. Fluid starts accumulating in the lungs due to the backlog of blood that cannot be satisfactorily pumped through the valves of the heart. The obvious result is that the person cannot breathe (cardiac dyspnoea). The homoeopathic use of Digitalis, however, is without these dangers. In fact, it is a very useful and good cardiac tonic.

The homoeopathic form of Digitalis works in every heart patient in whom the liver function has also been deranged and the pulse has become light and weak. It also has a beneficial effect on the function of the liver, spleen, as well as the lungs. Homoeopathic use of Digitalis should not be abandoned for the reason that its allopathic use is not completely successful. It must always be remembered in the **treatment of heart diseases**. According to Dr. Kent, who has been practising allopathy for a long time, the misuse of Digitalis has resulted in more deaths than saving lives. Its action is very short-lived. It deteriorates the heart muscles and knocks out the conducting system of the heart. This comment of his does not apply to the homoeopathic use of Digitalis but unfortunately, some homoeopathic doctors are still very fearful of using it.

One thing to remember is that in Digitalis, the patient does not have a fever, except occasionally. The pulse is slow; the liver is enlarged and tender to touch. Once the liver dysfunction has set in, the stools become either light-coloured or clay-coloured. The patient may have jaundice. There is a feeling of emptiness and a sinking sensation over the stomach. This particular symptom is noted only in a few remedies. The patient of Sulphur also feels weakness however, he will find relief on taking food. But in Digitalis, food does not relieve the symptoms. This particular sensation is not due to a stomach upset, but it is due to the weakness of the heart (sinking of the heart). It is an established fact that sometimes the pain due to the heart is perceived over the stomach or in the left, upper part of the abdomen, so much so that even the expert cardiologist may not be able to diagnose it in time. Similarly, some stomach problems may be referred to the heart and will not respond to treatment with cardiac medication.

If the food increases rather than decreases the discomfort at the stomach and the blood pressure rises, this is a symptom of a heart problem and of Digitalis.

In Digitalis, the patient is very **restless during his sleep**. He experiences nightmares in which he observes many frightful scenes, a sensation of falling down and a desire to run. He dreams of falling from heights. In fact, it is the sinking of the heart that results in the dreams of falling down. During his sleep, the **patient may feel jolted** due to the weakness of his heart and nervous system. As soon as he goes to sleep, sudden jolting wakes him up (similar to Grindelia).

In Digitalis, there is bluish discoloration on the face due to the disturbance of the blood circulation. The hands and feet also become cyanotic, while in Grindelia, there is no such symptom. However, blue coloration is found in Cuprum also, which is due to the other ailments rather than due to the weakness of the heart.

In Digitalis, the pulse is slow at the onset of disease, but later on becomes fast. If the basic symptoms of Digitalis are present it will be the most appropriate medication, even if the pulse is very rapid to start with. Its use should not be discarded due to the rapidity of the pulse. In general, the pulse is weak in Digitalis, yet it may be fast at times. In Arsenic, the pulse is rapid but thready and tense.

Digitalis is also useful in the treatment of heart problems arising out of grief. The heart flutters or may even be felt to be stopping altogether. There is intense restlessness. The feeling that the **heart is going to**

**stop** is typical of Digitalis. Digitalis would cure the cough due to heart failure (cardiac dyspnoea). It does not work on the cough arising primarily from lung diseases. Sometimes, the patient wakes up from sleep due to the feeling of suffocation even without any obvious jerking. This means that the sensation of the breathing being about to stop was due to the disturbance of the automatic system of breathing (Herring Breaur reflex). When the respiration rate starts decreasing progressively, the patient must be awakened periodically or he may die in the state of sleep. A progressive slowing down of the breathing is also a sign of the gastric patient. This is due to the build-up of pressure in the stomach, pressing on the diaphragm. The difference is that in a heart patient this condition is constant, while in a gastric patient the condition is occasional and noticed during gastric upset. A feeling of suffocation or choking is also seen in Lachesis, Phosphorus and Carbo Vegetabilis.

Unfortunately, the use of Digitalis has been attached to heart disease only, so most physicians do not consider using it for any other kind of ailment. Yet, it is a strong and effective treatment for an **enlarged prostate** in older age. The enlargement of the prostate at any age has been found to respond well to Sabal Serrulata and Chimaphila in Mother Tincture form. However, this form of treatment should be continued for a long period. Also, Belladonna, Arsenic and Thuja in high potency have also proved to be useful. However, if the prostatic problem is associated with a heart ailment then Digitalis should be the first choice. It makes the prostate gland gradually shrink back to normal size. In fact, very few medicines have the capability of reducing the size of enlarged glands. So, Digitalis should be used in low potency of 30 over a long period. Such conditions that establish and progress gradually will not respond to the high potency but will respond well to lower potency used over a longer period. The potency may, however, be increased later on. In my practice, I have used Digitalis in potency 30. I have not found it necessary to use a higher potency. But, if the original relief offered by Digitalis 30 has stopped, it should be tried in higher potency.

**Loss of appetite and intense thirst** are peculiar to Digitalis. Sometimes, as in Colchicum, even the smell of food may suppress the appetite altogether, yet in Digitalis, unlike Colchicum, there is no vomiting or tendency to become unconscious. The thirst flares up while the appetite gradually disappears. This symptom is common in the liver diseases and jaundice. If the constitutional symptoms of Digitalis are found in the patient, Digitalis alone may be curative.

The restlessness of Digitalis is even worse than that of Arsenic. The restlessness of Arsenic intensifies on lying down or remaining still in one position, while the restlessness of Digitalis is constant. It does not decrease by taking rest or by physical movement. If restlessness is due to the progressive weakness of the heart muscles, Digitalis alone should be administered. I am of the opinion that the deleterious effects on the heart resulting from excessive prolonged allopathic use of Digitalis may be treatable with high potency like Digitalis CM, although I have not experimented this in my practice. I suggest that if at all a homoeopathic doctor wants to try this, he may do so only on a patient in moribund state with no apparent hope of survival, and that too, after getting permission from the patient and his relatives.

Itching is also found in Digitalis. Red spots appear on the back. Symptoms are made worse on **sitting tiptoes after food or listening to music**, whereas the open air and empty stomach ameliorate the symptoms. Camphor relieves the ill effects of Digitalis. China is not compatible with Digitalis. So China and Digitalis should only be used one after the other with utmost care. Crataegus happens to be an important adjuvant medicine.

**Potency:** 30

# Dioscorea Villosa
## (Wild Yam)

Dioscorea is prepared from the thick voluminous root of the wild yam plant that commonly grows in Africa. Dioscorea is an important, commonly used medicine. It best works on the gall bladder, especially on **biliary colic associated with stones in the gall bladder**, if other symptoms of Dioscorea are present.

A peculiar sign is that the colicky pain may be over the gall bladder or on any part of the abdomen. It becomes worse on pressure, while yawning relieves the pain by decreasing pressure on the affected area. The **dysentery is associated with severe gripe**. The patient of Dioscorea feels better on walking about because it relieves the pressure inside the abdomen. The pain radiates towards the back and the shoulders like waves. In Dioscorea, **the pain is always of radiating nature**. The spastic pain of the gall bladder (colic) can be referred over the chest and to the shoulders or even on the arms and the hands. The pain of renal colic usually refers towards the liver. Similarly, the severe pain of the piles also radiates towards the liver. The colicky pain of the stomach radiates towards the heart. Dioscorea is useful in all such symptoms and ailments. Until the proper treatment for the gall bladder becomes known, I always include Dioscorea as an essential part of my formulary.

In Cactus too, the radiation of the undulating type of pain from the affected area to other organs is a essential symptom. But, the diagnosis of Cactus is based on different symptoms altogether, for example, waves of pain produced by spasm in the membranes of the brain or external organs radiating down to the big toe.

Dioscorea is a panacea for **the ill effects of the excessive drinking of tea**. A Dioscorea patient passes foul smelling gas. In the morning, the taste in the mouth is bitter along with the formation of white thick crust on the tongue. Dioscorea is also useful in the treatment of **neurogenic type of pain in the abdomen**. Its patient remembers and recalls the names of the objects incorrectly. There is mild pain over both the temples, which gets better on light pressure.

In Dioscorea, **bleeding piles** also occur. The piles are in the form of large bunches of red grapes. There may be diarrhoea, which is worse in the morning. There is a feeling of burning at the time of defaecation. The Dioscorea patient feels his chest is tight and tense. He cannot expand his chest to its full extent so his breathing is shallow. The fingernails are brittle and break easily. The symptoms of Dioscorea become worse in the evening, on lying on the stomach or on bending forward. On standing upright or on walking slowly, and with application of light pressure, the symptoms get better. Chamomilla and Camphor are its antidotes.

| **Potency:** 30 |
|---|

# DIPHTHERINUM

Diphtherinum is prepared from the toxin of Diphtheria. All such remedies prepared from the toxic material obtained from diseases are called Nosode. In general, the Nosode is not used to treat the sickness from which it has been derived; but rather for the treatment of similar types of ailments. Yet, the administration of Diphtherinum affects conspicuously on Diphtheria. In this way, it is a very important treatment for Diphtheria. So far no better medicine or remedy has been found as effective for Diphtheria. The traditional anti-Diphtheria vaccination is no match to it regarding prevention. During the epidemic of Diphtheria, a few doses in 200 potency not only dispel the immediate danger of contracting Diphtheria, but also may not be required for another eight years. The traditional vaccination is effective for three years at the most. A few doses of Diphtherinum 200 should be followed a few months later with Diphtherinum CM. This will offer protection against Diphtheria for life. Diphtherinum has been compared to the formal vaccination. It was found that some of the children who were given the vaccination still contracted Diphtheria or developed some ailment as a reaction to the vaccination itself, while in the case of Diphtherinum, not one child contracted Diphtheria nor were there any other complications or side effects.

Diphtherinum has also been found useful in the prevention of influenza. During an influenza epidemic, the combination of Influenzinum, Bacillinum and Diphtherinum is a potent preventive treatment. Diphtherinum has also been found very effective in weak and **paralysed muscles of swallowing**. Diphtherinum will also be useful in the treatment of the affliction of the heart due to influenza.

Diphtherinum is also of use in all those diseases which exhibit Diphtheria like symptoms. It is extremely beneficial in the treatment of enlarged tonsils, a thick red tongue, foul smelling excretions, difficulty in swallowing or, regurgitation of the food and water through the nose.

| **Potency:** 30 to CM |
|---|

# DROSERA ROTUNDIFOLIA
## (Sundew)

Drosera is a plant which is carnivorous in nature (it devours insects). Its leaves have a reddish, hairy structure on the surface, which produce a secretion to attract insects and helps to digest them. This secretion glitters like dew in the sunlight. The leaves remain spread on the surface of the ground. As soon as an insect comes near they immediately close and the insect becomes their food.

In the 16th century, Drosera became very famous in the treatment of tuberculosis, but it killed more people than it saved from the disease. Besides tuberculosis, it was also used for the treatment of toothache, insanity and problems related to childbirth.

In homoeopathy, the medicine is prepared from an extract of the plant and is commonly used for the treatment of cough. Its use has mostly been restricted to **whooping cough.** It has a much wider range of action in the **treatment of convulsive disorders**. Drosera is not only of use in coughs, but is also used for the treatment of convulsions related to other diseases. Therefore, it is also useful in the treatment of epilepsy. The Drosera patient becomes very worried and anxious after the convulsion and the subsequent unconsciousness. Drosera is a very highly effective remedy for the treatment of this confusion, perhaps an aftereffect of the convulsion.

Drosera should also be used in the treatment of **menopausal syndrome** because the symptoms of Drosera are very similar to that of menopause, such as flushing of the face, selective congestion of any part of the body and restlessness.

A Drosera patient **is afraid of being alone and suspicious**. He will not even trust his close friends. Such symptoms are also seen in the case of medicines prepared from snake venom. A patient of the constitution of Drosera is the **victim of superstitions**. He is restless, cowardly and a pessimist as well as extremely irritable. There is headache, especially over the **forehead**, which radiates outward through the cheekbones. The patient feels dizzy in the open and has a fear of falling on the left side. A feeling of severe cold and a stinging pain on the left side of the face while the right side of the face is dry and warm, are all typical features of Drosera.

Drosera may be of use to treat the cough arising out of irritation inside the windpipe after taking food.

An **epidemic cough** spreads wide during the formation of pods on the wild Acacia trees, Drosera is very useful in treating this cough. In Drosera, the windpipe feels tight and contracted. Drosera is very useful for the treatment of the cough associated with constant irritation in the throat, which is not relieved even after coughing. Any kind of cough which starts after midnight or which gets worse on talking will respond to Drosera. In children, bouts of **whooping cough** come on as soon as the child puts his head on the pillow, and then continue for two to three hours. Constant coughing makes them exhausted and there is no relief.

If such a patient contracts **fever**, he feels very cold and shivers. The face is flushed, while the hands become cold. There is complete absence of thirst. Typically, the Drosera cough becomes worse on lying down, laughing and singing or due to the warmth of the bed.

| | |
|---|---|
| **Antidote:** | Camphor |
| **Potency:** | 6 or 30 up to 200 |

# DULCAMARA
## (Bitter Sweet)

Dulcamara is prepared from a plant which grows abundantly in the continents of Europe and America. Its branches are quite long and spread out, bearing purple coloured flowers. Its stem and roots make the mouth bitter when chewed, but later on there is a sweet after-taste in the mouth. That is the reason why it is called bitter sweet. The homoeopathic medicine prepared from the extract of the fresh plant is called Dulcamara.

The main function of Dulcamara is on the inner linings (i.e. the mucous membranes). The most salient point is that any kind of sudden change of weather, from hot to cold or from cold to hot, from moist to dry and vice versa, affects the mucous membranes of the body, especially when the change is very prompt and sudden. For this kind of condition, Dulcamara would probably be the most appropriate treatment. The **common cold spreads far and wide during a change of weather**. Dulcamara would certainly be useful to treat a patient who catches a cold with every change of weather, even if the other symptoms of the patient do not give a clear picture.

After a vigorous game, some players change their clothes while the body is still hot. They develop nasal catarrh. Similarly, sudden exposure to hot weather from a cold situation also causes a cold. The symptoms get worse at night and on resting. The catarrhal changes can affect the kidneys, the intestines as well as the stomach, leading to frequent urination and the onset of diarrhoea, the reason being the same (i.e. irritation of the mucous linings of these organs). The symptoms aggravate in moist climate and wet weather.

If during summer a person contracts cold while visiting hill stations or coming back from the hill stations, Dulcamara would certainly be the indicated treatment. Some people develop **dysentery instead of diarrhoea on exposure to cold**. This type of dysentery would also be amenable to Dulcamara. Dulcamara given in high potency works as a sure preventive measure, so much so that sudden changes in weather would not affect such patients at all.

Dulcamara will also be useful in treating the symptoms which result from suppression of sweating on entry into a cold place.

The cold due to Dulcamara starts at the nose and settles in the eyes. The **eyes become heavy** and discharge yellowish liquid. The secretion is thin like water. The eyelids get swollen as well. If not treated adequately with Dulcamara, the cold becomes chronic. In Dulcamara, the **cold is usually of dry** nature, associated with blockage of the nose. The thick yellow secretion sticks in the nose. The nasal catarrh returns on exposure to even the slightest cold. The nose also bleeds.

Dulcamara is also the treatment for chronic ulcers of the inner linings (mucous membranes), as well as of the skin. The **eczema** like lesions develop on the skin of the face, which then spread rapidly and get covered with yellow scabs. Clusters of blisters develop and spread widely. The similar symptom is well seen in Arsenic also, though their nature is different. In Arsenic, the wounds can progress to the formation of **gangrene**, although there is no such tendency in Dulcamara. Dulcamara results in the formation of ulcers over the superficial bones, which are separated from the outside only by skin e.g., Shin bone. Regarding the wounds and sores of Arsenic and Dulcamara, the difference is that in Arsenic, there is formation of lumps similar to those found in plague. The **glands in the armpits** (axilla) also enlarge and pus forms in them. In Dulcamara, the enlargement of the glands does not lead to the formation of pus. They only get hardened.

In Dulcamara, **scabs form over the scalp** which can weep at the edges. This symptom is also found in Mezereum however, in Mezerum the eczema-type of lesion gets covered with a membrane-like structure. Under this structure, there is formation of pus, which obviously smells foul. In Dulcamara, the symptoms are not as severe and progressive.

The other remedies that produce eczema like signs are Sepia, Arsenic, Graphites, Petroleum, Sulphur, Calcaria salts and Rhus Tox. All these will have to be distinguished on the basis of their peculiar symptoms. Croton, Anagalis and Anacardium may also be very useful in treating such conditions. The **eczematous lesions** of Anagalis, Croton and

Rhus Tox are mostly on the **lower part of the body** and around the thighs, while in Anacardium, the **eczema affects the entire body**

In Dulcamara, the **headache** gets worse in the cold and wet weather. The patient feels light headed. The head is heavy, and there is **pain on the temple areas**. The **ears ache** and buzz, affecting the capability to hear. The glands around the ears become inflamed. The cheeks hurt badly and the pain spreads towards the ears, eyes and jaws. The tongue becomes dry and rough. Paralysis of the tongue is also prominent. The neuralgic pain on the face as described gets worse on exposure to cold.

The patient hates food. There is a non-ending urge to drink water. There is burning in the stomach, along with the tendency for **nausea and vomiting**. The vomiting contains white sticky secretions. During the act of vomiting, the patient feels very cold. On exposure to cold, the **bladder becomes inflamed and irritable**, leading to frequent urination. There is a constant desire to pass urine which comes in drops.

The ailments of Dulcamara are relieved by lying on the side, but become aggravated on lying on the back or bending forwards. Movement ameliorates the symptoms, which increase in the evening and at night. The symptoms also get worse during the change of weather or on getting wet in humid weather or taking cold beverages, etc.

| | |
|---|---|
| **Adjuvan:** | Baryta Carb |
| **Antidote:** | Camphor, Cuprum |
| **Potency:** | 30 to 200 |

# ELECTRICITAS

This homoeopathic medicine is prepared from waves of natural or industrial electricity. This remedy is related to patients who become affected by **thunder or lightning**. Before the onset of a storm or with the onset of stormy conditions, the patient becomes **asthmatic or develops catarrhal conditions**. The resultant depression, restlessness, despair, rapidity of pulse and headache, benefit from treatment with Electricitas. One should remember that that this medicine should not be administered to patients who already had the symptoms of cold before the onset of a stormy condition. The doctors who have such experience describe it to be a very dangerous practice.

Electricitas has been found useful in treating the body aches, chills, feeling of extreme weakness, tiredness, sleeplessness, catching fever and excessive sweating, all resulting from sudden change of weather. It is said that this medicine annuls the bad aftereffects of Mercury also.

This medicine is one of the most recently discovered, to which some homoeopaths give a great importance but personally I am of the opinion that in the above situation, the previously well-tried homoeopathic remedies should be further studied and mastered. However, I have entered this remedy in my book for those who intend to do further experimentation. If good well-experienced doctors, be they homoeopaths or allopaths, experiment on such medicines and then let the homoeopathic board know about their successful observations, this can be very useful for others. Some amateurs and lay Homoeopaths make lofty claims about the success of this remedy and keep writing to me. But, I have generally found it to be their own vain imagination only, I find it difficult to accept their reports as reliable.

| **Potency:** 30 or 200 |
|---|

# Electricity

This remedy is prepared from electricity rays but its preparation is different from that of Electricitas and so there is a difference in their working. It is used to treat **rapid heartbeat** (tachycardia) and the **paralysis affecting the upper extremities**. It is usually given to patients who happen to be sad and sallow, like those of Pulsatilla, they tend to heave sighs and are **frightened and depressed**. They get **extremely frightened at the onset of a storm** which aggravates their symptoms. **Long uncontrollable laughter, like that of an insane person**, is also a symptom of Electricity. Similarly, night blindness, involuntary bedwetting and asthma are also well within the effect of Electricity. I would advise the readers to study further on Electricitas as well.

| **Potency:** 30 to 200 |
|---|

# EUPATORIUM PERFOLIATUM
## (Thorough Wart)

Commonly, Eupatorium is known as Bone Set medicine because it has been in vogue for the treatment of bone pains for a long time. In the Eastern States of America, old ladies have been using it in the form of home-made tea for the treatment of the common cold.

It is very useful in the treatment of influenza, malaria and other fevers that cause **severe bone pains in the body**. It is one of the top most treatments for **Dengue fever**, which results from the bite of a tiny mosquito found in dry, hilly areas. Its peculiar characteristic is that there is severe pain in the bones all over and in the back, which is unbearable. Eupatorium does not offer complete cure but relieves the suffering to a great extent. This fever has to take its course of seven days in any case. Once the patient recovers from this, he develops antibodies and will never get Dengue fever again.

This medicine is considered to be one of the best against **influenza** and is also very useful in the treatment of the common cold. Eupatorium must be put to use when the common cold is associated with severe body aches and headache. It will protect the patient from further complications. In Eupatorium, the **bone pains are associated with a feeling of chills**. This symptom is also found in malaria so Eupatorium is also useful for the treatment of malaria. The chill is felt more from 6 o' clock to 9 o' clock in the morning. The symptoms of Eupatorium start with the sunrise while the symptoms of Natrum Mur usually get worse after 9 o' clock.

If **malaria** appears in the form of epidemic and Eupatorium is found beneficial in some patients, then most other patients will benefit from Eupatorium as well. To begin with, there is intense thirst. Even in the winter, the patient wants to drink extremely cold water, which will cause a chill in the body, but the thirst will still not get quenched. The patient keeps himself well covered. When the chill comes to an end and his temperature has risen, he starts vomiting and sweats profusely. However, this sweating does not lower the temperature. The vomited material contains bile. The severer the chill at the outset the more is the feeling of heat after getting fever. If the temperature is 103°F, the patient feels like it is 106ºF. In other words, his feelings for both cold and heat are equally enhanced. Once the fever is at its climax, the patient stops sweating. He starts sweating when the fever goes down. This sweating actually hastens the temperature to decrease. However the patient develops a severe headache which is a little bizarre because in the case of malaria, when the fever goes down due to profuse sweating, his headache also gets better. This peculiar observation, i.e. the fever is coming down but the headache is getting worse, is only found in the nature of a patient of Eupatorium.

Physicians have been warned previously regarding the treatment of malaria and it is repeated here once again. In malaria, no medicine should be given while the fever is coming on. Unless the fever starts subsiding, no medicine should be given. The best time for the treatment to be given is between two malarial attacks. If during that time, the properly indicated medicine is administered, either the patient will not get a new attack of malaria or the next one would be very mild. It may so happen for two or three days; every subsequent bout of fever will be milder and milder, so much so that the patient will be completely cured.

Eupatorium has also been successfully used in the treatment of **rheumatism**. In the patient of Eupatorium, the joints swell and lumps appear over them. There is pain along the course of the nerves. The gouty pain is mostly on the big toe. Rheumatism patients usually suffer from headache. They feel nauseated and become dizzy in the morning, The dizziness is reduced in the evening.

A patient of Eupatorium feels **pain behind the eyeballs**. For the treatment of pain in the eyes, Gelsemium and Bryonia can be useful adjuncts. When the patient develops diarrhoea, the stools are copious and greenish in colour and thin like water. There may be griping also. Sometimes, the stools are scanty to start with and then become plentiful causing severe dehydration and weakness. After that, the patient becomes constipated, which lasts many days.

In Eupatorium, the **cough** is very troublesome. There is pain over the chest and the whole body shivers. The patient is **oversensitive to cold**. Eupatorium, being a treatment for the common cold, is also effective on the lungs.

The patients of Eupatorium are depressed by nature. The body tends to be swollen (oedematous). If such oedema is noticed during the course of influenza or malaria, one should think of Eupatorium.

The ailments of Eupatorium recur once again after 21 days. The patient feels comfortable while kept busy in talking. Eupatorium has an effect on the mucous membranes of the stomach, liver and the air passages. Usually, it is useful in the treatment of ailments found in humid regions, but can also be found beneficial in completely dry weather (such as Dengue fever).

**Potency:** 30 to 200

# EUPHRASIA
## (Eyebright)

Euphrasia is a specific kind of plant called Eyebright. The Homoeopathic medicine is prepared out of it. As the name implies, it is **used in the treatment of cold affecting the eyes, which become extraordinarily red.**

The effect of Euphrasia is rather short-lived and certainly neither does it work for a long time nor does it have any deep effects. Hence, Euphrasia is useful in the kind of cold which, though severe, is but of a fleeting nature, especially with the effect being mostly on the eyes. Any kind of **cold, which attacks the eyes at the outset with excessive watering, burning and redness,** will respond to Euphrasia. During the daytime, while the eyes are watering and red, the patient does not have any cough. There is no burning or irritation in the throat either. As soon as the patient retires to bed, the excessive secretions of the eye divert towards the throat and injure the windpipe leading to **coughing**. At the outset, the cough is only at night, but after some time, due to persistent burning and irritation, sores develop in the throat and the cough lingers. It can remain during the day also. Along with the cold, there is an attack of severe headache. The eyes feel heavy as if somebody has put a heavy bandage over them. Ulcers form over the cornea. The secretion of the eye being acidic in nature shows its ill effects for a long time and can cause blurring of the vision.

A peculiar symptom of Euphrasia is the pain experienced over the nerves supplying the eyes. Although Euphrasia is an acute i.e. short acting remedy, however, the resulting eye condition may become chronic. It mostly afflicts the third cranial nerve (oculomotor).

Euphrasia has a distinct beneficial effect in the treatment of **German measles**. Measles are treated with Pulsatilla, but in German measles Euphrasia is a must. In this condition, the disease process starts at the eyes, which become extremely red. As such, German measles is not a dangerous disease but in pregnant women, it can produce severe bad effects on the foetus. If German measles attack women in the first trimester, the development of the foetus stops there and then, and the foetus does not grow. Pregnant women have to be extra careful during an epidemic of this disease because it is really very dreadful. In the first three months, the eyes may not form at all or there can be a serious maldevelopment of the heart. Similarly, the hearing can also be seriously affected. Sometimes, the child is born completely blind or completely deaf. Most of these children die in the first few months after birth. It may be taken as a blessing for the parents otherwise, if they survive, they become a cause of constant worry and anxiety. If a woman contracts German measles in the first three months of her pregnancy, she should be admitted into a well-equipped clinic and it should be ensured that the foetus has not been afflicted with German measles. If so afflicted, the doctors would certainly advise abortion for the benefit of the mother and the child.

In Euphrasia, there is extreme hypersensitivity to light. A similar kind of photophobia is seen in measles also. The ailments of Euphrasia become worse in the evening, in hot weather and in bright light.

**Antidotes:** Camphor, Pulsatilla, Causticum
**Potency:** 30

# FERRUM METALLICUM
## (Iron)

The homoeopathic physicians have noticed that when a person is given iron excessively, his colour becomes yellow or greenish. The face looks greasy, as if waxed. The skin over the entire body turns the same. There is a tendency to bleed, with the blood being thin and watery. Blood clots can also form, which are reddish in colour, whereas the blood clots formed as a result of poisoning are usually darkish in colour. The appropriate homoeopathic treatment for this kind of condition is Ferrum Metallicum, commonly called Ferrum Met.

One sign of Ferrum Met is that the entire body feels weak. Even mild physical activity causes tiredness. In Acid Phos, the body remains lethargic constantly. In the case of Ferrum Met, the **weakness** ensues suddenly after a trifling job, as if the torch containing old batteries may light up and then turn off abruptly. As long as the patient does not move, he is not aware of his state of weakness. Even if he walks a little or very slowly he will still become weak. But if he remains lying down or sitting for long time he may still feel weakness because by remaining in one state, the previous aches in the body flare up. On walking fast, both weakness and pain become pronounced. Even a long conversation can exhaust him physically.

In spite of being anaemic, the patient's face is somewhat **flushed,** which is known as a False Plethora. Both cheeks become flushed and especially in women, it resembles the blushing as a result of feeling shy. The menstrual bleeding continues over a long period and there may be only a day or two without bleeding. The bleeding is thin and light yellowish in colour. It may sometimes contain the shreds of the inner lining of the uterus. In spite of all this, strange it is that the face still has a reddish glow. Such women frequently abort due to the vaginal irritation. Similarly, the prolapse of the uterus is not unusual.

Like China, in Ferrum Met there is decrease in the number of red cells. The face however remains flushed and there may be redness and pallor on the face, alternating with each other. Similarly, the patient feels extremely chilly during the onset of fever.

Regarding the gastric symptoms, the patient has either a **voracious appetite** or no appetite at all. He hates sour things. On taking them, the patient develops diarrhoea. Soon after taking the food, he may regurgitate undigested food without the feeling of preliminary retching. Sometimes, vomiting is preceded by nausea as well. Such vomiting follows taking food, immediately or after midnight. The abdomen becomes bloated with wind. The patient will not be able to digest an egg. Even if he likes to eat eggs, they do not suit him. At night, he passes stools consisting of undigested food, but if he passes stools during the daytime, it is soon after taking food, which is not accompanied by pain. Sometimes, the stools are hard and there is associated pain in the back and gripe at the rectum. There is a tendency towards prolapse of the rectum. Some patients lose control over passing urine. This is more common during the day.

Regarding the symptoms pertaining to the lungs, there is a feeling of **pressure over the chest** and a difficulty in breathing. The voice becomes hoarse. The cough is dry and comes in the form of repeated bouts, sometimes associated with passing of red blood (haemoptysis). There are rheumatic pains in the shoulders as well as in the lower part of the back. Similarly, there is **pain over the buttocks**, calves or in the soles of the feet. All these symptoms become somewhat relieved on light movement.

| | |
|---|---|
| **Adjuvants:** | China, Alumen, Hamamelis |
| **Antidotes:** | Arsenic, Hepar Sulph |
| **Potency:** | 30 to 200 |

# Ferrum Phosphoricum
## (Phosphate of Iron)

Ferrum Phos is a compound of phosphorus and iron and is a natural component of the red blood cells. A deficiency of Ferrum Phos is also considered as a deficiency of iron in the blood. Ferrum Phos is the best remedy for **iron deficiency anaemia**. Open air causes discomfort to the patient of Ferrum Phos, thus the patient has a cold constitution. Due to the presence of phosphorus, some symptoms resemble those of this element. The patient does not have any specific fear but is usually somewhat restless, disgusted and in a state of mental confusion. There is a lot of weakness as well. Ferrum Phos given in homoeopathic potency works wonders in correcting a **lack of blood and associated weakness**.

The patient catches a cold when exposed to the cold weather. His face is flushed and feverish. There is distaste for meat and milk. The patient likes to eat those things that may enhance the appetite. Such a patient usually gets sour eructations. Piles develop at the anal margin and the stools are mixed with thin blood, there may be dysentery. If there is coughing, it causes stress and incontinence of the urine in women, which will dribble involuntarily. The phosphorus compounds are useful in patients with a thin, dilute blood who have the tendency to bleed. For Haemophiliac patients, there are three useful remedies: Phosphorus, Acid Phos and Ferrum Phos.

Phosphorus in homoeopathic potencies has the capability to thicken blood (haemoconcentration). If the blood becomes too thick, it can be dangerous and cause heart attack. It is very important that phosphorus should not be blindly continued for a long time. Patients who take Phosphorus, Acid Phos and Ferrum Phos must get their blood tested every two to three months. The normal coagulability (thickness) of blood prevents spontaneous bleeding. The thickness is however acceptable only to a limit. Once it becomes too thick, then the Phosphorus should be stopped to let the blood become thin and flow better. If the blood becomes too thin, this remedy should be restarted.

In the patients of Ferrum Phos, muscles on the back can get strained easily and result in permanent discomfort on lifting even a light weight. Millefolium has a similar tendency. Both are good to combat bleeding tendencies. The anaemic patient has a tendency to get angry easily. He starts sweating and the whole body trembles. His anger is directed towards himself. He becomes emotional very easily. Sometimes he is happy and at other times he starts talking nonsense. This symptom of unstable temper is due to the combination of phosphorus and iron. The patient of Ferrum Phos likes to remain alone and does not want to face other people. He cannot tolerate noise. Sometimes he yells out but this is not his normal temperament. Such patients usually talk less and like to remain aloof.

Cold air relieves the headache. The headache is more severe while going up the stairs, and sometimes the patient experiences temporary loss of vision due to the lack of blood (anaemia). When the patient tries to sit up suddenly or when he is climbing the stairs, the headache becomes worse due to lack of flow of blood to the brain. The headache is felt above the eyes. The nape of the neck and the temples ache as well. There is splitting headache affecting half of the head. The eyesight may be lost temporarily. This symptom is also found in the remedies associated with excessive blood accumulation such as Gelsemium. In Gelsemium it is not due to the lack of blood but due to the localised increase of blood pressure (congestion). Similarly, it can happen in the case of Belladonna. But in Ferrum Phos, it is due to a deficiency of blood, and not enough blood reaching the head. This is similar to the remedies causing vascular congestion leading to the loss of vision.

In Ferrum Phos, there is **catarrh of the Eustachian tubes**. (These are the tubes that lead from inside the throat towards the ears). The catarrhal secretions are mixed with blood, which is due to the bleeding tendency in the Ferrum Phos patients. The children usually get nosebleeds. If the patient of Ferrum Phos has bleeding from the lining of the mouth and the gums, it is red in colour as in Millefolium. The tonsils swell and there is irritation in the throat due to bleeding, burning and inflammation, causing difficulty in swallowing. These are the symptoms of Ferrum Phos. These symptoms are common in many other remedies, so the diagnosis for Ferrum Phos cannot be based on these findings alone. The patient has to be observed and studied overall.

Lack of blood or anaemia is a definite symptom. **During pregnancy**, Ferrum Phos should be administered to women **as a tonic**. For this purpose, the combination of Ferrum Phos, Calcarea Phos, and Kali Phos is very useful. In the first few months of pregnancy, the tendency of abortion is stopped and in the last two to three months of pregnancy, it helps in the development of the baby. These, however, should not be used continuously but should be resumed after an interval. This regimen does not cause any harm, rather it is useful. In Ferrum Phos, the appetite sometimes decreases a lot and at other times increases to the extent that it knows no bounds. These two extremes are the symptoms of Ferrum Phos. The pregnant women like to take harmful things, and dislike those that are useful for their body. There is a dislike for meat. In this situation, Ferrum Phos is useful.

After food intake, there is retching or nausea. The nausea of pregnancy is usually severe and obstinate. Ferrum Phos alone will help but rarely. There are many other remedies for nausea, particularly related to pregnancy of which one should have full knowledge. I have tried a new remedy called Pipli, which is prepared from the leaves and the burnt ashes of the tree called Pipal. This has proved very effective in the stubborn type of nausea of pregnancy.

In my view, the **nausea and vomiting of pregnancy** is sometimes caused by allergy. Some pregnant women develop an allergy to the baby developing in their wombs. Their nausea is very severe and prolonged. In the USA, it has been found during research that 40% of the women, who abort, do it due to an allergy against their own baby. In other words, the body's defences attack the embryo. If it was not due to the three coverings around the embryo i.e. the placenta, the uterine wall and the outer covering of the uterus, the embryos would be aborted. The Holy Quran has mentioned this saying: *We have placed the embryo in a safe and secure place under the three protective coverings (Chapter 39, Sura Al-Zumar: 7).*

If the defensive mechanism around the foetus is weaker than the attacking power, the pregnancy would certainly be lost.

In some institutions, the scientists have discovered ways to balance the internal and the external defence systems. At present, this treatment is very costly. However, a great majority of women who were able to receive this treatment delivered their babies successfully.

I have found Pipli to be very useful in controlling **nausea during pregnancy**. It may also prevent abortion by combating allergy towards the foetus. However, this needs further research and experimentation on a wider scale by homoeopaths all over the world. I would like Pipli to be tried in different potencies and carefully observed to see what kind of patients it works on, and on what kinds of patients it does not. I request the homoeopaths that whosoever experiments on this new remedy should inform the Ahmadiyya Muslim Central Homoeopathy Board at:
16 Gressenhall Road,
London
SW18 5QL
UK

The symptoms of Ferrum Phos aggravate by touch, jolt and movement. The cold applications offer relief.

| | |
|---|---|
| **Potency:** | Biochemic 3x to 12x |
| | Homoeopathic 30 or Higher |

# Fluoricum Acidum
## (Hydrofluoric Acid)

Fluoric Acid is a deeply rooted and vastly effective remedy. It is indicated in deep, slowly progressive ailments, which ultimately become part of one's life. It works slowly and does not produce its effect immediately. Fluoric Acid resembles Sulphur in one aspect and Natrum Mur in another. Some patients are labelled as Sulphur or Natrum Mur but do not respond to either of them. In fact, they are patients of Fluoric Acid. In this respect, it is a very interesting remedy. In Natrum Mur, the nails become unsightly, loose and grow rapidly, while their ends crack, shrivell and become lifeless. Similarly the hair loses its lustre and becomes weak and lifeless. It splits at the ends. These symptoms lead one's attention towards Natrum Mur, whereas the feeling of warmth, burning and sweating remind one of Sulphur. All these signs are found together in Fluoric Acid, which is a very effective remedy. If Fluoric Acid is ignored in this set of symptoms, the patient may be severely harmed. This kind of patient will not respond to any medication other than Fluoric Acid.

In those patients in whom the diseases progress to a stage where other remedies do not work, then certainly one has to look for profoundly acting remedies, Fluoric Acid is one of them. The deep illnesses, which pass on from one generation to another such as syphilis, gonorrhoea and leprosy, have been divided into three basic categories by many homoeopaths. Fluoric Acid exhibits the symptoms of all three. Tuberculosis of the lung is also passed from one generation to another, but it would need to be treated separately, as a fourth category.

In Fluoric Acid, symptoms of cold and warmth alternate with each other. At night, the patient feels intense heat while in bed and asks for cold water to be sprinkled on him as in Pulsatilla. In Sulphur, in spite of feeling hot, the patient still dislikes water.

The feet burn and the patient exposes his feet out of the covers. Both hands and feet sweat profusely. The web spaces between the fingers and toes soften and decay. Fluoric Acid is very useful in this situation. In contrast to Natrum Mur and Sulphur, patients of Fluoric Acid react badly to coffee and tea. They lose sleep or develop other symptoms. Fluoric Acid patients develop boils on the skin which do not heal easily. Often a boil develops on the face that does not soften for a long time. Silicea, which would ordinarily work on boils, will not be effective in Fluoric Acid patients unless Fluoric Acid is also used after the Silicea. If the boil still does not subside, symptoms indicating other remedies will show up.

If Silicea has been used by mistake, Fluoric Acid will abate its harmful effects, but not its useful action. In Fluoric Acid, the hair becomes weak and thin, with split ends, but it is limited to patchy areas of the scalp. But, in the case of Natrum Mur, the hair is affected all over the head. Such distinctive signs must always be examined, in order for a proper diagnosis and precise, timely treatment.

Typically in a Fluoric Acid patient, when the patient has the urge to pass urine but withholds, he will experience a headache associated with a sensation of warmth all over. Nevertheless, this feeling will subside after urination.

Fluoric Acid is one of the best treatments for patients who have been **afflicted with sexual misconduct**, and have virtually ruined themselves. Unfortunately, such patients will not give up their licentious behaviour. They can benefit from Fluoric Acid, Picric Acid, Lycopodium and Sepia, depending upon their constitution. In a Pulsatilla patient who does not respond to Pulsatilla anymore, Silicea or Fluoric Acid can be used to a significant advantage.

Fluoric Acid is the best remedy for **varicose veins and associated ulcers**. Women are very susceptible to developing varicose veins due to multiple pregnancies and childbirths, causing pressure on the deep veins in the lower part of the abdomen and pelvis. Varicose veins can bleed too, causing significant discomfort. In such a serious situation, Arnica, Aesculus, Lachesis, Sulphuric Acid, Nitric Acid or Fluoric Acid can be put to use for the treatment based on the symptoms and the signs as well as the constitution of the patient. If one is unable to think of a suitable remedy for varicose veins, one should try to diagnose on basis of the constitution of the patient. Many a time the constitutional remedy will also cure varicose veins.

In some patients, the **scalp feels numb** and senseless, especially the back of the head feels wooden. Fluoric Acid is the best remedy for this disorder. There can also be numbness of the hands and the feet. The numbness is absent in the areas under pressure of the body and weight-bearing areas. The backbone may also feel numb. Fluoric Acid should be promptly started to avoid the **possibility of paralysis**, which can occur suddenly. It must be remembered that Fluoric Acid is a slow-acting remedy and it should be continued for two to three months for better response. It should be ensured that the condition of the patient keeps improving.

**Eczema of the infants affecting their scalp** also responds well to the Fluoric Acid. In the adults, the hairy part of the scalp does not itch; only the hairless part itches severely. A peculiar sign of Fluoric Acid not found in other remedies is that the left side of the child's head is relatively small due to incomplete development of the skull bones. The left eye is also comparatively small, and depressed in appearance. Fluoric Acid, being **useful in bone development**, will prove useful in this condition. This useful effect has been found by experiments on many patients, although proper proving regarding this has not been done.

In Fluoric Acid, the patient desires to drink cold water and to eat as well. Usually, one loses one's appetite when thirsty, but this is not the case in Fluoric Acid. Fluoric Acid is beneficial for **chronic ulcers of the throat**. Thus it is compatible with Silicea and Mercury, which are not compatible to each other, and should not be used together. When switching from Mercury to Silicea, Hepar Sulph must be used in between. High potency Silicea can only be used to counteract the ill effects of Mercury if used in error.

In Sulphur, the patient experiences morning diarrhoea. In case of Fluoric Acid also, there is morning diarrhoea that tends to be chronic, intractable and debilitating. This will respond to Fluoric Acid only. Fluoric Acid is also very good for the relief of the swelling of the body due to **liver disorder**, with which there can be sensation of warmth, presence of bile in the stools and distension of the abdomen. Fluoric Acid symptoms aggravate on exposure to heat, with hot drinks and in the morning. The cold ameliorates its symptoms.

| | |
|---|---|
| **Adjuvant:** | Silicea |
| **Potency:** | 30 or higher as required. |

# GELSEMIUM

Gelsemium is prepared from jasmine bearing yellow flowers. It is a very frequently used Homoeopathic medicine. To an extent, it resembles Aconite and Belladonna; however, diseases of Gelsemium progress rather slowly compared to both Aconite and Belladonna. There is sudden rush of blood towards the head, causing headache. The mouth becomes dry. These three symptoms are common to Aconite, Belladonna and Gelsemium. In the case of Aconite, the face is flushed and warm, but there is no such warmth in case of Gelsemium. Constitutionally, it is a cold remedy. The mouth is dry, yet there is no thirst. Gelsemium symptoms do not appear until after two to three days after exposure to the cold. Gelsemium would certainly be indicated if a child contracts illness after having been exposed to the cold. If the illness comes on suddenly and severely from exposure to cold, then Aconite and Belladonna combined will be much more effective.

According to Dr. Kent, the symptoms of **nasal catarrh** set in a few days after exposure to the cold. One might presume that being a cold-natured medicine, Gelsemium's illnesses would be more prevalent in the winter and similarly the illnesses of Aconite would be more prevalent in the summer. In fact, the situation is the exact opposite (Aconite is used more often in the winter and Gelsemium more in the summertime). When one is exposed to cold in the summertime, Gelsemium will be of greater benefit. Thus, Gelsemium is most commonly used in dry, hot weather. However, when **acute dysentery** (along with the passing of lot of blood) is contracted in the drier part of the summer, Aconite will be the best treatment to work and does so equally well in the dry months of summer as well as winter.

Gelsemium is commonly used to treat headaches and catarrhal illnesses but not for the treatment of diarrhoea. However, it has been found to work extremely well for the **chronic type of diarrhoea** associated with the body being cold, a heaviness of the head and a complete absence of thirst in spite of the mouth being dry. Thus, it is a treatment of diarrhoea as well.

In spite of the fact that the Gelsemium ailments progress rather slowly, it is rarely used in the treatment of chronic diseases. Its use has been confined to treat diseases of limited duration. In Gelsemium, the blood rushes towards the face and head. The face becomes warm though the hands and the feet are cold. Similar is the case for Arnica. The calves feel cold or even ice cold. These symptoms are also found in Glonoine. However, the difference between Gelsemium and Glonoine is that in Gelsemium, the hands and feet become cold but there is no sweating, while in Glonoine, there is profuse sweating in addition to the hands and feet becoming cold. Due to the straining of the back muscles causing severe stiffness and spasms, the pain spreads over the shoulders and up to the back of the head. The **stiffness of the neck** causes great difficulty in turning the neck. The headache is mostly on the right side. Extreme spasm of the neck muscles (torticolis) at night, is better treated with Gelsemium and Belladonna combined. In case the rigidity of the neck resembles meningitis, the back does not feel cold but the hands and feet become cold. In addition to the severe muscular stiffness, the patient may become convulsive but there is no associated cyanosis. In this condition, one should not forget to use Gelsemium.

In Gelsemium, the patient is restless before going to sleep. He fears that he may not be able to sleep well. The head starts hurting, while still, there is no headache, per se. The headache becomes worse on sleeping (like Lachesis), though the overall picture of the patient is still Gelsemium. He does not sleep well. By the time the patient has got up in the morning, his headache has become very severe. The one difference between Gelsemium and Lachesis is that the Gelsemium pain does not remain confined to the head; instead, it radiates down the shoulders up to the back of the head and is most often on the left side.

Gelsemium is the antidote of Glonoine. Combined with Natrum Mur, it happens to become a complete immediate panacea.

Gelsemium is of great value for the treatment of women. It will immediately relieve the **tightness of the cervix of the uterus** as well as the associated lightning type of labour pains radiating to the back. The tightness of the muscles of the back becomes released and the child is delivered smoothly. It is also of significant use in relieving the severe backache accompanying the menstrual period, as well as the chills and relentless fever due to infection.

A **malarial fever,** which comes on every day with a tendency to be very high in the afternoon, will respond well to Gelsemium. Symptoms of Gelsemium become much worse in the evening. On the other hand, the symptoms of Arsenic are at their peak at midday and midnight. The pain of Kali Carb commences at about three o' clock in the afternoon while the symptoms of Gelsemium become worse between four and seven o'clock.

The **heartbeat is slow and weak**. Typically, the patient thinks that his heart will beat as long as he keeps walking and will stop as soon as he stops, as if the functioning of the heart is being sustained by physical movement. Over the heart area there is a feeling of vacuum and weakness. The patient believes that moving around is a must to keep the heart functioning or it will stop as soon as he sits down. Slow walking is good to strengthen the heart gradually while sudden rapid movement can do harm to it. The heart of a Gelsemium patient is weak and cannot bear sudden, severe physical stress. He will either faint or may even die. Gentle physical exercise gradually strengthens the heart muscle so that it may subsequently be able to take relatively rapid physical movement.

In Gelsemium, there is a feeling of **weakness and emptiness at the stomach**. Gelsemium can be of use in treating the diarrhoea of psychogenic origin. The stomach, like the heart, is subject to emotional stress. Fear, stress and bad news are known to upset the stomach. This is also seen in Argentum Nitricum although other symptoms are quite different.

Gelsemium can be compared also to Natrum Mur in some ways. The headache of Natrum Mur is as if being hammered, while the Gelsemium **headache generally begins as throbs over the nape of the neck**. Gelsemium is very effective in treating the left-sided headache that becomes settled at the nape of neck or radiates to the neck. In addition, Onosmodium may also be very useful. Both Gelsemium and Onsomodium combined can be used to treat **migraine**. At times, the headache may just be due to excessive heat but this may not come to one's mind, therefore all the symptoms should be considered carefully. It is essential to have a good working knowledge of the working of the disease as well as the nature of the remedy. Whenever the correct Homoeopathic remedy is used, the patient will have a good sleep or will start passing urine freely. In the case of Gelsemium, the urination is free and clear like water. Reduction in the severity of symptoms shows that Gelsemium was certainly the right choice. Often in Gelsemium, emotional stress and grief can induce physical illnesses.

Gelsemium is known for **eye troubles** also, such as temporary blindness. This kind of blindness is also found in other medicines, though not as commonly as in Gelsemium. If one eye is affected, Rhus Tox will suffice. In some cases, Lachesis may also be useful. In Gelsemium, there is drooping of the eyelids, which are difficult to keep open (ptosis). If this condition becomes chronic Gelsemium will not be of much use any more. It is useful in the beginning of the condition. The vision becomes blurred. One pupil happens to be dilated and the other constricted i.e. the pupils are unequal in size. The eye becomes red and swollen. Vision is foggy or the field of vision becomes occupied with spider webs. Gelsemium is also useful to treat the neurological weakness of the eye muscles. Hands and feet become partially paralysed. The limbs quiver and feel drawn. The patient does not wish to walk for want of physical energy.

Regarding the **catarrhal diseases** (affecting the inner linings/mucous membranes), the symptoms of Gelsemium resemble those of Natrum Mur. However, the patient of Natrum Mur is very thirsty and the patient of Gelsemium not thirsty at all. In Gelsemium the patient sneezes repeatedly. The tip of the nose becomes insensitive. **Ears may also become numb** over the skin surface. The skin is warm, dry and itchy. Gelsemium can prove effective immediately for these conditions.

**Boils form on the face and scalp**. Blisters form over the nerve ends, which can be very painful and even harmful. This is called Shingles (Herpes Zoster). Gelsemium is also of significant advantage in treating this condition. I usually prescribe a combination of Ledum, Arnica and Arsenic. Natrum Mur is also useful. Generally, I prefer to suggest a combination of any three, which proves very effective i.e. by substituting one of the first three with Natrum Mur or Gelsemium as indicated. By the grace of Allah, in my experience, within these five remedies (Ledium, Arnica, Arsenic, Natrum Mur and Gelsmium), most cases of shingles come under control.

Sometimes, **epilepsy-like conditions** can develop due to the disorder of the stomach. It is as if a flame or a flash erupts from the stomach and rises up towards the head or the heart. The patient may either become unconscious or very dizzy, losing balance. This is a symptom of Gelsemium. It results from gastric hyperacidity often seen in sportsmen. Gelsemium will be found very useful in treating this condition. Certainly, this is not epilepsy as such.

The Gelsemium ailments become aggravated in humidity and with emotional stress. Passing large amounts of urine freely and constant light movement in open air give relief.

| | |
|---|---|
| Antidotes: | China, Coffea, Digitalis |
| Potency: | 30 to 200 |

# GLONOINE
## (Nitro Glycerine)

Glonoine is also one of those remedies that, like Drosera, have been considered to be effective against only a few diseases although a great deal of benefit can be gained from it. Glonoine is trinitroglycerine. It contains hydrogen and oxygen elements and is a powerful explosive and combustible material. The formula of this compound was first invented by a scientist named Nobël. At that time, it was considered to be a very revolutionary invention. Although later on plastic and nuclear bombs etc. were also invented, the use of nitroglycerine has never been abandoned completely. In fact, it has been shifted more towards everyday use.

Nitroglycerine is also used in medicine. It is used either as such or in some other form for the treatment of **angina**. Glonoine also affects the human temperament. Sunlight makes one feel unwell. Just as nitro-glycerine is sensitive to heat, similarly, a patient cannot tolerate heat and the result is a **splitting headache**. One feels as if he is being hammered all over the head, or as if the head is exploding. Glonoine is a first class medicine for the **prevention of heat stroke**. It can also be used for the treatment of high blood pressure, but only when other signs of Glonoine are also present in the patient. The homoeopathic doctors often use Glonoine for the treatment of patients suffering from heat stroke and **blood pressure**.

I have prepared a **prescription for prevention against heat strokes** i.e. one dose of Glonoine, Natrum Mur and Arsenic combined in potency 30, taken before leaving the house. By the grace of God, this will protect a person from headache the whole day. However, once the headache sets in, it is difficult to stop it.

The symptoms of Glonoine include a **splitting headache**, which starts as soon as the head is rested on a pillow. There is a feeling of heaviness over the heart. There is sudden rush of blood towards the head or the heart, and the patient feels a kind of fluid passing through the body. The tendency of the rush of blood to the head originates either from the heart or the stomach.

Some symptoms of Gelsemium are also found in Glonoine. In Gelsemium, before falling asleep, **the patient feels faint signs of discomfort** centred in the head while still, there is no headache per se. After sleep the pain becomes clearly felt. By morning, it turns into severe pain. Symptoms of Glonoine are similar to that of Gelsemium. The difference is that in Gelsemium, the pain does not remain limited to the head only. Rather, it involves shoulder muscles and also reaches the lower part of the back. The pain is usually on the left side of the body, whereas in Glonoine, the entire head is affected, but the pain remains limited to the head and the eyes only, it has no relation to the other nerves.

In Glonoine, **palpitation** is very conspicuous. The whole body begins to throb. From the tips of the fingers down to the toes, one feels an uncomfortable pulsating. The patient is overcome by generalised throbbing of the body as soon as he retires to bed. He simply cannot sleep. A single dose of Glonoine can cure the ailment and the patient can sleep comfortably again. Glonoine is a very fast-acting medicine. In homoeopathy, the proving of Glonoine has been found to be a rapid process, therefore it should not be repeated frequently. Glonoine used in low potency a few times every five to ten minutes, will provoke a severe splitting type of headache, along with all other symptoms of Glonoine manifesting themselves. It does not need to be repeated more often or over a longer period. Proving with Glonoine is the best method for convincing the disbelievers of homoeopathy.

Another similarity between Glonoine and Gelsemium is that in both, the patient's hands and feet are very cold. However, in Gelsemium, there is no perspiration whereas in Glonoine, despite the hands and feet being cold, the patient perspires.

The tongue of a Glonoine patient is reddish in colour. The mouth is dry, but one does not feel much thirst. Despite having **high fever**, the patient still does not feel thirsty. The symptoms become worse in hot weather, in the sunlight and by sitting near the fire. The sensitivity to sunlight and heat is not limited to the head; the whole body is affected. The patient suffers from palpitation, shortness of breath, **nausea and vomiting**. Local pressure relieves the headache, while reading makes the headache worse. The eyesight is affected in such a way that the words appear small and the objects look only half-lit.

In Glonoine, the patient perceives **flashes of light and the stars shining in front of the eyes**. On bending over, dark spots appear in front of the eyes. The eyes feel under pressure and hurt. The eyes become congested with blood. The eyes of a Glonoine patient are rather retracted and yellow in colour. They are sensitive to light. Temporary blindness is also common. A characteristic feature of Glonoine is that during fever, the face is pale rather than being red.

Glonoine is very useful in the treatment of **meningitis** of children, contracted in the summer. The neck arches backwards (opisthotonus). The face becomes extremely hot and glares. The eyes become drawn upwards. The head and the upper part of the body are extremely hot while the lower part of the body becomes cold. The patient sweats profusely. The **overlying membranes of the brain become inflamed** (meningitis). If the malarial parasites reach the backbone, this may also cause inflammation of the linings of the brain. Glonoine would be ideal to treat this condition if it happens to be in the summer time.

Very often, one might experience a rush of blood towards the head while walking. The face becomes flushed. There is a feeling of choking of the throat as if the entire blood has pooled over the face and head. The body becomes cold and sweaty due to extreme weakness. The patient may become unconscious. This condition is called apoplexy in medical terminology. This type of fits of unconsciousness can be due to clotting of blood in the brain, while in Glonoine patients, these symptoms result from a temporary spasm (of the blood vessels going to the brain). If such a patient is not treated in time with Glonoine, the repeated fits of unconsciousness may result in permanent damage.

A Glonoine patient often **forgets the well-known routes** and does not know where he is and where he is going. The streets appear strange to him. These kinds of symptoms are also seen in Lachesis.

Glonoine is commonly used for **lowering high blood pressure**. Opium is also found to be useful in this respect. It is more effective than Glonoine. Dr. Kent is of the opinion that in the case of **high blood pressure**, one should prefer to use Opium over Glonoine because the effects of Glonoine are mostly temporary while those of Opium are long lasting.

Glonoine is very useful in treatment of **sudden stoppage of menstruation** due to exposure to cold, or due to fear resulting in neurosis. Cimicifuga and Bryonia are also useful in this condition. Aethusa may also be of use once the symptoms of **insanity** become evident. In general, Aethusa is ideal for the treatment of mental illnesses resulting from stomach disorder. Similarly, Aethusa can be useful to treat the **mental condition developing due to the sudden stoppage of menses**. In a Glonoine patient, the **throbbing of the ears** reflects the palpitation of the heart.

**The stomach and the intestines rumble**. It is only natural to experience **severe nausea and vomiting as a result of heat stroke**. There is a feeling of weakness in the stomach. The pulse is weak and slow. When walking, the pulse becomes rapid due to rapid heartbeat. There is a feeling of warmth and burning all over the body. The patient may **suddenly faint and fall**. One feels choked and froth comes out of the mouth. This is only a temporary resemblance to an epileptic fit.

**Itching** is also associated with Glonoine. There are **severe cramps** over the arms and the legs. **Pain in the fingers of the left hand** is the symptom of Glonoine. The symptoms are worse between six o' clock and noon. During summer, the severity of the headache varies with the sun. Even the slightest jerk would intensify the headache.

| | |
|---|---|
| Antidote: | Aconite |
| Potency: | 30 to 200 |

# GRAPHITES
## (Black Lead)

Graphite has commonly been described in reference to the treatment of heavy, strong and obese women. But I have not seen it effective in obesity. I have used it in various potencies but have not seen a single obese woman getting slim with it. However it has certainly proven useful in the treatment of other diseases mentioned in the chapter of Graphites. I always use it in potency 200 or over. I have never used it in potency 30. As far as the treatment of **obesity** is concerned, I have found the following three remedies most useful: Phytolacca, Phytolacca Berry and Fucus.

In Graphites the menses are **scanty**. The bleeding lasts for two or three days and the quantity of the blood loss is also much less. This is probably the reason for their tendency towards being obese. Perhaps Graphites is linked to the treatment of being overweight on this basis. Once the menstrual cycle becomes normal, one can hope to lose weight.

**The discharges of Graphites patient are usually very sticky. Eczema** of Graphites is recognized on the same basis. This eczema is usually found behind the ears, over different areas of the head and over the joints of the elbows and hands. There is always some sticky secretion coming out which subsequently changes into a hard scab. In Mezereum too, the discharge is sticky which then turns into a hard scab, making a sort of cover over the head. Some young children develop a severe type of eczema, which bleeds on scratching. The condition becomes really troublesome. The overall symptoms of their eczema resemble Psorinum as well as Graphites. This is due to the latent presence of some sinister substance of a deep-seated illness in their body. Whenever I gave Silicea to the children who, based on their symptoms require to be treated with it, without any exception the foul matter bursts open. This effect of Silicea is well established. However, if with the treatment of Silicea the foul substances only surface to the body but are not eliminated, then we must look for another suitable, similar related medicine. Next in order to Silicea are Psorinum and Graphites. Psorinum often dries up the eczema, yet sometimes it does not offer complete cure. The dry skin keeps on itching, although there is definitely some relief of symptoms, so much so that the child can sleep peacefully at night. However, the eczematous skin starts discharging again after some time. In this condition, Graphites should also be used as an adjuvant. It helps to a certain extent. Therefore, it is better that the resistant type of illnesses like eczema should be treated with a number of similarly acting remedies, complimentary to each other. If the itching amounts to restlessness, Arsenic 1000 will also be very useful. It is especially very effective against **dry eczema**. Even if all the symptoms are not present, the element of restlessness is such that Arsenic will benefit to some extent although the relief may only be temporary. No doubt, the proper use of Arsenic would be of avail where the patient exhibits most of the signs and symptoms of Arsenic.

It must be well remembered that the treatment is proper only when the nature of the medicine, as well as the constitution of the patient, are properly evaluated and matched. The assumption that a medicine that is effective against a particular disease will cure all the patients of that disease is only wishful thinking. At the same time it is not necessary that an effective cure for each disease has been discovered, or any doctor has full knowledge about the treatment of every sickness. Therefore it is not right to prolong the illness of a patient unnecessarily while the patient is not getting better under the treatment of one doctor. One should honestly admit that some other doctor may be able to offer a better treatment. There is no harm in accepting defeat. The patient should be referred to somebody more qualified.

Graphites is a very useful drug for its own specific kind of **eczema**. f the patient has other symptoms of Graphites, then this drug alone will suffice. Otherwise, in cases of various types of eczemas (with super-added infections) Graphites is only used as an adjuvant remedy. If the skin becomes raw and red, as is the case with early symptoms of Psoriasis, then Graphites should be prescribed. This symptom of the skin is also associated with Silicea. However, the indication of Graphites is the sticky exudate oozing from the skin.

Graphites is also very useful for the treatment of **cancer**. The tendency towards the formation of a cancer is in the nature of every carbon compound. Having healed, some wounds burst open again and again and ultimately become cancerous. Even after surgical removal, they tend to recur after some time. In such cases, one should always remember Graphites. Graphites should be given in potencies 200 or 1000. The treatment must be repeated until the positive effects of treatment become apparent.

Graphites also has an effect on the muscular system in the body. Particularly, it has significant effect on the back of the thighs (hamstring muscles). The patients who feel difficulty in standing or sitting are of two kinds. In one group, the movement becomes difficult due to backache and paralytic symptoms. Graphites has no effect on this group. In the other group, the **muscles have become tense and contracted**, as if they have become shrunk and are neither stretchable not contractable without discomfort. There is severe tightness on the back of the thighs. This group is amenable to treatment with Graphites. Graphites must definitely be tried in this group even if other particular symptoms of Graphites are absent. Such kind of partial treatment becomes necessary on and off.

Graphites is associated with severe **constipation**. Faeces pile up in the distal part of the intestines (rectum) as large hard masses packed in layers. When there is generalised inflammation of the intestines, often, such a patient may get temporary relief from Bryonia. The difference between Bryonia and Graphites is that in Bryonia, the faeces are generally hard in the beginning and then become somewhat softer. In the case of Graphites, the faeces are and remain hard and very dry. The patient remains constipated for several days. If diarrhoea starts, the stools become very watery, black and happen to contain undigested food.

**Herpes** is a disease in which blisters form along the course of the nerves. The skin becomes raw. The patient feels severe burning sensation, discomfort and pain. Herpes is of two types. Herpes Zoster or "shingles" appears due to the affliction of nerves with the virus. The blisters burst open and promote further spread of blister formation. The other type of herpes is genital herpes, which results from improper sexual behaviour. It tends to recur frequently and is related to external genitals. It is a very painful disease. Once established, the disease lasts forever. Graphites has a special merit for the treatment of this type of herpes. However, Graphites alone is not enough. Some other medicine also needs to be used along with Graphites. I have devised a standard formula for the **treatment of all kinds of herpes**. This includes Arnica, Ledum and Arsenic. This formula also offers cure for snakebite. The prescription is very useful when the pain has started in the previously afflicted snakebite wounds, associated with burning, sensation of heat and the involvement of nervous system. With these medicines, herpes gets cured fast. The genital herpes being very obstinate with the probability of recurrence, the treatment must be continued for about six months with intervals of seven to ten days in between.

The patient of Graphites is of cool temperament like that of Psorinum and Silicea. When the medicines of similar temperament and efficacy are used one after the other, they do not lower the efficacy of one another. The drugs help each other in curing the disease.

The patient of Graphites does not like the open air, yet leaves the windows open. Despite the body being cold, the draft of cold air does not bother him, while in most patients; the draft of air is also unbearable. The Graphites patient dislikes cold. He feels comforted with heat, but the internal body heat resulting from exercise, jogging or walking intensifies his symptoms.

The symptoms of paralysis are also found in Graphites. Like Causticum, the paralysis of Graphites affects only certain organs, especially the lower part of the body. Graphites is very effective in the treatment of the **paralysis of legs**. It is also of great use in the treatment of epilepsy. Epilepsy develops as a result of some serious deep-seated illness of the body. Naturally, its treatment also requires to be conducted with an appropriate remedy of matching nature and profound effectiveness. Graphites is certainly one of those drugs.

Graphites being pure carbon, resembles Carbo Veg. Each carbon compound may exhibit symptoms of spasms/convulsions. Carbo Veg is the best treatment for the **painful muscle cramps of the legs**. Once these cramps lead to the development of epilepsy, and the other specific symptoms of Graphites being present, Graphites would certainly work. The distinctive beauty of Graphites is that if it is effective against a disease, it will produce excellent results. The disease may either completely disappear or rendered so mild that the epileptic attacks may never recur. Graphites is an excellent treatment for **depression**. But this symptom alone cannot be enough to arrive at proper diagnosis, because depression is so common that everybody seems to have suffered from it at one time or another. A Graphites patient is always anxious, sad and dejected. His mind gets confused. He loses the ability to think, understand and make decisions. **On getting up in the morning**, the patient becomes dizzy. The mind is dulled and the light becomes unbearable. **The eyes burn and become red with watery secretions**. The sense of smell becomes very sharp. The patient cannot tolerate the smell of the flowers. The nose is painful and dry. The nasal secretions dry up in the form of scales. The patient feels as if his face is covered with cobwebs. Itchy kind of blisters form on the skin. A wet type of eczema develops around the mouth and on the chin. The **mouth smells foul. Blisters with burning sensation appear on the tongue**.

A patient of Graphites usually dislikes meat. Sweets provoke nausea. The patient tends to **nauseate and vomit** after every food. Women feel nausea in the morning, during menstruation. There is a **feeling of pressure and burning sensation over the stomach**, increasing the appetite. In Graphites, there is **severe pain over the neck, shoulders, back and upper arms**. The backache causes severe weakness. The left hand becomes numb and the left arm too. The fingernails become thick, black and ugly. Over the **toes, there is a feeling of stiffness and pinching**. The **nails become thick, deformed and are very painful**.

The Graphites ailments become more intense with heat, at night, as well as during and after the menstruation. Darkness and covering with a piece of cloth relieve the symptoms.

| | |
|---|---|
| Adjuvants: | Argentum Nitricum, Causticum, Hepar Sulph, Lycopodium, Arsenic, Tuberculinum |
| Antidotes: | Nux Vomica, Aconite |
| Potency: | 30 to 1000 |

# GRATIOLA

Gratiola, though rarely used, is notably important in some diseases. It is known for causing profound nervous, mental and physical weakness. If there is nervous exhaustion, mental and physical weakness along with other specific ailments, the administration of Gratiola in such cases will promptly cure the symptoms. In Gratiola, there is a type of stinging irritation of the eyes. The eyesight is hazy like looking through a cobweb. There is a peculiar type of colour blindness, in which green appears to be white. The patient complains that it is as if sand particles are irritating the eye.

Melancholia in women is probably related to Gratiola. Gratiola presents a unique paradox that women apparently feel weak, but deep down they may experience passionate excitement of sexual organs. Young girls, if so afflicted, tend to be immodest and shameless. They must be treated to control their passions and desires. Gratiola will work if other associated symptoms are not very complex.

In responding to heat and cold, the constitution of Gratiola patient is like that of Pulsatilla. Gratiola works better on left-sided ailments like Lachesis. Its sexual excitement resembles that of Taraentula. However, Taraentula is good for right-sided symptoms. Gratiola symptoms are mostly localised, while in Lachesis symptoms shift from left to right.

Gratiola is useful in some kinds of colds. If nasal secretions enter the stomach, it causes severe spasms, in the form of twisting and curling of the stomach. Gratiola is useful in common stomach problems associated with the swelling of the upper lip and this is true about Pulsatilla as well.
Sometimes Gratiola annuls the effect of Coffea. Similarly, Coffea works the same way against Gratiola. The symptoms of both these remedies are similar. Although the nervous infirmity peculiar to Gratiola is not as pronounced in Coffea. Yet, it is said that Gratiola resembles Coffea. One thing is clear that if one cannot sleep in the early part of the night and other symptoms of Coffea are not present, then this indicates Gratiola. In Gratiola, typically, **swallowing relieves the throat's discomfort**. But in Gratiola, swallowing

ameliorates the pain. Therefore, Gratiola patient drinks fluids in sips so that the discomfort at the throat may be relieved.

The Gratiola patient feels dizzy while eating, more so after having finished eating. Closing the eyes, reading, and getting up suddenly also produces dizziness, showing that the patient is anaemic or has low blood pressure.

Another type of stomach upset is associated with nausea and distension of the stomach due to gas. In Gratiola nausea disappears as soon as food is taken. Usually in nausea, one does not feel like eating, but in Gratiola, strangely enough, the treatment for nausea is eating food. Acidity of the stomach can be relieved by food intake, but returns after a short while. Acidity of the stomach is not necessarily due to Hydrochloric acid (HCl). Very often, due to a lack of hydrochloric acid, food remains undigested, producing various other acids. In the case of hyperacidity of the stomach, nausea or belching cause a reflux of the acidic contents of the stomach into the distal part of the food pipe (oesophagus). The patient feels burning behind the breast bone (sternum) and feels tightness of the chest, as in angina.

In Gratiola, there is a feeling of burning all over, but an inflammation and a burning sensation of the reproductive organs, male and female both, can provoke unusual and unnatural physical reactions. In the Gratiola patient, typically there is palpitation after passing stools.

Homoeopathic physicians must prepare a library of similarly acting remedies, store them in their memory and then sub-classify them according to their peculiar, distinctive features. Then alone will they be able to make proper diagnoses. If they do not do so, they will always remain confused and find difficulty in treating their patients properly.

| | |
|---|---|
| Potency: | 30 to 200 |

# GUAIACUM

Guaiacum is a profoundly effective and very powerful remedy. However, homoeopathic doctors rarely use it. Only a few experienced doctors have used it and even then once in a while, otherwise, the drug has remained unknown. Usually, it is used for the treatment of **rheumatic pain and gout**. If the symptoms of hereditary tuberculosis are found in a patient, Guaiacum must be kept in mind for the treatment of such a patient. In a patient of Guaiacum, there is a tendency towards diarrhoea. Furthermore the white ropy structures called tendons, which attach the muscles to the bones, become contracted and then shrink, resulting in the contracture of the joints, meaning that they cannot be fully stretched, and hurt on such an attempt. There is a feeling of pain and tiredness over the muscles of both the shoulders. Guaiacum is useful in treating this condition.

The symptoms of Guaiacum aggravate with heat while they ameliorate in cold. From this point of view, it is similar to Ledum, Pulsatilla, Lac Caninum and Iodum. However, there are clear-cut symptoms of each of these remedies, by which they can be distinguished; a proper diagnosis can be arrived at and the optimal treatment may be given.

Due to the multiple joint pains, the patients of Guaiacum **stoop forward while walking.** Their **knee joints become weak**, and the hands and feet become stiff. The person may become completely disabled physically. Besides Guaiacum, these symptoms can be treated with Colchicum. The significant feature of Colchicum is that the pain starts at the big toe. The salient sign of Guaiacum is that the affected area is hypersensitive to any kind of touch. The symptoms become worse with the application of heat. The swelling of the joints may lead to the formation of ulcers and abscesses. Guaiacum is deeply related to the bones as well. The **bones become soft**, **bend** and become porous like a sponge (osteoporosis). This condition often reminds one of Calcarea Carb. However, if there is the tendency towards joint pains, Guaiacum will be found more effective. Another sign of Guaiacum is the feeling of extreme tiredness. On the slightest movement, the patient feels weak. The weakness then involves the nerves leading to further physical weakness. The body then starts wasting.

Guaiacum is very useful in the treatment of **tuberculosis in its early stages**. If the tuberculosis bacteria are present in the blood and the patient suffers from rheumatism along with the tendency to development of boils, and there are generalised body aches, then Guaiacum will be found very effective.

Guaiacum is also an antisporic remedy i.e. it is very effective against **skin diseases** related to psoriasis and leprosy. Sulphur and Psorinum are also top class antisporic medicines. The nature of Sulphur is hot whereas that of Psorinum is cold. However, Sulphur and Psorinum alone cannot cure all types of psoriatic diseases. When such diseases have afflicted the mucous membranes also, several other medicines need to be used. If the developing condition is of eczema, the appropriate analogous remedy will need to be given according to the type of the eczema. If a condition develops out of psoriasis and the appropriate remedy administered, but the recovery stops after a little beneficial effect, then it will become necessary to use other antisporic drugs in high potencies. If the associated symptoms can be directly linked to a particular remedy, then certainly that alone will be the most effective. Sometimes the picture is not clear. In this condition, they will serve as a general cure for psora facilitating the beneficial effect of similar homoeopathic remedies.

There is many a kind of skin conditions, which require to be treated with their constitutional remedy. If the drugs selected after careful thinking, do not benefit the patient, then it becomes necessary to use antisporic drugs. They will reduce the aggressiveness of the sickness so that it becomes responsive to the overall treatment. Besides Sulphur and Psorinum, these medicines include Merc Sol, Tuberculinum and Syphilinum. Similarly, Guaiacum is also antisporic.

Guaiacum is also related to **facial neuralgia**. In Guaiacum, there is a pinching type of pain on one side of the face. It is very annoying. Spigelia is more effective in the treatment of facial neuralgia on the left side while Silicea and Mag Phos are more useful on the right side.

In Guaiacum, the **eyes become swollen**, the pupils are dilated and the eyelids are contracted. Small boils appear around the eyes. Once in a while, the ear also hurts. This, however, is not due to any infection or epidemic disease. Apparently, there is no swelling or external redness. When the pain in the ears is about to disappear, the patient feels pinpricks over the head. If a patient is suffering from **severe cold** along with a runny nose and feels pain over the nasal bones, he can get relief with Guaiacum. With this kind of cold, the patient feels pain in the jawbones. Eupatorium Perfol is famous for the treatment of **bone pains.** However, its effectiveness is limited. It has commonly been found useful in the treatment of influenza like fever. There is a small insect called "kutri", found in the dry areas. Its bite produces severe burning sensation and inflammation. It causes Dengue fever, associated with severe bone pains. Eupatorium Perfol is very useful for the treatment of this fever. The aches and pains associated with Guaiacum are precisely timed. The bone pain, especially the pain in the roots of the teeth, often gets worse at night. Pains starting at six o'clock in the evening and continuing up to four o'clock in the morning, should be treated with Guaiacum. In the presence of its other symptoms, Guaiacum will be found effective and fast. Along with the joint pains and gout, there is a tendency of contracting sore throat. With the sore throat the entire body starts hurting. Sometimes, toothache can also cause severe body aches. In allopathy, the doctors usually advise the extraction of the tooth or the surgical removal of the tonsils, but the aches and pains may still persist. Timely treatment with Guaiacum will obviate the need for such surgery.

In Guaiacum, the patient has a **constant urge to pass urine**, but cannot ease himself. The repeated fruitless effort makes him restless. There is a kind of piercing sensation at the end of urination.

Women suffering from rheumatism **develop permanent inflammation inside the uterus**. They may develop complete cessation of the periods or other conditions due to uterine dysfunction. There is a feeling of hissing over the mammary glands. The overlying skin shrinks and small pimples develop over it.

**Rapid heartbeat** is also a symptom of Guaiacum. Furthermore, a dry cough and fever develop. Sometimes, rheumatic **types of pains develop in the muscles of the chest wall**, which become worse in winter. There is a feeling of pain over the heart. If the rheumatic fever and the associated joint pains are suppressed with some strong medication, the toxic material of the infection will afflict the valves of the heart (rheumatic carditis). The patient feels discomfort over the heart, like joint pain. When the heart gets afflicted secondary to the suppression of flu, this will be best treated with Spigelia. Spigelia is also of use to treat the aftereffects of the forcefully suppressed gout. However, Guaiacum is more useful for treating the gout as well as its deleterious effect on the heart. These pains may be on the back of the neck and when associated with tightness and stiffness of the neck; Guaiacum should be remembered. Guaiacum is also useful in the treatment of the pain over the upper arms, thighs, as well as the finger joints.

In Guaiacum, the patient may also suffer from **kidney problems**. Usually, the patients sweat a lot, which in fact is beneficial to them. As long as the patient perspires, the symptoms of kidney dysfunction do not appear. As soon as the patient stops perspiring, kidney symptoms will ensue. If such a patient develops renal pain in the winter, he will benefit from sweating induced by heat treatment. It simply means that the sweat, as well as the kidneys, helps eliminate similar kinds of toxic materials from the body. Guaiacum helps in elimination of these toxic materials and the salts from the body to keep their balance in the blood.

The symptoms of Guaiacum aggravate with movement, heat, pressure and on touch. The symptoms ameliorate on the application of external pressure.

| | |
|---|---|
| Antidotes: | Nux Vomica and Sepia |
| Potency: | 30 or sometimes higher potency. |

# HAEMATOXYLON

Basically, Haematoxylon is used for the treatment of **angina** associated with a peculiar type of constriction and tightness. The patient feels as if someone has placed a heavy slab of stone on the chest. The feeling of constriction is also found over other parts of the body. The stomach feels full of gas, hurts and has a feeling of internal scraping. This feeling extends up to the throat and there is a feeling of internal pain and cramp at the heart. Touch aggravates the discomfort. The head feels heavy. The effect of Haematoxylon can be annulled by Camphor.

| | |
|---|---|
| Potency: | 30 |

# HEDEOMA

This medication plays a significant role against the diseases of both men and women. Its ailments are aggravated by mental stress.

**In the morning, the patient's head feels heavy** or there is pain over the head as if somebody has physically assaulted him. He feels very weak but feels better on lying down. The stomach becomes inflamed and hypersensitive and hurts on eating or drinking anything. A white coating on the tongue, nausea, distension of the abdomen and bellyache are all the symptoms of Hedeoma.

This is an extraordinarily effective medicine for the treatment of **urinary symptoms**. The patient is unable to hold water and wants to pass it out immediately. The pain (colicky in nature) begins at the kidney and then it radiates down to the ureter, bladder and then along the urethra. Hedeoma is deeply related to this kind of urinary complaint. Even in the absence of other symptoms it proves to be extremely effective to relieve these symptoms.

For women who feel **pain over the uterus** radiating downwards, or tightness over the ovaries accompanied by spasmodic type of pains, this is a very useful remedy. The **leucorrhoeal discharge causes burning** and severe itching.

I have found Hedeoma and Pulex Irritans very useful in the treatment of **cancer of the uterus.** Both have a very beneficial effect on the health of the inner lining of the uterus (endometrium). However there is no mention of this for these two remedies in any literatures. My statement is based on my experience, and I am sure that whoever tries these remedies will not be disappointed by them.

| | |
|---|---|
| Potency: | 1 or any other low potency |

# HEKLA LAVA

Mount Hekla is a volcanic mountain. The medicine prepared from the lava of this mountain is called Hekla Lava. I do not know of any other kind of lava used for the preparation of a homoeopathic medicine. The contents of all the lavae are probably identical, however, the effects of lava may differ from area to area. Therefore, the lava of other volcanoes should also be experimented upon.

Hekla Lava mainly affects the bones, especially the **bones of the face and the jaw**. However, it has an effect on the other bones of the body as well. Hekla Lava can be of useful in the treatment of tooth decay associated with a lot of pain and which refuses to respond to any other treatment.

Sometimes, the jaw becomes very swollen and may apparently exhibit all general signs of Hekla Lava, yet does not benefit from the treatment with Hekla Lava. In that condition, the most important and effective treatment is Sulphur. Sulphur is found to be very effective against certain dangerous conditions that the doctors have labelled as incurable. For example **cancer of the jawbone** that has advanced significantly and causes severe discomfort, affecting the ears. Once, a woman was in severe pain due to the cancer of the jaw. One side of the face was extremely swollen causing pressure over the eyes. She used to scream due to the severity of pain. She remained in one of the best hospitals for a long period, but the doctors found no effective treatment for her disease. Ultimately, she was discharged from the hospital with the pronouncement that her disease was incurable. I gave her one dose of Sulphur CM, which decreased the severity of the pain and within two weeks, there was marked decrease in the size of the swelling of the face. After this, I treated her with one dose of Silicea CM. With this the process of recovery, which had previously slowed down, was restored. Sometime later, I gave her another dose of Sulphur CM. The disease completely disappeared. Several years have passed since the treatment of this patient and until today, she is completely healthy. My reason for mentioning this in relation to Hekla Lava is that she had apparently all the symptoms of Hekla Lava but did not benefit at all with Hekla Lava. This shows that Hekla Lava may be effective against other diseases of the bone but is definitely ineffective against the cancer of the bones.

Hekla Lava must be a really good remedy but personally, I do not have experience of its effectiveness. However, some homoeopaths adore it.

The specific symptom of Hekla Lava is stated to be the **pain in the jawbones**. There is considerable swelling around the jaws and the jawbones become thickened and enlarged.

Regarding the treatment of the deep-seated bone diseases, in addition to Sulphur, I have found Calcarea Carb to be much more effective than Hekla Lava. I have used Calcarea Carb in the treatment of bone cancer that had been histologically proved. Within a few months of the treatment with high potency Calcarea Carb, the disease was overcome significantly. Such patients should doubtless be treated carefully, over a long period. One should not just rely on using Calcarea Carb, some other adjuvant treatments will also be required keeping in view the overall symptoms of the patient. Thus, the focus of the treatment would obviously be Calcarea Carb, however, several other medicines may also prove to be very useful.

Calcarea Carb is particularly very useful in the treatment of bone diseases due to a lack of calcium (osteopenia). Sulphur is also effective. Calcarea Carb is chronic of Sulphur. Generally, Calcarea Carb is more effective in the diseases of the bones of the lower legs than Sulphur. Calcarea Carb is also effective against the cysts of the hands.

In my practice, I have not been able to use Hekla Lava much, possibly due to the fact that I was not fully conversant with its signs and symptoms. I do not mean to discourage other homoeopaths from using it. I would advise them to go over the writings of other doctors about Hekla Lava and then use it on their patients in different potencies. It is just possible that they may successfully use it for the treatment of many more diseases, in spite of my failure to use it much.

Some doctors have found Hekla Lava very useful in the treatment of teething problems of children. I do not have much experience of that myself. Instead, I have found the following prescription effective, without any doubt, in teething problems:

Kali Phos + Ferrum Phos + Silicea + Calcarea Phos + Calcarea Fluor

Additionally, the above prescription has been found very effective against certain kinds of bone cancer and the diseases of the covering membrane of bones (periosteum).

In the homoeopathic literature, the conditions which can be effectively treated with Hekla Lava are: the thickening of the skull bone behind the ears, the thickening of the outer surface of the bone, ulcers on the nasal bones, neuralgic pains over the face resulting from the extraction of the teeth or the caries, and neck glands which have somewhat receded after initial enlargement. The symptoms of Hekla Lava aggravate in humid weather.

| | |
|---|---|
| Antidotes: | Camphor, China |
| Potency: | 30 or above. |

# HELLEBORUS NIGER

## (Snow Rose)

Helleborus Niger is prepared from a flowering plant called Snow Rose. It is prepared by grinding the roots of the plant.

The most important characteristic of a Helleborus Niger patient is that of becoming disorientated and being **out of his mind.** This results in a lack of coordination of the functions of the body. Moreover, the inflammation of the membranes of the brain and the spinal cord (the meninges) leads to the dysfunction of the nervous system and then **insanity**. Helleborus Niger is that medicine which, by the grace of God, relieves all these symptoms and restores the person to mental health once again. In the diseases of Helleborus Niger there is no voluntary control over the functioning of the limbs and the muscles, and their response to the message from the brain is delayed. The mind is clear and active, but the muscles do not respond properly in time because the basic nervous system has been affected. When something is said to a patient he does not react to it at all. It becomes necessary to jolt him in order to make him aware. His thoughts are scattered and he needs to be reminded again and again to make him do something or he will simply do nothing. The patient exhibits a strange type of drowsiness and insensitivity, which may lead to unconsciousness.

Sometimes, the Helleborus Niger patient starts **viewing Satan and evil spirits**. He becomes fearful of having committed an unforgiveable sin. Such scary ideas are also noticed in Aurum, Lachesis and Stramonium.

Several remedies may be used in the treatment of hydrocephalus, which means an **increase in the size of the head due to build up of pressure inside the skull (secondary to excessive accumulation of cerbro-spinal fluid)**. The most effective, of course, is Silicea. Helleborus is also useful in treating this condition. When the head of the child becomes enlarged and the eyes apparently sink, the child may suddenly make dreadful screams. This symptom is distinctively present in Apis. In Apis, the headache is of a stinging nature. Apis would make the child feel better in this kind of pain associated with hydrocephalus, but Apis is relatively slow acting medicine. In contrast, Silicea is a fast-acting medicine. Helleborus Niger is very effective in the treatment of excessive production of cerebrospinal fluid and thus decreases the build-up of pressure in the skull (intracranial pressure). Even if it may not cure, it would certainly benefit to some extent.

**In the kind of epilepsy (petit mal) where the patient does not lose consciousness and his eyes remain open**, Helleborus is very useful. After the fit is over, the patient feels extremely weak and drowsy.

In a patient of Helleborus, the **headache** moves from inside out, causing pressure on the eyes and forehead. The eyeballs move upwards and squint. The patient is very sensitive to light. The head feels heavy and hot deep down. The patient groans with pain. Despite being hungry, he cannot eat or drink anything. There is a sensation of burning in the oesophagus, **gas in the stomach and rumbling over the stomach area**. There is a feeling of pressure over the stomach. The stomach hurts on walking and coughing. **General weakness** is a prominent feature of Helleborus, which may result in paralysis.

Helleborus is very effective in relieving the pressure inside the urinary bladder, which results in the inability of the child to pass urine. The urine is dark coloured. Helleborus is also famous for the treatment of continuous uncontrolled movements in the arm and leg on one side of the body (chorea and athetosis). The thumb becomes tightly contracted into the palm. Blisters form between the fingers of the hand and toes of the feet. All these symptoms need to be treated immediately with Helleborus.

The relationship of Helleborus to hydrocephalus has already been described. The screaming of the children during sleep resembles that of Apis. However, in the Apis patient, there are no involuntary movements affecting one side of the body. In a patient of Helleborus, there is soft pitting oedema of the skin with the formation of blue spots. Hair loss on the scalp and breaking of the nails is also amongst the symptoms of Helleborus Niger.

| | |
|---|---|
| Antidotes: | Camphor, Cincona (China) |
| Potency: | 30 to 1000 |

# HELONIAS

Helonias is a very important drug specifically linked to women's diseases. It has a strong association with the **cancer of the cervix of the uterus**. Carbo Animalis can also be a useful medicine for the treatment of this cancer if its symptoms related to other parts of the body are also present. However, Helonias has a direct association with cancer of the uterus. It definitely produces some results. Prompt treatment with Helonias on the appearance of the swelling and redness of the cervix uteri will be very effective. If the patient is not fully cured with Helonias, the treatment should be followed by Carbo Animalis. Hopefully, by the grace of God, with the combination of these two drugs, the patient will be fully cured.

After a woman has miscarried, her **uterus sags down**. She feels pressure on the front as well as the back. On walking, the discomfort increases, and the uterus tilts from its place to the left or to the right. In these conditions, Helonias makes the muscles strong and thus would revert the uterus to its original position.

The symptom of deflection of the uterus from its normal position has reminded me that it may be of use to correct the position of a foetus in the uterus, which happens to be mal-positioned. I hope it would be beneficial. In case the **baby is upside down** (breech position), Pulsatilla 30 or 200 is very effective. In poor countries, facilities for immediate surgery are not available, women with this kind of pregnancy (foetal mal-position) suffer a lot, and some even die. In those areas, it becomes imperative for a homoeopath to remember well the medicines that may be of use on such occasions, such as Pulsatilla, Caulophylum and Helonias. In addition, Gelsemium, Kali Carb and Arnica are very useful at the time of childbirth. They prevent against the possible complications of delivery such as **puerperal fever**. If during or after delivery uterine infection has set in causing high fever, then Sulphur and Pyrogenium 200 should be given together three times a day till the fever subsides, and then once a day for a few days. This happens to be the best treatment in this kind of situation.

Helonias is very effective against **diabetes** also. In women who suffer from diabetes along with the diseases of the uterus, Helonias can be effective against both. The treatment should be continued for at least one month. If the diabetes seems to be coming under control Helonias alone may be enough, otherwise some other remedies should be looked for to treat the diabetes.

Another symptom of Helonias is that the **periods are too frequent** or may cease for many months. The patient gets fits of severe depression and becomes very lazy. Severe kind of leucorrhoea associated with itchiness sets in.

Helonias is also linked to the **kidneys. They become congested with blood**. There is a feeling of severe burning, which may also be felt externally on both sides over the skin (kidney areas). The patient can clearly outline the course of the pain with his finger. Such patients may also pass albumin in the urine. If this happens during pregnancy, then Helonias must be considered.

The Helonias patient feels better if her attention is kept diverted from her illness. Movement aggravates the symptoms.

| | |
|---|---|
| Potency: | 30 to 200. |

# HEPAR SULPHURIS CALCAREUM

## (Calcium Sulphide)

Hepar Sulph is another name for Calcium Sulphide. Dr. Hahnemann prepared it from the shells of the oysters (a sea animal) and performed different types of experiments on it. It is a compound of Calcarea Carb and Sulphur, possessing some of the characteristics of both of its components. However, most of its symptoms are different from both Calcarea Carb and Sulphur. In the olden days, Calcium Sulphide was used externally for the treatment of itching, joint pains, gout and the swellings associated with tuberculosis. It was also considered to be useful against asthma and tuberculosis of the lungs.

Hepar Sulph is a common remedy of daily use. It is deeply related to Silicea. Wherever Silicea becomes ineffective, Hepar Sulph may be found useful. It is also very **effective against common contagious diseases**. In case Silicea is unsafe to be given, Hepar Sulph may be used as a substitute without any fear. Hepar Sulph is often used in between the usage of Mercury and Silicea. To avoid serious untoward symptoms, it is not proper to use Silicea by itself after the treatment with Mercury. It is imperative to give Hepar Sulph after treatment with Mercury and before starting treatment with Silicea. Similarly, if it becomes necessary to give Mercury after treatment with Silicea, Hepar Sulph must be used in between to avoid the danger of incompatibility between Silicea and Mercury.

Hepar Sulph is of great use for **throat conditions**. If the phlegm sticks in the throat and it is difficult to expel despite coughing, Hepar Sulph will be found very effective. The patient of Hepar Sulph coughs a lot, especially in the morning. The **cough** aggravates in the cold and is mostly painful.

In Hepar Sulph the **patient feels as if something is stuck in the throat,** which despite effort, cannot be expelled. If, in fact, there is something stuck in the throat, it will come out easily with Silicea since Silicea is known to expel foreign bodies lodged in the body. In Hepar

Sulph, there is nothing sticking in the throat, it is just an uncomfortable feeling.

A patient of Hepar Sulph is **extraordinarily sensitive** and reactive to his surroundings. Every kind of pain is felt magnified. He is short-tempered and angry by nature. Even though he may be a gentle person, during the disease he becomes very impulsive, so much so that he may even kill his close friend. So far, I have not known such a patient myself. This description mentioned in literatures may apply to mental patients but seems like an unbelievable exaggeration in regard to ordinary patients.

The swelling and **hardening of the glands** is known in relation to many remedies and also in Hepar Sulph. If the hardening and swelling of the glands becomes persistent, it is treated with various remedies according to the circumstances. Once the glands start suppurating (pus formation) then Hepar Sulph should be used without any further delay. Calcarea Sulph is also very useful.

Some **children have the habit of biting their nails**. This results in tearing of the pulp of the fingers causing discomfort. The slightest touch produces severe pain. The child chews the pulp and then tears it apart. This habit then becomes firmly established. Besides Natrum Mur, Hepar Sulph is also very useful in treating this condition.

Sometimes, **pus forms around the nail** (paronychia). The nail becomes loose and is uprooted. The new nail replaces it. Here, the drug of choice is Hepar Sulph. If a **nail becomes dark and begins to deform**, then Psorinum should be tried first. If it happens to be ineffective, other remedies should be sought. Nail deformities are also found in Antimonium Crude. If warts ulcerate and start bleeding, Hepar Sulph will be useful. If they happen to crack open and fungate like cauliflower, then the best treatment is Nitric Acid.

The skin of Hepar Sulph children looks dirty and may not look clean in spite of the child having taken a shower. With Hepar Sulph, the skin becomes neat and clean. At the same time the dirty appearance of the face disappears.

If during a cold, the **phlegm sticks inside the nose or throat**, causing sneezing, Hepar Sulph should be administered. Sneezing due to feeling cold is another symptom of Hepar Sulph. If a person starts sneezing on entering a heated room during winter, Pulsatilla is the appropriate treatment for this condition. If the sneezing occurs on moving from a hot area into a cold area, then one should think of Sabadilla, Silicea, Natrum Mur and Hepar Sulph. The onset of severe sneezing while sleeping with the hands or feet exposed in the cold is a characteristic symptom of Hepar Sulph. A patient of Hepar Sulph cannot tolerate even the slightest draft of cold air. Noise is also unbearable for such a patient.

Hepar Sulph may also be useful for treating **ear problems**, like Chamomilla, Pulsatilla, Belladonna and Allium Cepa, which are more commonly used.

Hepar Sulph is also related to the **eye ache**. If the eye becomes intensely red due to the cold then Euphrasia will be found more useful. However, Hepar Sulph is very useful in the common eye conditions associated with a lot of watering and stickiness.

Belladonna, Arsenic, Hepar Sulph and Ipecac are useful in the treatment of day-to-day coughs. Please remember the distinction between Ipecac and Hepar Sulph. The phlegm in the case of Ipecac is relatively soft and can be expectorated easily. If the phlegm is thick and sticky, then Hepar Sulph, Kali Bichrome or Coccus will be more useful.

Hepar Sulph is a deep acting remedy. In the case of sudden and severe attack of an illness, the patient would benefit with high potency of Hepar Sulph. The high potency can even be repeated again and again without any possible harm. To curtail the severity of the disease, Hepar Sulph 1000 can be given twice a day. Once the disease comes under control, it becomes necessary to use the doses in intervals. One should learn to use the homoeopathic medicines in different potencies from one's own experience. One gradually learns the exact potency to be used with experience. If the disease becomes prolonged and chronic, one should not expect immediate cure with one dose of high potency. For the satisfactory treatment of chronic illnesses, the body has to make deep adjustments, which can never happen instantaneously. In particular, if the defensive system of the body of the patient has already weakened tremendously, with the resistance being very low, a homoeopathic remedy given in high potency may produce serious adverse effects or may even prove fatal.

Since Hepar Sulph contains Sulphur, it has some similarities with Sulphur. Sulphur has the capability of curing the **old scars of tuberculosis in the lungs**. If the bacteria form tiny little lesions in the lungs (miliary Tuberculosis), Sulphur helps to destroy them. One should not give Silicea in this condition. Sulphur attenuates the tuberculous bacteria, which then become expectorated with cough. It is important to know that one should never administer Sulphur in high potency unless and until one is sure that there are no enlarged glands near the arteries in the lungs. Tuberculosis patients, who have such lumps in the lungs, may bleed from ruptured blood vessels in the lungs as a reaction to Sulphur or Silicea, given in high potency. In this kind of patient Sulphur works as potently as Silicea. The better way to treat these patients is that first of all, Sulphur should be given in moderate potency for some period and then the patient should be put on Calcarea Carb. Calcarea Carb helps to make protective shells around the tuberculous lesions, like the shell around the egg. The bacteria become imprisoned in these protective shells.

Hepar Sulph is very useful for the **treatment of tuberculosis of the lungs, intestines or anywhere else in the body**. Hepar Sulph will be found effective irrespective of the site of the tuberculous infection.

Hepar Sulph has elements of Sulphur and Calcarea both. The element of Sulphur is more dominant. So, it shares a similarity to Silicea, like Sulphur.

Hepar Sulph is effective against all sorts of skin wounds. They may have started to **discharge pus and bleed,** or have become putrid with new boils forming around them, or have become like a non-relenting abscesses that do not heal. Hepar Sulph is effective against all of them. But Hepar Sulph and Nitric Acid are similar in the way that the small wounds or sores may develop individually or in the form of clusters, which spread out from one side. Both Hepar Sulph and Nitric Acid can be used for the **treatment of ulcers in the intestines**. Mercury is similar to both remedies in the treatment of the intestinal ulcers.

Hepar Sulph is useful in the **treatment of warts** that do not heal. The skin starts to **itch** and pimples form over the body. Scales and thick scabs also form resembling eczema. If these scabs form behind the ears and around the neck, and they discharge a gum-like sticky exudate, this can be treated with Graphites. For scabs that do not respond to any other medicine, one should not forget to try Hepar Sulph.

| | |
|---|---|
| Antidotes: | Belladonna, Chamomilla, Silicea |
| Potency: | 30 to 1000 or sometimes up to CM. |

# HURA BRAZILIENSIS

This remedy is useful against **leprosy** as soon as it is felt that the skin has become thick and contracted. Thus, it is also useful against **Lupus**. In Hura, the skin becomes tense and drawn. Besides, Hura and Hydrocotyle, Madura is also useful against diseases like leprosy and Lupus. In Hura, the patient feels as if he has splinters under the fingers as a result of the disease whereas actually, there is nothing under the fingers. In it there is itching over the bony prominences. The neck becomes stiff and the back aches. Although, homoeopaths use it in potency 6, it is my experience that whatever is effective in potency 6 must be more effective in potency 30 and 200, rather more so. It is possible that the physician may have found it effective in potency 6 only, because there are some diseases in which a particular potency is most ideal. Therefore, one should try it and then note down what dose is most effective against a particular disease. Camphor and Opium annul the effect of Hura.

| | |
|---|---|
| Potency: | 6 and 30 up to 200 |

# HYDRANGEA

This remedy is prepared from a tree called Seven Barks. It is related to the **diseases of the kidney**, though it is not very commonly used. One of its most prominent symptoms is the presence of excessive amounts of salts in the urine and the formation of sediments, which settle in the form of a thick white layer. Besides this, the patient may start passing blood in the urine (haematuria), small stones or crystals, which injure the urethra and cause severe burning pain. For these symptoms, Hydrangea is very useful. Passing reddish coloured urine, a burning sensation, and the presence of gravel in the urine, are also found in Lycopodium. Hydrangea is also very useful in the treatment of senile **enlargement of the prostate**. If the prostatic enlargement is non cancerous and there is evidence of deposit of salts in the urine, one must use Hydrangea.

| | |
|---|---|
| Potency: | up to 30. |

# HYDRASTIS

The medicine Hydrastis is prepared from the roots of orange tree. It is very important in the treatment of **liver diseases**. It is also related to the skin and inner linings (mucous membranes). Amongst its superficial symptoms, **skin ulcers** are very conspicuous. When these ulcers change into **cancer**, and do not respond to any other treatment, Hydrastis must not be forgotten. By the grace of God, Hydrastis is known to control these dangerous kinds of ulcers growing out of hand.

Hydrastis is very effective **against the deep-seated cancerous masses** and **chronic ulcers of the eye**. Honey is the best form of local treatment for these chronic ulcers. The local application of pure honey two to three times a day will initially increase the exudation of the fluid, following which the ulcers start to heal. Recent research has shown that cancerous wounds that do not respond to any other medicines are cured with local application of honey.

Being deeply related to the **liver diseases**, Hydrastis affects the appetite. A very peculiar symptom is that there is a feeling of strong craving and weakness while hungry, even though there is intense dislike for food. However, there is no associated nausea. These symptoms are also found in some other diseases, though in slightly different form.

The **cold** in a patient of Hydrastis is associated with **constant presence of sticky yellow thick exudates in the nose, which then dries up**. On picking the nose, the children develop sores, from which blood may ooze. Hydrastis is the best remedy for these kinds of sores in the nose. The symptoms of Hydrastis are relieved with rest. When the ailment aggravates, the face shows signs of **jaundice**. It becomes yellowish. The **eyelids swell and sores develop** on them (Blephritis). **Thick offensive smelling material forms in the ears** causing deafness.

While the patient with symptoms of nasal catarrh stays inside the room, the nose stops running but the discomfort increases when in the open again. Due to the extreme dislike for food a Hydrastis patient has to live on milk, which he zealously drinks and can also digest easily. The patient suffers from stiffness and cramping of the muscles.

Hydrastis is also useful in the treatment of **chronic piles**. There is a lot of wind in the stomach. The **urine is scanty but offensive**. The **leucorrhoeal discharge** in women also smells foul. There is itching in the trachea (windpipe) causing cough. In Hydrastis, like Phosphorus, even a gentle laugh provokes severe coughing.

In a patient of Hydrastis, apart from the aching of the body and the legs, there is increasing weakness, which improves on slow movement. In this regard, it resembles Rhus Tox. Although, in Hydrastis rest gives general relief to the patient however, gentle walking relieves his **aches.** The feet of such a patient swell. The swelling or oedema due to liver disorder usually affects the face and the abdomen before involving the feet.

Hydrastis is in general a very effective remedy for the old, frail and those who get tired easily. The **patient remains depressed**. He believes he is going to die soon. In fact, he desires to be dead. He is both lazy and cowardly. The **pain over the forehead** is a prominent symptom, which is often due to constipation. There is pain over the head and in the muscles of the neck. A streak of **eczema** forms along the hairline over the forehead.

The patient remains **constipated**. There is **pain over the lower part of the abdomen,** which becomes worse after defaecation. The stomach aches. Digestion becomes poor. The taste in the mouth is bitter and the tongue becomes whitish. In women, there is a tendency towards the **formation of lumps** in the breasts, and if these lumps persist for a long time, they can transform into cancer. After the periods finish the discharge increases, leading to the formation **of ulcers over the cervix** associated with severe itching.

Hydrastis is also useful in **smallpox**. It ameliorates its symptoms, shortens its duration and minimizes the potential bad aftereffects.

| | |
|---|---|
| Antidote: | Sulphur |
| Potency: | 30 to 200. |

# HYDROCOTYLE

Hydrocotyle is very effective against **leprosy** and it can also cure several other **skin diseases**. Leprosy progresses very slowly. The disease does not spread immediately but it slowly flourishes in the blood. Only after long close contact, the disease can transfer from the patient to another person. On noticing early signs of leprosy of the skin, the patient should be immediately treated with Hydrocotyle. Once the disease has well advanced and the affected areas have become riddled with deep sores and ulcers, it is too late for Hydrocotyle to work. I have used Hydrocotyle to treat many patients and by the grace of God, I have always found it very effective. Sometimes, the disease was fully eradicated, while at other times, the disease was rendered very mild.

**Lupus** is another skin disease, which along with leprosy is thought to be incurable. Lupus appears in several different forms. In addition to the formation of blisters or sores and itching, in Lupus the skin starts to become tense and then shrinks. There is a lot of pain and anguish. Hydrocotyle is very useful against this disease also. Hydrocotyle has been found to be effective against the common itch without formation of swellings on the skin or the appearance of pimples and wounds. Similarly, another drug, Dolichos, is also very effective for the treatment of a dry, obstinate type of itch.

If the skin becomes thick and scaly like that of a fish, this is the symptom of Psoriasis. These symptoms should not be confused with leprosy. Instead the patient should be treated for Psoriasis. Psoriasis requires a lengthy, careful treatment with very deep acting medicines. There is another skin disease similar to Lupus, in which fish-like scales start to appear, when the patient should be given Psorinum 1000 or Arsenic 1000. The basic difference between Psorinum and Arsenic is that in Psorinum, the discharges have a strong bad smell. If an **offensive smell comes from the mouth, armpits and feet**, without any obvious underlying disease, for this problem Rhus Glabra in potency 6X is very effective. I have also used it in homoeopathic potency 6 and found it quite useful.

Hydrocotyle is very useful in **Psoriasis** also. If the Psoriasis is more prominent on the palms of the hands and the soles of the feet, for that also, Hydrocotyle should be used. Even if the itching on the palms of the hands and soles of the feet is not due to Psoriasis, Hydrocotyle is still useful against this type of itch.

Another extremely dangerous disease is the **cancer of the cervix of the uterus**. The detailed account is given under Helonias and Carbo Animalis. According to cancer experts, there is no cure for this. The disease can recur even after the surgical removal of the uterus. Hydrocotyle is extremely useful in alleviating the pain due to this cancer but it does not offer complete cure. However, if there is a formation of ulcers, redness or inflammation at the mouth of the uterus (cervix), one should not forget Hydrocotyle.

| | |
|---|---|
| Potency: | 30 to 200 |

# HYDROCYANIC ACID

This is an acid that develops in bitter almonds and cattle fodder due to extreme drought and it produces extremely dangerous convulsions. Even the slightest taste of Hydrocyanic Acid can cause severe intestinal colic. If tasted a little carelessly, it can cause severe laryngeal spasm (constriction of the throat), causing suffocation and immediate death. Since the amount of Hydrocyanic Acid found in the bitter almonds is very little, the consumption of almonds may not even cause colic in the abdomen or spasm of the larynx, although some possibility still remains. It is present in the fodder in a relatively large amount, so the cattle fed on this kind of fodder will definitely contract severe abdominal colic, and sometimes it is impossible to save them. In such situations Colchicum 200 is the best remedy to treat the **abdominal colic**.

Most physicians have restricted the use of Hydrocyanic Acid to severe abdominal distension and severe colic, although it is extremely useful in the **treatment of asthma, epilepsy and whooping cough**. All these three conditions may be associated with constriction of the throat muscles. If a patient of asthma or whooping cough becomes unconscious due to the constriction of the upper respiratory passage, the patient can be saved from serious possible complications with the immediate use of Hydrocyanic Acid, otherwise due to the constriction of the air passages, the oxygen supply to the brain would be depleted, which sometimes results in permanent brain damage. Sometimes severe constriction of the throat may cause immediate death. In this condition, Hydrocyanic Acid is the top most remedy. When given along with Hydrophobinum 200, it happens to work much better than the inhalers used in the allopathic system of medicine. Moreover, possible side effects of the inhalers are also avoided.

It is extremely useful in the treatment of **hysterical fits and epileptic seizures** in women. There is a condition called Catalepsy, in which there is impediment of the blood flow to the brain and flushing of the face, after which the patient either loses consciousness or his memory is lost. The memory can sometimes slowly recover or be lost forever. Hydrocyanic Acid is very useful for the treatment of this condition.

Some patients develop cramps in the abdomen after taking food and others before taking the food. Hydrocyanic Acid is indicated in those patients who feel a colicky type of pain on an empty stomach, or a marked weakness and sinking sensation over the stomach, or experience a rumbling sound in the abdomen after taking food. Their heart beats very fast, their pulse is weak and irregular, their hands and feet become cold, their jaws become tightly closed during a severe convulsion, they froth at the mouth, their lips turn blue, and there is a feeling of tightness and pain over the chest. All these symptoms require to be treated with Hydrocyanic acid, in particular.

| | |
|---|---|
| Antidotes: | Ammonium, Camphor, Opium |
| Potency: | 30 to 200 |

# HYDROPHOBINUM

This homoeopathic remedy is prepared from the saliva of a rabid dog. It is a very important anticonvulsive medicine, especially in treating the **laryngeal spasm (constriction of the throat)**. Its onset of convulsions is related to hypersensitivity to light and water. The patient goes into severe convulsions at the sight of bright light, shining objects or upon seeing water. Even though the convulsions and fear are related to seeing water, the patient cannot sip water even if he closes his eyes out of fear. The saliva of the patient is like sticky threads as in Coccus Cacti and Kali Bichrome. Though in Hydrocotyle, the saliva may or may not be sticky and thready.

A Hydrophobinum patient has **difficulty in swallowing** things. He keeps on attempting to swallow even without eating or drinking anything. The froth forms at the mouth and the patient keeps on spitting continuously.

This medicine is also useful in the treatment of **sex-related diseases**. In women, it is especially useful in the **treatment of pain and discomfort related to the prolapse of the uterus**. Due to extreme hypersensitivity, the sound or even the thought of running water can aggravate the symptoms. A slight draft of air can also aggravate the symptoms.

| | |
|---|---|
| Antidote: | Hydrocyanic Acid |
| Potency: | 30 to 200 |

# HYOSCYAMUS
## (Henbane)

Hyoscyamus is prepared from a plant that in appearance resembles the Belladonna plant. Apparently it is harmless, but its seeds are extremely poisonous. The medicine prepared from this plant is called Hyoscyamus. It profoundly affects the mind, especially in relations to the sexual functioning.

In Hyoscyamus, there is total disarray of mental functions. The patient feels as if his mind is under the control of a supernatural power. The patient is **delirious and acts insanely**. Sometimes, a patient develops the symptoms of Hyoscyamus during the typhoid fever. He talks while sleeping and constantly crimps and pinches the bed sheet. He **talks unabashed obsceneties** due to the inflammation of the sexual organs. It is not unusual for a decent person to talk obscenely when sick, whereas he would never utter such foul things under normal circumstances. If a girl happens to be sick her parents will not, out of embarrassment, even call the doctor to see her. Nevertheless, the use of obscene language is no reflexion of her desire in sexual misadventure. It is a typical symptom of Hyoscyamus, which causes inflammation of the sexual organs affecting the mind. The patient talks in an absurd way that he would never do in the state of normal health. This excitement is due to the sickness also found in Cantharis, i.e. the inflammation of the sexual organs. (For further differentiation between Hyoscyamus and Cantharis, please refer to Cantharis).

A Hyoscyamus patient talks obscenely during sleep or while he is semi-conscious. This condition disappears when the patient is awake and conscious.

In a patient of Hyoscyamus there is a generalized twitching of the muscles. The nerves are irritable, causing severe muscular contractions. The patient feels a piercing type of pain. **Muscles become tense and contracted with tonic convulsions**. There are fasciculation's over different parts of the body. The patient becomes very weak and his head slips and sags from the pillow due to the weakness. This symptom is also found in a patient of Muriatic Acid. In women, **severe convulsions develop at the time of childbirth**.

All sorts of mental diseases can be found in Hyoscyamus, but there is no tendency towards committing physical violence. Physical violence is very common in Belladonna. The patient has a very suspicious mind. He believes that somebody is standing next to him, and he starts conversing with him. Sometimes, he thinks that somebody is standing behind him, thus he will often turn back to look at him. He is extremely **suspicious** like the patient of Lachesis. He presumes that his close relative has poisoned his food. This symptom is present both in Lachesis and Hyoscyamus. If a patient is afraid of taking the remedy through suspicion of being poisoned, a drop or two mixed in a large amount of water may be administered.

When semi-conscious, a patient of Hyoscyamus talks to himself. He then screams and may become totally unconscious. Quite a few normal people have the habit of talking to themselves. However, the Hyoscyamus **patient talks to himself** only during the sickness.

One of the ideas imprinted in the mind of the patient is that he can never be forgiven for his sins. In fact, in his own thoughts, he believes himself to have committed murder or some other heinous crime, though in reality, he never committed such a crime.

One symptom of Hyoscyamus, which resembles Glonoine and Lachesis, is that the **patient feels lost while on a journey**. While at home he still thinks that he is not at home. He remains similarly disorientated outside the home also. He feels himself a stranger everywhere.

The Hyoscyamus patient develops **fear of water** (hydrophobia). Even the sound of running water bothers him. He cannot swallow water due to severe constriction of the throat. According to Dr. Kent, Belladonna, Hyoscyamus, Cantharis and Hydrophobinum are all excellent medicines to treat this condition. In my experience, I have found Stramonium and Hydrocyanic Acid capable of totally uprooting this condition. They are very effective against the **constriction of the throat developing on swallowing water**. **Hydrophobia develops after being bitten by a rabid dog.** Stramonium is the best treatment for Rabies. In the olden days, some doctors used to treat the patients with Stramonium. In homoeopathy also, Stramonium has proven to be very useful. The patients who develop symptoms of Rabies should be treated with Stramonium and Hydrophobinum combined. By the grace of God, they work very well. In case the anti-rabies vaccine is not available, and one is not sure whether the biting dog is rabid or not, Stramonium and Hydrophobinum combined must be administered immediately. These remedies should first be given daily for a few days, then twice a week for a few months and then gradually tapered off. This will, by the grace of God, prevent against the onset of Rabies and obviate any further dangers forever.

If the **eyesight becomes weak due to the dysfunction of the nerves**, then Hyoscyamus will be of good use. In case the vision becomes intermittently blurred and does not focus properly, then also Hyoscyamus must be used. Sometimes, during a high fever, the patient goes into a **severe convulsion with the locking of the jaw**. The mouth becomes dry and smelly, the tongue becomes red or brown, dry and fissured; the movement of the tongue becomes sluggish or it is not under voluntary control anymore, resulting in frequent interruptions of speech. The tongue becomes insensitive and liable to be cut between the teeth while eating food. If all these symptoms are due to **stomach upset**, then Pulsatilla and Carbo Veg can also be used.

In Hyoscyamus, the stomach becomes flaccid and dilated. The **stools** (as in typhoid) are granular in appearance or may be watery and mixed with blood. Another troubling problem is that the patient has no control over passing urine or opening the bowels (urinary and faecal incontinence).

If women are unable to pass urine after **childbirth**, then Causticum is the best remedy. Causticum will be much more effective when given along with Arnica. If this treatment is ineffective, then Hyoscyamus must be used. Hyoscyamus is very useful in the **treatment of urinary tract infections and inflammations**.

In Hyoscyamus, there is **severe griping pain in the abdomen** and the patient feels as if his abdomen is going to burst open. The patient vomits frequently, has **hiccups** and screams due to pain. He feels dizzy and also has a **burning sensation in the stomach**.

Before their periods, women become **hysterical** and develop cramps. Even during their periods they experience stiffness in the muscles and sweat profusely.

There is a feeling of tightness over the chest as well as suffocation. The patient bends over due to the severity of the pain. At night, the patient develops a **dry cough**, which worsens on lying down and is relieved on sitting up.

At night, a Hyoscyamus patient may develop **epileptic convulsions** in which the toes become very stiff. The child cries and graons, while asleep. The patient feels very uncomfortable at night and cannot sleep. There is widespread twitching of the muscles. The patient does not like to cover himself.

The suffering of a Hyoscyamus patient aggravates at night, after taking food and on lying down. The patient is afraid of being alone. The symptoms improve on bending over.

| | |
|---|---|
| Antidotes: | Camphor, Belladonna |
| Potency: | 30 to 1000 |

# IGNATIA

Ignatia is an excellent treatment for **depression**. Women who have the constitution of Ignatia are very sensitive in nature. Although extremely pleasant and affable, they are very frail and tender. They become easily stricken with grief, which affects their mind, resulting in various diseases and physical ailments. It is not surprising that women who have the nature of Ignatia become mentally ill due to grief. Sometimes, such a patient becomes **hysterical**. Under these circumstances, the patient should be treated with Ignatia.

One obvious symptom of Ignatia is that the patient cannot drink coffee. Since the patient's mind is already very sensitive and delicately tuned, coffee amplifies her symptoms. It becomes extremely difficult for the patient to take even one or two sips of coffee. When mentally agitated, the patient cannot express her anger openly. Instead, she torments herself in solitude or becomes extremely sallow. Staphysagria patients also tend to keep their anger suppressed. When the condition becomes out of control, this results in physical ailments. Similar is the case in Ignatia. If an Ignatia patient is taunted or laughed at in a social gathering, she will quietly tolerate it. But when she returns home, she will develop severe headache, mental anguish and restlessness. In this situation, a single dose of Ignatia will relieve her anger and save her from the ill effects of her suppressed emotions.

In Ignatia, the patient **feels the grief of the death of a child or a dear one very strongly**, resulting in far reaching bad effects on the health of the person. Ignatia can be very useful to avert this from happening. In my experience, I have found Ignatia to be very useful in the **treatment of recent grief or bereavement**, as well as to prevent its long lasting ill effects. However, if the ill effects have already been well established, then Ignatia is of no use. Under these circumstances, Ambra Grisea, Silicea and Natrum Mur will prove to be more effective.

Sometimes the woman quivers or may shudder when nervous. This may lead to convulsions followed by unconsciousness like hysteria. This unconsciousness is not a sign of epilepsy but a sign of their nervous weakness. This unconsciousness, superficially resembling epilepsy, is merely an indication of her being high-strung and is a reaction to grief and sorrow. In hot countries, often women may fall unconscious amidst a thick crowd. A very strange symptom of Ignatia is that a patient reacts overjoyed when she was expected to be angry, and behaves angrily when in fact she was expected to be happy on hearing good news. Similarly surprising is her reaction to physical ailments. For instance, if her joints have become stiff, red hot and swollen, she does not feel any discomfort. In short, Ignatia will be the essential part of the treatment of a **woman expressing conflicting forms of response to mental and physical stresses.**

In a patient of Ignatia, **swallowing relieves the throat discomfort**. Local pressure relieves the pain. The patient tends to sleep on the painful side. The headache feels as if a nail has been driven into the head. Pressing the painful side over the pillow also reduces the pain.

In Ignatia, like Cocculus, the patient **vomits** but there is no nausea or retching before it. It is amazing about Ignatia that if the patient happens to feel nauseated, he feels relieved on eating something hard and indigestible. A light soft diet will however, aggravate the condition. The cough resulting from the irritation of the throat further aggravates the problem, which in turn makes the cough linger on for a long time. If during the cough, the patient is given a dose of Ignatia, it will stop the cough surprisingly fast. It is my experience that if Ignatia is going to be effective in a given situation, it is so immediately.

An Ignatia patient may sometimes develop **constriction of the throat**, producing a noise like snoring. Ignatia works wonderfully well in this condition. As soon as a few pellets are placed in the mouth, the spasmodic constriction of the throat disappears at once. In other words, Ignatia is full of surprises regarding its action as well as its ailments.

The Ignatia patient is often in **despair and depressed**. She does not want to see or meet anybody. She **loses her memory**, develops **hysteria** and has a suspicious mind. She firmly believes that something dreadful is going to happen to her. She remains fearful of the death of her relatives or may even have such visions. If such a patient is not treated with Ignatia in time, she may become completely insane. Once, she becomes insane, Ignatia is useless. Instead, Natrum Mur works better.

Like some other homoeopathic remedies i.e. Pulsatilla, Helleboris, Aurum, Hyoscyamus, Lachesis, etc., the Ignatia patient believes that she is guilty of having committed grievous sins that are absolutely unforgivable.

The body of the Ignatia patient is always cold, yet she desires to drink cold water. The patient is disinterested in taking regular food. Rest provides her comfort.

In an Ignatia patient, all sorts of complaints related to vision may be present. **Spots appear before the eyes**. Irregular lines wave in front of the eyes. The eyesight becomes weak and the eyes begin to hurt. The neuralgic pain over the face is also susceptible to treatment with Ignatia. The facial muscles twitch. The taste of the mouth becomes sour. The patient may suddenly become thirsty or lose thirst unexpectedly.

One should never argue with an Ignatia patient. The patient will respond to a positive argument with irrelevant talk, and will keep on prolonging the conversation unnecessarily. It is best to leave her alone.

Ignatia patients do not sleep soundly. As soon as they retire to sleep, either the **muscles start to violently contract** or the grief and worries dispel their sleep. Such a woman may often stop menstruating altogether or the periods become tardy, due to grief and mental shock. The patient feels painful cramps in the abdomen. The hands and feet go into spasm, while the feet and ankles hurt.

The Ignatia ailments become worse in the morning and in the open, while they subside on eating, resting or changing sides.

| | |
|---|---|
| Adjuvants: | Natrum Mur, Silicea |
| Antidotes: | Chamomilla, Coccus |
| Potency: | 30 to 200 |

# INSULIN

Insulin is a natural substance present in the body for controlling sugar levels in the blood. It is produced in the pancreas. When given in the required dose, it normalises the blood sugar. The homoeopathic Insulin is prepared from this substance. Like regular Insulin, it is useful in the **treatment of diabetes.** The homoeopathic Insulin has also been described to be useful to certain diabetics. In case it cannot offer a complete cure, it eradicates the danger of the harmful effects of diabetes. It has a certain beneficial effect regarding the treatment of ulcers, blisters, bedsores and carbuncles that result from uncontrolled diabetes. Insulin is also useful in the treatment of **chronic intestinal conditions** associated with a tendency of soft-stools, and enlargement of the liver, etc. For the irritatingly itchy eczema associated with liver dysfunction, which is not amicable to any other treatment, one should use Insulin. Similarly, it benefits patients who tend to pass urine frequently or suffer from skin diseases, boils and abscesses.

If the **lymph glands at the neck** tend to develop pus, then Insulin is given in potency 30. Insulin is also useful when the blood sugar is high, but there is no passage of sugar in the urine. It has also been found to be useful in the **treatment of gout**.

| | |
|---|---|
| Potency: | 30 |

# IODUM

Iodum is a remedy of very hot nature. Its patient feels extremely hot and very hungry, yet despite eating a lot, remains thin and lean. The patient is very talkative and cannot sit still. He keeps on moving around constantly. The lymph glands in the body become enlarged and hard, resembling that of Conium. The skinny appearance of Iodine patient reminds one of Abrotanum and Natrum Mur. However, both these remedies are of cold nature.

The restlessness of an Iodum patient is due to the **anxiety neurosis**. Unlike Arsenic, the irritability of the nerves is due to availability of more energy for the nerve function. Since the patient eats a lot and the food is not converted into fatty acids, the unused surplus energy does not let him keep still. Therefore, he is in constant motion and consumes his energy by running around. If such a patient is forced to sit, he reacts very angrily, and is ready to beat or even kill the person. If he is not treated with Iodum during childhood, then on becoming an adult, he may become a very dangerous criminal, ready to kill without any reason or provocation. Although the tendency of violence and killing without reason is also found in Natrum Mur and Hepar Sulph, their other symptoms are very different. This dangerous tendency is also found in Nux Vomica. A Nux Vomica woman may develop an uncontrollable urge to throw her child into fire or kill her husband despite loving him immensely. She then becomes extremely fearful of such desires but cannot get rid of such thoughts sticking in her mind and following her like a shadow. If the patient also becomes extremely frightened, these symptoms may turn into insanity. If other symptoms of such a patient demand Iodum, it would prove extremely useful.

Some symptoms of Iodum are also found in Kali Iodide. A Kali Iodide patient walks a lot but does not feel tired. On the day that he does not get a chance to walk, he feels uncomfortable. His constitution is also hot. However, there is one difference and it is that in Kali Iodide there is a tendency to develop sores and deep ulcers, while in Iodum, the **glands become simply inflamed and hardened**. There is a tendency to develop tuberculosis also.

A special symptom of Iodum is that the glands throughout the body become swollen and hard. However, in women, the mammary glands shrink to a thin membrane. This symptom is an exception, otherwise generally, when the body is wasting, the glands enlarge in size. A patient, whose body is wasting while the glands are enlarging, needs Iodum. In Iodum, the glands and the body do not enlarge simultaneously. Usually, the glands inside the abdomen become markedly swollen and hard. The glands in the armpits (axilla) also become swollen and indurated.

Iodum being a hot natured remedy, its **cough aggravates in hot weather**. On entering a heated room, the patient starts coughing but this symptom alone is not enough for making the diagnosis of Iodum. Other symptoms also need to be present. In Iodum, the liver, spleen and throat are inflamed. Generally, such inflammation and glandular affection results in diarrhoea. In Iodum, there is throbbing all over the body. This sign is common to Belladonna and Iodum both. Iodum being a remedy of hot nature resembles Apis. Both Apis and Iodum also affect the kidneys. Like Apis, in Iodum, the swelling appears under the eyes. However, the swelling is not restricted to the area under the eye; the eyelids also swell. If the **entire eye becomes swollen**, Phosphorus is also found to be very effective. The swelling of only the eyelids is a symptom of Kali Carb. The patients who become weak and anaemic due to chronic illnesses develop bags under the eyes, which make them look prematurely old. For this condition, Chininum Ars and Sarsaparilla, etc. can be benificial. The diagnosis should, however, be arrived at carefully.

A distinctive feature of an Iodum patient is his excessive appetite. In all the Iodum ailments, the increased appetite is disturbing and aggravates the symptoms. The intensity of appetite and illness are closely related in Psorinum also, but in Psorinum the appetite increases at night and its patient is usually cold. Therefore, it is not difficult to distinguish between the two remedies.

Iodum plays an important role in **kidney disorders** also. Due to the kidney dysfunction, the hands and feet become swollen (oedema). Timely administration of Iodum will safeguard against numerous incurable and painful diseases. Kali Iodide is also useful in the treatment of kidney diseases, but in Kali Iodide, there is a tendency towards the formation of ulcers that is absent in the case of Iodum.

In Iodum, the internal organs like **spleen and liver become swollen and hard**, while the entire body begins to waste. Despite this, the patient retains his appetite. Later on, the stomach fails to function and diarrhoea sets in. The diarrhoea due to tuberculosis is worse in the morning and gets better with Sulphur. If tuberculosis of the lungs becomes severe, the toxic substances are then excreted naturally through the stools. Thus suppression of diarrhoea which will result in dire consequences, therefore it should be handled very carefully. According to the homoeopathic system of treatment, Sulphur will not only benefit the lungs but will also stop the diarrhoea. In such patients, if only the diarrhoea is controlled, it will result in further damage to the lungs. In this condition, if Sulphur does not work, then Iodum will be found very useful. In fact, if other symptoms of Iodum are also present, Iodum alone may offer a complete cure. Therefore, Iodum is not just for temporary relief. Some of its illnesses resemble those of Sulphur, such as the formation of whitish blisters and ulcers.

All sorts of **blisters and ulcers** developing on the mucous membranes can be cured with Iodum, provided the patient is of Iodum constitution. Despite being of hot constitution, an Iodum patient develops catarrh on exposure to cold. It is not necessary that the patient develop catarrh due to heat only. The nasal membranes in an Iodum patient become extremely weak, and vulnerable to catch cold easily. The secretions dry up in the nose making breathing difficult. A slight cold or change in the food habit causes cold. Some of the medicines used for the treatment of a cold are of cold and hot nature, each having its own separate symptoms distinct from Iodum. However, if the nose remains stuffy due to constant catarrh and bleeding, along with excessive appetite, then by the grace of God, Iodum will cure all of the symptoms

Iodum is also very effective in the **treatment of tumours of the uterus**, especially if other symptoms of Iodum are also present. In Iodum, the leucorrhoeal discharge is very thick and burning in nature. Iodum is also useful in the treatment of joint pains. An Iodum patient gets relief with local cold applications. The ailments related to Iodum aggravate on remaining quiet, working hard and being in hot weather. After eating food the patient feels comfortable for a short period. He also feels comfortable while strolling in the open air.

| | |
|---|---|
| Adjuvant: | Lycopodium |
| Antidotes: | Hepar Sulph, Gratiola, Sulphur |
| Potency: | 30 to 200 |

# IPECACUANHA

## (Ipecac-Root)

The Ipecac is prepared from the dried-up roots of the Ipecac plant. In allopathy, it is used to induce vomiting, while in homoeopathy, Ipecac is used to control **nausea and vomiting**. Its patient has a persistent feeling of nausea even after vomiting.

Ipecac is a very important **anti-malarial treatment**. Malaria is strongly connected with nausea and also attacks the stomach. From this point of view, Ipecac is naturally related to malaria. A distinctive feature of Ipecac is that the patient feels severe cold in his back with constant waves of cold up and down. The pain also undulates similarly in the back. A child struck with malaria obviously cannot explain the symptoms himself. However, the symptoms of feeling severe cold, shivering and chattering of the teeth will indicate the need for Ipecac. If such a child presents other symptoms of Ipecac also, then there should be no delay in treating him with Ipecac. A severe stabbing pain is felt over the stomach, moving from left to right. The patient feels as if the stomach has been cut with a knife. The patient becomes riveted in one position. However, the pain disappears after a short while. Pains that are not of a permanent nature, which come on fast like a spell of lightning and then leave the patient weak and exhausted, typify Ipecac. In every ailment of Ipecac, nausea is a must. Even coughing provokes nausea. Ipecac ailments become worse in hot and humid climate.

Ipecac is the best **treatment for bleeding**. The bleeding is of a sudden and forceful nature. In Ipecac, bleeding is always associated with a feeling of nausea. The patient does not feel thirsty at all. Like the patient of Arsenic, the Ipecac patient may feel very weak and restless, but other symptoms of course are different. Every ailment comes on in the form of an attack, whether in the form of weakness or feeling cold. Similarly, there can be an episode of bleeding which will end after some time. These attacks are usually not that long. The Ipecac ailments do not stay permanently. However, there is a possibility of rapid progress of the disease. Whenever an ailment starts, it progresses rapidly and then goes away equally fast.

In Ipecac, **convulsions** occur. Like Cicuta and Dioscorea, the body tends to bend backwards due to severe muscular contractions (opisthotonus). Ipecac is one of the best treatments for stomach disorders, such as **distension of the abdomen** and **dysentery** associated with severe cramps and frequent motions. In the **dysentery of children**, the stools contain greenish mucus. Stools may also be mixed with blood and there is a definite tendency of nausea and vomiting. There is a kind of pinching sensation around the navel. The entire body becomes stiff. Ipecac is useful in the treatment of all these symptoms.

Ipecac is also closely related to **asthma**. Its patient has a full face, glowing with good circulation, while in Antimonium Tart, the asthma patient is very weak and has near-death appearance. This difference is only arbitrary and manifests in later stages. Instead of waiting for this clear distinctive appearance, one should be able to distinguish between the two at the outset of the disease. In Ipecac, the illness is sudden, progresses rapidly, and the face becomes flushed. But in Antimonium Tart, on exposure to cold the child becomes weak slowly and steadily, and once the disease has well established the symptoms become extremely aggravated, more than in Ipecac. Moreover, the defensive body response does not develop. In Ipecac, the entire body of the patient reacts to the illness, but in Antimonium Tart, even if the chest is full of phlegm and there is difficulty in breathing, the patient does not have the desire to expel the phlegm. The result is that the patient becomes overwhelmed by the severity of the disease. If initially, the diagnosis for Antimonium Tart has been made the treatment should be started without any delay. Once the symptoms aggravate, the condition becomes dangerous. One distinctive point between the two is that if there is nausea but no vomiting, then it is probably due to Ipecac. However, if there is a tendency to vomit with or without nausea, it is a symptom of Antimonium Tart, except in the case where the chest becomes full of secretions, which the patient cannot expel due to marked weakness.

Ipecac is also useful in the **treatment of uterine conditions**. Ipecac is very effective to treat the excessive red **menstrual bleeding associated with nausea**. It is also useful in the vomiting of pregnancy. If the placenta happens to be partially retained in the uterus after the childbirth and if the patient has other symptoms of Ipecac, then it will help in the expulsion of the placenta. If the patient develops Puerperal Fever after childbirth, then Sulphur and Pyrogenium should be considered.

The **nasal catarrh** of Ipecac gets rooted in the nose. The nose becomes stuffy at night and the patient sneezes a lot. The nasal discharge drips into the throat and the chest, causing pain and tightness of the chest. **Asthma** develops. The cold starting at the nose and then affecting the throat and the chest, leading to asthma, can be cured with Ipecac. The standard formularies are mostly meant for those who do not understand much homoeopathy. At the same time, it is difficult to think of a unique prescription keeping in view the detailed symptoms of the patient. After the attack of asthma is over, the illness should be studied, keeping in mind the constitution of the patient. An asthmatic should be very careful about his diet. He should make every effort to avoid contracting nasal cold or sore throat.

When the **kidneys become infected**, the patient feels severe chills. So in the beginning of the disease, the patient should be well covered and given hot fluids to sip. Many a time, the symptoms of kidney infections and the onset of malaria resemble each other therefore undue haste should be avoided. Initially, symptomatic treatment should be given and once the symptoms have been clearly defined, then the proper treatment should be started.

Ipecac is also useful in the **treatment of whooping cough** in view of the associated symptom of **spasmodic constriction of the air passages**. If during a convulsion, the entire body becomes stiff, the face becomes flushed and there is nausea, then Ipecac will prove to be extraordinarily beneficial. One may think of Belladonna in this condition, though Ipecac should first be tried.

Ipecac is also related to tetanus.

| | |
|---|---|
| Adjuvants: | Cuprum, Arnica |
| Antidotes: | China, Tobaccum, Arsenic |
| Potency: | 30 to 200 |

# IRIS TENAX

The homoeopathic medicine Iris Tenax comes from a plant. In 1885, Dr. George Vig experimented with this medicine. He tested it on patients suffering from severe **intestinal colic associated with vomiting of greenish material.** Iris Tenax is somewhat similar to Iris Versicolor. However, there are differences and each has its own specific characteristics. Iris Versicolor is ideal for the treatment of hyperacidity of the stomach, whereas in Iris Tenax the hyperacidity of the stomach is associated with symptoms related to the throat and mouth cavity. Iris Tenax is considered to be the best **treatment for appendicitis**. Therefore, in general, its usage has been restricted only to appendicitis. In fact, it is also very useful in the treatment of other day-to-day problems.

In Iris Tenax, the patient feels a **burning sensation inside the mouth**. The **surface linings of the tongue, throat and mouth are affected**. The throat becomes dry and drinking cold water does not help. When the condition becomes worse, severe headache sets in. Often, the headache settles on the right side, but it may be felt on the left side as well. It is associated with bilious vomiting. The patient suffers from severe abdominal pain, associated with the feeling of being tense and distended. There can be severe cramping as well as diarrhoea. In Iris Tenax the patient remains depressed and pessamistic. He feels homesick. Sometimes, the tendency to become depressed may alternate with happiness. There are no associated mental symptoms. His mood changes suddenly. Sometimes, he feels happy and at other times very sad. At about midnight, he feels extremely sad and lonely. The temple areas hurt. There is burning and itching over the scalp. This itch is not the usual kind but merely a temporarily associated burning sensation. This is certainly not a permanent ailment. The burning usually settles over the right eye. The **headache comes once a week**. The vomit is of a green colour and sour in taste. The eyes also itch. There may be associated feeling of burning and pricking. There is **pain over the teeth of left upper jaw**. However, in my opinion, Iris Tenax may also be used for the treatment of pain affecting any tooth presenting the symptoms just mentioned.

Iris Tenax is also associated with **diarrhoea**. There is pain and severe cramping in the lower part of the abdomen. Being more closely

**related to the right side**, it is considered the best treatment for **appendicitis**. Dr. Vig himself never mentioned the use of Iris Tenax for appendicitis. But in view of its symptoms, subsequent experimentation with Iris Tenax has found it to be very useful in the treatment of appendicitis. I have often used Iris Tenax with Arnica and Bryonia in potency 200 for the treatment of appendicitis, and found it very useful and amazingly effective. If cramps are the salient symptom, then instead of Bryonia one should use Belladonna. Very often, appendicitis can become complicated and lead to a very dangerous situation. The triad just mentioned can bring the situation under control. I often would get sick with appendicitis and used to get better with this prescription. Once, while travelling, I felt uneasy right from the beginning of the journey. I used these three medicines. We travelled the whole night. The next day, I drove the car myself for 400 miles and we reached Karachi. The pain had remained under control throughout the journey. The next day I was taken to a hospital and examined by a surgeon. He was amazed to find that my appendix had burst open, discharging pus. The surgeon could not comprehend that not only was I alive but had also driven the car for 400 miles. Naturally, I underwent the surgical removal of my appendix, but I did not take penicillin; instead I used homoeopathic antibacterial drugs.

My advice to homoeopathy students, as well as to the patients, is that they should not totally depend upon these three remedies and keep postponing the need for surgery. Once the appendix is diseased, the homoeopathic remedies may only be used temporarily but the removal of the appendix by surgery is still the best treatment.

The pain of appendicitis can start during any time of the day or night. However, the usual time described for appendicitis is the night. According to my experience, there is no such restriction on the time of the onset of appendicitis. In Iris Tenax, the pain starts on the right side and then spreads in the entire abdomen. There is a tendency towards severe vomiting.

On waking up in the morning, the Iris Tenax patient has a sinking sensation over the stomach. There is severe pain in the abdomen, moving from the right to the left. Many a time the patient develops diarrhoea at night, which aggravates further by midnight. Hyperacidity of the stomach may lead to frequent urination. If the patient happens to feel a burning sensation during frequent urination and the colour of the urine is brown, then this is a symptom of Iris Tenax. Arsenic and Natrum Phos are also useful in the treatment of this condition, though their individual symptoms should also be kept in mind. In Natrum Phos, the urine is somewhat pale in colour. **Hyperacidity of the stomach**, which causes the urine to turn yellow in colour, is also found in relation to other medicines. **Excessive and frequent urination** leaves the patient very weak and makes it difficult for him to walk. Such patients should be treated with Iris Tenax.

The Iris Tenax patient loses sleep. In spite of decrease in pain and extreme weakness he is unable to get up in the morning.

| | |
|---|---|
| Potency: | 30 to 200 |

# IRIS VERSICOLOR

Iris Versicolor is the best remedy for the treatment of **hyperacidity of the stomach**. It also affects the internal linings of the intestines as well as the stomach. It has all the symptoms of **migraine** i.e. the acidity of the stomach, the tendency towards nausea, a one-sided headache and the feeling of tightness, etc.

The **ear symptoms** are also very prominent in Iris Versicolor. The patient hears noises and humming sounds, leading slowly to deafness. Since it affects the ears, it proves effective against **the vertigo, secondary to ear problems**. In this condition, mostly Cocculus is very effective. However if Cocculus has failed, then Iris Versicolor must be used. Iris Versicolor is also the best medicine for the treatment of the vertigo resulting from problems of the eardrum and imbalance from the fluid inside the ear (middle ear). Nux Vomica and Bryonia Alba are useful against the giddiness due to stomach upsets.

The symptoms of Iris Versicolor include: **facial neuralgia**, which begins after taking breakfast, a burning sensation on the tongue and inside the mouth, thick string-like saliva like Coccus, and a burning sensation throughout the digestive system due to hyperacidity. Excessive wind forms in the stomach causing pain. Sometimes, the patient suffers from constipation and at other times develops diarrhoea. This drug is also useful against **herpes** related to the gastrointestinal upset.

Any skin disease may be associated with Iris Versicolor. However, it is difficult to pick this remedy on the basis of skin signs alone. Iris Versicolor is diagnosed mainly on the basis of symptoms pertaining to the stomach. The ailments of Iris Versicolor aggravate while resting, during the night and ameliorate with movement. Nux Vomica annuls the side effects of Iris Versicolor.

| | |
|---|---|
| Antidote: | Nux Vomica |
| Potency: | 30 to 200 |

# KALI BICHROMICUM

## (Bichromate of Potash)

Kali Bichrome is deeply related to the mucous linings of the trachea and the upper respiratory passage. Kali Bichrome, Kali Carb, Kali Iodide and Kali Sulph have one thing in common, their illnesses and pain are specific to certain areas of the body.

Sometimes, the affected area may just be the size of the thumb. Even the nasal cold begins from pain over a tiny localised area, mostly on the left side. These symptoms of Kali Bichrome are now well known and proven. Long ago, I also used to suffer from headache, felt mostly at a tiny specific point, such as the temple. It could be alleviated with the pressure of a thumb. Similarly, the cold also used to start from a small area inside the left nostril. Both were cured by Kali Bichrome.

In Kali Carb, the pain and the sickness affect larger areas. In Kali Bichrome, there is widespread throbbing from the head to the toes. Whichever side the patient rests his head on a pillow, the throbbing follows. The patient cannot sleep. This is the characteristic of all potassium salts, much more so in Kali Bichrome.

The bones hurt as if scraped or badly beaten. In Eupatorium, all the bones hurt deep inside. In Kali Bichrome, the **bone pain is superficial** like a graze. Catarrhal conditions alternate with joint pains. These rheumatic type pains should be handled carefully. In case these are suppressed with some strong allopathic medicines, it will prove harmful instead of being beneficial. A more serious illness may ensue. Kali Bichrome is also useful for the treatment of rheumatism. This medicine should be used to treat those patients in whom catarrhal conditions appear, when the body aches get better. If the cold is suppressed with some powerful medicines, rheumatic pains return. Kali Bichromeshould be remembered, wherever this alternating situation is found.

Kali Bichrome is very good in the treatment of **diphtheria**. However, it cannot be compared to Muriatic Acid, which of course is the best treatment of diphtheria and also alleviates the profound physical weakness of the patient. The feeling of weakness is associated with all Potassium salts. For example, Kali Phos is used as a nerve tonic. Similarly, analogous use of Kali Carb is unique in vitalizing the muscles and the body. The heaviness of the legs disappears and it becomes easy to sit down and get up. Kali Bichrome is also of similar nature. If the patient presents the symptoms of Kali Bichrome, he will immediately respond to Kali Bichrome in that the body will feel light and active. All Potassium salts are a useful tonic for the muscles and nerves. In all these salts, there is a tendency to develop sores. One tends to develop ulcers in the stomach when the acidity is too high. Whenever ulcers are found in the stomach or intestines or anywhere in the body, one must try to correlate the patient's symptoms to some Potassium salt. There was a patient who had an old deep ulcer on his foot. I treated him with Kali Iodide. The ulcer healed in no time. Before this treatment, the patient had been treated in the best military hospitals without any success. I had also prescribed Potassium Iodide, since all his other symptoms were those of Potassium constitution.

Kali Bichrome is also very useful in the treatment of the **diseases of the stomach**. The peptic ulcer and cancer rarely present in a patient at the same time. Either the patient is suffering from the ulcer or cancer of the stomach. The Kali Bichrome patient usually suffers from stomach ulcers. If the symptoms of Kali Bichrome are found along with the stomach ailments, then the patient should be treated immediately with Kali Bichrome in order to preclude any grave situation.

The ulcers of Kali Bichrome are very deep and their edges are raised. However, this symptom is not diagnostic per se. This symptom is found in other remedies also. One particular symptom of Kali Bichrome resembles that of Causticum i.e. the cracking sound from the knees on walking, standing or sitting. Cracking is painless, though, definitely worrisome. Causticum is considered to be the most effective treatment for this problem, though Kali Bichrome is equally good. However in Kali Bichrome, the patient feels a burning sensation and feels the cold. The feeling of cold and the burning sensation is found in all Potassium salts.

Like Belladonna, the symptoms of Kali Bichrome come on suddenly and disappear equally fast.

Kali Bichrome is also very useful in the treatment of **infectious fevers**. Since the body of the patient is cold, he feels comfort when confined to a warm bed. The symptoms aggravate during the latter part of the night and exacerbate at about the same time the next day also.

Kali Bichrome is famous for the treatment of **epilepsy**, especially when the sputum is of the patient is thready.

The **headache** associated with Kali Bichrome is relieved by taking hot drinks. The headache aggravates at night and becomes most intense after midnight. The **thready discharge from the eyes**, being a symptom of Kali Bichrome, will also respond very well to it.

In Kali Bichrome, the aches and pains are mostly on the left side, though they may also occur on the right side. However, the headache and the neuralgic pain of the face invariably affect the left side. The headache is associated with nausea and returns after a lapse of a few days. Kali Bichrome is also very beneficial in the treatment of **migraines** (hemicrania).

Kali Bichrome is useful in the treatment of **eczema over the scalp**. Though, if the eczematous area is scaly and the discharge is yellowish and offensive, then these are the symptoms of Mezereum. Another resemblance to Mezereum is that when the nasal symptoms subside, the eczema flares up and vice versa.

In Kali Bichrome, the nasal cold begins at a small specific area deep inside the nose. The bacteria settle at the junction of the nose and throat (nasopharynx), resulting in the production and emission of a foul smell. These symptoms are common to both Kali Bichrome and Mezereum, though the latter works only locally, while Kali Bichrome affects the entire body. Moreover, in Mezereum, the symptoms of feeling hot or cold do not exist.

Kali Bichrome is also useful in the treatment of **various eye conditions**, such as photophobia, the appearance of spots of different colours before the eyes, blurring of vision, affection of the retina and formation of corneal ulcers. The wounds and ulcers of Kali Bichrome pulsate. If the corneal ulcer pulsates painfully, Potassium Bichrome must be administered at once for immediate relief. Kali Bichrome is also very effective in the treatment of boils forming on the upper eyelids and the puffiness of the lower eyelid due to swelling.

The symptoms common to ear, nose, jaws and lips (i.e. face area) are as follows:

The ears discharge sticky material along with a throbbing sensation in the ear. When the condition becomes chronic, the eardrums may perforate. The sense of smell also becomes dull. When the discharge settles inside the nose, it causes pain as well as difficulty in breathing. The symptoms aggravate with humidity. A piercing type of discharge runs from the nose. Persistence of this discharge results in the perforation of the septum of the nose (the dividing wall between the two nostrils). One strange symptom is that when the discharge sticks to this septal bone and then hardens, and scraping it affects the eyesight. Furthermore, there is pain over the forehead and the eyes; the nose bleeds, and upon coughing, the molar teeth (i.e. large hind teeth with deep roots) hurt. During the headache and nasal catarrh, the lower molar teeth on that particular side hurt as if these are the root cause of the pain, though in fact this is caused by the nerve root pain.

Kali Bichrome is also beneficial in the treatment of **ulcers of the lips and inside the mouth.** Cistus is also of use in this condition, especially for the ulcer of the lower lip. Dulcamara is effective against ulcers of both the upper and lower lips as well as against skin conditions that tend to spread quite fast. It also affects the sweat glands (pyretic glands).

In Kali Bichrome, the nose tends to bleed and blebs (polyps) form over the lining of the nose. It is also beneficial in the treatment of the tuberculous infection of the facial skin and the mucous membranes. By the grace of God, both these conditions have been successfully cured with it.

In Kali Bichrome, the tongue becomes covered with a thick coating, which is whitish near the tip and yellowish at the back, with some dirty patches here and there. The tongue exhibits a peculiar type of glare, not found normally. Sometimes, near the gullet, small nodules form resembling a strawberry in colour and shape. The resulting roughness of the surface of the tongue can be felt in the throat. Kali Bichrome is also very useful in the treatment of ulcers over the tongue, inside the cheeks and the roots of the teeth. Along with the inflammation of the throat, sores develop causing pain in the nasal passages, as well as the part of the throat behind the nose. The tenderness is localised to one area, though the pain is felt over a much larger area.

The important homoeopathic remedies used in the **treatment of inflammatory swellings** similar to those of Kali Bichrome are Lachesis, Kali Iodide, Nitric Acid, Phosphorus and Sulphuric Acid.

There is a strong tendency towards the **formation of ulcers**. Swelling of the tonsils, when severe, causes a lot of pain with the swelling and redness becoming externally visible in the upper part of the neck. The patient feels as if a hair is stuck in the throat. In Tarentula, such a feeling is widely spread in other parts of the body. In Hepar Sulph, the feeling is of something sticking. The ailment concentrates at the root of the tongue causing severe pain and the formation of hardly visible sores.

**There is a tendency towards nausea and vomiting:** The vomited material consists of undigested food mixed with bile and blood. The expectorated phlegm is in the form of sticky threads. Kali Bichrome is considered to be the best treatment for the nausea of alcoholics. Kali Bichrome may also be used for the **treatment of ulcerative colitis**. Chronic ulcerative colitis is a very obstinate condition for which no effective cure has been discovered so far. Kali Bichrome is also useful in the treatment of gastritis resulting from exposure to cold. The stomach becomes weak and hypo functional. The secretion contains a lot of mucus. The patient feels indisposed.

In Kali Bichrome, the **liver pain is referred to the right shoulder**. It is an ominous sign found in cancer of the liver and the gall bladder. The patient complains of severe pain at the shoulder, which must be treated with Kali Bichrome. Kali Bichrome is of great use in the treatment of this vexing pain caused by **stones in the gall bladder** or cancer of the liver, and referred to the shoulder. The shoulder itself has no problems of its own. The gall bladder stones and the liver disorders must be treated with Kali Bichrome without any delay. Often, it dissolves and then expels these gallstones, obviating the need for surgery. Stones of the gall bladder result from increased viscidity and the altered composition of bile. Once the chemistry of the bile is restored, it gradually dissolves the stones. I happen to come across many patients suffering from gall bladder stones. Due to the scarcity of time, I cannot afford to achieve an individual diagnosis of each and every patient. I, therefore, treat them with a combination formula, rather than using one single homoeopathic remedy. By the grace of God, the prescription has proven to be very effective in most of the patients.

Kali Bichrome is one component of that formulary, which is detailed as follows:

Kali Bichrome, Lycopodium, Cholesterinum and Natrum Sulph, all in 30 potency.
Besides these, Mag Phos 30, Colocynth 30 and Diascorea 30 combined toghether may be used to relieve the associated biliary colic.

In addition to these, a herbal medicine, Ospafell, available from Germany, is also famous for the capability of dissolving the stones in the gall bladder. For additional benefit, it may also be used in homoeopathic form as an adjunct.

In Kali Bichrome, a patient **feels pain at the time of passing stools or even on movement**. The peristaltic movements of the gut at the time of defacation cause piercing pain over the liver as well as over the spleen. A lot of wind forms in the belly, causing distension. The entire body aches lightly while the intestines feel sore. A feeling of weakness and sinking sensation over the stomach precede diarrhoea. Nausea, vomiting and then diarrhoea; this is the pattern in Kali Bichrome. Diarrhoea starts in the morning (like Sulphur). Kali Bichrome is very useful in the treatment of **morning diarrhoea** in which the stools are clay coloured.

Sometimes, **rheumatic pains alternate with dysentery** instead of nasal catarrh. With the onset of dysentery, body aches disappear and the body feels light. There is cramping before, during and after the passage of stools. The **rectum also prolapses**. Piles become swollen and painful. Kali Bichrome should also be remembered for treating **backache** associated with the passage of **blood in the urine**. In Kali Bichrome, the urine may contain strings of mucus and urination is preceded by pain over the coccyx (tail end of the spine). This is typical of Kali Bichrome.

In women patients of Kali Bichrome, **the uterus related ailments aggravate during the summer**. The menstrual discharge becomes acidic and causes burning. Periods start before time. Kali Bichrome should be remembered to treat the passage of **thread-like strands in the milk while breast-feeding**. If the **milk tends to clot**, then Phytolacca would be the best remedy, which is also useful in the treatment of vomiting during pregnancy.

Kali Bichrome is very useful in the **treatment of permanent loss of voice**. Kali Bichrome is very effective in relieving wheezing due to the retention of sticky phlegm and constriction of the trachea and upper respiratory passages, commonly seen in asthma. Kali Bichrome is also useful in the treatment of whooping cough. The catarrhal complaints of Kali Bichrome become worse in the wet, wintery season. The patient develops diarrhoea in the summer during the rainy season. He feels comfort lying down in the bed. The phlegm is greenish in colour and contains blood clots. Both Kali Bichrome and Kali Carb are very useful in the **treatment of tuberculosis of the lungs**. Potassium salts are very deeply related to the formation of cavities in the lungs and coughing of blood in the sputum.

In Kali Bichrome, like Kali Carb and Ipecac, there is a **feeling of chill over the back**. In Kali Carb, this feeling is confined only to the lower part of the back, while in Ipecac and Kali Bichrome it stretches all the way up to the neck. The rheumatic pains aggravate on movement, like in Bryonia. The pain is worse in the morning. On getting up and walking, the pain gradually dissipates. Rest at night offers relief, though by morning, the pain becomes concentrated in one area from where it then scatters on movement.

All sorts of skin diseases may be found in Kali Bichrome, such as eczema, blisters and boils. If skin conditions are forcibly suppressed with some strong ointments they may affect the mucous linings of the intestines. Therefore, in a patient exhibiting symptoms of Kali Bichrome, one should desist from external use of medicines.

| | |
|---|---|
| Antidotes: | Arsenic, Lachesis, Pulsatilla |
| Potency: | 30 to 200. |

# KALI CARBONICUM

Kali Carb is a white compound made of Carbon and Potassium. In olden days, it was obtained from the ashes of wood, leaves and seaweeds. Besides Potassium Chloride, Kali Carb was the most important compound that was prepared for commercial purposes. Later on, the chemical, instead of being prepared from charcoal, was extracted from mineral deposits found under the ground. The largest source of the compound was the salt mines in Germany. Nowadays, the compound is being manufactured in different ways for industrial use.

In homoeopathy, it is used in the form of a very dilute solution, prepared from the powder of Potassium Carbonate. An in-depth comprehension of Kali Carb is extremely difficult because of a number of contradictions in its nature. The patient is sensitive to both heat as well as cold. His mind is very much preoccupied. Even if the diagnosis is correct but the constitution of the patient happens to be different, its use will be harmful instead of being beneficial. Generally, it is the incorrect selection of a remedy that causes harm, but in case of Kali Carb, even if the selection is correct, the patient may still be harmed due to a mismatch with the nature of the patient. For example, even if correctly selected, the usage of Silicea in very high potency may prove extremely harmful.

In **gout,** nodes form at the fingers and wrist joints causing disfigurement of the hands, and deformities of the fingers. To give Kali Carb in high potency in this condition even if appropriate to the constitution of the patient, is very dangerous. It amounts to torturing the patient to death. Indication being correct, the medicine will command the body to prepare for immediate cure for which the body is not ready. Even if Kali Carb is prescribed after arriving at the correct diagnosis in **gout**, one has to be very cautious. Carbo Veg should always be given before giving Kali Carb. Carbo Veg prepares the patient for proper response to Kali Carb and serious reaction to Kali Carb is then prevented. Kali Carb must first be given in the low potency of 30 and then in a high potency, as the patient becomes acclimatized.

Besides **joint pains**, Kali Carb is strongly linked to **chronic backache**, especially the one starting after childbirth. Very often, the back pain starting after the delivery becomes chronic and not curable until treated with Kali Carb. Kali Carb is also very effective in the **treatment of tuberculosis**. Kali Carb has the capability to heal the lung cavities resulting from a tuberculous infection. It is also very effective in controlling all types of bleeding. Ulcers of the intestines result in the passage of blood in the stools, like Antimonium Crude. In Kali Carb, the stools are soft, while in Antimonium Crude they are hard. Occasionally, the patient of Kali Carb may be **severely constipated** and pass blood in the stools. It is not that common however.

In Kali Carb, besides **severe stomachache**, discomfort and cramps, the patient occasionally passes blood in the stools. Several types of aches and pains are associated with Kali Carb. Severe abdominal discomfort, cramps and blood in the stools are common to many drugs used to treat dysentery. Therefore, it is essential that each one of them should be identified based on its specific symptoms. Sometimes, Kali Carb is used to cure the bad effects resulting from the wrong use of Nux Vomica, especially diarrhoea or the headache following an overdose of Nux Vomica. Kali Carb is best for the treatment of **diarrhoea,** and Gelsemium for **headache**. If diarrhoea starts suddenly after taking Nux Vomica, then a dose or two of Kali Carb will cure the patient, with God's grace. However, it should not be used over a long period of time, or it will cause constipation. Once the patient has benefited from one or two doses of this medicine, the treatment should be stopped.

The **irritability** is a prominent symptom of this remedy and is often present in mental illnesses. **Fear of loneliness** is also its symptom. The patient is very **superstitious**. The superstitious ideas have nothing to do with the loneliness of the patient. Imagination becomes a part of the patient's life. However, the loneliness definitely perturbs the patient. The patient is sensitive to both heat and cold. In general, the Kali Carb patient is of very short temper and is easily enraged.

Both hot and cold things hurt the teeth. Sometimes, the teeth become oversensitive to cold. The symptoms of **Pyorrhoea** are common. There is **swelling of the gums,** which start to decay exuding pus.

Such patients are extremely sensitive to cold. However, when these patients of Kali Carb are fomented with ice-cold water, the nerves become numb and relaxed. The relief is temporary because the symptoms recur as soon as the effect of the cold is gone. The heat also bothers the patient. It increases the burning sensation and becomes intolerable. In Merc Sol also, **toothache** becomes worse with both heat and cold. When the **gums decay** and start discharging offensive pus and blood, Kali Carb can still cure the condition if other general symptoms of Kali Carb are present, or Merc Sol may also offer a cure.

Both localised as well as migrating type of pains are found in Kali Carb. The backache usually remains localized in one area. However, during childbirth, the pain starts to move from one area to another. If, during sleep, the quilt slips off from the body and a backache starts on exposure to the cold wind, Kali Carb is very effective. I have tested the remedy on myself and on many others, time and again. Once while travelling I woke up around three or four o' clock in the morning with severe backache, even though by the grace of God I rarely suffered from backache. I took one dose of Kali Carb 30. It immediately alleviated the pain and never did I have this problem again.

In Kali Carb often the ailment becomes worse during the winter, yet the affected parts of the body feel hot (and do not feel comfort from the outside cold). A draft of cold wind sometimes produces a blazing sensation along the course of the nerves with the appearance of prickly heat on the skin. It is one aspect of Kali Carb that the external cold, instead of having a cooling effect, enhances the feeling of heat. Heat ameliorates the symptoms.

Once the nasal cold begins, it also causes **headache**. Light-headedness along with the headache is a specific symptom of Kali Carb. By the way, it should be remembered that the **sinus** headache resulting from flu often gets cured by just one dose of Nux Vomica 1000. Sometimes, the irritable bladder (cystitis), causing **frequency of urination**, may respond to Kali Phos better than Kali Carb. However, in Kali Phos, the frequent passage of urine is during the daytime while in the case of Kali Carb, the patient has to wake up repeatedly during the night, especially between three to four o' clock in the morning, to ease himself. Frequency of urination at night other than due to diabetes can also benefit from Arsenic in addition to Kali Carb, provided other symptoms of Arsenic also exist. One particular symptom of Arsenic is more common in women i.e. they lose bladder control so much so that they may not even be able to make it to the lavatory. A similar condition can also develop in men due to various diseases and this becomes definitely more difficult to treat. The reason is the difficulty in finding the appropriate remedy out of the scores of remedies available.

Kali Carb patients, often have a **sore throat**. The tonsils become inflamed and enlarged. Swelling of the glands behind the ears, (parotid glands) is not as dangerous as the swelling inside the throat due to the inflammation of both tonsils, which then become hard. The exudates solidify in them and prevent the glands from shrinking in size. Kali Carb is an effective treatment for this condition if its other symptoms are also present.

In the diseases related to Kali Carb, there is a tendency to develop widespread swelling and inflammation in various parts of the body, but especially the **swelling of the upper eyelids** is very prominent. Like some other medicines, the symptoms of feeling a pulsation on the side on which the patient lies down is found in Kali Carb also. Furthermore, the patient feels anxious and cannot sleep. If the throbbing is too severe due to an increased rush of blood towards the head and does not respond to Kali Carb, then Belladonna will be found to work very well.

Since in Kali Carb, often the patient feels **pain and heaviness on the left side of the chest** over the area of the heart, it may be well to suspect it is due to the heart disease, even though heart pain is often felt in the middle of the chest, radiating to the back, the arms and upto the fingers. Although the pain of Kali Carb makes one suspicious of possible heart disease, other symptoms can help to make the distinction clearer. The cardiac pain (angina pectoris) becomes worse on walking fast. On the other hand if the pain, becomes less on walking or on changing the side, it cannot be due to a heart problem. Homoeopaths, in general, do not have access to instruments and machines to test the heart, so they must critically examine each symptom. Besides neurologic ailments, Kali Carb is also useful in the treatment of heart pain (angina) especially the unusually strong palpitations.

In Kali Carb, **piles** are like hanging tags instead of being in rounded masses, which give an intense burning sensation. Cold water comforts only temporarily, reducing the burning sensation. In the abdominal complaints of Kali Carb, cramps are a must, such as in **dysentery**. However, the **diarrhoea**, which often alternates with constipation, is without pain.

The **burning sensation after urination** responds favourably to Natrum Mur. However, if the burning sensation is experienced before, during, as well as after urination, then Natrum Mur will be ineffective because this condition relates to Kali Carb.

Kali Carb is an excellent treatment in women, especially for the treatment of the complications arising from childbirth. One should remember Kali Carb as the first choice. It indeed is the best remedy to treat these complications and the ones arising after D&C (dilatation and curettage).

Kali Carb is also related to the **enlarged glands of the uterus (uterine fibroids).** Other symptoms being present, it can be used for the treatment of **vomiting of pregnancy**.
Kali Carb is an ideal remedy in difficult labour with weak labour pains that radiates to lower back and thighs in **difficulty in delivery of the child**.

Kali Carb is very useful in the **treatment of severe cough associated with vomiting**, as well as the **cough following measles**.

Kali Carb is a very powerful remedy for **neuralgic conditions.** It is also deeply linked to the bones because carbon has a powerful influence on them.

Kali Carb patients suffer from general weakness. In these patients, the pulse becomes slow. There are sharp pricking type of pain and **burning sensations along the course of the nerves**. Furthermore, such patients have a sensation of burning inside their internal organs (viscera). The severity of the disease increases at night between two to five o' clock in the morning and which becomes worse on turning onto the left side or lying down on the affected side. Hot weather ameliorates the symptoms. A distinctive character of Kali Carb is that sometimes, there is a severe burning sensation over tiny circular areas, the size of a fingertip or a thumb.

| | |
|---|---|
| Adjuvants: | Carbo Veg, Nux Vomica |
| Antidotes: | Camphor, Coffea |
| Potency: | 30 to 1000 |

# KALI MURIATICUM

## (Chloride of Potassium)

Kali Mur is extremely useful in the treatment of **catarrhal diseases**. One of its prominent symptoms is the deposition of grey coloured material over the tongue of the patient. As the deposits of Diphtheria inside the throat are also grey coloured, Kali Mur is used in the treatment of Diphtheria. In fact, some physicians include it in the standard remedies for Diphtheria.

In Kali Mur, infants develop **eczema over the scalp (cradle cap)**. Kali Mur is also useful in the treatment of dandruff and **chronically discharging ears** (chronic otitis media). The glands around the ear become inflamed. Noises and sounds are heard in the ears.

Blisters with **whitish material form inside the mouth**. There is catarrh with blocked nose and formation of large amount of whitish discharge. Kali Mur is also useful in the treatment of diseases of throat and **Tonsillitis**. I however, do not use this alone but combine it with Silicea, Calcarea Fluor and Ferrum Phos, each in 6X. The combination proves immediately effective in most of the throat conditions.

In Kali Mur, the patient has wind in the stomach. Kali Mur is useful in the treatment of **intestinal worms,** which cause lot of itching. Whenever there is **constipation**, the liver also becomes afflicted. The stools become clay coloured or very light and pale coloured. One must not forget to use Kali Mur in these conditions. External **piles** also develop and bleed.

In the women of Kali Mur constitution, the **periods are either** delayed or stop altogether. In this case, if Kali Mur does not work, Natrum Mur must be used. The **leaucorrhoeal discharge is milky in appearance**. It is harmless and does not cause any burning. The vomitus during the pregnancy is also of a white colour.

In Kali Mur, the **voice also becomes hoarse**. Symptoms of asthma, as well as cough, associated with stomach upset, are common. Kali Mur is useful in the treatment of **Rheumatic fever** and pains getting worse at night. These pains become worse on retiring to bed and radiate like waves of lightning.

**Skin diseases** are also manifest in Kali Mur. The peculiar sign of eczema associated with Kali Mur is that the skin sheds whitish dry material like thick dry flour. The ailments of Kali Mur become worse with heavy fried food and on movement.

| | |
|---|---|
| Potency: | Biochemic, 3X to 12X<br>Homoeopathy, from 30 upwards |

# KALI PHOSPHORICUM

## (Phosphate of Potassium)

Potassium Phosphate is an important element found in the secretions of the human body and glands. In the brain, nerves, muscles and blood especially, its mere presence is not enough, rather, it has to be in a state of equilibrium. It plays an essential, prominent role in the development of human life. While its deficiency causes numerous neurological and mental disorders, its excess, too, is sometimes extremely lethal. Its chemical name is Potassium Phosphate, though in homoeopathy it is known as Kali Phos.

Kali Phos is a renowned **nerve tonic**. It is an antipsoric remedy, meaning that it is effective against skin conditions which, when forcefully suppressed, can inflict the inner linings of the body and the nervous system. Though homoeopaths classify it as antipsoric, yet it is mainly related to the nerves. By nature it gives strength to the nerves and on the same basis, it has antipsoric effects. For example, if any illness remains suppressed due to the weakness of the nerves, and the body is too weak to expel it, Kali Phos will throw it out on the skin.

Kali Phos **works on the brain**, the nerves and the blood. It is surprisingly effective in the treatment of mental and physical fatigue. It is useful for the treatment of ailments resulting from anxiety, confusion, overwork and mental anguish. By nature, a patient of Kali Phos is **lazy and fearful**. He feels nervous to meet people, **loses his memory** and becomes indifferent to his work.

In Kali Phos ailments become aggravated by resting in the cold and humid weather. These symptoms are also seen in Rhus Tox, but in Rhus Tox the patient tosses and turns all night because of the increasing discomfort. Whereas, in Kali Phos, the sufferings build up all night and then forcefully express themselves in the morning when the patient wakes up. So the discomfort is at its peak in the morning and then gradually abates. The gradual increment of the disease is an important sign of Kali Phos. In a patient of Rhus Tox, the discomfort is worst at the onset of movement and gradually improves on walking. A patient of Kali Phos gets relieved with slow movement. Like Rhus

Tox, there is a tingling and **numbness of the hands and feet** as well as the flaccidity of the muscles. All kinds of body excretions have a foul odour in Kali Phos. In Rhus Tox, however, there is no such foul odour. Rhus glaba and foul odour are very deeply related. Many antipsoric medicines are used for treating the foul smelling secretions of the armpits (due to the infected sebaceous glands in the axilla). But Rhus Glabra in potency 3X or 6X and Kali Phos in 6X are extremely effective when given together. Kali Phos is also deeply related to foul smell.

Kali Phos is also very useful in the treatment of **gangrene**. In the allopathic system, the treatment of infected indolent **ulcers** that become necrotic and gangrenous is amputation. But amputation is usually performed through a healthy area of good circulation, well above the gangrenous area. In many such patients, I have successfully obviated the need for amputation with the use of Kali Phos and Silicea.

Allah, the Almighty has created a very elaborate immune system in our body against diseases. The cure is not obtainable without these antibodies. When a disease has knocked down the body defence to the extent that it cannot react any more, any amount of antibiotics given will be ineffective because body can no longer react. Similarly, in the case of gangrene, the immune system of the body is completely damaged. Kali Phos revives the immune system and empowers the tissues to defend. Consequently, the body starts defending itself against the gangrenous process. Silicea also works well once the tissues become strong again.

Kali Phos is also useful in the treatment of **inflamed lymph glands**. Sometimes the glands become inflamed on both sides of the neck. This also happens in the case of tuberculosis and cancer. In these patients, Silicea alone can lead to serious consequences. Therefore, many other medicines are given before or along with Silicea. One of them is definitely Kali Phos. Kali Phos streamlines the reaction of the body towards Silicea. In my opinion, this method is very effective. It is also possible to give Kali Phos before Silicea and prepare the patient for proper reaction. In this situation, it is better to give Kali Phos 1000 and wait for a few days. Sometimes this alone produces miraculous results, and a single dose starts decreasing the size of the lymph nodes. At this time, we do not even need to give Silicea.

Another dose of Kali Phos can be repeated after eight to ten days. As long as the size of the lymph nodes is reducing, we do not need to add another medicine. Kali Phos is not only effective in the treatment of superficial glands, but it also affects the glands of the internal organs and uterus. When the glands look like they are transforming into cancer, Kali Phos must be kept in mind because of its beneficial effect on the **healing of cancerous ulcers**.

Kali Phos resembles Agaricus to some extent. The twitching of the muscles of the face may require Kali Phos, Agaricus or similar medicines.

**Kali Phos, like Ambra Grisea, is also useful to alleviate the ill effects of a serious accident or a bad news**. The development of such a mental shock is an important sign of Kali Phos. Kali Carb is the best remedy for any gastric or heart ailment resulting from sad news. Natrum Mur is also useful for the mental disturbance consequent upon sad news. Sad news or grief due to shock does not affect everybody uniformly. In Kali Phos, sudden shocking news afflicts the mind and the patient suffers from sadness and weakness for a long, long time. In a patient of Natrum Mur, the grief results in **insanity**.

Kali Phos is very useful in the **treatment of mental stress and severe fatigue**. My late father had a prescription devised for nervous weakness and this should be remembered i.e. Kali Phos 6X and Calcaria Phos 6X, Mag Phos 6X, combined and taken two to three times a day. This can relieve all kinds of nervous exhaustions.

In Kali Phos, the **memory can be affected temporarily** without the narrowing of the blood vessels of the brain. This is not permanent. While someone is seriously thinking over a particular matter and then suddenly his attention gets diverted to another focus, he fails to recall the desired name or word that he is looking for. The reason is that the mind, being busy in another thought does not concentrate on the new thought immediately. This is due to the mental stress and not due to arteriosclerosis (narrowing of the cerebral blood vessels). Besides Kali Phos, Caladium is very useful in the treatment of this transient ailment. In Kali Phos, the patient may feel dizzy suddenly, reminding one of Bryonia. The dizziness on sudden standing up, lowering of the head or movement of the head from side to side is a sign of Kali Phos,

Bryonia and many other homoeopathic remedies. Nux Vomica is also very good for the treatment of dizziness. Sometimes the head feels heavy and there is loss of balance and unsteadiness on walking. Movement of the head leads to the sensation of vertigo. Similarly, when the distension of the abdomen suddenly jolts the stomach, this movement can also lead to unsteadiness and dizziness. In this situation, Nux Vomica works immediately and effectively. If the **dizziness is only because of nervous exhaustion**, Kali Phos should be the top priority.

If any ailment is aggravated by motion and there is **dizziness during travelling**, both Cocculus and Bryonia are useful. When unsteady, the patient of Kali Phos tends to fall forwards. Some just tend to bend backwards. This tendency of theirs to bend back, sometimes changes to the tendency to fall forwards. The patient of Kali Phos is in general very intelligent and adapts to bending forwards for the fear of falling backwards, which results in a forward fall.

In the **neurogenic pains** of the face (trigeminal neuralgia), besides Kali Phos, Phosphorus, Silicea, Spigelia and Magnesium Phos are also very useful. Mag Phos is also deeply related to the nerves. For the treatment of restlessness and **muscular cramping**, it is more useful, compared to Kali Phos. Kali Phos is also associated with tonic contractions of the muscles, which it relieves in homoeopathic and biochemic forms. The convulsions of Kali Phos are usually related to the lower parts of the body, namely the thighs, calves and feet. The muscular spasms of Mag Phos are more generalised and can affect the intestines as well. Kali Phos also works well on the infections of the kidneys. In Mag Phos, in addition to the hyperexcitability, there may be other factors that lead to violent muscle spasms.

In **typhoid**, deep **ulcers form inside the mouth**. The tongue looks filthy and smells foul. These signs are also seen in Kali Phos. Lack of body immunity leads to the spread of toxins into the blood, sepsis, and **oral thrush** (fungal infection of the tongue). Another sign of Kali Phos is that the patient feels hungry but does not want to eat anything. This is common in very sensitive types of people. Slim, skinny boys and girls, who are over-sensitive and are teased by others, react against food, refusing to eat important nutrients. These children become **anorexic** because of hypersensitivity. Kali Phos is the best remedy for such children. Initially, it should be given in potency 6X.

After it has shown some beneficial effect, another dose in high potency will show surprisingly good results. For the anorexia, due to a stomach or liver disorder, Nux Vomica is the best. The effect of Nux Vomica on sleep is similar to that of Kali Phos. Nux Vomica is useful in treating the **insomnia** and restlessness arising from drinking tea or coffee, but in case of insomnia due to nervousness and anxiety, Kali Phos should be used.

The patients of Kali Phos and Arsenic are usually very neat and tidy but unfortunately their body secretions become very foul smelling and putrid during the severity of the illness and fever. Because the foul smell of secretions is common in other medicines too, one should not consider the foul smell as a diagnostic sign for Kali Phos. Most bodily secretions happen to be foul smelling in contagious diseases and infections. Kali Phos ranks high in the cure of such a patient. Ferrum Phos 6X and Kali Phos6X combined given five to six times a day along with Pyrogenium 200 and Typhoidinum 200, work very well in a **typhoid** patient who has a tendency towards constipation. The patient of Kali Phos likes cold and sour drinks.

Kali Phos is very effective in the **inflammatory conditions of the liver and the intestines**. It also works for irritable bowel syndrome (an intestinal disorder of psychological origin). One or two doses of Kali Phos are very effective in the treatment of **acute dysenteric symptoms** associated with severe cramps in the abdomen (tenesmus). It should be remembered that Kali Phos and nothing else will work for gastro-intestinal disturbances associated with nervousness and anxiety. Kali Phos should especially be used when all other similar medicines have failed. Kali Phos is usually used as a tonic in combination with Mag Phos and Calacarea Phos. But if the symptoms of Kali Phos are obvious, then the effect of Kali Phos would diminish in the presence of other medicines. In this situation, one should keep in mind that if the diagnosis is correct then that one particular medicine could hit the target, with the blessings of Allah. One or two doses can cure the patient, and if by chance it does not help, then other appropriate medicines should be sought.

Regarding the disease pattern of some medicines, the symptoms shift from right to left or from left to right. In Kali Phos, like Lachesis, the symptoms move from left to right. In Kali Phos, it is not the disease itself which transfers from left to right but simply the pain moves from left to right, while in Lachesis, the disease itself tends to shift from left to right.

In the **diarrhoea** of Kali Phos associated with **fear and anxiety**, the stools are watery and foul smelling causing weakness. The **dysentery** in Kali Phos is associated with the passage of mucous without blood, but sometimes there could be fresh bleeding. It is the irritation of the nerves in the walls of the intestines that increases their mobility. The adjacent loops of the gut rub against each other, causing inflammation, production of mucous and then bleeding.

Kali Phos works on the **bladder rendered irritable due to exposure to cold**. Some people suffer from frequent urination, more so in cold weather. On exposure to the cold, the bladder becomes irritable, leading to the frequent passage of urine but there is no associated burning. The urine is clear like water, showing that there is no infection. Instead it is mere irritation of the bladder. As in the common cold, there is excessive running of the nose but no physical discomfort. It is the frequent wiping of the nose that causes inflammation inside the nose. If this bladder condition of a Kali Phos patient does not abate soon, inflammation will ensue; even infection can set in. Sometimes in a patient of Kali Phos, the headache resulting from mental fatigue may apparently get better but the associated mental stress becomes directed towards the kidneys. As a result of this, the patient passes an abundant amount of urine every few minutes or so (polyuria). Such episodes occur in people involved in serious literary work. Highly intellectual work and mental anguish may cause migraine or headache or sometimes frequent urination.

Kali Phos is also the remedy for **sexual weakness resulting from nervous tension**. Kali Phos should also be remembered in **women who tend to abort**. In general, in the beginning of pregnancy, Viburnum Opulus Q is used to prevent the abortion. In the second and third month, Sabinais used, while in the fourth and fifth months, Kali Carb is used. However if the abortions occur because of the patient being highly-strung and anxious, Kali Phos would be the best treatment.

Kali Phos is deeply related to the aborting tendency secondary to mental stress. These women should be made to take Kali Phos 1000 (even when not pregnant) once or twice a month. At the onset of bleeding during pregnancy, Kali Phos should be combined with Ferrum Phos.

Kali Phos is also worth remembering in the treatment of **angina**. In angina, it should be combined with Mag Phos but other appropriate medicines may be used.

The **acne and boils of Kali Phos** are more on the abdomen and the back rather then on the face or other areas. Initially Kali Phos alone should be used for this, but other medicines should be looked for if there is no relief.

**When the skin diseases become suppressed and migrate to the deep internal organs**, the nervous system becomes inflicted and loses its normal function. The body becomes cold and unable to defend itself. Kali Carb and Psorinum are among those homoeopathic remedies that can immediately warm up the body and surface the disease out onto the skin. Kali Phos would certainly be indicated when diseases like measles and chicken pox, originating from the deep organs do not manifest their signs on the skin due to the suppressed nervous system. Kali Phos is completely different from Psorinum and other such medicines in its action.

Some homoeopath physicians warn that Kali Phos and other potassium salts should not be used during a fever, but this is only true when the **temperature is rising** in the early stage of the disease. Once the fever starts lowering, any proper medication can be given to its advantage.

Regarding the **loss of memory** and nervous breakdown, Kali Phos should be used in potency CM.

Kali Phos, Calcarea Phos and Ferrum Phos combined in 6X potency are useful for the correction of **anaemia** and the general well being of children. If the child is congenitally weak, then one should also add Silicea. In the case of premature children, most of their organs, which were supposed to develop in the uterus, remain weak. Silicea is very useful to strengthen them. It is a very good remedy to improve such congenital weaknesses.

Kali Phos is also useful in the treatment of **Puerperal fever** alongside Pyrogenium and Sulphur.

| | |
|---|---|
| Potency: | 6X to 30, 200, 1000, 10 0000 or 100 000 as indicated |

# KALI SULPHURICUM

## (Sulphate of Potash)

Kali Sulph is a biochemic medicine, which contains the elements of Potassium and Sulphur. Sulphur and potassium being profoundly effective medicines, their compound i.e. Kali Sulph, also has quite a profound action. It affects each and every part of the body.

It is difficult to include in one chapter the large number of diseases, which can possibly be cured with Kali Sulph. Everybody should try to find out which diseases or symptoms can be treated with it. During a preliminary study, one could feel that Kali Sulph is a panacea for every kind of disease, yet its nature is not going to be a match for every kind of illness. Numerous illnesses are described in relation to Kali Sulph; however, the proper diagnosis of all of them is difficult, and so would be the treatment. This medicine should be studied at least ten to fifteen times. Despite this, the physician would be at a loss to comprehend its effectiveness or non-effectiveness, in reference to the diseases mentioned under Kali Sulph in literatures. The mere presence of symptoms is not enough because the constitution of the patient also has to exactly match that of the remedy. Once a complete match is arrived at, Kali Sulph can totally uproot even the most dangerous of diseases.

According to Dr. Kent, this medicine can offer complete cure from **epilepsy**, but it is not necessary that a single dose may produce that effect. Sometimes, it has to be repeated over a long time (with some intervals in between). During these interval periods, other types of treatments have to be administered. The difficulty about Kali Sulph is that there is no given detail about the kind of epilepsy amenable to Kali Sulph, because complete proving has never been done with that purpose in mind. This is why most homoeopaths do not give much importance to Kali Sulph. Had the proving been done, it would obviously be known what kind of epilepsy should be treated with it. Under the present circumstances, we can only say that if an epilepsy could not be treated with any analogous remedy, Kali Sulph should also be tried.

In addition to **skin diseases,** Kali Sulph is also useful in the treatment of diseases affecting the mucous membranes. It is said that some patients of **Lupus** can be totally cured with Kali Sulph. Similarly, **malaria** going out of hand can be treated very well with Kali Sulph, provided it fits the constitution of the patient.

Kali Sulph must be used in the treatment of **chronic catarrhal conditions**, especially when the discharge becomes green.

Kali Sulph is called the Pulsatilla of biochemy because most of its symptoms resemble those of Pulsatilla, for example, the worsening of the symptoms with heat, and getting relief with the cold and open air. This feature is very important regarding the diagnosis for Kali Sulph. The full clinical picture of Pulsatilla would, however, distinguish it from Kali Sulph. In other words, the presence of most but not all of the symptoms of Pulsatilla would be taken as the indication for Kali Sulph. In this situation, it will be found an effective treatment for almost all of the diseases mentioned under the chapter of Kali Sulph.

In Kali Sulph, the muscles tend to be flabby and without proper tone. Kali Sulph would be useful in the treatment of patients with **liver disorder and dilatation of the muscles of the heart**. It will tone the cardiac musculature but has to be administered in a low potency over a long period. Within a few months, the patient feels much better. He feels invigorated and to a large extent the fatty degeneration of the liver and the excessive amount of fat under the skin starts to melt away. These kinds of symptoms are more common in women, especially after childbirth. The liver becomes fatty, the muscles become flabby, the heart becomes weak, and the patient becomes short of breath. The legs of the women become heavy and swollen. Light touch bothers them while deep pressure offers relief. In such patients, Kali Sulph being the proper analog would offer great relief.

In Kali Sulph, the **headache** becomes worse on movement and is relieved in the open air. The pain spreads to the eyes, forehead and on both sides of the head. The head feels tight and there is a feeling of being suffocated. The **eyelids stick together** due to a yellowish discharge. There is lot of itching and watering from the eyes. Small pimples form over the eyelids. The cornea becomes hazy. Once again, if Kali Sulph is the proper match for the disposition of the patient, it will cure all these eye ailments.

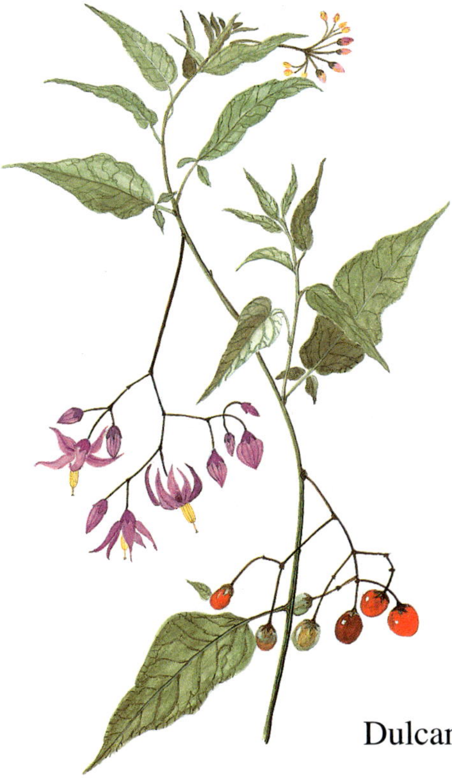

Dulcamara

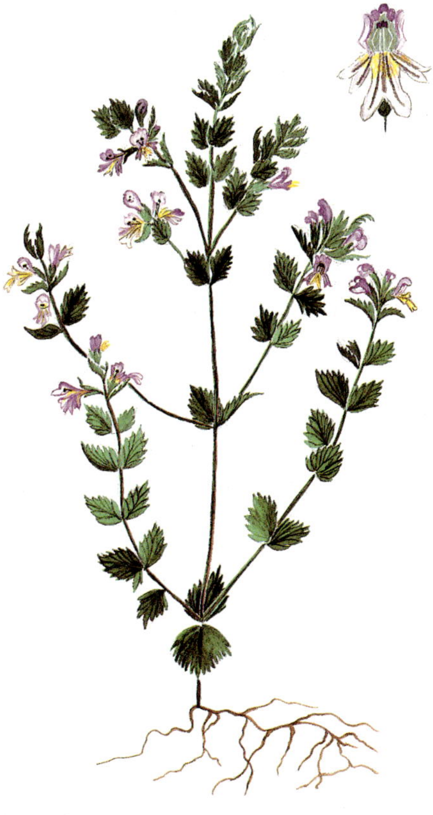

uphrasinum

Ferrum Phosphoricum

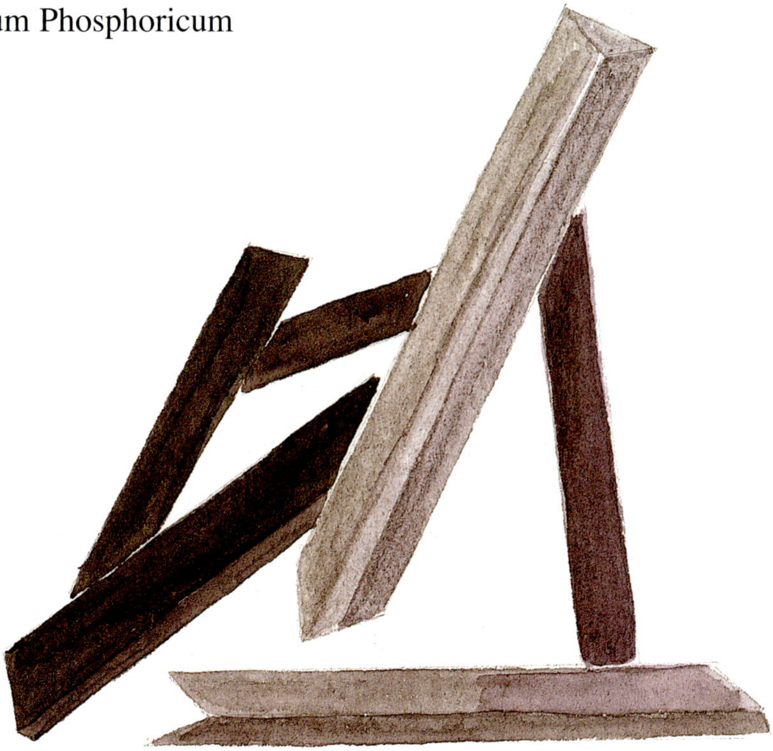

Gelsemium

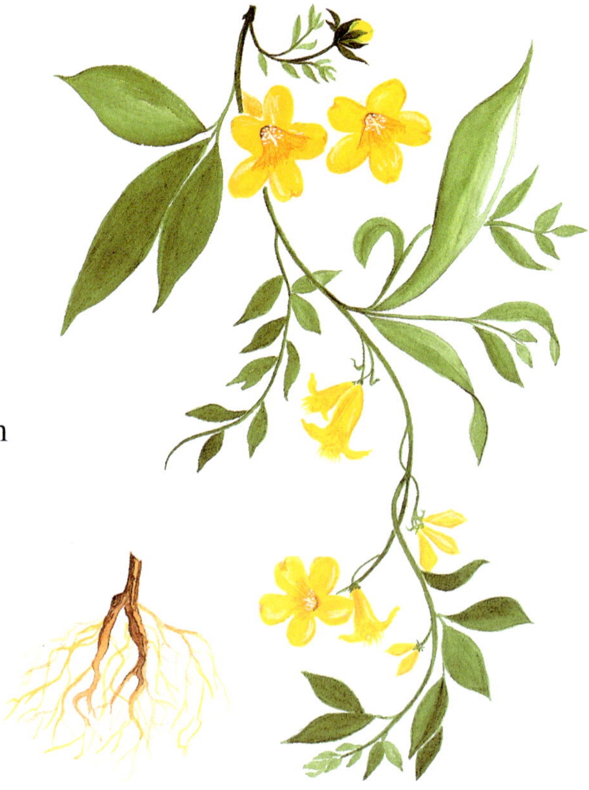

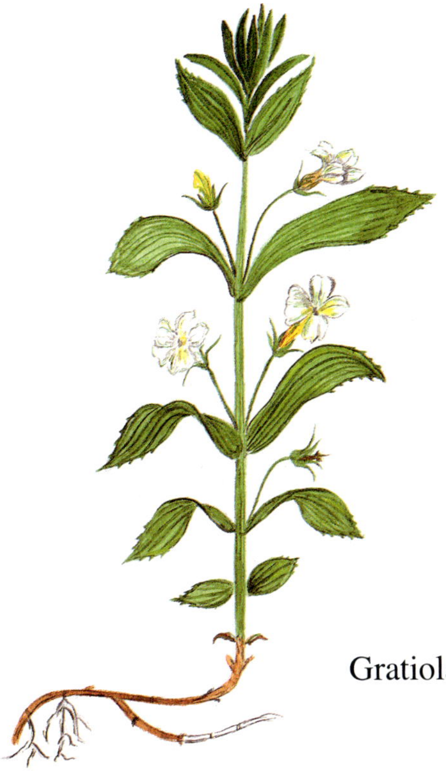

Gratiola

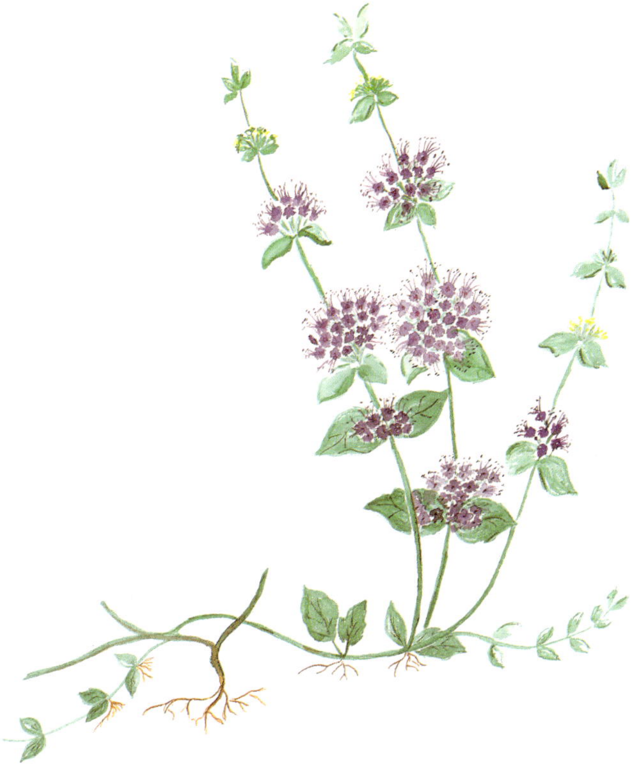

Hedeoma

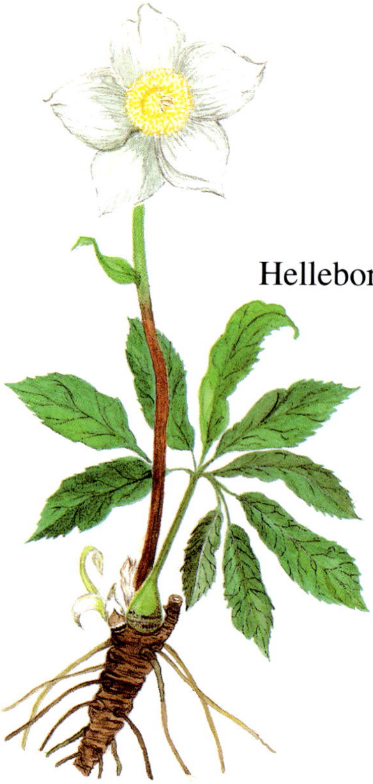

Helleborus Niger

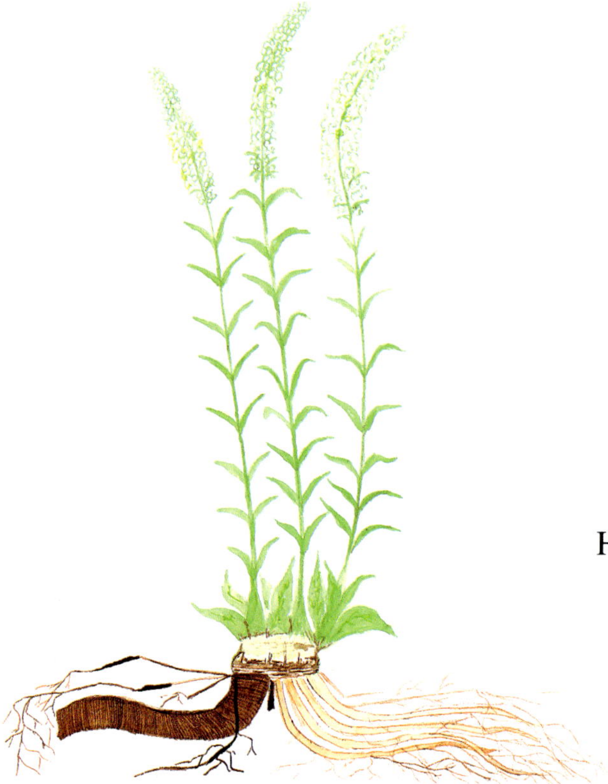

Helonias

Hydrangea

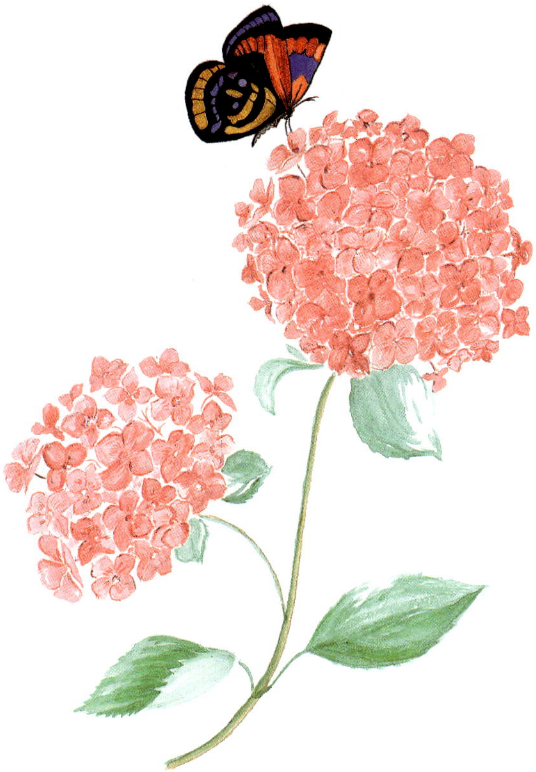

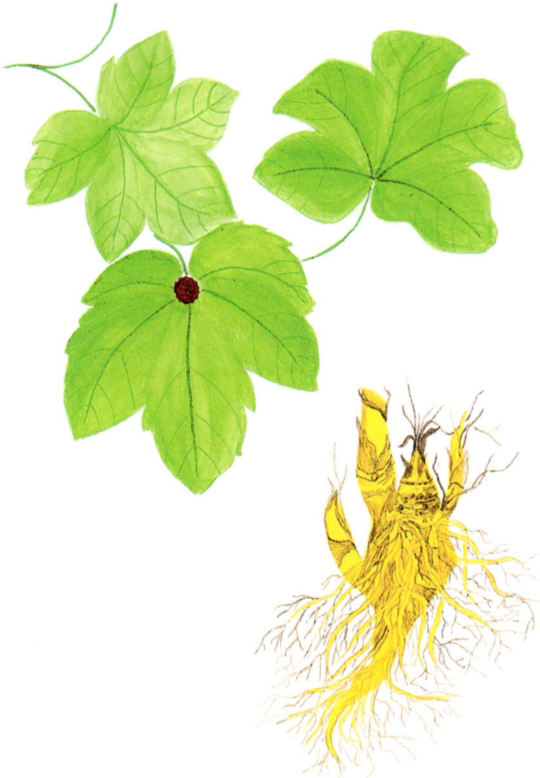

ydrastis

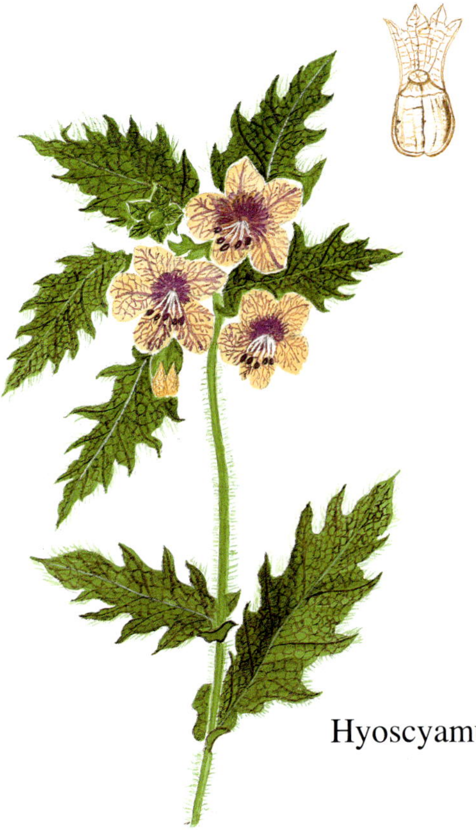

Hyoscyamus

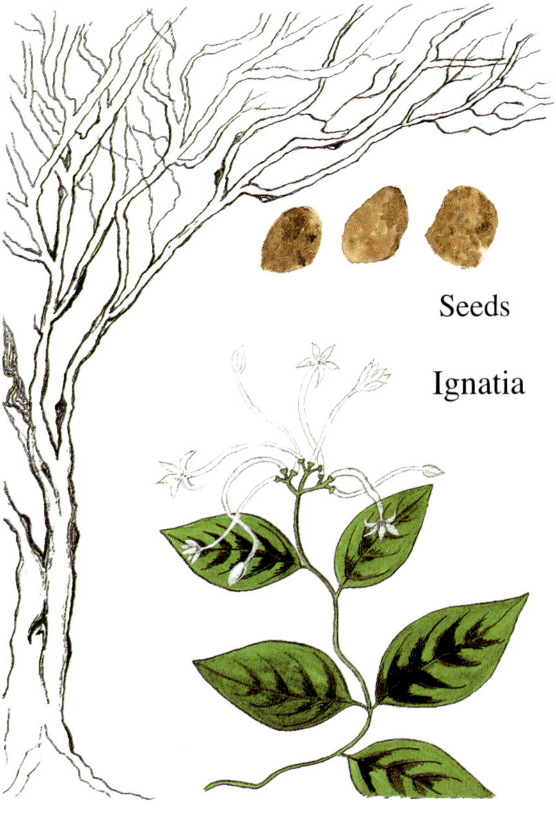

pecacuanha

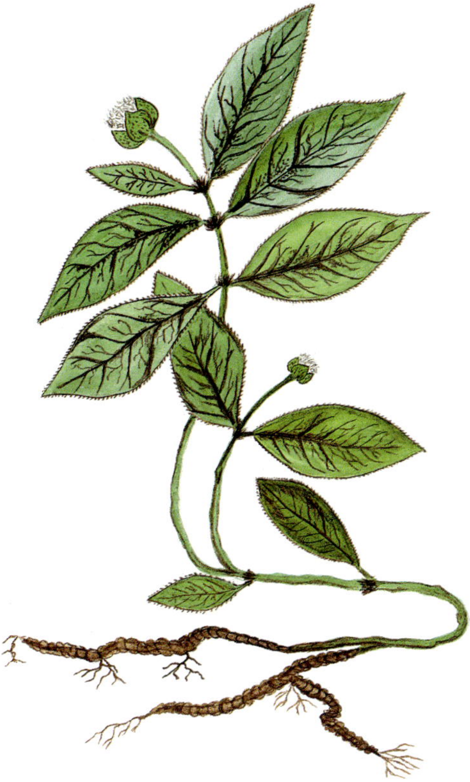

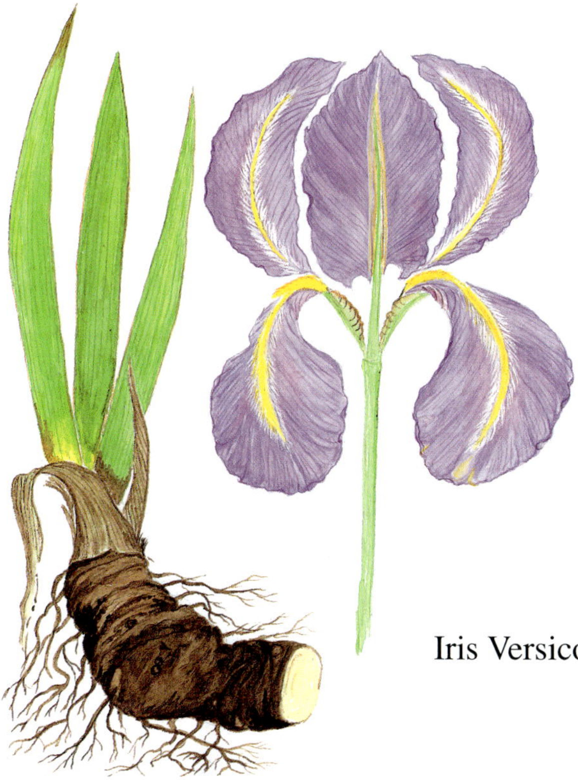

Iris Versicolor

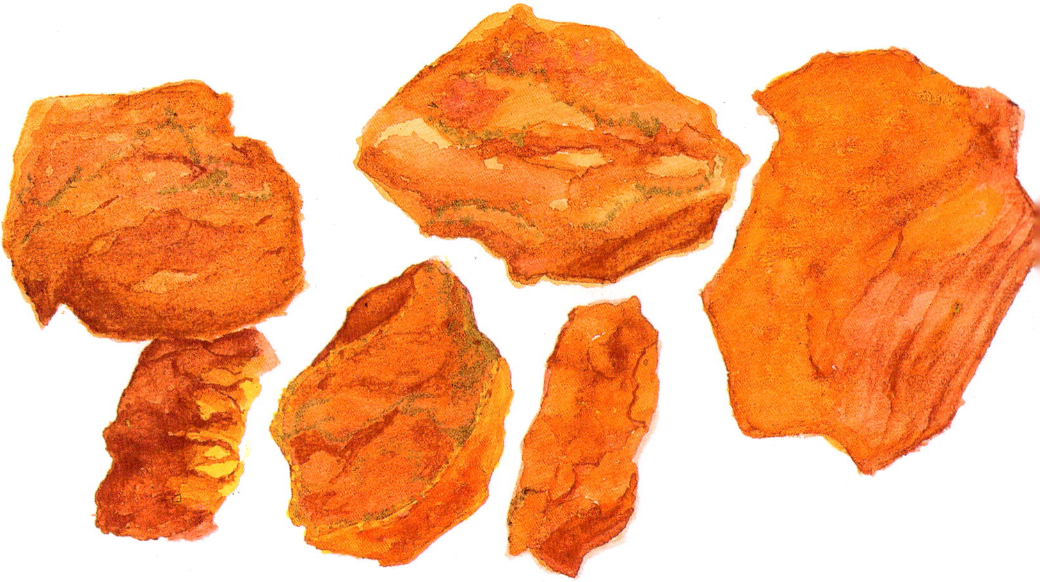

Kali Bichromicum

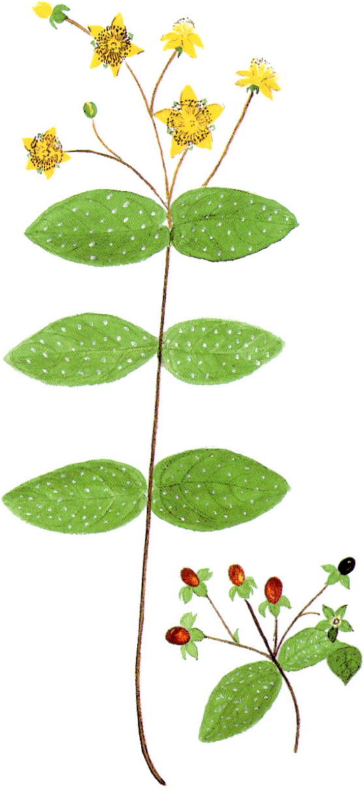

Hypericum

The **ears discharge a yellowish coloured, offensive smelling liquid**. There is dryness in the middle ear. At the outset, the discharge is watery, which then becomes thick and yellowish in colour. Once the disease is well established, the discharge becomes greenish and smells terrible. There is bleeding from inside the ears. These complications gradually keep on progressing and after many years, the drums (tympanic membrane) become thick, the discharge becomes extremely foul smelling and **deafness** develops. If Kali Sulph happens to be the appropriate matching remedy, its use in the beginning of the disease will prevent all these complications. In Kali Sulph, there is intense **itching** inside the ears and behind the ears with lots of noises being heard.

In the **eczema** associated with Kali Sulph, boils and blisters develop. There is a feeling of burning. The skin looks like frog's skin i.e. yellow in colour and without any healthy lustre. It commonly happens in the **diseases of the liver and the spleen**. Anaemia and tuberculosis also make the face look yellow and without natural glare. This facial appearance helps in making the proper diagnosis. It is an art to make the diagnosis based on the facial appearane and the symptoms pertaining to the eye. In Germany, a number of such experts can be found. Kali Sulph is very effective in the treatment of all such **infectious diseases**, provided it is analogous to the nature of the patient.

In the nature of the Kali Phos patient, there is chronic irritation of the bladder; **urination is very frequent**, and especially worse at night. The patient sees distressing dreams. Sleep is not peaceful. The patient feels dizzy in a heated room after dinner. The head feels tense. The **hair tends to fall** and there is dryness over the scalp. The lips become fissured. According to Dr. Kent, Kali Sulph is useful in the **treatment of warts over the lips**. Kali Sulph is also useful in the treatment of the skin cancer called Epithelioma. Blisters form inside the mouth. The tongue is covered with yellow sticky secretions. The chest rattles though the cough is dry. The tongue becomes dry. The **tonsils swell** and cause difficulty in swallowing. The patient dislikes eating eggs, bread, meat, hot food and hot drinks. After taking food, there is a feeling of **pain, burning and cramping over the stomach**. On coughing, the patient vomits; the vomit contains undigested food and the sputum from the lungs. The abdomen becomes bloated with gas and is tense. The patient cannot pass flatus. The soft pitting swelling, common in liver diseases is noticed on the face and over different parts of the body. The abdomen hurts at night. Diarrhoea and severe constipation alternate with each other. The **piles** happen to be inside as well as on the outer surface of the skin and tend to bleed.

In Kali Sulph, the patient feels **severe griping after having been to the lavatory**. This is also common in Merc Corr. In Merc Corr, the pain starts during defacation and continues afterwards. The **stools** are thin, darkish in colour, cause tearing pain and smell terrible. In Kali Sulph, there is severe **itching**. The lining of the kidney tubules becomes inflamed and is associated with a light to severe kind of piercing pain over the kidneys. Sometimes the patient also passes **albumin in the urine**. The urine is deep coloured, abundant and causes burning. Sometimes, it is in the form of a continuous dribble. It looks as if the kidneys are constantly producing offensive smelling infected urine.

Kali Sulph is also very useful in the treatment of **sexual impotence and weakness** in men. It is also useful in the treatment of continuous **vaginal discharge**, inflammation and burning. The **uterus moves away from its normal position**. During menstruation, there is a feeling of pain over the uterus, as well as a feeling of downwards pressure.

Inside the windpipe (trachea), the expectoration may be green, yellow or sometimes mucoid. There is a feeling of dryness and scraping inside the throat which is worse on taking food and when the person is in bed. There is a sort of hissing inside the trachea. Other symptoms of Kali Sulph are **hoarseness of voice**, repeated common cold, the onset of **asthma** in a closed room and difficulty in breathing which gets worse on coughing, lying down, walking and in the evening. In the open, the suffering becomes less. The cough becomes worse in the presence of nasal catarrh. On being exposed to cold, the chest rattles. There is a feeling of choking, burning pain and unease. The **cough at night is dry while in the morning there is a lot of expectoration with it**. The ailments become aggravated with a sudden change in weather or if it becomes too cold. However, normally, the symptoms of Kali Sulph become worse in hot weather like Pulsatilla, as if this remedy is full of contradictions. Regarding the nature of the patient and the severity of thirst, it shows the same kind of contradiction. It can be of great use for patients of the soft and sallow temperament of Pulsatilla, as well as for patients with the nature of irritability and anger. Again, like in Pulsatilla, thirst may be absent or sometimes very severe and non-relenting. The mouth remains dry and the stomach is constantly on fire. In view of this bizarre nature of Kali Sulph, I have already warned the readers that to understand Kali Sulph is not an easy job. In biochemy, Kali Sulph is normally used in low potencies while in homoeopathy, high potencies are more beneficial.

| | |
|---|---|
| Potency: | Biochemic 6X<br>In homoeopathy, high potency as needed |

# KREOSOTUM

The patients of the constitution of Kreosotum exhibit three prominent symptoms. Firstly, all their **excretions and discharges are burning and corrosive in nature, which is very irritative**. The second symptom is that there is a feeling of pulsation all over the body as in Cactus but there is no associated pain or convulsions. The third symptom is **frequent bleeding**. The slightest pressure leads to bleeding. The swollen eye bleeds as soon as it is touched by the physician. If this condition affects the uterus, women suffer from constant bleed. Bleeding continues even after the menstrual period. A light needle prick causes the outpouring of blood. Sometimes, the tears are also mixed with blood. Bleeding frequently due to trivial causes, and the tendency to spontaneous bleeding from any part of the body, are the typical signs of Kreosotum. The **gums recede** from the teeth. The gums bleed even on cleaning the teeth by hand. Mostly, the blood is of red colour, but it may sometimes be darkish in colour. The angles of the mouth are peeled. Dry and fissured lips are typical of Kreosotum. The margins of the nose are abrased and injured. This is usually seen in bad catarrh and is a definite feature of Kreosotum. There is a tendency of frequent bleeding from the orifices like nose, eyes, kidneys and uterus.

In Kreosotum, like Chamomilla, the patient is of a **hot temper** and easily enraged. The Chamomilla patient is furious by nature, however in Kreosotum, the condition is short-lived. The patient becomes irritable due to the severity of the illness therefore the symptoms like that of Chamomilla become apparent. Whether he is sick or healthy Chamomilla patient is always irritable and bad tempered.

In Kreosotum, the affected area becomes raw and burns due to bleeding. Once the discharges become dark in colour, they start smelling. Kreosotum is the best remedy for **children's bedwetting**. The urgency to pass urine is so severe that the patient may not be able to reach the bathroom. The use of Kreosotum over a period of time will gradually decrease the urgency. The patient will be able to regain control. Pertaining to the stomach, there is a tendency towards **acidity, nausea and vomiting**. The vomited material causes burning and irritation in the throat. The taste in the mouth becomes bitter after drinking water. The stomachache is relieved on eating something. It is followed by vomiting. Hot food makes the patient feel better, while cold food aggravates the discomfort. The stomach feels tense and cold.

Kreosotum is also of used in preventing against the tendency to develop cancer. It offers significant relief when given with Conium in the early stage of **cancer of the stomach**. Once the symptoms of Kreosotum become evident it must be started immediately, otherwise, once the cancer has set in, it is impossible to control it. Appropriate treatment can make the patient somewhat more comfortable but does not cure him of the cancer. It makes the life of the patient comfortable to the limit destined by God. Some physicians say that the proper treatment may add years to the patient's life. We know that we cannot prolong anyone's life. However, he may be permitted to live as much as possible, limited by the final time decreed by Allah, the Almighty. This is the gist of the philosophy of sickness and cure. Sickness shortens the life span of a person, while health prolongs it to the limit destined by God.

The patient of Kreosotum also suffers from summer **diarrhoea** in severely hot weather. Similarly, Kreosotum has the capability to completely cure **diabetes**. Kreosotum is extremely useful in the treatment of **teething problems in children**, especially when the teeth become dark coloured or tend to decay and rot with the formation of cavities, and if the gums become black. Then Kreosotum proves curative. In Kreosotum, there is a deposit of white crust over the tongue. The lips are red and tend to bleed. The taste is bitter. The symptoms become aggravated in the open air, cold weather, from drinking cold water or on taking a shower or by lying down, while heat commonly relieves the symptoms, except for the diarrhoea caused by extremely hot weather.

| | |
|---|---|
| Antidote: | Nux Vomica |
| Potency: | 30 to 1000. |

# LAC CANINUM

Lac Caninum is prepared from the milk of a female dog. For this very reason, most people scorn it and hate to even touch it. Yet, other medicines like Psorinum and Syphlinium are prepared from much more loathsome and dangerous materials.
Dog's milk converted into homoeopathic form becomes a purely clean remedy. One must not hesitate to use it.

Initially, Dr. Reisig and Dr. Bayards, on proving, found the extreme usefulness of this medicine. After their death, Dr. Dyer pursued their course. After him, Dr. Kent took over the use of this medicine, which he used successfully on a vast array of diseases. Its most prominent feature is **mental anguish and mental confusion**. The nerves become extremely excitable. It is in the nature of dogs that they jump around imaginary objects and start barking. Probably, that is the background of storywriters' claims that the dogs can see ghosts and spirits. The above-mentioned doctors did not have any background of this sort of knowledge. However, when the homoeopathic potency was prepared from this milk, it was found on proving that a person given Lac Caninum starts seeing imaginary things (hallucinations) and feels as if those things will jump over him and endanger him. This is in the nature of the dog and through the supply of her milk, the human mind and the nervous system can be made to express certain illnesses. If such ailments already exist, the homoeopathic form of the canine milk has the capability to cure them.

This medicine has significant mental symptoms. It also affects the glands. It takes care of the **enlarged glands**. When the glands become inflamed, the overlying skin becomes shiny but unattractive and tense. Lac Caninum cures such wounds.

In Lac Caninum, the **skin is extremely sensitive**, more prominent in women as a result of which they keep their fingers spread apart. If by chance, one finger happens to touch the other, they scream. Even the lightest touch of a cloth is unbearable. This kind of hypersensitivity is also found in Lachesis. Sometimes, these two medicines can be used in the place of the other. Another factor common to both Lachesis and Lac Caninum is that their feelings become very sharp and they are scared of even imaginary things. In spite of these commonalities, there are definite differences between the two. A patient of Lac Caninum cannot be left alone, while the patient of Lachesis likes solitude. The ailments of Lachesis get aggravated after sleep and move from the left to the right.

**Mental and psychological symptoms:** A prominent feature of Lac Caninum is that while walking the patient feels as if he is floating in the air. He believes that whatever he is saying is a total lie and considers himself to be a liar. One specific symptom of a Lac Caninum patient is that he believes that the nose he has on his face belongs to somebody else, or that his body is not his own, or as if somebody else is talking instead of himself.

Lac Caninum is also useful in the **treatment of joint pains**. The fleeting muscle pains migrate from one place to another like a quick jump-over. The pains are less in cold weather. A beneficial response to cold is also seen in Ledum and Pulsatilla. Pulsatilla is of a hot nature while Ledum is not. However, joint pains belonging to both respond very well to cold application to the extent that the patient would like to put ice in the water to make it colder and then dip his feet. Joint pains associated with Ledum begin in the lower part of the body and then migrate upwards.

In Lac Caninum, there is extreme sensitivity to light and noise. While reading, vision becomes slightly blurred. Sounds appear to be coming from a far off distance. Nearby sounds also feel as if they are moving away. This condition is specific to Lac Caninum.

Lac Caninum is one of the best remedies for **Diphtheria**, especially when associated with the pain migrating from one tonsil to the other and then to the first one again and so on. Diphtheria used to be a very common disease and its treatment was also very difficult. But now, preventive vaccination has enabled us to overcome this disease. In third world countries, however the sickness still persists. It is a very dangerous disease, associated with greyish deposits in the throat, which become thicker layer over layer with deposits of more material, so much so that it can block the air passage. There is great difficulty in breathing, while eating and drinking becomes almost impossible. Diphtherinum has been prepared from the toxic matter of Diphtheria. It should first be given in potency 200 and then gradually increased. For further details, please refer to the chapter on Diphtherinum. If

Diphtheria is associated with the jumping of the discomfort from one side to the other and then back to the first side again, Lac Caninum would be the most optimal treatment. Sometimes, even if Diphtheria has been cured, the patient is left with **permanent paralysis of the muscles for swallowing**. Lac Caninum is very useful in the treatment of this condition. In case somebody develops a heart problem after a cold or Diphtheria, Spigelia should be used first. It controls the sickness there and then. Some patients become unable to swallow due to the paralysis at the throat of the muscles for swallowing. In children, a similar condition can develop due to the weakness of the muscles rather than paralysis of the muscles. In this condition, Lac Caninum is very useful. Its beneficial effect however, is only on the paralysed muscles, and not on muscles weakened due to some other condition.

Lac Caninum is also related to many diseases of women. There is pain over the uterus and both ovaries. Once the menstrual blood flows freely, most of the gynaecological troubles of the patient get better. In this respect, it is different from Cimicifuga in which as the menstrual bleeding flows freely, the ailments become aggravated. Lac Caninum is useful in the treatment of those ailments that persist throughout the month but disappear at the onset of menstrual bleeding. The throat trouble starts with the onset of the period and disappears at the end of it. This is a **typical sign** of Lac Caninum that must be kept in mind. In all the systems of medical treatments other than homoeopathy, such symptoms are not given much weight, but are considered imaginary and useless. However, in the field of homoeopathy, these odd symptoms do point to one homoeopathic remedy or another. Therefore, it is necessary to remember them. For example, irritation of the throat, starting before the onset of the periods is a sign of Magnesia Carb. This throat condition will not automatically get better on the cessation of the periods. Instead, it will have to be treated separately. The close relationship of the trouble of the throat and the periods is a special feature of Lac Caninum. In Calcarea Carb, like Cimicifuga, the ailments become worse at the onset of the free flow of the period. However, in Calcarea Carb, the ailment is related to the throat itself. It does not originate from the affliction of internal organs.

In the case of Lac Caninum, the menstrual blood contains big clots as if containing the shreds of the lining of the uterus, like Kreosotum.

Menstruation starts rather early and is plentiful. There is soreness over the mammary glands before menstruation or during lactation. They get inflamed. **To stop lactation for any reason**, Pulsatilla and Lac Caninum combined, are very useful because in this respect, they are similar to each other.

| | |
|---|---|
| Potency: | 30 or above. |

# LAC DEFLORATUM

Lac Defloratum is said to have been prepared from skimmed milk. I do not agree with this statement. I believe that the milk will still have some fat particles in spite of being apparently skimmed. The milk definitely becomes dilute after the removal of fat, but, a little bit of fat must remain. Based on the homoeopathic view, if the medicine is prepared from ordinary milk, it should have the same features as that prepared from skimmed milk because of the residual amount of fat in it.

Lac Defloratum is very useful in children who are **allergic to milk**. They cannot digest milk and instead they develop diarrhoea. Most often, one dose of Lac Defloratum CM may prove effective, so much so that they will not get the allergy again. Sometimes, the allergy may partially remain, or it may not respond to the treatment after some time.

Lac Defloratum is of a cold nature, while Lac Caninum is of a hot nature. The patient of Lac Defloratum is very cool minded. He feels cold even while clad in warm clothing in hot weather. Blowing lightly on the face will make him feel cold. This kind of strong feeling for the cold is different from that associated with Arnica, Lachesis and Psorinum. The patient feels extremely cold all over. He is sensitive to the even the draft of cold air and will start suffering from rheumatic symptoms. He hurts all over the body, but more so over the head. This pain is not the result of any infection but is rheumatic in nature. There is pain along the course of the nerves on the face and the head. If the patient feels extremely cold, Lac Defloratum must be kept in mind for his treatment.

The symptoms become relieved with warmth. However, the patient will never feel warm enough; he stays cold. The symptoms become relieved with rest and local pressure. The skin is very sensitive, as in many other homoeopathic remedies. The hypersensitivity of the skin is due to the irritability of the nerves, but in Lac Defloratum, it is due to the sensitivity towards the cold.

Lac Defloratum has mostly been overlooked in the treatment of **diabetes**, even though its singular use can cure the diabetic, if other symptoms of Lac Defloratum are also present. A single dose in high potency may cure the patient. I have seen diabetics getting better many times. Diabetes is not the kind of disease that must need continuous treatment for every patient. A suitable homoeopathic treatment can cure the diabetes completely, but in some patients the treatment may have to be continued. Some symptoms of diabetes may be present in a patient of Lac Defloratum even if he is not an established diabetic i.e. the frequent passage of thick urine and intense thirst.

Homoeopathic remedies are related to specific groups of diseases. Once the basic symptoms of a disease are taken care of, other diseases with similar group of symptoms may also be cured.

When a patient **hates milk,** or his symptoms become worse on taking milk, or he develops nausea, vomiting, headache, eructation and gas in the stomach etc; a single dose of Lac Defloratum CM can cure all these symptoms. At times, it may have to be repeated after a while. If two such doses, one after the other, do not benefit, it should be abandoned. If it is going to be effective, it is effective immediately, or not at all. When the first dose has offered some relief but the symptoms have recurred, a second dose may be tried but no more.

The symptom complex of Lac Defloratum also includes the aftereffects of **malaria**, such as lack of blood (anaemia), swelling (oedema), symptoms of diabetes and weakness of the heart etc. Instead of trying to remember all the symptoms, one must remember that the nature of this remedy is very cold. The skin is very sensitive to cold. Whenever there is hypersensitivity to cold, and any of the symptoms pertaining to the heart, malaria or diabetes appear, then Lac Defloratum will most probably be found more useful in the treatment of all these diseases as well.

I have no personal experience of using Lac Defloratum for the treatment of heart problems, so I cannot say for sure as to what potency would be ideal. However, while dealing with the heart, the treatment should be started in low potencies. If the patient starts getting better, this should be repeated and the potency should gradually be increased. The heart responds in a very slow and steady way; therefore, only low potencies are safe.

The Lac Defloratum patient **loses his memory** and avoids intellectual work. This medicine is also useful in the **treatment of fatty degeneration of the heart and the liver**. This condition is commonly found in alcoholics but may be found in people who consume too much fat. Streaks of fat start depositing in the liver, which gradually increase with age. The affected part of the liver loses its function and cannot produce chemical secretions in the required amount. The usefulness of this remedy in the treatment of fatty degeneration shows that it dispels the bad effects of fatty disease.

A Lac Defloratum patient is usually very **sad**. He wishes to die and looks for a simple straightforward way to achieve it. He is not aggressive. He is sad, with no sign of explosion. He wants an easy way to die without much trouble. Perhaps the poet Ghalib was also of Lac Defloratum disposition. He said: "I wish somebody would sing to me in such a beautiful and enchanting way, with the voice having the speed and radiance of lightning so that I may die without any discomfort". What a lovely death! Alas, he did not get such a singer to solve his problem.

The patient of Lac Defloratum feels dizzy even on raising his arm. His **dizziness** is like that of Conium. In Conium, the patient feels dizzy on lying down or closing his eyes, while the bed spins around him. In Lac Defloratum too, the situation is somewhat similar, while in Lac Caninum, the patient feels dizzy while walking, and he finds the entire world swinging around him. He finds himself in a fantasyland. Similarily a patient of Cannabis has his own imaginary world, in which he feels like he is flying or floating in the air. Its prominent sign is that perception of the passage of time is affected. Sometimes the passage of time seems to flow rapidly, while in the state of grief and sorrow, time stands still for him. There is a kind of strange situation in Lac Defloratum time is prolonged with the feeling of joy, whereas normally, a good time passes away rapidly. The mind of a Lac Defloratum patient is not focused on something in particular but goes astray. He trusts nothing.

In Lac Defloratum there is one particular characteristic that the women suffer from headache before and after the periods. The headache occupies the nape of the neck, the forehead and the temples. **Yellowish offensive leucorrhoeal** discharge, before and after the periods, is also a solid sign of Lac Defloratum. Once both these symptoms are present, the treatment becomes very easy. Lac Defloratum is also useful in the treatment of vomiting during pregnancy.

When a female patient with a cold body who has a tendency towards being overweight develops **diabetes,** Lac Defloratum may be a possible treatment for her. If a woman delivers an overweight child, while on normal food intake, it may very well be that her diabetes may be passed on to the child. If she is of a cold constitution, and her body remains cold then Lac Defloratum can offer a complete cure. Therefore, it must be used without any delay as soon as the diagnosis is made. Obese ladies with the feeling of cold all over and who are unable to digest milk will find this medicine very useful. It will also cure the vomiting during pregnancy in any woman who does not have a natural distaste for milk, but in pregnancy is unable to digest it. All the symptoms pertaining to the stomach dysfunctions result from the inability to digest milk. If the indigestion is due to not being able to digest milk or due to fatty food, the commonly used remedy is Pulsatilla. The nature of Pulsatilla is very hot, while that of Lac Defloratum is very cold and this is the **main distinguishing factor** between the two.

A patient of Lac Defloratum has extreme **photophobia**. He feels a gritty sensation in the eyes. The vision is blurred.

A patient of Lac Defloratum grinds his teeth at night. The grinding of the teeth may also be due to an infestation with worms or due to the swelling of the gums. Similarly, stomach upset and the indigestibility of the milk can also result in grinding of the teeth even in the absence of worm infestation. These three possibilities must be kept in mind. In the presence of worms, the child develops a severe itch over the nose, and the margins of the nose as well as the margins of the lips become yellowish. The second symptom is that the patient feels very hungry. Both these symptoms can be best treated with Cina, while Sabadilla is also very useful.

The third symptom of Lac Defloratum is **nausea**, however there is no vomiting, except very rarely. In this respect, it is somewhat similar to Ipecac but in Ipecac the vomiting is relatively more frequent.

The **constipation** in a patient of Lac Defloratum is very severe; even more severe than in Silicea. Sometimes straining may lead to rupture of the veins but the stools are not passed. Such patients can develop piles or hernia.

In Lac Defloratum, the patient passes urine freely, and has a headache, like Gelsemium. Gelsemium also is of a cold nature, but the difference between Gelsemium and Lac Defloratum is that in Gelsemium there is no thirst at all while in Lac Defloratum there is severe thirst. In Lac Defloratum, the urine is abundant and light yellow in colour, but it may also be thick and darkish in colour indicating that albumin is being passed. Lac Defloratum will be found very useful in treating this condition if other symptoms of Lac Defloratum are also present.

A strange sign of Lac Defloratum is that when exposed to extreme cold, there is loss of control over passing urine. This is more common in women than in men. There is **incontinence**. The small muscles (sphincters) become insensitive due to exposure to the cold and become temporarily non-functional. A similar situation occurs in Causticum but there, it is due to permanent paralysis. Gradually worsening incontinence of the urine can also be found in Kali Carb. In Lac Defloratum, the condition is temporary. As soon as the exposure to cold is over, urination comes under voluntary control.

Lac Defloratum is also useful in the treatment of **backache associated with menstruation**. While menstruating, the patient happens to dip her hands in extremely cold water, the periods will cease immediately, and some other ailment may ensue. Therefore, such ladies had better take the precaution of refraining from using very cold water during their periods.

Lac Defloratum is also useful in the treatment of heart disease especially the **cardiac asthma** in which the heart is weak and there is a shortness of breath. On breathing, the lungs press on the heart. Similarly, this symptom is found in Spongia in its own form.

In a patient of Lac Defloratum, only the fingers may be cold rather than the whole hand and will not warm up at all. The one exceptional situation is that its headache gets better only in the cold, even though the patient is already feeling extremely cold, like in Phosphorus. But the Phosphorus patient would want to protect himself with warm clothing except for his head, which he would like to keep cold. Nothing but only the cold can offer him relief. Other symptoms of Phosphorus are quite different from Lac Defloratum.

| | |
|---|---|
| Potency: | 30 to CM |

# LACHESIS

## (The Venom of the hooded cobra called "Surucucu")

The Surucucu is a very poisonous huge and long snake. Its skin is of reddish colour, with dark grey coloured spots. The homoeopathic remedy prepared from the venom of this snake is called Lachesis. The venom of this snake has been subjected to homoeopathic proving on a very large scale.

The venoms from different kinds of snakes are not too dissimilar from each other. Broadly speaking, these venoms can be divided into two groups. One group affects the circulatory system, while the other one affects the nervous system. The kind that affects the nervous system also influences the blood circulation, although its main function is on the nervous system. It paralyses the nerves as well as afflicting the heart directly. Similarly, the kinds of venoms affecting the circulatory system also affect the heart indirectly. They clot the blood within the blood vessels and thus affect the functioning of the heart.

The Snake venom as such is not dangerous if taken by mouth. The poisons derived from all animals consist of large protein molecules. They are completely harmless when taken by mouth. That is the reason why the treatment of snakebite has traditionally been the immediate suction of the poison from the snakebite by mouth. As long as there is no open wound inside the mouth, the venom has no harmful effect because it is not absorbed into the blood circulation directly. The human body reacts violently against the entry of a protein directly into the blood. The blood itself is a mixture of so many proteins. These proteins are classified into different groups and each group is named separately. During the transfusion of blood, these groups have to be kept in view. Human blood is also a kind of poison, like snake venom, or it may prove to be even more dangerous. On the transfusion of an unmatched blood group, the recipient may die immediately.

The proteins of snake venom accumulate in the glands inside the mouth of the snake. With the passage of time, they become more and more concentrated. The system of the snakebite is not a mere coincidence but it has been well planned and devised by the Almighty God. It is impossible that this system could have evolved on its own or that it could be the result of a mere coincidence.

Along the canine teeth of the snake, there are two additional curved teeth (fangs) that have a very thin hole in them, connected to the glands containing the venom. When the snake bites, the venom does not enter the body immediately. However, when the snake retracts his head to pull the teeth out, the venom from the glands squeezes out through the minute holes in the additional teeth (fangs) and then enters the blood. Further reaction is the result of entry of the venom in the body.

Out of all kinds of snake venoms, Lachesis is the most important for homoeopathic use. No other venom or poison has been put to use like Lachesis and it has been found extremely beneficial. According to Dr. Kent, Lachesis has been found useful all over the world. The evil and acrimony of the Lachesis venom is also found in all malefactors and people of wicked mind and bad character. Intense jealousy, mischief and trouble making in a severe form are found in Lachesis. Thus, Lachesis may be called the universal poison. The snake venoms become more concentrated in the spring. In winter, the snakes hibernate and during this period, their venom becomes more concentrated and dangerous. The spring season is the time when the snakes come out of their holes and places of hibernation. In this season the snakebite is extremely dangerous.

The timing of the symptoms of snakebites happens to be very precisely punctuated. In whichever season the snakebites, the symptoms and bad effects recur exactly in the same season the following year. If a person is bitten by a snake in the spring season and happens to survive, then he has to face the symptoms of snakebite in every spring season. Patients may presume that they have probably been bitten by the snake again. This is especially so because the wound of the previous snakebite also becomes swollen and congested. In other seasons also, the symptoms of snakebite can recur but not that severely and the patient does not feel that he has been bitten again.

**The sudden onset of a violent type of sneezing in the spring season** is also a sign of Lachesis. I have tried Lachesis 1000 on the patients who suffered from hay fever for many years. A single dose relieved their problem forever. About ten percent of such patients got significantly better like this, just with one dose of Lachesis 1000. Once the allergy becomes controlled and then recurs, in that case it should be repeated after two weeks or a month. If Lachesis fails, then Natrum Mur and Sabadilla also work well. So the proper diagnosis of the patient should be arrived at carefully.

For any such patient who is predisposed to fall sick as a result of moving from the cold to a relatively warm temperature, due to the change of weather or a geographic change of place, Lachesis must be kept well in mind for his other ailments also. However, Dulcamara is the only one remedy that can be used in treating sneezing in any season. Bryonia is also of great use during the change of cold weather into warm weather.

A peculiar symptom of Lachesis is that its ailments definitely get worse after sleep. Most of the patients bitten by snakes exhibit the same feature, but Lachesis is the most prominent of all snake venoms. Although it proves to be beneficial for the treatment of such patients whose ailments aggravate after sleep, it does not mean that every patient who shows this symptom must have been bitten by a snake. It simply means that it is a commonly shared symptom in which Lachesis is certainly useful. If indeed a person has been bitten by a Lachesis kind of snake and then goes to sleep, he may not wake up and thus will be untreatable. Every physician must remember that whenever he is called upon to see a patient bitten by a snake, he must make sure that the patient be kept awake under all circumstances, even if he has to be repeatedly slapped on his face. Once he remains awake or can be made to wake up, the chances of his survival become bright. The symptoms of a patient of Lachesis keep aggravating during sleep in which he observes scary dreams and by the morning, his illness has become very severe. He is extremely restless in the morning his head feels warm and hurts. His heart beats fast. Besides that, he becomes badly stricken with grief, which is typical of Lachesis. A patient of Gelsemium also wakes up with a headache but he sleeps comfortably at night without seeing any frightful dreams. In Gelsemium, the patient develops a headache if due to some reason, his routine of waking up in the morning or his timing for breakfast changes. In a headache of this kind the proper treatment is Gelsemium and not Lachesis.

The patient of Lachesis is very cold especially his feet are ice cold. However, hot water aggravates his symptoms especially the headache. The pressure of the blood rises inside the head. The patient feels as if his head might explode. In Lachesis like Belladonna, the rush of blood is more on one side. In Belladonna, the rush of blood may be directed to any part of the body while in Lachesis, this tendency is only limited towards the head. There is rush of blood towards the head while the feet become cold. The person feels riveted due to pain as if somebody has tightly tied a cloth over his head. Patients showing the symptoms of Lachesis may also sometimes faint while taking a shower with hot water.

Another prominent symptom of Lachesis is that **purple or darkish spots form** on the body, much more so on the face. Similar spots are exhibited by the patients who experience severe **heart attack**. Such patients who have the tendency to develop such spots should be periodically, treated with Lachesis. Lachesis prevents the clotting of blood in the circulation and potential heart attack. Lachesis is the best remedy against such happening. For this purpose, when given along with Arnica, it is much more effective.

Lachesis is also proved to be very useful in the treatment of **swollen lymph glands**. The wounds bleed severely; the **colour of the blood is dark** and it clots in the form of grass weeds. In Lachesis, like Kreosotum and Phosphorus, there is a tendency towards copious dark bleeding. In Kreosotum, slight pressure can cause bleeding. The gums, which apparently look healthy, will start bleeding with finger pressure or when there is a minor ailment, the local application of pressure will start bleeding. In Phosphorus, the bleeding is brisk and of red colour. In Secale Cor and in Lachesis, the blood is darkish is colour and the configuration of their wounds is also similar. In Lachesis, like Secale, there is a tendency towards the **formation of gangrene over the wounds**. Dark blood keeps on oozing from the wounds. The margins of the wounds become swollen. The surrounding skin shrinks and becomes dark and wrinkled. However, other symptoms of Lachesis are quite different from those of Secale. In Lachesis, the patient is very cold and feels severe cold, while the patient of Secale feels intense heat and gets relief with cold applications on the affected areas.

Another symptom of Lachesis is the formation of **Varicose Veins** (the veins become engorged and tortuous). The blood clots inside the veins and makes lumps and bumps that may rupture. Varicose Veins are a serious and troublesome illness. In general, it affects women during pregnancy or after their delivery, involving the legs and feet. Sometimes, it is so severe that walking around becomes difficult. Lachesis alone is not effective against the varicosity of the veins. In such a condition, other symptoms of the patient must also be observed to arrive at a proper diagnosis and to devise the optimal treatment. If the proper diagnosis cannot be established, then Arnica and Lachesis together may be given routinely to get some relief. However, the best routine treatment is Aesculus.

For the so-called **piles of the eyes,** in which the eyes become intensely red and swollen, Aesculus is very useful. It is also effective in the treatment of the piles, which become purple and cause severe pain. A characteristic symptom of Aesculus is that although it seems that the wounds will soon mature, form pus and then rupture, they neither suppurate nor burst. The constant presence of these non-healing piles is a great menace. Aesculus is well known to offer cure in this painful condition although it does not succeed alone. It has to be supplemented with Arnica, Lachesis and similar adjuvant remedies. One must constantly examine one's feet to control this problem at the outset. The appearance of bluish marks over the ankles and the heels is indicative of impending varicosity of the veins. The blood can clot in them. Once the veins become swollen and tortuous, the disease may get out of control. Blood clots can form within the tortuous veins, which can dislodge themselves and lead to heart attack by embolism. In the early stage of this condition, Arnica and Lachesis, by God's Grace, are very effective for the prevention of serious consequences.

In Shingles, as already mentioned in various chapters the remedies Arnica, Ledum Pal, Lachesis and Natrum Mur happen to be very useful.

In Lachesis, the hands and feet of the patient become cold and patient suffers from weakness of the heart. The head feels warm and the veins pulsate. During a headache, the patient cannot rest his head on the pillow because whichever side he lies on, the head starts throbbing due to excessive rushing of blood.

Lachesis affects the emotional state as well. On hearing sudden sad news or due to some other emotional upset, the heart sinks, the body sweats and the head becomes warm but the feet become very cold. While the **feet are cold** and the usual symptoms of Lachesis are also present, a single dose of Lachesis will offer magical relief. The patient, previously shivering with cold and covering himself in layer after layer of quilts with the feet feeling unbearably cold, will notice in just a few minutes after administration of this remedy, a sudden flow of heat waves emerging from the upper part of the body spreading downwards. I infer from this that Lachesis disperses the excessive blood from the head towards the rest of the body, resulting in the warming up of the feet in no time. Psorinum also possesses this quality, though with some difference. The patient of Psorinum is always cold all over. Even in the summer, he keeps himself covered. His skin becomes dark in colour and the body discharges are offensive. However in Lachesis these signs are absent due to stress, sudden shock or sometime for no apparent reason, his body may suddenly turn cold yet the head remains warm.

In the case of Lachesis, the **ailment attacks the left side** though it does not remain localised there. It shifts towards the right side of the body after some time. This is a very clear symptom, which, if associated with worsening of the condition at night, definitely warrants the use of Lachesis.

Lachesis is also very useful in the treatment of **conditions related to the ovaries**. If the discomfort or pain begins in the left ovary and then shifts towards the right ovary, it will respond best to Lachesis. If the condition originates in the right ovary, Lycopodium and Tarentula will be more beneficial. In Lachesis, **throat conditions also begin on the left side** and then migrate towards the right side. In Lycopodium the situation is reversed. In Pulsatilla, the pain radiates in any direction (migratory) as found in Lac Caninum.

In Lachesis, the **headache** also **starts on the left side** and then spreads over to the nape of the neck. The temple feels under heavy pressure, while the lower jaw may also be involved. Gelsemium may also be very useful in the treatment of such a headache although the headache typical of Gelsemium descends from the nape of the neck towards the shoulder blades in the muscles of the back. In other words, it is not confined to the nape alone.

Another characteristic of Lachesis is that its pain tends to change sides when it originates in the upper body and then migrates to the lower body. For example, if the patient has pain over the heart or feels pressure over the left side of the chest then this pain may travel to the right hip or groin, or sometimes it may affect both sides simultaneously. Many a time, the pain remains on the left side from top to bottom, especially when associated with paralysis. However, one thing is sure that the sensation of pain and muscular stiffness in the upper part of the body must be associated with similar discomfort on the right lower body. This is **typical** of Lachesis.

Symptoms of Lachesis include **large swelling of the tongue** and numbness over the lips resulting in a difficulty to speak properly. Any patient with this symptom, whose head remains warm and who develops purple spots on the skin, should ideally be treated with Lachesis. In fact, the swelling of the tongue and numbness of the lips indicate the onset of paralysis inside the mouth and throat, which, if not promptly treated with Lachesis, will definitely result in the paralysis.

Another salient symptom of Lachesis is the **feeling of tightness around the neck**, so much so that the patient cannot even tolerate a collar. In Glonoine, there is a similar feeling with the addition of the feeling of tightness around the head and intolerance to wearing a cap. The feeling of being strangulated is indicative of Hydrophobinum. In Lachesis, the patient feels tight and constricted at the upper part of the neck but cannot say for sure, if it is from within or from outside. In Hydrophobinum and Hyoscyamus, there is a feeling of constriction inside the throat while in Lachesis, there is no such feeling of internal constriction. He just cannot tolerate anything around the neck.

Lachesis patients by nature are **extremely suspicious**. They believe that everybody is talking against them or that their food has been poisoned. They distrust even their near relatives. The symptoms then gradually become worse. Such patients must be treated with Lachesis and soon. In my experience, Lachesis benefits to some extent, but not for long. Other remedies must be sought after the psychoanalysis of the patient. Lachesis will offer cure only if the other basic symptoms of Lachesis are also present.

A Lachesis patient has the constant fear of bleak future for himself, or of having committed a sin which is unforgivable, or having been possessed and being manipulated by a superpower. Once a small girl, who was similarly sick and who had the habit of stealing was brought to me. On being asked, she would reply that she did it under divine command. Such patients should be treated with Lachesis. Those who disobey God on "His command" will start obeying Him on the command of a snake i.e. Lachesis. The women of Lachesis disposition have a constant fear of being chased by someone or they may become religious fanatics. Both these symptoms are characteristic of Lachesis. The situation becomes worse when they start thinking of killing somebody with the firm belief that God wants them to do it. Such patients may in fact kill somebody, or will at least try to do so. If they are religious fanatics, they become extremely talkative. They are disorganised and impatient in all matters and do not even talk properly, changing the topic halfway through and fail to convey what they intended to say. They themselves may yell and scream at full volume but cannot tolerate external noise, which stuns their nerves. They tend to think of committing suicide, though practically are very afraid to do so. They feel like jumping from a high place but dare not do so. When a patient becomes frightened at the thought of high places, he may benefit from Arsenic or Argentum Nitricum. In general, Lachesis works well on such kinds of mental patients. It must be given in at least potency 200. In my practice I have found it much more useful in potency 1000. Many times, I have used it in potency CM and found it definitely effective.

**A Sore throat** contracted in winter is a peculiar symptom of Lachesis. In Psorinum too, the patient catches cold right at the onset of winter. Psorinum is useful in the treatment of sore throat as well, though it is more useful in the treatment of cold. Another peculiarity of Psorinum is that when the nasal discharge stops, a headache sets in i.e. the headache and runny nose alternate with each other. Such is not the case in Lachesis.

Another sign of Lachesis is the **extreme skin sensitivity**, so much so that the patient may not even tolerate touch with a light cloth. The simultaneous presence of discomfort in a particular area and extreme sensitivity of the overlying skin, causing severe restlessness and worsening of the headache, is characteristic of Lachesis. This symptom is also found in Kali Carb. Strong pressure is soothing, while light touch hurts. Light touch causing severe discomfort is well pronounced in Lac Caninum. If the fingers seem to hurt, the patient keeps the fingers open (straight). On bending the fingers, he cries out with pain. In case the armpits are extremely sensitive to touch, the patient keeps his arms away from his sides.

Lachesis is also deeply related to **jaundice**. For jaundice, I usually prescribe the combination of Sulphur, Bryonia and Carduus Marianus, which by God's grace have been very successful. In the case of failure, one can use Chelidonium, Lachesis, Berberis and Lycopodium etc., all being very useful in the treatment of **liver diseases**, though they need to be used with extreme caution. Phosphorus is also related to liver disorders, especially **liver cancer**. Its repeated use in high potency, or its unnecessary use, can bring about dangerous consequences. Sometimes, the jaundice becomes chronic. This will respond very well to Lachesis. The **jaundice** of Lachesis is **associated with nausea** similar to Chelidonium. Ipecac may be of some use in some cases of jaundice but it is not deep-acting remedy. However, it works in certain cases. Lachesis would be ideal in treating jaundice and **stones in the gall bladder** provided the patient also exhibits general symptoms of Lachesis.

Generally, a **mild soreness of the throat** causes severe pain in the eyes when pressed locally. The examination of the ear with an instrument provokes cough, showing that the ear, nose and eyes are very much interconnected. When any one of these is disturbed, the other may also be affected. Lachesis, specifically, can by God's grace, relieve the ailments pertaining to all three.

Sometimes, the glands of the eye that make tears (lacrimal glands) become painfully sore. Lachesis will cure this condition also. Here Lachesis will be recognised by an eczema-like condition of the face, swellings and blisters. Probably this facial condition is transferred to the eyes. Eyesores alone are not diagnostic of Lachesis. In the presence of facial symptoms, Lachesis would be the best treatment to cure eyesores. It is the topmost remedy of the **fistulae of the eye**, as is Kali Bichrome.

In Lachesis, the nose bleeds during the symptoms of cold. The correct diagnosis is only made by the proper scrutiny of symptoms. In Psorinum and Lachesis both, the **nasal discharge** is very offensive. The **cold may lead to eczema of the scalp**, which becomes covered with a thick shell under which germs flourish. When this shell bursts, it emits an offensive smelling discharge. When the eczema is forcefully suppressed with some local treatment, a severe form of resistant nasal catarrh develops. In such conditions, **Mezereum** is much more effective than Lachesis and Psorinum. Once a child was brought to me who had a severe cold of a resistant nature. It did not respond to any kind of treatment. The nose smelt awful. It just so happened that just then I had read about Mezereum. I gave him Mezereum and it cured the cold immediately but he developed eczema on the scalp, which by the grace of God also cleared with Mezereum in a few days.

Lachesis and Psorinum are both anti-psoric. Lachesis is the **best remedy for blisters containing blood** i.e. haemorrhagic blisters. This kind of skin condition occurs on and off. Generally in Lachesis, like in Arnica, the bleeding is of a darkish colour. However, the blood-filled blisters on the face are related only to Lachesis. The gums bleed. The tongue becomes dry and leathery in consistency. The mouth is dry yet there is no thirst. The dryness of the mouth and tongue is like Gelsemium. So the diagnosis of Lachesis will be made on the basis of its other symptoms. In Lachesis, sputum resembles soap-lather in appearance but not in taste. Sometimes, the saliva exudes like thick hard threads of yellowish colour. This sign is more pronounced in Kali Bichrome.

In Lachesis, **fluids tend to get stuck in the throat**, especially hot fluids. Almost all snake venoms cause constriction of the throat, resulting in difficulty of swallowing food and water. In Lachesis, hot fluids make this condition still more difficult while cold drinks offer some relief. This symptom is contradictary to the usual nature of Lachesis i.e. the body of the Lachesis patient is cold and he cherishes heat. Regarding the **constriction of the throat**, Lachesis resembles Belladonna in which the suffering gets worse in heat, while cold offers relief. Apis ailments also become worse with heat and get better in the cold. This symptom is common to Lachesis, Belladonna and Apis. However, in Lachesis, a cold drink relieves the condition. In fact, the patient likes cold drinks, though nausea immediately follows. This is typical of Lachesis.

Belladonna also relieves a **dry cough** like that of a Lachesis patient. The cough resulting from the misuse of Lachesis or in a patient bitten by a Lachesis kind of snake, who luckily survives but is left with a persistent cough, will significantly benefit from Belladonna. Belladonna is not a very long acting remedy but is considered to be an intermediate kind of remedy. Nonetheless, it cures the persistent type of cough, following the misuse of Lachesis. Likewise, Lachesis annuls the bad effects of Belladonna.

Lachesis is also useful in the **treatment of gas in the abdomen** (flatulence). The abdomen becomes distended with gas. Once the constitution of the patient is recognised, it becomes so much easier to find the appropriate cure. If the patient is very cold in cold weather and his abdomen is full of gas, then Psorinum will be useful. It will restore the expulsion of the blocked up foul-smelling gas. In Lachesis too, the passage of flatus softens the belly, though the flatus is not very malodourous.

| | |
|---|---|
| Adjuvants: | Lycopodium, Hepar Sulph, Nitric Acid |
| Antidotes: | Arsenic, Mercury |
| Potency: | 30 to 1000 |

# LACTICUM ACIDUM

Lactic Acid is an excellent remedy for the **treatment of diabetes**, but it has not been used much. If some diabetics do not respond to the commonly prescribed medicine, addition of Lactic Acid 200 is helpful in controlling the diabetes.

Lactic Acid is useful in the **treatment of morning sickness**, perhaps due to pregnancy or diabetes. The nausea gets better on eating something. There is a feeling of tightness at the lower end of the food pipe (oesophagus), as if a ball is stuck there, which the patient tries to swallow downwards. Lactic Acid is also useful in women who happen to be **anaemic** and whose faces look pale. It is also effective in the treatment of chest problems.

Lactic Acid may also be of good use in the **treatment of enlarged glands in the axilla**. Silicea is equally good. Silicea, in high potency makes the glands soften and melt inside. If the glands are about to burst open, then Silicea or Hepar Sulph should be administered in a low potency.

In some Lactic Acid patients, the body becomes tremulous. Urination is not only frequent, but also in large quantity. Shoulders, wrist and knee joints hurt. The Patient feels extremely weak and cold. The tongue is dry. The patient feels very thirsty and hungry. Saliva pours from the mouth. In spite of drinking water, the thirst is not quenched.

| | |
|---|---|
| Antidote: | Bryonia |
| Potency: | 30 |

# LAUROCERASUS
## (Cherry Laurel)

This remedy is frequently used in the **treatment of heart conditions**. When somebody starts to tremble due to sudden fear, terror or intense grief, Laurocerasus will offer immediate relief. Its patient **starts trembling** when terrified in a dream or on the sudden appearance of a stranger before him. He becomes overwhelmed with fear when excited. The body becomes cold and bluish. Sometimes, such a patient may develop **epileptic fits**. The vision becomes blurred. Evidently, such a patient is a coward and weak at heart. Laurocerasus happens to be a cardio-tonic for such patients. In particular, it is relatively beneficial in older people. These patients have a weakening of the heart muscle, which results in accumulation of fluid in the lungs (i.e. pulmonary oedema), and causes difficulty in breathing. Generally, doctors give such patients inhaler treatment or strong asthma medicines. These help by relieving the constriction of their air passages and facilitates breathing for some time. However, on prolonged use, these medicines lose their effectiveness even if given repeatedly. The patient may, in fact, die during this attack of cardiac asthma. Laurocerasus helps to eliminate the need for using the inhaler. Laurocerasus is a very effective treatment for combating **difficulty in breathing, (dyspnoea), suffocation, and tightness of the chest as well as the sudden feeling of being choked and sinking of the heart**. It increases the efficiency of the valves of the heart and is very helpful in the treatment of heart murmurs. It also tones the heart musculature and thus relieves the backlog of blood in the lungs and the oedema of the lungs. It is particularly useful in the **treatment of a cough arising from the failing heart** which causes congestion of the lungs. Spongia also helps such patients. The face of a Laurocerasus patient turns bluish (cyanotic) due to the relative lack of oxygenation of blood in the lungs. Not all of its patients necessarily become cyanotic. In fact, some have a pale complexion. Such patients will need a different kind of therapy. Laurocerasus is famous for the **treatment of cyanotic diseases of the heart.**

In Laurocerasus, the chest muscles become weak (expiratory muscles). Sometimes, the diaphragm becomes weak and fails to expel air from the lungs i.e. expiration while breathing in (inspiration) faces no such difficulty. This type of symptom complex reminds one of Laurocerasus i.e. the chest muscles continue to help breathing in, though, breathing out is difficult and laboured.

A Laurocerasus patient feels very cold. Attempts to warm him up externally do not help either. Sometimes, there is **severe pain in the stomach**, so much so that the patient may not even be able to talk. The muscles on the face become tight and contracted, giving a grim appearance. Thirst is severe and the mouth is very dry. **Small swellings form at the nails** of the fingers and toes (clubbing of the fingers related to cyanotic diseases of the heart). There is a feeling of the hips and ankles being painfully sprained. The fingers become deformed and the dilated veins become visible on the hands.

In Laurocerasus, **drowsiness and dizziness** are not unusual. The patient may also faint. **Mental infirmity induces loss of memory**. Thoughts are no longer streamlined. **Severe headache** is associated with a cool feeling on the forehead. The patient feels very thirsty but his appetite is lost. The stomach feels contracted and hurts badly. The stools are watery, greenish in colour and associated with severe griping pain.

The ailments of Laurocerasus subside on sitting down. On lying down, **coughing** starts. There is a feeling of a big ball rolling from the stomach towards the back. On bending forwards and moving, all the symptoms become aggravated.

| | |
|---|---|
| Potency: | 30 |

# LEDUM
## (Marsh Tea)

Ledum is prepared from a plant, with a distinctive strong smell. In traditional medicine, the extract of the plant is used in the treatment of headache, heart attack and for expulsion of phlegm from the lungs. In homoeopathic form, it has been found very useful in the **treatment of insect bites and joint pains**.

The poisonous effect of Ledum very much resembles snake venom. Like Lachesis, its ailments begin on the left side, are more intense in the upper part of the body than the lower, start mostly at the feet or the leg and then spread from below upwards.

Like Arnica, Ledum is also closely related to **injuries**. Particularly, when used along with Arnica and Hypericum it proves to be much more effective. Ledum is of special use in the treatment of old injuries, leaving deep residual effect, or in the **treatment of injuries caused by pointed objects** like nails and thorns, etc. Ledum-susceptible wounds emit a lightning type of pain, even after having apparently been healed for years. In this situation, if the patient happens to get **convulsions or severe muscular spasms**, Ledum proves to be the best remedy.

Horse dung is notorious for causing tetanus. However, if the horse itself should step on a sharp rusty nail, and sustain a deep wound in the hoof which then happens to dig into the bone, the convulsions of tetanus can rapidly be cured with Ledum 200. Ledum has the capability of curing tetanus resulting, even after many years, from wounds inflicted with sharp weapons. Ledum is also very useful in the treatment of injuries penetrating through the surface linings of the bone (periosteum). However, for the associated damage to the nerve fibres around the bone, Hypericum is much more effective. Similarly, if the nerves are damaged following surgery and the pain continues then Hypericum is found to be more useful than Ledum. Arnica in a high potency is useful in treating the **sprain at the heel**, but not for the residual pain due to injury to the nerve fibres. Ruta and Bellis prove to be of much greater advantage in this situation. **Persistent swelling and chronic pain of the ankle** resulting from repeated ligamentous sprains responds better to Equisetum. Ledum may also be very beneficial if the chronic swelling is due to the involvement of the joints. **Chronic ill effects of repeated ankle injuries** are better treated with Ruta, Bellis and Equisetum.

Some homoeopathic remedies have been found useful on clinical evidence, though they have not been described in literature. At one time, proving had been the standard for establishing the efficacy of homoeopathic substances, which obviously is the best method. However, in view of the scarcity of conscientious and impartial volunteers, clinical evidence has definitely played an important role in the advancement of homoeopathic knowledge.

Sometimes, the effect of **injury to the ankle** does not remain localised. It may also result in the cramping of the legs, which becomes worse on walking or excessive movement, causing severe discomfort. The cramps may affect the knees and hip joints. No ordinary treatment seems to relieve them. Only, on specific treatment, will the discomfort start receding towards the original site, where it will become localised. The appropriate analogous therapy will prevent the spread of discomfort from here.

The swelling of Ledum originates from the joints of the feet, like the onset of gout. Gout has its own specific nature and is easily diagnosed, i.e. relief of discomfort in the cold or by pouring cold water over the affected area, while the discomfort increases in the hot weather. This kind of pain in the foot also gets better with Ledum very quickly. All conditions related to Ledum will be relieved on cold applications.

**Phantom pains** in which a diseased or injured part has been amputated and yet the patient feels the original part of the limb existing and continuing to hurt, is an extremely troubling condition. For example, a person's leg has been surgically removed (amputated) for some incurable condition, but he feels as if the big toe (that does not exist any more) is hurting. Arnica and Ledum are very effective to relieve this condition. If the treating physician comes to know of the existing condition that required the amputation in the first place, then he should treat that very condition. The phantom pain is the pain along the nerve fibres that have been sensitized by the sickness. In case the analogous treatment of the sickness is administered, the affected nerve fibres will receive the message of reverting to their normal state. Arnica, Ledum, Hypericum and Symphytum, etc. can be useful in the **treatment of phantom pain**, provided that the original disease i.e. before amputation, is the focus of treatment.

The Ledum patient is cold and feels very cold both inside and out, yet his **joint pains** feel better with cold applications. They become worse on the application of heat. It is strange, yet real in the case of Ledum.

The face of a Ledum patient, like that of Lachesis, appears swollen. Similar symptoms are also found in heart patients. The face of a Ledum patient is somewhat bluish. The **legs and feet also, are swollen** (oedematous) and bluish in colour. The Ledum patient is generally stout and well built.

Ledum may also be useful in the **treatment of chronic pain of the knee joints**, in addition to the ankles, provided the pain seems to be relieved with cold applications. As in Gelsemium, the patient passes plenty of colourless urine freely.

In female patients of Ledum, periods are frequent, excessive and of deep red colour. These symptoms being present, Ledum will cure the uterine dysfunction also. Remember however, that symptoms of Ledum subside with cold applications.

One symptom is common to Pulsatilla and Ledum yet it is not difficult to differentiate between the two. In Ledum the limbs that become the seat of chronic pain, gradually become weak, contracted and shrivelled, in comparison to the non-affected side. The clear distinction is that a Pulsatilla patient feels hot and gets relief with cold, while the patient of Ledum feels cold yet gets relief with cold. Moreover, his ailments still get better in cold weather.

Ledum is also useful in the **treatment of eye conditions.** Injury to the eye, blood shots, and simultaneous onset of gout and cataract respond beautifully to treatment with Ledum. In Ledum, tiny red pimples form on the forehead and cheeks, which are painful to touch. Acne appears on the nose and at the mouth. The nose burns. There is a **suffocating type of cough** and the **phlegm** is mixed with blood. The trachea feels sore and constricted, causing difficulty in breathing. The innate body temperature of a Ledum patient is low (sub-normal), yet he cannot tolerate the warmth of the bed. Heat aggravates his symptoms. Instead he likes to keep his feet dipped in cold water.

| | |
|---|---|
| Potency: | 30 to 200 |

# LILIUM TIGRINUM

## (Tigor Lily)

Lilium Tig is considered to be the friend of women. It is particularly very useful in the **treatment of women of hysterical and impulsive nature** who chronically suffer from uterine and heart conditions. Their mind is occupied with doubtful thoughts, fear and anxiety. They have a feeling as if their uterus and internal organs are sagging down, which they unknowingly keep on trying to push up. The **periods in such patients begin before time**, are scanty but quite foul. They may also pass dark blood clots. Bleeding increases on movement and stops on resting and on lying down.

A Lilium Tig patient happens to be a **religious fanatic.** If she is a sadist and of hysterical nature, she can best be treated with Lilium Tig. While behaving in a stubborn or hysterical way, a Lilium Tig patient talks nonsense; whereas in her normal life she is quite rational. The patient indulges in useless argumentation only under the influence of this disease. Generally, young boys and girls continue to argue even if they know that they are wrong. People who diet excessively may also develop this tendency, although they are not Lilium Tig patients. Excessive dieting can affect thinking temporarily. However prolonged scrupulous dieting can leave permanent ill effects on their mind for life. Therefore, it is extremely important to avoid over dieting. A balanced diet and suitable exercise, rather than starvation, are the best means to control body weight and achieve good health, or the person will acquire the stubborn nature and illogical argumentation of Lilium Tig due to starvation.

Like Hyoscyamus and Cantharis, there is a **tendency towards sexual ecstasy**. However, in Lilium Tig, unlike Hyoscyamus and Cantharis, the sexual urge becomes a chronic illness that is very difficult to overcome.

Regarding the response to heat and cold, Lilium Tig resembles Pulsatilla i.e. the heat aggravates the symptoms with a burning sensation of the hands and feet.

In Lilium Tig, the **headache** is mostly localised to the forehead. Light is unbearable. The **eyesight becomes weak**. The patient may even become **temporarily blind**. The room appears pitch dark and shadows dance before the eyes. The eyes become inflamed. If the inflammation becomes chronic, then the eyes become swollen forever. One symptom resembles that of Merc Cor e.g. the **dysentery** in which the patient continues to feel discomfort and griping even after having passed the stools. In Merc Cor, the patient has only the feeling of incomplete opening of the bowels, while in Lilium Tig the patient continues to feel like going to the lavatory all the time. Like Merc Cor, the patient also feels a **burning sensation even after having passed the urine.**

Once the scary **thought of becoming insane becomes set in the mind**, it is indelible. The patient begins to think himself of being something or somebody else. He cannot avoid this supposition. This is typical of Lilium Tig. The patient frequently goes into severe sadness and depression. I have, by God's grace, successfully treated many such young men. In addition to the medication, the patient also requires counselling with love and affection. In general, psychological and physical ailments are very intimately related, even to an inseparable extent. If during homoeopathic practice, one can diagnose the psychological condition, the treatment of the related physical condition will help cure both. If the mind is at peace, the body will also feel relief. Some of the Lilium Tig patients believe that they have not been properly understood. It becomes very difficult to avoid them and their useless continued argumentation. One cannot make them understand in any way. They should just be given the appropriate treatment. If the treatment becomes effective, they will return to normality, otherwise they will forever insist that nobody has been able to understand them properly.

In Lilium Tig, **heart conditions** also exist i.e. sudden feeling of the heart being caught in a vice. This feeling is even stronger than that of Cactus. The pulse is very rapid and irregular. Over the area of the heart, the patient feels cold and heavy. The patient feels suffocated amongst a crowd and in a heated, closed room.

In Lilium Tig, there is a lot of **gas in the stomach**, with a feeling of heaviness. The patient feels very hungry and especially desires to eat meat. He also remains very thirsty. **Urination is frequent**, but scanty. The urine feels warm and milky white in colour.

Lilium Tig ailments aggravate in a heated room and with outward superficial consolation. The patient feels better in open air.

| | |
|---|---|
| Antidote: | Helonias |
| Potency: | 30 to 200 |

# MAGNESIA CARB
## (Carbonate of Magnesia)

In allopathy, Mag Carb is used in the treatment of hyperacidity of the stomach and diarrhoea. The prolonged use of Mag Carb can result in serious ailments and bad aftereffects, which can luckily be treated with the homoeopathic form of Magnesia Carb in high potency.

The ailments of Mag Carb recur after twenty-one days. Even if the symptoms apparently seem to be getting better, they will definitely show some aggravation after twenty-one days. The patient aspires to be in the open, even in cold weather. Normally, cold is harmful to the patient of Mag Carb. The patient likes to keep himself wrapped. Hot drinks induce sweating. The patient feels severe pain along the course of the nerves supplying the teeth (dental neuralgia).

Mag Carb is very useful in the **treatment of toothache during pregnancy.** The toothache may last till the child is born. A similar kind of toothache may be experienced during menstruation, which disappears after the periods are over.

The neuralgic pains of Mag Carb subside on a light stroll, especially the toothache. The neuralgia usually begins at night. In Lachesis, the movements do not relieve the pain, unlike Mag Carb. In Mag Carb, like Natrum Mur, the nails and hair become damaged. The teeth and gums become hypersensitive as also found in Antimonium Crude. This hypersensitivity can be treated with Antimonium Crude, Mag Carb or China.

Any patient with the **symptoms suggestive of tuberculosis** and having a sallow face may be treated with Mag Carb, if other symptoms are not pointing to another specific remedy. In Mag Carb, the **stools are clay-coloured** and quite foul, indicative of liver disorder. The stools are exuberant but in small bits, which float in water. In the cancer of the stomach and intestines also, the stools contain lot of gas and being lighter, float in water. However, the stools floating in water are not necessarily diagnostic of cancer. One has to be very careful before labelling a patient with the diagnosis of cancer. If other symptoms are also suggestive of cancer, then of course the doctor must feel seriously concerned. Mag Carb stools may sometimes be greenish in colour.

All the ailments of Mag Carb are known for dryness. The **stomach contents are sour**. The throat irritates. The face looks sallow as in tuberculosis. The **cough, usually dry**, may be associated with small amount of phlegm.

In Mag Carb patient, the shoulders hurt, especially the right shoulder. The entire body feels tired. The skin loses its lustre and is pale and wrinkled. The cold is unbearable. The symptoms aggravate in warm bedding. The patient feels better in changing weather and in the open.

| | |
|---|---|
| Adjuvant: | Chamomilla |
| Antidotes: | Arsenic, Mercur |
| Potency: | 30 |

# MALANDRINUM

Malandrinum is prepared from the material obtained from the lesions of horses suffering from the disease called Horse Grease. An experienced veterinary surgeon found that in areas where horses suffered from this disease, the cows and other cattle contracted a condition like smallpox by sitting on the grass. It is an established fact that in homoeopathy, Malandrinum has been used very effectively in curing smallpox. It is also famous for its prevention. It has also been found very useful to annul the ill effects of the smallpox vaccination. A group of doctors experimented on four children. They gave Malandrinum to three of them but not to the fourth one. All were then vaccinated against smallpox. The child who was not given Malandrinum exhibited the most severe reaction to the vaccine while the other three did not. Another doctor vaccinated one child but did not vaccinate another. To the latter, he simply gave Malandrinum. The vaccinated child contracted smallpox while the non-vaccinated child did not. Once during an epidemic of smallpox, another doctor continued treating the patients and himself using only Malandrinum 30 in repeated doses. He and others who had taken Malandrinum remained safe from contracting smallpox.

With the use of Malandrinum, even after having been afflicted with smallpox, the patient makes rapid recovery without any serious damage. Doctor Burnett is of the opinion that Malandrinum is a profoundly active and effective homoeopathic remedy, and as such it should not be repeated unnecessarily. It may be repeated but only during an acute illness. As a preventive measure it should only be repeated after a long interval.

Malandrinum is also useful in the treatment of eczema developing after a smallpox vaccination. However Thuja is known to be much better regarding the control of bad side effects of the smallpox vaccination.

Malandrinum has an effect on the **bones** also. If the bones become deformed and bent, causing knock-knees (genu valgum), then Malandrinum will be helpful in correcting the deformities. No doubt, Calcarea Carb is the most useful for strengthening the weakened bones. Malandrinum also works well, though.

Malandrinum is also useful in the **treatment of skin conditions** including different forms of eczema, blisters and pustule formation. Its blisters/pustules appear gradually in the form of crops, one after the other, over a long time. Malandrinum is also found useful in the treatment of similar diseases of cattle. One doctor successfully cured a dog riddled with pustules on his neck with Malandrinum.

Malandrinum is also useful in the **treatment of joint pains** associated with inflammation of their inner linings (synovitis). Usually, it is more effective on the lower half of the body such as the legs, from the knees down to the ankles. Malandrinum is also of use in treating backache due to muscle injury. Malandrinum is also reported to be useful in the **treatment of uterine conditions** causing deep itch, inflammation and discharge of **greenish leucorrhoea**.

Like Kreosotum, it may also be useful in the **treatment of bleeding gums** that begin to bleed on trivial pressure.

**Children who forget everything whatever they have learnt previously,** benefit significantly with Malandrinum in low potency, used two to three times a week for a few months.

| | |
|---|---|
| Potency: | 30 and higher. |

# MALARIA OFFICINALIS

Malaria Officinalis is useful in the **treatment of malaria and its aftereffects**. Headache, nausea, generalized body aches, and irritation of the stomach, are its unique symptoms. It is used for the treatment of malaria as well as fevers of similar nature i.e. the body feels hot, yet the patient shivers with cold and there are severe body aches.

Malaria Officinalis is also very good for the **liver**. The pain and tightness over the liver, the dysfunction of liver, spleen and kidney, anaemia, pallor, feeling of cold and generalised debility and weakness should be treated with Malaria Officinalis. It is also useful in the treatment of chronic malaria, which is untreatable otherwise. With the use of Malaria Officinalis, the patient either starts feeling better in a few days or his symptoms become clearly delineated, so they can be diagnosed correctly.

| | |
|---|---|
| Antidotes: | Bryonia, Nux Vomica, Arsenic, Rhus Tox |
| Potency: | 30 |

# MANGANUM ACETICUM

## (Manganese Acetate)

The homoeopathic form is prepared from the Acetate of Manganese. Dr. Hahnemann has done its proving. It works profoundly on haemopoeitic system (i.e. blood formation), but for certain reasons has not been used much. Its main effect is on the voice box (larynx). Manganum is very useful in the **treatment of accumulation of tuberculoses matter, causing gradual reduction of voice** and constant coughing. It also dispels other effects of tuberculosis. The symptoms of Manganum described in literature present a very horrible picture. Therefore, most doctors fail to benefit from its use because they do not use it until and unless the symptoms manifest in their vividly dreadful form.

In Manganum, the skin becomes greasy and pale while the patient feels extremely weak. But all these signs do not appear right from the beginning of the disease. Once the symptoms appear in their severe form, it is too late and very difficult to treat. Manganum should be used as soon as a symptom suggestive of Manganum is noted. If the patient's **voice box (larynx) seems to be getting afflicted** and there are other symptoms of tuberculosis present (i.e. fever and cough), then Manganum should be started without delay. If the patient is that of Manganum, other remedies may reduce the cough but will not have a profound effect. Manganum is also intimately related to the function of the outer layer of the bone (periostium). Thus, it is also beneficial in the treatment of chronic sinuses originating from the bone (osteomyelitis).

**Menstrual disorders** are also common in Manganum. It is better to treat a short scanty flow of thin watery fluid with Manganum rather than with any other remedy to promote the menstruation. Here, the problem is the lack of blood (anaemia). Remedies other than Manganum will further aggravate the anaemia. I have noted that if the treatment chosen is precisely appropriate, then the periods will cease for a few months in order to conserve blood. Once the anaemia is corrected and the body strength restored, normal periods will then commence. In case the periods have stopped in the absence of anaemia, then some other suitable treatment should be started to restore them.

Manganum is very useful in the **treatment of leg cramps, stiffness and insensitivity of the legs, as well as shin pains**.

In Manganum, **skin conditions** are also not uncommon. The edges of the sores and ulcers become thickened. Most of the ulcers fail to heal. Manganum has been reported to be useful in the **treatment of Psoriasis**. Psoriasis, that has previously been suppressed, will at first forcefully express itself on taking Manganum, and then gradually get better with its prolonged interrupted use. Therefore, if psoriasis shows up with the use of Manganum, it should not cause concern. Dr. Kent was strictly opposed to the suppression of psoriasis with powerful medicines in order to avoid the development of cancer in the intestines or any other internal organ. Most of the statements of Dr. Kent are true; therefore this one may well be true as well. Psoric symptoms of Manganum are also found in Phosphorus and Dulcamara.

Manganum adversely affects the blood cells. There is a tendency towards the inflammation of the voice box (larynx) and the wind pipe (trachea), which extends from the voice box to the lungs and is made of multiple circular elastic rings. Every successive attack is stronger than the previous one, so much so that it ultimately brings about the flare-up of the previously suppressed tuberculosis of the lungs. Timely use of Manganum saves the patient from grave complications in the future.

In Manganum, ulcers become indolent. This is a pre-cancerous condition that may lead to the formation of cancer if suppressed forcefully. A mere light touch may cause the patient to suffer. When the bones hurt on walking and do not respond to Arnica or Bryonia, then Manganum may be used. It has more profound effect than Arnica and Bryonia. In a similar way, the pains like that of Baptisia may be experienced by the patient of Manganum. In Baptisia, the pains are due to the dysfunction of the stomach and toxic putrefaction of Typhoid. In case, Baptisia stops working, Manganum should then be remembered.

The patient of Manganum is **very depressed** and is fearful of some impending mishap. Generally, women suffer from this condition.

They have superstitions about their dear ones. Once the mental symptoms are well advanced, the patient may lose the ability to understand and comprehend. The eyesight becomes weak. Manganum will not only cure all the symptoms but also other related conditions of the patient.

In Manganum, the symptoms aggravate on movement and on walking, yet do not get better on sitting either. However, if the patient lies down, the entire suffering disappears as if it was never there. Obese women, who suffer permanently from body pains and tend to keep lying down constantly, may well be cured with Manganum provided other salient symptoms of Manganum are also present. Sometimes, a person becomes sick and tired of just sitting down and likes to get up and stroll around, but walking makes the pain worse. In this condition, one may think of Arsenic and Rhus Tox. Their main symptoms are different, of course.

Regarding tuberculosis, symptoms similar to those of Manganum are also found in Argentum Metallicum, Phosphorus and Graphites. In a tuberculosis patient, the **headache due to the associated anaemia** will benefit from Manganum. The pain of Manganum is sharp, prickly and piercing type. Red painful pimples appear over the scalp. There is inflammation of the eye and the eyelids, with hypersensitivity to light. Looking at near objects causes pain in the eyes. That is why the eyes hurt on reading a book and doing needlework. This symptom somewhat resembles Ruta.

In Manganum the **ears discharge foetid material**. Ammonium Carb also is very effective in treating this condition. In Manganum, the ears may feel temporarily blocked and heavy. Blowing the nose, which increases the pressure inside the ears, helps restore the hearing. The Outer Ear (Pinna) is painful to touch. The nasal catarrh with cold and sore throat affect the ears, causing pain. Similarly, toothache may also be referred to the ear. Therefore, one should always remember Manganum for treating the **nasal catarrh, which causes heaviness in the ear** and impedes hearing. In cold and humid weather, even without infection, one may temporarily become hard of hearing. If there is irritation in the ear, which then affects the throat on the application of local pressure, and the patient begins to sneeze, then Manganum can be beneficial. These symptoms, most often, become aggravated in cold and wet weather.

When the face is pale, listless and without natural glow, Manganum can play an important role in treating the condition.

**Boils associated with fever** can also be treated with Manganum. Manganum is also useful in the **treatment of all sorts of stomach disorders**, especially if there is complete loss of appetite (as in **anorexia**). This remedy restores the appetite. The abdominal pain of Manganum gets relieved on bending over as in Colocynth. In Manganum, the patient definitely suffers from a stomach upset of one sort or the other. He will either be constipated or have diarrhoea or dysentery. The digestive system is never completely normal. Hot flushes due to the **menopause** or simply due to anaemia are treatable with Sulphur, Graphites and Lachesis, though Manganum is also a good remedy.

Manganum also **prevents against the fatty degeneration of the liver**. It is also useful in the **treatment of jaundice and stones in the gall bladder**. The patient feels light dragging pain below the navel. A severe pain is suggestive of Plumbum.

The constant hawking needed to clear the throat can benefit from Manganum. This symptom is also noted in other remedies such as Wythia, Argentum Met, Silicea and Phosphorus, etc. The cough in Manganum, like its other symptoms, subsides on lying down. Conversely in Hyoscyamus the patient starts coughing on lying down. This symptom is more common in young girls of a sensitive nature. In Argentum Metallicum also, the cough subsides on lying down. A cough which becomes severe on talking and laughing responds better to Phosphorus than Manganum. Manganum helps restore the strength of patients who are progressively getting weaker.

In Manganum, the symptoms become worse in cold and humid weather as well as during the calm before a storm.

| | |
|---|---|
| Antidotes: | Coffea, Mercury |
| Potency: | 30 to 200 |

# MEDORRHINUM

Medorrhinum is prepared from the toxic substances of Gonorrhoea. It has proved to be very useful in the treatment of **inherited Gonorrhoeal diseases**. The role of Syphilinum in the treatment of hereditary Syphilis is similar to that of Medorrhinum in hereditary Gonorrhoea. If these remedies are not used, then these diseases become a permanent part of the person's life, flaring up every now and then and become difficult to get rid off. Some eminent doctors are of the opinion that syphilis and gonorrhoea have been present in human society since ancient times and their toxins have been passed on from generation to generation. The sufferer does not have to contract the disease personally. His/her symptoms of syphilis and gonorrhoea may very well be hereditary in nature.

Previously, the treatment **of syphilis** was considered to be very difficult. It consisted of mercury compounds. Nowadays, penicillin given continuously for a month is considered to offer a complete cure. According to homoeopathy, syphilis is incurable. It simply disguises itself in different forms. It becomes dormant, only to reappear when the conditions become favourable. Modern research in allopathy is also supportive of this homoeopathic view. During research on AIDS in America, it came to be known that many AIDS patients suddenly showed signs of syphilis, although previously they had no trace of it. On retracing their family history, it was observed without a shadow of doubt, that the ancestors of at least some of them suffered from syphilis, which was treated with Mercury compounds. However the Syphilis was only suppressed and persisted in dormant form. Similar is the case with gonorrhoea. This also gets passed on from generation to generation. Unless completely uprooted, the treatment of gonorrhoea and resultant diseases would only prove superficial. The **diseases of the reproductive organs in men as well as in women**, due to the result of gonorrhoea having been suppressed, may present in two different forms i.e. over-excitement or total palliation. There may be complete loss of libido. In short, the sexual behaviour of the patient is extreme, either one way or the other, but nothing in between. Medorrhinum is considered to be the most highly valued **treatment of suppressed gonorrhoea** (latent gonorrhoea). In fact, most of the doctors advise using it first and foremost. Medorrhinum in high potency will surface the symptoms of latent gonorrhoea, which can then be treated appropriately. Furthermore, dangerous consequences will also be thus avoided.

Asthma also is related to Medorrhinum. **Marasmus** (the wasting disease of the children), **asthma, chronic nasal catarrh, ringworm and special forms of warts** remain dormant in the body as sequelae of suppressed gonorrhoea, only to express themselves on and off. The warts of any kind and form not amenable to Thuja may respond to Medorrhinum.

Some women, who suffer from **irregularity of periods, pain or nervous weakness** after marriage, may need to be treated with Medorrhinum. Patients feel extremely cold yet sweat profusely. The palms of their hands may feel like burning, though the right and left hands may become cold alternately, or sometimes both hands at the same time.

**Multiple joint pains and rheumatism** provided other symptoms of Medorrhinum are also present, benefit significantly from Medorrhinum. Although, most of its ailments present from sunrise to sunset, some become especially pronounced at night such as seeing ghosts or dead people in frightful dreams all night. Urinary symptoms also become more severe at night, such as frequent urination or urgency to the extent that the patient may not be able to make it to the lavatory. Such patients also have some swelling or inflammation of the prostate glands.

Thuja also resembles Medorrhinum in certain respects. Most of its symptoms worsen after midnight. In **multiple joint pains**, Medorrhinum will surface the true symptoms of the latent disease so it may be treated easily.

Another symptom of Medorrhinum is the sensation of pins and needles all over, along with **urticaria**. Noise, especially a loud noise, causes mental anguish and then urticaria. In Medorrhinum, swelling of feet and legs is usual. The lower legs (below the knees) become cold. Sometimes, the soles of the feet are extremely sensitive; so much so that the patient will is not able to walk on his feet. He will either crawl on his knees or walk extremely carefully, putting minimum pressure on the sole of the feet. On walking a little, the feet become warm making the walk easier. But afterwards, the discomfort in the soles becomes more intense.

Another salient feature of Medorrhinum is that the time seems to pass very slowly. Young boys and girls feel as if somebody is standing behind them. They become **frequently startled** and look back to see if somebody has quietly approached them from behind. They believe that they are being watched. Medorrhinum, as well as Phosphorus, is very useful to abate this feeling. In Phosphorus also, the patient has a feeling as if somebody is peeping over him. The toxic effects of certain diseases cause this feeling.

In Medorrhinum, the patient is **afraid of the dark** and has a fear of falling. The Scalp feels tense and tight. Medorrhinum has also been very successful in the **treatment of skin conditions and dandruff**. Its symptoms pertaining to the hair are similar to those of Natrum Mur. Both of these remedies are related to gonorrhoeal diseases. In Natrum Mur, the **hair becomes dry** and brittle along with severe dandruff. In certain cases, Medorrhinum alone can cure these conditions.

Some people become nervous easily. **Objects start to dance before them**. The vision becomes blurred and does not focus. Black or brown spots appear before the eyes. The patient may have **double vision**. If these symptoms become chronic, then Medorrhinum will be found very useful. Hallucinations, tension in the eyes, mental anguish and **falling eyelashes** can also be successfully treated with Medorrhinum. Also in Medorrhinum as in Apis, there are bags below the eyes. In Apis, the swelling hangs, while in Medorrhinum the swelling is rather diffuse.

Medorrhinum, given in very high potency, is also useful in the **treatment of chronic nasal catarrh**. It shows that there is a deep-seated residue of gonorrhoea, which is out of the reach of common remedies. Medorrhinum is useful in chronic catarrh as the disease is deep-seated it will only respond to high potency of Medorrhinum CM or at least 10000. It proves to be extremely valuable in this condition. Medorrhinum is very useful if the patient feels extremely hungry and craves to eat insatiably when nervous, or similarly if his severe thirst becomes unquenchable. Extreme hunger is also known in Psorinum, but it mostly bothers at night.

Medorrhinum has been found useful in the **treatment of ascites** (accumulation of water in the abdomen due to liver disease), as well as the swelling and inflammation of glands in the groins.

The **constipation** of Medorrhinum is characterised by stools in the form of dry rounded droppings. The urine is scanty, brown in colour, very pungent and less frequent. It is possible that Medorrhinum may also be helpful to patients who have been rendered **physically disabled and limp due to chronic joint pains**. It is also useful in the treatment of frequent urination due to neurosis but not due to diabetes.

Medorrhinum is also closely linked to conditions related to the **kidney, urinary bladder and prostate gland**. The first and foremost **treatment of kidney pain** (renal colic) is Aconite 1000 and Belladonna 1000 combined, two doses given ten minutes apart. The patient will, by the grace of God, get better immediately. If the kidney pain gets worse with cold, then Mag Phos 6X repeated a few times or simply one dose of Colocynth CM will offer magical relief. After the relief of pain, its root cause i.e. the kidney stones, must be treated appropriately. If the kidney pain is caused by inflammation or infection rather than by stones, the proper curative treatment should be sought, and this could be Medorrhinum.

Medorrhinum is also related to **deafness**, especially nerve deafness, in which the patient feels no pain. Medorrhinum is useful in chronic and progressive deafness. However, Sulphur should not be overlooked. In fact, I have treated patients who had developed deafness due to the thickening of the bone around the auditory nerve (otosclerosis) with Sulphur CM. The thickening tendency of the bone disappeared and hearing did not deteriorate any further.

In Medorrhinum, the **teeth being very sensitive** hurt on chewing food. **Ulcers,** having jagged margins, also **form in the mouth**. Medorrhinum has also been found beneficial in the **treatment of chronic ankle pain.**

Medorrhinum is deeply related to **asthma** also. Generally, Nat Sulph is considered to be a very effective remedy for asthma. Natrum Sulph is often found useful in the treatment of children presenting symptoms of a familial type of gonorrhoea, but sometimes Medorrhinum may also be required, so as to better express the latent symptoms of gonorrhoea. Calcarea Sulph is also reported to be very effective in the treatment of gonorrhoea. If phlegm **becomes deeply seated in the lungs** and is difficult to cough out, and other homoeopathic remedies have proved ineffective, then Medorrhinum may offer substantial cure. Kali Iodide and Arsenic Iodide are also useful for the expulsion of deep-seated phlegm from the lungs. For the treatment of deep ulcers resulting from the dislodgment of thick sputum or phlegm, Kali Iodide is better, but for relatively superficial ulcers, Arsenic Iodide is better.

Medorrhinum is considered very useful in the **treatment of lightning type of joint pains** associated with severe pain in the chest. Like Lachesis, its pain and burning is also over the left side of the chest. Slip disc with resulting nerve root pain (sciatica) should be thoroughly investigated before treatment. If the investigation is inconclusive then Medorrhinum can be given in high potency and then wait for seven to ten days. I happened to treat one such patient with Colocynth based on his symptoms. He responded well, but after a while, the condition stopped improving any further. So I gave him Medorrhinum instead of Colocynth CM wherupon his original symptoms returned including the severe pain. Had I continued to treat him with a high potency of Medorrhinum, he might have been completely cured. The patient was rather impatient, so I gave him Colocynth, instead of Medorrhinum as I had proposed. This time, Colocynth proved to be much more effective. I failed to follow him further and do not know whether he was fully cured or not.

Sometimes, the **legs may feel very heavy due to pain in the back**. The legs become stiff. This is suggestive of Medorrhinum. At times, the **spasm impedes circulation**. This remedy also shows sign of cramp especially in the **calves of the legs**. If a person feels cramps in the legs on standing for a long time, then Mag Phos 6X may also be useful. In Medorrhinum however, cramps also affect the under surface of the feet, which tend to be drawn and turn inwards.

Many of the symptoms of Medorrhinum become worse in the heat of the sun. Humidity and the seaside offer relief. Some of the symptoms become worse at night, as detailed above.

| | |
|---|---|
| Potency: | 30 to CM |

# MERCURIUS (MERCURY)

Mercury in general is an important deep-acting remedy. It affects each and every part and cell of the body. Once Mercury has settled in the body it is extremely difficult, if not impossible to eradicate its ill effects. Like Arsenic, it too produces deep and permanent ill effects, however, Arsenic does not get carried into the next generation. Its ill effects remain confined to the person poisoned, though they last throughout his life. Arsenic embedded in the body gets buried with the person. Mercury however, is extremely dangerous because its ill effects pass on from generation to generation.

Syphilis also behaves the same way. That is why Mercury happens to be a top class **treatment for syphilis**. Syphilinum too, given in very high potency, is very useful in the treatment of syphilis; it is prepared from the syphilis lesions. However in case it does not benefit, it will at least enhance the action of other remedies, especially the Mercury compounds. The above basic feature of Mercury must be well remembered that its poisonous effects last throughout one's life as well as getting passed onto the next generation. In an ironic sense, Mercury is a dangerous poison with ever-lasting effects. In fact, it tops the list of dangerous poisons. It affects the bones as well as the nerve cells. It percolates through the blood, skin, heart, inner linings and nerve fibres and then settles in the bone and brain tissue. In olden days, the doctors used to treat syphilis with Mercury. It offered temporary relief but resulted in long-lasting deleterious effects on the body. The syphilis simply got suppressed and transmitted through reproduction to future generations. Besides this, past physicians used Mercury fearlessly for other conditions as well. Excessive, unnecessary use of mercury produces syphilis like symptoms. Mercury kills the nerve cells and causes decay of the nasal bones and fingers, like leprosy. The homoeopathic use of Mercury, on the other hand, has the capability to cure these symptoms.

**Excessive salivation, profuse sweating, sore throat and pungent smell are the common symptoms of Mercury,** well known to doctors. A Mercury patient always smells putrid, unbearable to others. It is difficult to explain the nature of this smell. One has to personally experience it. Proper use of Mercury will surface the illness to the skin. Sometimes a severe itch, **discharging sinuses and**

**ulcers covered with whitish matter** develop. White spots appear on the skin. Once I saw a patient who had widespread painful **whitish ulcers** on and around the thighs that were intractable. With the use of Mercury, he was, by the grace of God, completely cured within a month.

When the **sores** developing on the skin turn into ulcers with raised edges, and there is a fear of **gangrene** formation, then Merc Cor instead of Merc Sol is a better remedy. The difference between the two, it that Merc Sol is relatively mild but long acting compared to Merc Cor. The ailments of Merc Cor happen to be severe and of acute nature. Merc Cor is distinctively a fast-acting remedy in acute as well as chronic conditions. **Chronic dysentery associated with passage of mucus and blood** should be treated with Merc Sol. If, however, the dysentery is of acute onset and is associated with severe gripes (tenesmus) and continuous bleeding, then Merc Cor will be found more effective.

In Mercury ailments, the **gangrenous process** involves the lips, the inside of the cheeks and the gums (cancrum oris). The overlying skin becomes dark and looks horrible. In **syphilis**, a similar affliction is noted on these areas. The nose may also be affected with the resultant decay of the nasal bones. **Chronic ulcers of the mouth** are also suggestive of Mercury ailments.

One sign of Mercury is the formation of white specks on the skin resembling leucoderma. This condition is neither leucoderma, nor do the spots spread and coalesce like leucoderma. But, if the constitutional symptoms of Mercury are also present, then Mercury can effectively cure even leucoderma. Another tine, a patient had widespread leucoderma affecting the entire body and also had the general symptoms of Mercury. A single dose of Mercury 1000 resulted in the disappearance of his white patches for good, within the week. When Mercury benefits skin conditions, it does not afflict any damage to deeper glands, but, while it primarily works on the deep glands and organs, it may surface some kind of skin condition. This shows that the Mercury has rendered the glands healthy by pushing the disease from the inside, out to the skin.

The Founder of the Ahmadiyya Community is believed to be the Second Coming of the first Messiah by the Ahmadiyya Community.

He put forth a unique discovery, to enhance the faith of homoeopathic physicians in homoeopathy. He claimed that it was revealed to him that if the diseases of the glands can be expressed to the exterior of the body i.e. in the skin, then the deep glands are spared from some grave conditions. He mentioned Mercury and Sulphur in this respect. In homoeopathy also, these are the two remedies, which are commonly used for this purpose. He further said that he had a strong desire to proclaim the extreme usefulness of these two potentially curative medicines.

Mercury is useful in the **treatment of chronic bone pains**, especially of the superficial bones that are devoid of any muscle padding under the skin. Mercury should not be forgotten while considering the treatment of chronic sinuses connected to the bones or glands. A peculiar symptom of Mercury is that joint pains tend to be associated with pus formation. The constitution of a Mercury patient is like that of syphilis. Therefore the bones, when inflamed, develop sinuses and produce pus. Conventional therapy consists of aspirating the pus with a syringe. On the other hand, Mercury when started in a low potency and then gradually increased, can in fact produce better results. However, a high potency, right at the onset of the disease, can prove dangerous. In chronic diseases, the potency should be increased gradually. The safest way is that the treatment should be initiated in a low potency and then gradually increased.

Another characteristic of Mercury is that **arthritis** and rheumatism are associated with swelling and inflammation. Suffering increases with the warmth of the bed and on sweating. The patient sweats profusely yet gets no relief. His restlessness continues in spite of frequent sweating. In acute tonsillitis, when the fever subsides on sweating, the patient's condition further deteriorates. In this condition, two to three doses of Mercury will first bring back the **fever** and then make it subside gradually. The patient sweats profusely once instead of sweating repeatedly. In this fever, susceptible to Mercury, one sign is that the child's eyes appear glossy as if painted with varnish. In measles and chicken pox too, the eyes have a similar appearance for as long as the rash has not appeared. Their breath has a foetid odour. The child may develop **meningitis** and have visual delusions. In this condition, if Mercury becomes ineffective, Hepar Sulph should be used. If this also fails, then Silicea will be found effective by God's grace. Usually this condition is within the range of these three remedies. I also use a biochemic prescription for such conditions and that is Natrum Phos, Ferrum Phos, Silicea, Kali Mur and Calcarea Phos in 6X. For **inflamed tonsils**, Calcarea Fluor should also be added and the mixture administered repeatedly. This prescription has often proved very useful. If the illness is still not controlled and the patient has the symptoms of Mercury, then Mercury must be used, after Hepar Sulph of course.

Mercury has a fluctuating nature. Its ailments show ups and downs in their severity. Blood pressure and fever can also behave the same way. In other words, Merc Sol should be used for the treatment of any inconsistent type of condition.

When the symptoms of Mercury become severe, the hands tremble and become weak. One becomes incapable of even holding a cup of tea.

Mercury may possibly be of benefit in the treatment of **epilepsy-like conditions** in children as well as neurological diseases associated with **spontaneous involuntary movements of the limbs** (chorea, athetosis).

A Mercury patient has an **impulsive nature**, speaks rather fast and is **impatient**. He wants to do things at the spur of the moment. His anger knows no bounds. The tendency towards insanity may be very strong. When emotionally excited, he is very dangerous. He may commit a serious crime or kill himself. He remains tense and is extremely restless. He is fearful of becoming insane and of death. He becomes a coward and possesses a suspicious mind. He loses hope in life. When questioned, he replies carefully and slowly. **Memory and the mind become weak**. The headache in a Mercury patient is connected to the suppression of body discharges. For example, the suppression of sweating of feet or the sudden stoppage of nasal secretions will precipitate the headache. A **sudden cessation of menses will also provoke the headache**. The head feels tied up with a bandage. On lying flat on the back, the patient feels dizzy. The Skull feels tightly squeezed and under pressure. Burning and itching are also common.

Mercury ailments intensify in the cold as well as hot weather. Gusty wind is unbearable. If **after measles etc.,** the **head seems expanding,** then Mercury can put a stop to this tendency immediately.

The skin of Mercury patients has a clay-like appearance. Secretions from the **itchy and eczematous skin** are offensive and start bleeding. The edges of the ulcers are rounded in shape and covered with white exudates. Skin conditions aggravate at night. The warmth of the bed aggravates symptoms.

The **eyes become inflamed and red along with a burning sensation**. There is a lot of watery discharge from the eyes. Black dots appear before the eyes. On looking towards the fire, the eyes become red and swollen. There is pain around the eyes and at the temples. The vision becomes blurred. The cornea becomes inflamed. Eyes become hypersensitive to light. All the eye symptoms of 'pink eye' at the onset of summer are also found in Mercury. If the eye symptoms are not clearly identified, then Merc Sol should be used. Seeing the **sun during its eclipse** can seriously **damage the retina of the eye**. The effect may not become apparent right away. Damage shows up years after the incident. Black dots appear in the visual field. Sometimes the right eye gets blinded and at other times, the left eye. The patient then gradually becomes totally blind. This blindness is not amenable to any kind of conventional therapy so far. However, two to three doses of Merc Cor CM given monthly seem to be of benefit, by the grace of God. The process of being blinded stops there and then. It is not possible to repair the detached retina that definitely needs to be treated with laser surgery. Some doctors are of the opinion that Merc Sol, in a low potency, may benefit many retinal conditions. I have no such experience. I suggest more research should be carried out.

Stinky, white or dark green pus discharging from the ears is a typical sign of Mercury. The **inner as well as the outer ear become infected**. The ear-drum (tympanic membrane) may perforate causing deafness.

Sometimes, Merc Sol can quickly control the **common cold**, although this is only a superficial treatment. Since Merc Sol is not a long acting remedy, one should not depend on it. Instead, for a persistent common cold, one should use Kali Iodide. Kali Iodide is intimately related to the conditions affecting the mucous membranes.

Nevertheless, Kali Iodide alone may not be sufficient for catarrhal conditions. Several other remedies can also be used.

Dr. Kent has warned against the repeated use of Mercury for skin diseases, lest it causes permanently serious ill effects. It is possible that Mercury may only be related to certain skin diseases and may not have any similarity to the overall constitution of the patient. The result would be that some diseases might get better while the majority would merely be suppressed or rendered latent.

Mercury is very useful in the **treatment of diseases of the teeth**, especially when they become brittle and the gums recede, along with the formation and collection of offensive discharge (**pyorrhoea**). Teeth turning black and decaying at their root can be treated with Kreosotum as well as Merc Sol. If the roots of the teeth have become black, then Staphysagria works better than Merc Sol. In congenital syphilis, the teeth of the children decay at an early age and become black. The tongue appears to be thick and expanded with teeth markings on its margins. **Deep ulcers form inside the mouth**. The gums hurt on eating or on touch. **Extremely foetid odour from the mouth** fills the entire room. In Mercury, the taste of the mouth becomes metallic. The throat is red and swollen. Due to excessive salivation, the patient needs to constantly swallow it. Any change of weather results in inflammation of the throat. A worsening of the discomfort on drinking hot fluids, the difficulty in swallowing liquids and the persistent feeling of something being stuck in the throat (as in Hepar Sulph), need to be treated with Mercury.

The appetite of a Mercury patient is either markedly increased or it is totally lost. There is aversion to meat, coffee and fatty food. There is an intense feeling of weakness along with increased appetite. Milk and sweets produce hyperacidity in the stomach. The patient has a strong desire to drink cold liquids. The **stomach feels inflamed, burns inside and is tender to the touch**. The patient experiences hiccups as well as belching. The stomach becomes tense. There is a feeling of a pin pricking over the area of the liver. The patient feels uncomfortable while lying on the right side. **Dysentery and a stinging type of abdominal pain** are also the symptoms of Mercury. In Merc Cor, there is irritation and inflammation of the bladder also. **Urination becomes frequent and interrupted, associated with scalding**. Dysentery also sets in. In the presence of all these symptoms, Merc Cor proves to be almost a sure shot remedy. **Acute summer dysentery** can also be effectively treated with Aconite and Ipecac.

One symptom of Mercury is that the heart starts beating fast on the slightest physical exertion. There is a feeling of weakness over the heart. The symptoms become worse at night. The **limbs tremble**, but especially the hands and the feet. There may also be sudden jolting of the muscles (tonic convulsions). The body feels unusually heavy, weak and tired. The stiffness becomes worse at night in the warmth of the bed.

Regarding the diseases of women, such as stinging and burning the ovaries, **excessive menstrual bleeding**, abdominal pain, the abrasive type of **leucorrhoea** getting worse at night, morning sickness and **scalding** urination, followed by itching which gets relieved on washing with cold water; are all the signs of, and effectively treatable with, Merc Sol. **Abortion,** in the early months of pregnancy, resulting from weakness can be treated with Merc Sol. Merc Sol removes the weakness and provides the strength to carry the pregnancy through.

Mercury cannot cure the **cancer of the uterus or the breast**, but definitely ameliorates the pain and relieves the suffering. Non-cancerous lumps can however be cured with Mercury. One Mercury compound called Proto Iodide has proved to be very useful in the **treatment of breast cancer**. Dr. Kent used to prescribe Proto Iodide 100 for the treatment of pain due to cancer of the breast. It helped every time it was used. Dr. Kent had noted an egg-sized cancerous lump of the breast was resolved or dissolved completely with the use of Proto Iodide of Mercury. It benefits more on the right-sided tumour, while another compound of Mercury-bin-Iodide, works better on the left-sided tumour.

Merc Sol is very useful in the **treatment of spasmodic stiffness of the neck,** on exposure to the cold. If the suffering is noted as first thing in the morning, then Belladonna should be used first. If it fails, then use Merc Sol.

In certain **paralytic conditions**, there can be **spontaneous jerky movements of the limbs**, bending them. These too may possibly be treated with Merc Sol. Its **Eczema** and the ulcers are associated with a burning and piercing sensation. The exudating smells are extremely foul and nauseating. In this type of symptom complex, any homoeopathic remedy of which the main constituent is Mercury will be found useful with rare exceptions.

The symptoms of a patient of Mercury aggravate at night, like Syphilinum and Sulphur. In Sulphur, the aggravation is due to the warmth of the bed, while in Mercury it is the time of the night, that aggravates whether the patient is asleep in bed or not.

| | |
|---|---|
| Antidotes: | Hepar Sulph, Aurum, Mezerium |
| Potency: | 30 up to CM |

# MILLEFOLIUM

## (Yarrow)

Millefolium is especially related to **bleeding**. Usually, the bleeding of Millefolium is reddish. Dr. Boericke has also restricted this medicine to the out-flow of bright red blood only (arterial), without mentioning its relationship to the venous blood. However, Dr. Kent right from the start describes Millefolium as the top class treatment for varicose veins. Therefore, he does not describe Millefolium's blood as always bright red, but rather describes it as generally red. Anyhow, Millefolium is the best treatment for any bleeding, be it of bright red or darkish colour. Perhaps there is no other drug that has more symptoms related to bleeding than Millefolium. Millefolium may also be effective whenever there is increased bleeding from **cancerous wounds**, in stopping such a bleed. It is now well established that repeated local application of pure honey on the wounds helps healing.

One symptom of Millefolium is that the **eyes become red** and there is a strong feeling that a lot of blood has accumulated in the eyes. The eyes get congested with blood before the onset of **headache**. Sometimes, this condition develops on reading for a short while. Millefolium is the cure for all these ailments.

Millefolium will also be useful when the **eyes become red due to the increase in local blood flow**, the vision becomes blurred and there is a strong tendency of **nosebleed**. Millefolium 30 given in combination with Phosphorus 30 proves to be much more effective against this ailment.

In women, **excessive and prolonged menstrual bleeding** and cramps over the uterus and lower part of the abdomen are a specific symptom of Millefolium. The triad of these symptoms occurring simultaneously in a patient will, by the grace of God, immediately benefit from the use of Millefolium, with rare exception. Similarly, Millefolium is also useful to avert a **threatened abortion,** i.e. the tendency to bleed on slight activity, which stops on taking rest. Women who tend to bleed right in the beginning of their pregnancy, and are predisposed to abortion (habitual abortion) should take one dose of Millefolium CM before the expected pregnancy. Quite often, a single dose of Millefolium may cure them of this problem forever. Similarly, I found the astonishing efficacy of this remedy in 100 000 (CM) potency in a person who was thrown from a horse cart due to a sudden jolt, and suffered from continuous spitting of blood for weeks. By God's grace, just one dose of Millefolium in 100 000 potency completely cured him,

If patients who have the **tendency to bleed** are given one dose of Millefolium in 1000 potency before a surgical operation, they will be saved from the complications of excessive bleeding during the operation. Another benefit of Millefolium is that it prevents the formation of blood clots. On the contrary, allopathic drugs that are used to stop bleeding usually make the blood thick, whereas homoeopathic remedies stop the bleeding while keeping the blood flowing healthily. From this point of view, Millefolium is an excellent remedy as it stops bleeding without making the blood unnecessarily thick and prone to clotting.

Millefolium is also very good in controlling the **excessive blood flow towards the heart**. Generally, this happens when the patient is very excited. Aconite is generally useful for this condition; however, Millefolium also produces good results.

Millefolium is generally useful in the diseases of the old and the weak, as well as of women and children. Its symptoms are as follows: usually the patients feel **increased blood flow towards the head**, pressure on the right side of the head and there is contortion in the muscles of the eyelids and the forehead. Movement causes giddiness and the patient feels as if his ears are clogged; whereas, at the same time the patient feels cold air coming out of the ears. The head feels heavy after sleeping in the afternoon. The patient always thinks that he has forgotten something. The face feels hot and flushed. The mouth becomes very dry, **sores form over the gums and in the throat**. There is pain over the left side of the throat.

There is always a feeling of burning and scraping in the stomach. There is pain over the liver. The flatus is stinky and there is bleeding from the intestines. Severe dysentery with loose **blood-mixed stools** develops. The **urine also contains blood**. The patient develops inflammation of the bladder and there is a feeling of pain over the left kidney area.

The onset of **severe cramps or epileptic fits due to the stoppage of menstrual bleeding** from the uterus or the onset of bleeding due to severe hard work will benefit from Millefolium, which should also be used for the **treatment of bleeding piles**.

If phlegm sticks inside the lungs and tuberculosis becomes chronic with the spitting of **blood on coughing** (haemoptysis), and there is a feeling of tightness in the chest, Millefolium can also be a very helpful adjuvant, given along with other appropriate remedies.

Where other medicines have failed, Millefolium works miraculously against the following ailments: hernia resulting from repeated excessive weight lifting, bleeding after the surgical removal of stones (lithotomy) and the high continuous fever due to an unknown cause.

While the conjugal relationships between husband and wife are normal in every aspect and the sperm are also healthy, yet there is a problem with the ejaculation of semen preventing pregnancy, then Millefolium is a very important treatment for this unusual condition.

| | |
|---|---|
| Potency: | 30 to 200 or even 1000 |

# MORGAN CO

Morgon Co is a new type of remedy prepared from the putrid material produced in the intestines. It is very effective against the **chronic diseases of the intestines**. When, apart from the intestinal problem, there is swelling of the feet and legs, and the skin has also become affected, splitting on slight rubbing and then excoriating, the homoeopaths appreciative of Morgon Co claim it to be very useful and fast acting in treating this condition.

| | |
|---|---|
| Potency: | 30 or higher potency, based on the experience. |

# MURIATICUM ACIDUM

Muriatic Acid, i.e. Hydrochloric Acid, is a common acid deeply linked with our digestive system. Most homoeopathic doctors draw a very scary picture of Muriatic Acid, i.e. a patient whose muscles have become completely useless and his head constantly rolls off the side of the bed, with death only moments away. Such a patient is typical of Muriatic Acid. In fact, Hydrochloric Acid is routinely secreted in our stomach on a daily basis. The amount secreted varies. When the acidity increases in the stomach, it is possible that the quantity of Muriatic Acid has increased. However, the situation may be exactly the opposite in the sense that the level of Hydrochloric Acid in the stomach has decreased (hypochlorhydria). This also, can produce the symptoms of hyperacidity, because when the gastric lining make less hydrochloric acid, then due to a lack of the antiseptic effect of Hydrochloric Acid, the food inside the stomach starts to decompose, leading to the formation of other acids and producing gases in the stomach. The normal acidity of the stomach does not weaken a person. However, when the acidity increases above or decreases below the normal level, it produces the ailments that we commonly call "acidity". Anyhow, one has to decide after carefully observing the symptoms. As soon as the **digestive system is noted to be upset**, the patient should be given Muriatic Acid in homoeopathic potency **so as to normalize** the acidity in the stomach.

In Muriatic Acid patients, the mind remains absolutely clear and alert, even if the nerves and muscles have been afflicted. However, the symptoms of a patient ameanable to Acid Phos treatment are exactly opposite to those of Muriatic Acid patients. In Muriatic Acid, the body is affected first and the mind last, whereas in Acid Phos patients, the state of mind deteriorates first and physical ailments appear later on. The patient's ability to think and understand is badly affected. The intellectual capacity slowly decreases and memory deteriorates. After some time, these symptoms gradually lead to the weakening of the muscles. The Acid Phos patient takes a while to develop the symptoms of the muscular weakness. If the mental symptoms are treated with this remedy, then the muscles may not be affected at all.

It is relatively easy to take care of the Muriatic Acid patient. As long as the mind remains alert and the mental faculties have not been affected, the patient will be cured by just one or two doses even if he is at the point of death. The profound weakness due to the "acidity" is very dangerous but at the same time can be very easily reversed, without leaving any long-lasting bad effects. The same is the situation with Sulphuric Acid. So, it is most essential to understand and compare the nature of the various acids.

In Muriatic Acid, there is **severe headache** that may also **blur the vision**. On straining the eyes, the headache becomes worse. Furthermore, pimples appear on the face. The lips become dry and crack. The tongue becomes pale, dry and swollen. Quite often, **ulcers develop in the mouth and over the tongue**. **Gums become swollen** and may also bleed while **teeth become loose**.

Some Muriatic Acid patients do not even like the sight of meat, however, most of them enjoy eating it. Sometimes, the patients feel severe hunger and thirst. Some patients are so sensitive to touch that they do not even like to cover themselves with a sheet. The ailments of Muriatic Acid get worse during humid weather. The disease aggravates shortly before midnight. The patient finds comfort on lying on the left side.

The headache starts from the nape of the neck and **vision becomes blurred**. Sometimes, the **field of vision becomes half** (hemianopia). Either the upper half or the lower half of a thing becomes invisible. Similarly, either half of the left side or half of the right side becomes obscure. In the latter condition, Muriatic Acid is very effective. For **quivering vision in one eye**, Rhus Tox is very useful as it also protects against many dangerous conditions.

One symptom of Muriatic Acid is that when the child passes stools, a **portion of the intestine prolapses out** (rectal prolapse).

In the conditions associated with **formation of blisters and sores in the mouth,** and cuts developing on the tongue, there is a need for vigorous treatment not only to cure the mouth problems but also to cure the fever and its bad effects. Sometimes, in Muriatic Acid, the **tongue becomes paralyzed**. There is no problem of the voice mechanism, but only the tongue is non-functional. For such paralysis, Muriatic Acid is very valuable. The tongue is usually dry.

In Muriatic Acid, despite the skin being sensitive, the paralytic effects are more manifest internally. All these kinds of contradictions help in identifying the remedy. Though, the body appears lifeless, yet the **slightest touch on the skin produces shudders**. Such hypersensitivity is also found in Agaricus, Staphysagria and Oxalic Acid. Similarly, Picric Acid is also a very sensitive remedy. In all these remedies, strong pressure is bearable, although a light touch is unbearable and the patient pushes the hand away with a jerk.

In Muriatic Acid, the legs and arms become cold and feel heavy. Most of the excretions (i.e. urine, stools) are no longer under voluntary control. The pulse is rapid but weak.

| | |
|---|---|
| Antidote: | Bryonia Alba |
| Potency: | Usually up to 30 |

# NATRUM CARBONICUM

## (Carbonate of Sodium)

Natrum Carbonicum is composed of Sodium and Carbon elements, and exhibits the symptoms of both. **The Natrum Carb patient quivers even on the slightest noise** so much so that the heartbeat becomes irregular, even with the rustling sound of paper. The Natrum Carb patient is recognized through these peculiar symptoms. It is strange that, no matter how loud the noise is, if the level is constant it does not bother the patient. However, any change in the volume level badly affects the nerves. The ups and downs in noise level become unbearable. A sudden explosion or loud noise is very harmful for Natrum Carb patient. If such a patient is scared suddenly, his heart may stop. Therefore, one should be very careful around him.

When the ailments of Natrum Carb become chronic, the patient starts to feel indifferent, even towards his own family members. **The patient feels indifferent.** The circle of friendship and relationship shrinks. The situation worsens to the extent that the patient becomes disgusted and disconnected from the whole of humanity. The patient cannot tolerate anyone. Disgust is more prominent than fear.

**The urine of a Natrum Carb patient smells like horse's urine.** This symptom is found in Benzoic Acid also. The patient **needs to urinate again and again**, while the patient may also wet the bed during the night. Urination is associated with a scalding sensation.

In the skin diseases of Natrum Carb, swellings develop at the edges of the fingers and of the toes, but especially over the finger joints. On the rest of the body the spots are itchy areas of raised circular shape (Urticarial). This remedy is also useful against **herpes**, though it is not easy to pick this remedy specifically from the symptoms of herpes alone. If the symptoms of Natrum Carb are present in a patient and the other remedies have not been effective against herpes, then Natrum Carb should also be tried. Both Sodium and Carbonate are linked with nerve tissue. Since herpes is basically a disease of the nerves, the herpes patient can benefit from Natrum Carb.

Natrum Carb plays a prominent role in the treatment of **bad aftereffects of heatstroke**. Sometimes, after a heatstroke, **nasal catarrh starts dripping in to the throat** and becomes a permanent menace (Post-nasal drip). For this condition, Natrum Carb is very useful. It is also very effective against bouts of headache and sensitivity to heat. In Natrum Carb, **raw-looking sores start to appear at the tip of the nose**. A peculiar symptom of this remedy is that the tip of the nose always exhibits a skin disease of one kind or the other. It is also valuable in the treatment of **boils on the nose**. Once, a patient was not benefiting from Natrum Carb and so I treated him with a Propolis ointment. (Propolis is a bactericide that the honeybee prepares for herself). His wounds became fully healed in less than a week. Honey is extraordinarily effective against cancerous wounds and chronic sores of the eyes, etc. Propolis is a powerful medicine, but chemically it is very light. Once, research was carried out in France to find out the types of bacteria various insects carry. All the insects in the world are supposed to carry some bacteria. The scientist who conducted the research on honeybees was surprised to discover that there was no trace of any kind of bacteria on the body of the honeybee. He found that the honeybee was absolutely free of bacteria. This was an astonishing discovery and it led to the beginning of a new era of research to find out why the honeybee is free from all sorts of bacteria. The words of the Holy Quran "**feehi shifaa-unnaasi**" (In it lies cure for mankind) carry a deep meaning hidden within them. During the research in France, it was discovered that the honeybee likes cleanliness so much that it puts a chemical called Propolis at the edges of each honeycomb. The honeybee prepares Propolis from the wax exuding from the white eucalyptus and other trees and rubs it at the edges of her honeycomb. Whenever the honeybee enters the honeycomb, it puts its feet on the edge of the honeycomb and does the same when it comes out of the honeycomb. In doing so, the antibacterial material (Propolis) sticks to the feet of the honeybee and keeps it free of bacteria. This is the reason why bacteria cannot enter the honeycomb. After this discovery, a wise and able farmer in Denmark prepared a special farm and bred the honeybee. From this farm, he used to collect Propolis in large quantities.

Propolis mixed in glycerine or vitamin E cream is very useful against common pimples and boils.

In Natrum Carb, sores not only form on the surface of the nose, but also inside it. The **nasal catarrh is quite foul smelling** and becomes chronic. It produces constant irritation in the throat. The sense of smell is also lost.

Usually, the face is pale. Circles develop around the eyes. **Sores and blisters form inside the mouth**. Natrum Carb is particularly effective against sores inside the mouth of nursing mothers. It is also effective against the **infertility** of women who suffer permanently from leucorrhoea. These symptoms are also found in many other remedies. However, a special symptom of Natrum Carb is that the woman patient is of a cold constitution, has been sterile for a long time and suffers from **persistent leucorrhoea**. If all these symptoms are present together in a patient, then by the grace of God, Natrum Carb will be found very effective in curing her infertility.

In Natrum Carb, there is a tendency of permanent weakness of the ankles (flail ankles). In such patients, feet usually twist easily. Such a weakness is a part of the patient's constitution and not due to any kind of accident or injury. For this condition, Natrum Carb is a very useful remedy. However, the most effective treatment for **sprained ankles** is Ruta or Bellis. To abate the bad effects of severe sprains, Arnica given in a high potency, combined with Belladonna, shows positive effects immediately and the symptoms of the disease completely disappear. However, if these are not used in the beginning of the disease, then Ruta will relieve the residual bad effects. Sometimes, it becomes necessary to treat the patient with Bellis or Rhus Tox also. Natrum Carb alleviates the tendency of ankle sprains due to structural weakness.

Natrum Carb **patient remains sad and worried most of the times**. The patient remains deeply occupied with sad thoughts, is cowardly and loses the power to think and understand. The mind feels fickle. The cold, and any change of weather, becomes unbearable. The patient becomes very **restless** when the **clouds thunder**. **Music aggravates his symptoms**. The patient has no tolerance for certain people. The patient becomes bad tempered and irritable after eating food. The slightest mental fatigue leads to **severe headache**, which worsens in the sunlight or the lamplight. He also feels dizzy. Physical as well as mental hard work, make the symptoms worse. He feels very weak and staggers while walking. The patient feels cramps in the muscles and the glands become hard and swollen. The patient dislikes the cool breeze. Apparently, these symptoms should not appear due to heatstroke; however, in some patients of Natrum Carb, these are the permanent symptoms following a heatstroke. One should remember that Natrum Carb is a cold remedy by nature.

In Natrum Carb, **black spots appear before the eyes**. On waking up, the vision is blurred. There is a feeling of pinpricks and burning in the eyes. There is a kind of piercing pain inside the ears. **Brown moles, yellow spots and acne appear on the face**. Furthermore, the upper lip appears swollen to the touch, the face becomes pale, blue circles develop around the eyes and the eyelids become swollen.

The **stomach** of the Natrum Carb patient **is very sensitive to touch** and appears to be swollen. Drinking cold water aggravates the symptoms. The patient feels hungry in the morning at five o' clock. The digestive system becomes very weak. The patient feels very sad after eating food and the mouth tastes bitter. Drinking milk causes diarrhoea and the patient needs to rush to the lavatory.

The cough of the Natrum Carb patient is a **dry cough**, which worsens when the patient enters a heated room. The feeling of cold on the left side of the chest increases the cough. The heart palpitates quite fast when lying down on the left side at night and also on climbing the stairs. The patient wakes up very early in the morning and his **suffering is worse by five o' clock in the morning**. The patient sweats a lot in the morning and feels burning of the soles of the feet.

| | |
|---|---|
| Antidotes: | Camphora, Arsenic |
| Potency: | 30 to 200<br>However, Dr. Boericke has described its use only in potency 6 |

# NATRUM MURIATICUM
## (Sodium Chloride)

In homoeopathy, Natrum Muriaticum is a wide acting remedy, despite the fact that it is simply the homoeopathic potency of the common table salt we consume daily. Sodium Chloride is abundantly present in the human body. It plays an important role in maintaining the normal physiological functions of our body. Its deficiency results in different kinds of diseases. It is strange that a large variety of salts are always present in our mouth, Sodium Chloride being probably the most abundant. In spite of this, when even a minute dose of homoeopathic potency of Sodium Chloride is dropped into the mouth, it provokes an immediate body reaction. The salt already present in the mouth does not interfere with the body's response.

One of the diseases related to the excessive use of salt is high blood pressure (hypertension). Therefore, it is generally thought that to protect against high blood pressure and related heart problems, one should not consume too much salt. However, the research done by heart specialists in England and America does not support the general impression that those who consume less salt will not develop high blood pressure, and those who consume more, must develop high blood pressure. High blood pressure is an independent disease with its own specific causes. However, if someone is suffering from high blood pressure, it is better that he or she abstains from eating too much salt. A healthy person, however, may eat as much salt as he likes. The excessive salt is automatically excreted from the blood, through the urine or sweat. People who do not sweat due to some problem or have abnormal kidney function should abstain from consuming an excessive amount of salt. Excess salt in the blood increases the blood volume by retaining water, which will naturally lead to rise in blood pressure.

Salt is an essential part of human body. Its imbalance produces diseases. Excessive intake of salt will not produce any ill effects in those who have the habit of exercising daily, sweat profusely and also excrete the salt in their urine i.e. their kidneys are functioning normally.

Natrum Mur is a profoundly active, long-acting medicine. No part of the body is beyond its influence. Generally, the skin of a Natrum Mur patient is very shiny. Due to the increased content of water in the blood, the skin feels greasy as if oil has been rubbed over it. However, one should remember that every patient may not necessarily exhibit all the symptoms or that all the relevant symptoms must appear in each and every part of the body. For a remedy to be the exact match, the basic as well as distinctive symptoms must be present in a patient. However, it is not essential for every symptom to be expressed fully.

A patient of Natrum Mur feels **tired and weak**. Weakness, either physical or mental, is always found in Natrum Mur patients. This is due to the imbalance of Hydrochloric Acid, resulting in episodes of sudden severe weakness.

Natrum Mur is deeply related to malaria. In swampy areas, malaria spreads through mosquitoes. Malaria causes breakdown of red blood cells, resulting in anaemia and the resulting relative dilution of the blood (haemodilution). These signs require the usage of Natrum Mur, which otherwise, has no special affinity to wet marshy areas. The real connection of malaria is with the mosquitoes. Wherever mosquitoes are present, malaria must also exist. Generally, the mosquitoes are found in swampy and coastal areas. In such areas, naturally, Natrum Mur would also be required to treat malarial fever and is one of the best remedies against it. However, it should never be given to the patient while the malarial fever is still rising, because under these circumstances, Natrum Mur may produce serious ill effects or an immediate severe reaction. Several different ways have been described to use Natrum Mur. One is that either one should wait for the temperature to drop and then give the remedy, or it should be given in high potency during the interval between the two bouts of fever. In the case where Natrum Mur becomes effective, it will change the timing of the fever. The fever will either come on earlier or later than its usual time. If only the timing of the fever alters, but there is no decrease in the duration or the severity of the fever, it proves that the remedy has not been effective. In this situation, one must find another remedy without further delay. The appropriate remedy should either result in immediate disappearance of fever with no return, or will alter the timing and decrease the duration of the fever. The fever may not then return, or will be much milder. If so, the treatment should be repeated after the fever has subsided.

The mental signs of Natrum Mur are strange. In the beginning, the **patient feels victimized** and is always obsessed with the feeling of being a victim of some wrongdoings. Despite this, the patient does not like sympathy. Furthermore, the **patient gets captivated with imaginary love**. Even some old women get captivated with this kind of hypothetical love. If love could ever be cured with a medicine, then probably Natrum Mur will be the most appropriate.

If the fever does not subside for a long time and affects the brain, then Natrum Mur should be tried. Natrum Mur has been found to be specifically effective against the **bad effects of grief and sadness on the mind**. Ignatia and Ambra Grisea are the best and promptly effective remedies during the early stages of bereavement. Ignatia is a fast acting remedy, but its effect is very short-lived, so it needs to be given repeatedly. Once the deep grief becomes embedded into the mind of a patient, then he goes out of the range of Ignatia. Ambra Grisea works better in these patients. Next, comes Natrum Mur. It is my personal experience that with Natrum Mur, even the **totally insane** patient can be cured. Natrum Mur patients are not aggressive; rather they either sit quietly or **become indifferent to the world** altogether and then gradually become physically weak. They **get very angry**, yet do not show violence. Their mind becomes slow and weak. The patient, while talking, forgets and does not remember what he wanted to say. Concentration is lost. Break in the continuity of thoughts in the midst of talking is the symptom of Natrum Mur. However, if while listening, someone fails to understand or there is a delay in understanding, then, Plumbum will be more appropriate.

One symptom of the Natrum Mur patient is that **reading causes tiredness**. He tends to cry like a chronic Pulsatilla patient. The Pulsatilla patient tends to cry repeatedly, though mentally he is absolutely normal. The hands and feet of the Natrum Mur patient remain cold, and he is also weak. He is inclined to cry with or without a reason. If the **ill effects of grief** on the patient are not cured with Natrum Mur and the disease appears deep-seated, then Silicea might be helpful in such cases (Silicea is chronic of Natrum Mur). Silicea is also chronic of Pulsatilla. Natrum Mur should not be used repeatedly without good reason, because its excessive use can cause an imbalance of the salts in the blood. There is no harm in the occasional repetition of this remedy, but it should not be repeated too often in one day. The Natrum Mur patient feels very thirsty. During the **headache**, the patient feels as if being hit with a hammer over various parts of the head. Light hurts the eyes. Movement aggravates this condition. From this point of view, Natrum Mur resembles Bryonia. **Constipation** in Natrum Mur is more severe than that in Bryonia. Natrum Mur is the chronic, as well as the antidote of Apis.

The Natrum Mur patient suffers from **chronic backache**. He feels weakness in his arms, legs and particularly the knees. The **skin around the nails of the hands (cuticles) becomes fissured due to dryness** and the legs become insensitive.

The Natrum Mur patient does not like to eat bread or oily food. The patient feels very hungry but after eating food, he feels tired and weak. He feels burning sensation in the chest, also hardness and a piercing sensation over the liver. After taking food, the stomach becomes heavy and distended. Hunger pangs cause a fainting sensation over the stomach.

The Natrum Mur patient is highly strung and does not tolerate even the slightest noise. A sudden sound causes a headache. The patient is intolerant even to the rustling sound of paper.

The Natrum Mur patient is very cold. However, his symptoms aggravate in a heated room. He likes the open air. From this point of view, half of the constitution of Natrum Mur resembles that of Pulsatilla. Despite feeling cold, the patient likes to go in the open air. In the open, physical ailments ameliorate but the mental ailments aggravate. One must keep in mind these subtleties in the nature of this remedy. The constitution of a Natrum Mur patient changes frequently and rapidly. When the patient sweats, he catches cold, which however gets better in the open.

Natrum Mur affects the skin also. **Eczema, itching and inflammation** are found mostly at the hairlines. This is typical of Natrum Mur. Both dry pimples as well as discharging boils form. There is itching as well as a pins and needles sensation on the skin. Pus exudes from the itchy spots. Scabs also form, which then peel off in pieces. One symptom of Natrum Mur that resembles Sarsaparilla is that the patient starts **ageing prematurely.**

In Natrum Mur, the **headache** starts either after midnight or in the morning after nine o' clock. Severe morning headache is a symptom of Gelsemium. Usually in Natrum Mur, the ailments, which either start due to heat stroke or during malarial fever, continue from nine o' clock in the morning till night. The **headache usually starts at the nape of the neck** and spreads to the backbone. Natrum Mur is related to several back conditions. Especially if there is a sudden attack of "lumbago", then Natrum Mur works very well in the early stages. The symptoms of a Natrum Mur patient usually become worse on lying down in a soft bed. The backbone becomes relatively very sensitive. There is discomfort and pain along the nerves (sciatica). The patient feels comfort, when lying on a hard surface.

Symptoms related to the prostate gland are also present in Natrum Mur. There is considerable delay in the onset of urination. The urine comes in drops followed by the feeling of discomfort and unsatisfaction because of incomplete evacuation of the bladder. Sometimes, the patient feels pain either at the end of urination or afterwards. During walking, laughing or coughing, **urine may be passed involuntarily (stress incontinence).** For bed-wetting at night, Natrum Mur with Kali Phos is very useful. Usually this problem i.e. bedwetting is found in children during deep sleep.

In Natrum Mur, either there is **severe constipation** or diarrhoea. In Natrum Mur, the patient, despite having an excellent appetite, remains slim and thin. Along with a **burning sensation in the stomach**, there is palpitation. While eating, the patient sweats. The patient craves salt. He feels better on an empty stomach. After eating food, **there is heartburn and the acidity increases,** along with excessive salivation from the mouth.

As it has already been mentioned, Natrum Mur is an excellent treatment for **malaria**. Every type of malaria is included i.e. whether with daily fever or with relapsing fever. The most dangerous type of malaria is the one in which the fever returns every third day. This type of fever does not easily leave the patient. Natrum Mur is very beneficial in this kind of fever. Repeated use has proven that by giving Natrum Mur, the fever starts coming on the second day instead of the third day, and then slowly disappears completely in eight to ten days.

If the diseases of Natrum Mur have become very complicated or have become chronic due to the wrong treatment, then Sulphur 200 will be found very effective in delineating the underlying symptoms of these patients clearly. Sulphur, being a profoundly active remedy, may also cure some of these diseases. Natrum Mur also clearly brings out and clarifies the symptoms of the patients with complicated fevers that have gone out of hand. When the fevers become complicated, they may adopt different forms. **When malaria deteriorates further**, the symptoms become very complicated. Sometimes the symptoms appear as pain and at other times, they may appear in some other way. A very eminent English doctor has said about malaria that with the exception of pregnancy, it can mimic any disease. It complicates the symptoms so much so that doctors may not arrive at the root cause of the disease. In this regard, both Natrum Mur and Sepia play a very important role. When given in high potency to a healthy person, Natrum Mur sometimes proves to be very useful in protecting against the general tendency towards malaria. Similarly, Arnica 1000 (or higher potency) along with Arsenic 1000 (or higher potency) has often been found to be very effective when given as a precautionary measure against malaria.

In Natrum Mur, like Hepar Sulph, the patient feels as if something has got **stuck inside the throat**. The patient tries unsuccessfully, again and again to remove the entrapped thing from the throat. He feels as if a thorn is stuck inside. However, if something like fishbone or something else is really stuck in the throat, then Silicea has the ability to expel it. Sometimes, in Natrum Mur, the throat becomes very dry and ulcers develop.

Soft **swellings**, which pit on pressure, resembling those resulting from a honeybee sting, are also found in and are treatable with Natrum Mur. That is the reason why Natrum Mur is very effective in **treating the symptoms of bee-sting**. If Natrum Mur is used in combination with Arsenic and Ledum, it benefits the patient astonishingly fast. Furthermore, Carbolic Acid is very famous as the fast acting antidote of bee-sting venom.

Natrum Mur is chronic of Apis. Chronic means that if a remedy, which works for a short while and then stops working, then another remedy takes its benefits further. The second remedy is called the chronic of the first. The swelling of the Apis, if not fully cured with Apis, will completely disappear when treated with Natrum Mur. Similarly, some other diseases, which are not completely cured with Apis, will also be cured when the patient is treated subsequently with Natrum Mur. Therefore Natrum Mur is called the chronic of Apis.

Natrum Mur is a good **treatment for weakness following childbirth**. If a woman's general health weakens after delivery, apart from Kali Carb, Natrum Mur is also very effective. Natrum Mur restores the health of the woman. If **post-childbirth backache** is not cured with Kali Carb, then it can be cured with Natrum Mur.

If there is some kind of deficiency in the mother's milk, due to which the child is not thriving normally or the milk dries up too soon, Natrum Mur should be used. Natrum Mur rectifies the internal defect due to which the child does not grow properly, as well as increasing the quantity of milk according to the need of the child. Natrum Mur is the best **treatment of the emaciating, underfeeding and wasting disease of the children** (Marasmus). The emaciation process starts from the upper part of the body and then spreads downwards. Sometimes, this disease is secondary to some disease of the mother; therefore the mother should also be treated.

**Irregularity of periods**, excessive bleeding, **leucorrhoea** causing burning and itching, depression and sadness before the onset of periods, heaviness in the lower part of the abdomen getting worse in the morning, are all the symptoms of Natrum Mur. The **gums become swollen** and bleed. **The teeth become loose and sensitive to cold and cold air**. Teeth hurt after eating food and at night, and the pain may also spread to the ears. A layer of dirty foam-like material deposits over the tongue. There is a feeling of hissing, as if a hair is stuck on the tongue.

The heart beats fast on going up the stairs or lying on the left side. Furthermore, there is a feeling of cold over the heart. There is a feeling of tightness and suffocation in the chest.

**Whooping cough with watering of the eyes, severe headache and also worsening of the cough on movement** on taking deep breathing and upon getting warm in bed are common symptoms of Natrum Mur. The symptoms of Natrum Mur aggravate in the coastal areas.

| | |
|---|---|
| Adjuvants: | Apis, Sepia, Ignatia |
| Antidotes: | Arsenic, Phosphorus |
| Potency: | 6X to 30 or even to CM |

# NATRUM PHOSPHORICUM

## (Phosphate of Sodium)

Natrum Phos is a compound present in the blood, muscles, nerves, brain tissue and various secretions of the human body. It keeps the sugar level balanced and is very good for the **treatment of high blood sugar**. However, its general symptoms include nervous tension and its related ill effects, mental disposition, fear and anger. Furthermore, Natrum Phos is very **effective against the diseases resulting from moral transgression and inappropriate sexual conduct during the youthful years**. Usually it is given in 6X potency. If the desired results are not produced with 6X, then it becomes necessary to give the remedy in potency 30 or 200 or sometimes even in higher potency.

Natrum Phos has a deep relationship with the formation of red cells in the blood, although Ferrum Metallicum or Ferrum Phos are the actual remedies for treating the deficiency of red blood cells. However, sometimes these remedies by themselves are not effective. When Ferrum Phos and Ferrum Met are given in combination with Natrum Phos, this becomes a very good treatment for **iron deficiency anaemia.** For the treatment of iron deficiency, at the beginning, Ferrum Phos, Kali Phos or Calcarea Phos should be given. These are the best treatment for iron deficiencies in pregnant women. However, they should not be used continuously. After being used for some time, they should be stopped and then given again. If this formula does not work and the blood deficiency in women, whether pregnant or not, needs to be corrected, then Natrum Phos should also be added. Natrum Phos is very useful in the treatment of both blood deficiency and diabetes.

One symptom of Natrum Phos is that the patient does not like open air. The patient of Natrum Phos, like that of Sulphur, dislikes taking a bath and there is a **tendency to permanent nasal catarrh**. Hunger is unbearable and satisfied only by taking a lot of food. The patient does not like greasy heavy foods, vinegar, fruit and milk, etc. The dislike for fatty foods resembles Pulsatilla.

When due to prolonged illness, the **body secretions dry up** and the **digestive juices decrease**, Natrum Phos does an excellent job of rectifying them. However, China has clear superiority over Natrum Phos.

Sometimes a **part of the body becomes numb**. If the hand, finger or a part of the ear becomes numb, Natrum Phos is a good remedy. Similarly Natrum Phos is useful, if the blood rushes to a particular part of the body. **Sudden body shakes at night** and associated sharp pain along the course of the arteries is also one of the symptoms of Natrum Phos. But in all these conditions, Natrum Phos will be effective only if it matches the constitution of the patient. Otherwise, these conditions may resemble several other remedies, though every one of them cannot be a match. Sometimes, while lying in the bed, the body may suddenly start to shake violently.

Natrum Phos is very effective in the treatment of **weak musculature and nervous tension especially affecting the eye**, as well as in the treatment of muscular twitching. Since the patient of Natrum Phos suffers from hyperacidity in the stomach, it also reflects in the sourness of their perspiration and on their person. This pungent type of smell does not remain unnoticed by others.

**Sometimes, on hearing some bad news, a patient becomes totally mute.** In this condition besides others, Natrum Phos produces an immediate benefit, safeguarding against future dangers. Otherwise, the patient may either become insane or start having fits of hysteria. The **scalp starts itching** with yellow pimples. Natrum Phos is also **effective against eczema** over the forehead. If the head feels heavy and hairs start falling, then Natrum Phos is also useful. In general, there is no cure for baldness, however, **if hair loss is due to a particular deficiency**, then the hair loss may start to improve by itself when that deficiency is treated. In particular, there is a specific formulary that has shown extraordinary success in homoeopathy for **Alopecia**. In Alopecia, the hair on the head starts to come off in bunches. With appropriate treatment, the hair starts growing rapidly in a very short period of time.

In Natrum Phos, the **headache** becomes worse on mental exertion. The pain begins in the eyes, at the nape of the neck and temples with pins and needles and burning sensation. Natrum Phos is very beneficial **for the eyes** as well. If while reading, the right eye starts to twitch, Natrum Phos will be especially effective. If some other symptoms of Natrum Phos are also present, then Natrum Phos will be effective against **squint** also. If on being tired during the day, the patient sees stars dancing before his eyes, then Rhus Tox is the best, although Natrum Phos may also be effective. In Natrum Phos, yellowish fluid starts to flow from the eyes, and the eyes also become yellowish. The eyesight becomes foggy. There is an itching and burning sensation in the eyelids. The distant vision becomes weak.

The **patient hears all sorts of noises in his ears**. The hearing either increases or decreases. There is earache and a pins and needles sensation behind the ears. Only one ear becomes red, hot and itchy.

The Natrum Phos patient generally **suffers from cold and catarrh**. Thick secretions stick inside the nose. There is a **tendency to sneeze**. The sense of smell becomes sharp. There is irritation in the left nostril causing sneezing and the eyes start watering. Natrum Phos may be effective to treat the post-nasal drip of yellowish colour. In Natrum Phos, the **gums bleed**. A yellowish crust is formed on the tongue. The palate becomes yellowish while the mouth and tongue become dry. **Children grind their teeth at night**. The teeth decay, the **cavities in the teeth due to excessive consumption of sugar**, respond well to Natrum Phos.
Natrum Phos may be useful in the treatment of **peptic ulcers of the stomach**, resulting from hyperacidity, associated with throbbing pain and a piercing sensation over the stomach.
The symptom of diarrhoea alternating with constipation is common to many drugs. If the constitution of such a patient resembles Natrum Phos, then Natrum Phos alleviates the problem. **Intestinal worms** are also treatable with Natrum Phos.

Some **children urinate on the bed during the night**. For this symptom, Natrum Phos, when given in combination with Kali Phos and Natrum Mur, is very effective. If one sweats a lot, then the urine output decreases. However it is strange that in Natrum Phos both sweat and urine increase. Natrum Phos may be useful for the **treatment of the diseases of the reproductive organs of both men and women** that are due to diabetes. If the uterus happens to sag from its normal position, hindering pregnancy, then Natrum Phos can restore the uterus to its original place and thus promote pregnancy.

Natrum Phos is also good for the treatment of a **dry hacking cough**, which starts with a hissing sound in the chest and trachea. A special symptom of Natrum Phos is that a 'bubble'seems to originate from the heart region and he has a feeling of constriction and tightness in the chest. The patient feels uncomfortable due to fullness in the upper part of the chest. Sometimes, there is pain also. After eating and on deep breathing, the blood vessels of the heart are compressed and the heart symptoms can develop. The heartbeat becomes rapid with anxiety. The noise aggravates the symptoms. Lying on the left side also aggravates all the symptoms, which are a prelude to heart disease. The palpitations increase on climbing the stairs.

The **backache during menstruation** responds very well to Natrum Phos. However, according to my experience, Natrum Phos given in combination with Kali Phos and Mag Phos is much more effective.

Natrum Phos is very useful when the symptoms of tightness at the back, pain and sweating are more prominent. Natrum Phos may also be useful to control the cardiac pain felt on both sides of the neck. During menstruation, the hands and feet become cold especially during the day. Cramps on writing, the feeling of ants crawling over the arms and legs, the limbs feeling heavy and numb are all the symptoms of Natrum Phos. There is pain in the joints and a feeling of cramps and weakness in the legs. The joints crackle (crepitus). Joint pains usually start from the right shoulder and may sometimes remain limited to the shoulder area only. The whole body feels abrased. While walking, a leg may suddenly give way temporarily.

Dry pimples with burning sensation form on the skin, with golden yellow scabs. Red or yellow spots become visible on the body, as in Ferrum Phos. In Natrum Phos, the skin becomes pale. There is swelling of the affected area and the skin. There is a feeling of ants crawling. **Moles** also form.

Although the Natrum Phos patient sleeps a lot, the sleep is never deep. The patient sees worrisome dreams and may drop asleep while seated in a chair. Sleep overwhelms the patient after eating food.

| | |
|---|---|
| Potency: | 6X and 30 up to 200 |

# NATRUM SULPHURICUM

Natrum Sulph, which is made of two elements i.e. Sodium and Sulphur, has the ability to produce important internal body changes. It is intimately related to the liver and is very useful in **diabetes**. Natrum Sulph given once or twice a week, in potency 200, along with Calcarea Phos, Kali Phos and Natrum Phos, three to four times a day in 6X potency, has proven to be a widely effective formula for diabetes. Sometimes all these four remedies can be given in 6X potency with good results.

The symptoms of Natrum Sulph appear before midnight. In wet weather the symptoms become worse. Natrum Sulph patients are of very sensitive nature, physically as well as mentally. They are extremely sensitive to pain that is relieved on movement. The entire body seems to be hurting. The **catarrhal conditions** become more pronounced during spring. Natrum Sulph is an excellent homoeopathic remedy to protect against deep internal ill effects of a head injury. Natrum Sulph, in combination with Arnica, is very useful for the **treatment of an old head injury**. During **birth**, sometimes, the baby's head comes under severe pressure. Such babies must immediately be given Natrum Sulph through the mother's milk, so that the ill effects of the pressure may be averted and the child saved from becoming mentally deficient.

Natrum Sulph is also the best remedy for **asthma**, particularly in those patients, whose asthma becomes worse in humid weather. It starts with the nasal catarrh, which soon becomes worse and then invades the chest, leading to the onset of asthma. The cough with a lot of phlegm is accompanied by severe difficulty in breathing. The phlegm (expectoration) is whitish and sticky. The patient becomes short of breath on slight movement or walking.

In Natrum Sulph, there is a **tendency of mole formation** on the entire body. **Eczema over the head** is also a characteristic symptom of Natrum Sulph. Red spots form too.

**Eyes sensitive to light** respond well to Natrum Sulph. The eyes tend to water. If water flows out of one eye, associated with pain at the nape of the neck on the same side, this is an early sign of **glaucoma**.

For this, Calcarea Phos and Gelsemium are the best remedies. However, if the water flows out of both eyes and the eyesight has become weak then Natrum Sulph is the best treatment. If the eyes become yellowish and badly infected, with the formation of greenish coloured pus making the eyelids stick together, even then Natrum Sulph can be effective. **Noises in the ear**, associated with a feeling of pressure in the ear will also benefit from Natrum Sulph, if the patient is of Natrum Sulph constitution.

In Natrum Sulph, the ailments are more prevalent on the right side of the body than the left. If there is a tendency of **nosebleeds**, either before or after the menses, Natrum Sulph is well worth a trial. Natrum Sulph is also used during an **epidemic of influenza**. It may also be of significant use for the **treatment of the gums receding from the teeth;** infection of the throat, with the formation of thick **sticky phlegm and the feeling of suffocation or shortness of breath on walking fast**. Natrum Sulph is also useful in the treatment of goitre. Natrum Sulph is deeply related to the tonsils. If the glands have become enlarged and swollen inwardly and the patient vomits sour greenish material, then Natrum Sulph happens to be the unique homoeopathic remedy.

Natrum Sulph given regularly can even dissolve **stones in the gall bladder**. The other important remedy for this disease is Lycopodium in 200 potency, which with Chelidonium 30, should be given three times a day. If the **stomach becomes distended with gas and there are griping pains** or the abdominal glands have become enlarged and hardened, then also, Natrum Sulph is very beneficial.

When person contracts **sudden diarrhoea** on exposure to heat and the stools are copious offensive and greenish in colour and explosive; then besides many other possible remedies, Natrum Sulph can also be useful.

Natrum Sulph is considered to be one of the best **treatments for liver disorders**. Frequent nocturnal urination that is not due to diabetes may well be treated with Natrum Sulph.

Sometimes, either due to nervousness or due to change in weather, the **patient urinates several times during the night**. For this problem, Arsenic and other nerve related remedies could prove to be more beneficial. If one fails to work, then based on the situation, other remedies should be tried.

If the **prostate gland becomes enlarged** and other symptoms of Natrum Sulph are also present in the patient, then Natrum Sulph alone is sufficient to cure the disease. However, it would be better if Natrum Phos 30 or 200 potency is also given with Natrum Sulph.

A rattling of the chest due to sticky phlegm, deep severe pain in the chest on **coughing**, and a cough having become chronic, may all well respond to treatment with Natrum Sulph. The patient aspires to be able to take a deep breath. The chest hurts, especially on the left side.

Natrum Sulph is an excellent treatment for **meningitis** or swelling of the brain (encephalitis). If a child develops meningitis, then first of all he should be treated with Ferrum Phos, Silicea, Kali Mur, Mag Phos and Kali Phos in 6X potency. At the same time, Natrum Sulph in 200 potency should also be given two to three times a day. This prescription has proven to be very effective in the treatment of meningitis. If meningitis is not treated promptly, epileptic fits may ensue which may even become permanent. Especially if the fever is suppressed with antibiotics, then there is danger of long-lasting effects on the brain. Therefore, only the above stated prescription for meningitis including Natrum Sulph should be used. Meningitis may be cured within a few days.

**Body aches** generally become worse during humid weather. Natrum Sulph is also useful in the treatment of joint pains, which aggravate during winter and also against **severe body aches due to fever**. Natrum Sulph can also be useful to treat the warts on the hands and arms. Natrum Sulph in 6X potency has proven to be an extraordinarily useful treatment of eczema on the palms of the hands and the wet eczema between the fingers. Even if a disease has become chronic, it can be cured with low potency Natrum Sulph. However at times, based on the symptoms and constitution of the patient, it becomes necessary to change the potency of the medicine. Like Sulphur, in Natrum Sulph, there is a feeling of intense heat on the top of the head. After eating there is severe pain over the forehead, characterized further by **the heaviness in the head, pain at the nape of the neck and dizziness.**

One symptom of Natrum Sulph is that the **roots of the nails become inflamed (Paronychia)**. There is a burning sensation over the heels, and tightness and stiffness of the knee joints. **Pain in the hip joints, hands and feet** aggravate during humid weather. Natrum Sulph plays an important role in maintaining the fluid imbalance in the body (i.e. between the blood and intra-cellular and interstitial compartments).

| | |
|---|---|
| Adjuvants: | Arsenic, Thuja |
| Potency: | 6X and 30 up to CM |

# NUX VOMICA
## (Poison Nut)

Nux Vomica is prepared from the seeds of an evergreen plant. The scent of its flowers is rather unpleasant. Its fruit is of orange colour. The seeds of the plant remain wrapped under soft hair. The remedy is prepared by grinding the seeds. In traditional medicines, it has been used in the treatment of extremely serious conditions, like plague, hysteria, rheumatism and rabies. Since Nux Vomica seeds contain many poisonous substances, therefore the homoeopathic medicine produced from the seeds is extensively used as an antidote to many poisons. Patients who have used different medicines in large quantities should be treated with Nux Vomica in order to dispel their ill effects and to give the patient's body a fresh start.

Nux Vomica is very intimately related to Sulphur. While restoring the natural body responses, Sulphur produces painful **skin diseases**. Nux Vomica cleanses the body of these skin diseases without suppressing the diseases back inside the body. Thus, Nux Vomica works as an extremely potent adjuvant of Sulphur. It ameliorates the skin diseases without impeding the useful functions of Sulphur. If haemorrhoids need to be treated with Sulphur, then Nux Vomica should also be used with it. Nux Vomica proves to be the best adjuvant in abating the discomfort of **haemorrhoids**.

Nux Vomica is also useful in the treatment of different allergies. Some people develop an **allergy to rice or meat** and develop hyperacidity. By the grace of God, with the use of Nux Vomica, the patients find instant relief. Nux Vomica has not been mentioned in any of the literatures as a specific treatment for rice allergies but based on its symptoms; I have tried Nux Vomica on such patients. In spite of the fact that Nux Vomica is of a hot nature and the rice allergy is related to a humid climate, it relieves the symptoms of allergy to rice.

Indigestion produces **hyperacidity in the stomach**. The patient becomes peevish and easily enraged. Such patients are usually thin and skinny. However, sometimes even fat people can develop hyperacidity in the stomach. For them, there are many other remedies available. Nux Vomica is the ideal homoeopathic remedy for the treatment of rather skinny, peevish and irritable type of people. Such patients have certain habits that make their symptoms worse. For example they remain awake late at night, they work for a long time in a sedentary state and they do not exercise regularly. Excessive drinking in the western culture or eating too much oily food in the eastern culture produces hyperacidity. All such patients benefit from Nux Vomica.

Apart from the digestive system, Nux Vomica does not have any profound effect on other major internal organs. However, it does affect the external musculature, mucous membranes and the skin. A **backache developing from sitting for too long** can be cured with Nux Vomica. The Nux Vomica backache is usually localised at one particular area. If other symptoms of Nux Vomica were present, including **gastric hyperacidity**, then the profound weakness which appears suddenly in such patients would also be cured with Nux Vomica. During this weakness, the person may not even be able to move his hands. The patient feels instantly rejuvenated with Nux Vomica. It should be given in potency 30 to be repeated every few minutes.

The Nux Vomica poison slows down the peristaltic movement of the intestines. In healthy people, after taking food, the peristalsis beginning at the stomach must continue to the end of the intestines, so that the semi-digested food may be passed on. Normally this cycle should complete in fourteen hours. After fourteen hours, the contents remain inside the large gut to allow for the absorption of excess secretions. Thus a healthy person normally has one motion in twenty-four hours. If the system of peristalsis slows down the person becomes **constipated**, and if it becomes too speedy then **diarrhoea** develops, or sometimes the patient may have frequent solid motions, one after the other. Nux Vomica is an effective treatment specific for this condition.

**Gastric dysfunction** can often aggravate **asthma**. So asthmatics should avoid eating food that may upset their stomach and also food causing irritation of throat. Such foods would always precipitate their asthma. Extremely cold or sour things like pickles can also be very dangerous to asthma patients. Nux Vomica is very beneficial in the **treatment of asthma due to hyperacidity**. To prevent against the asthma related to the nasal cold, one should keep taking prophylactic

Lachesis

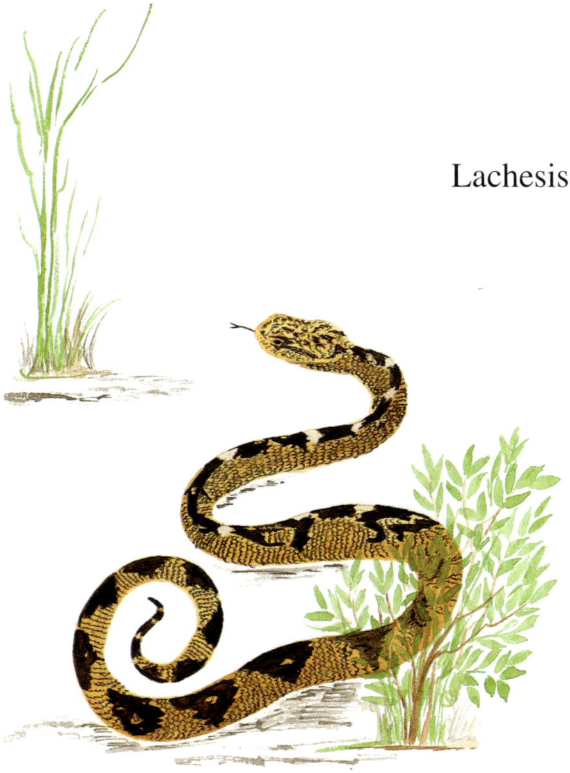

Laurocerasus

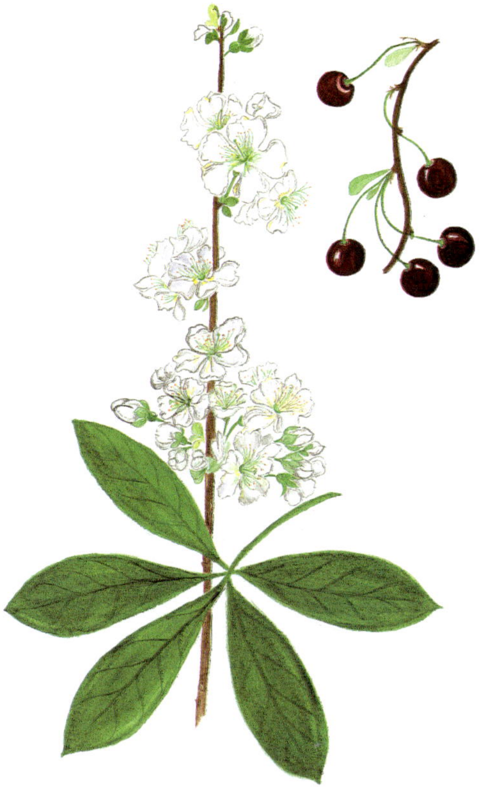

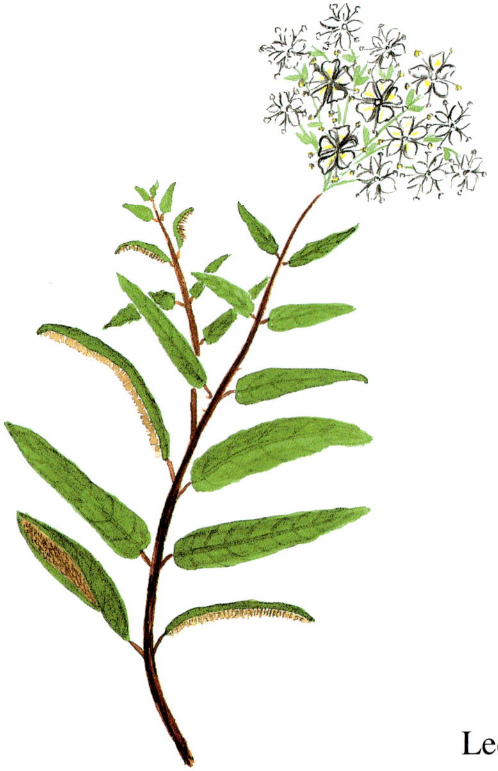

Ledum

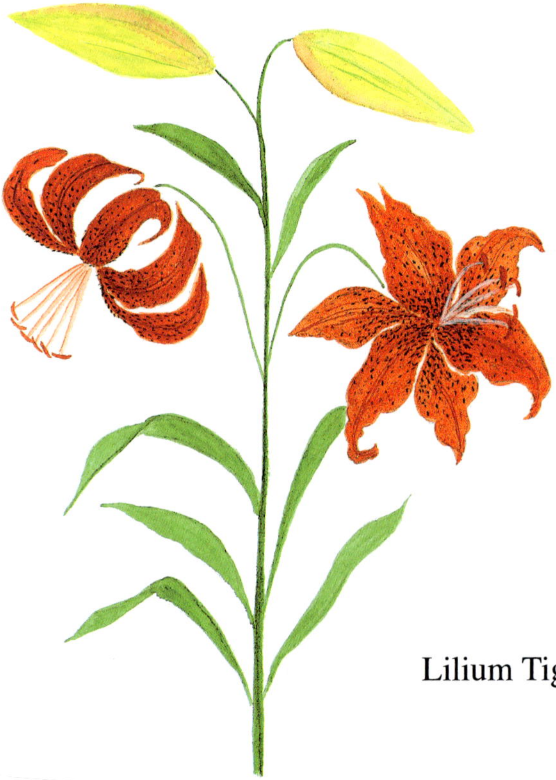

Lilium Tigrinum

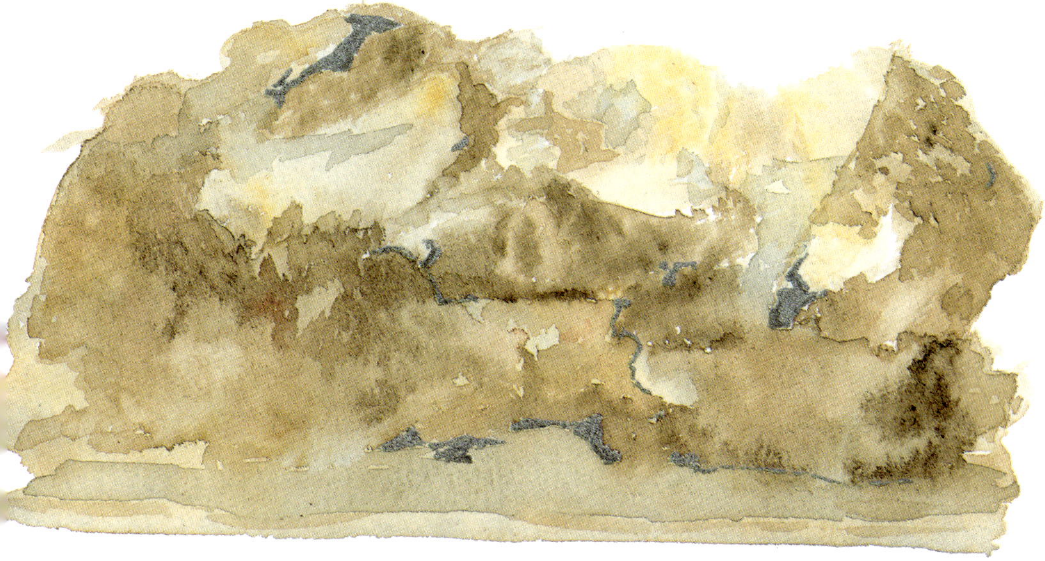

Mercurius

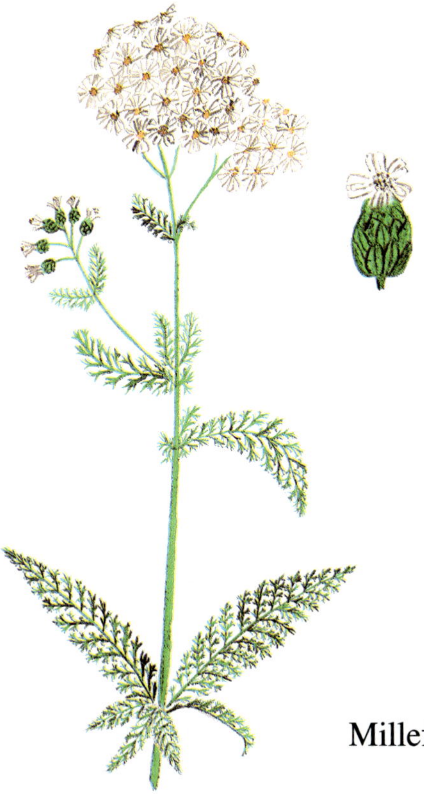

Millefolium

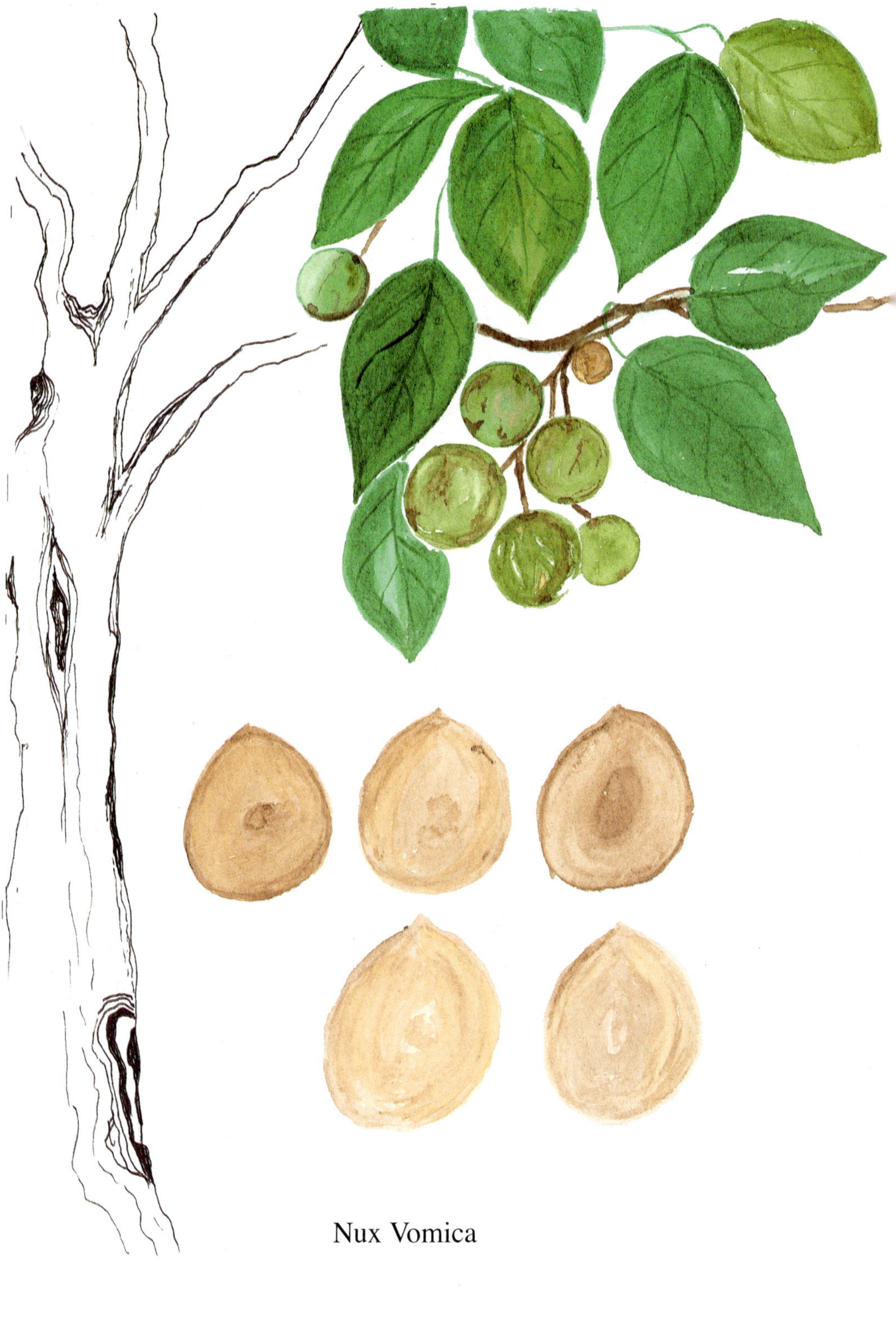

Nux Vomica

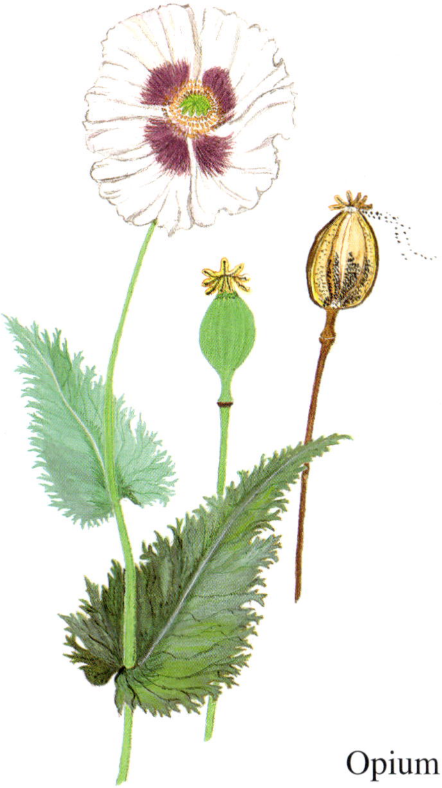

Opium

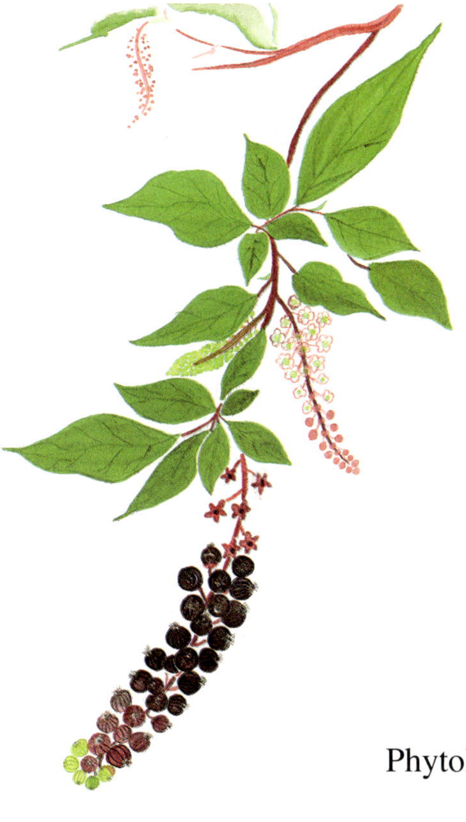

Phytolacca

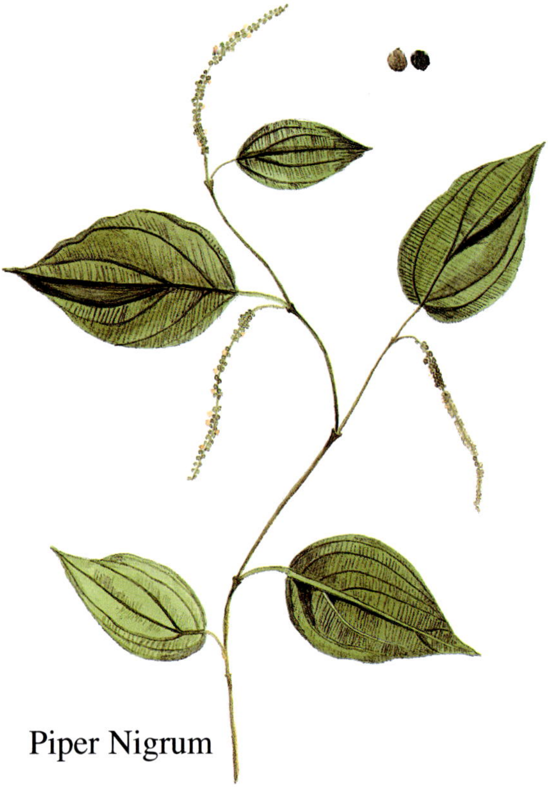

Piper Nigrum

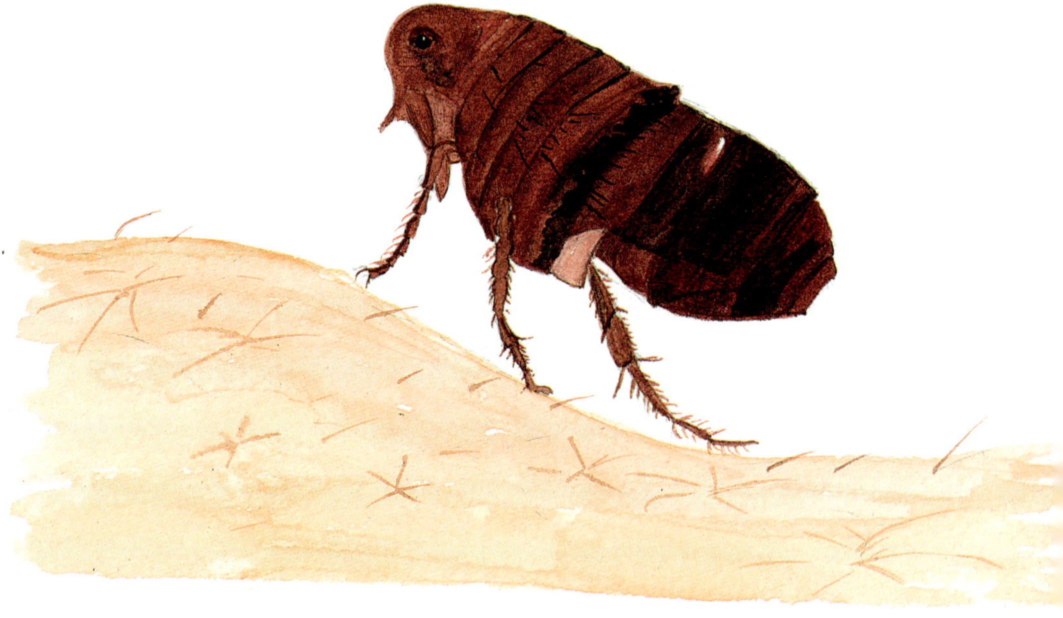

Pulex Irritants

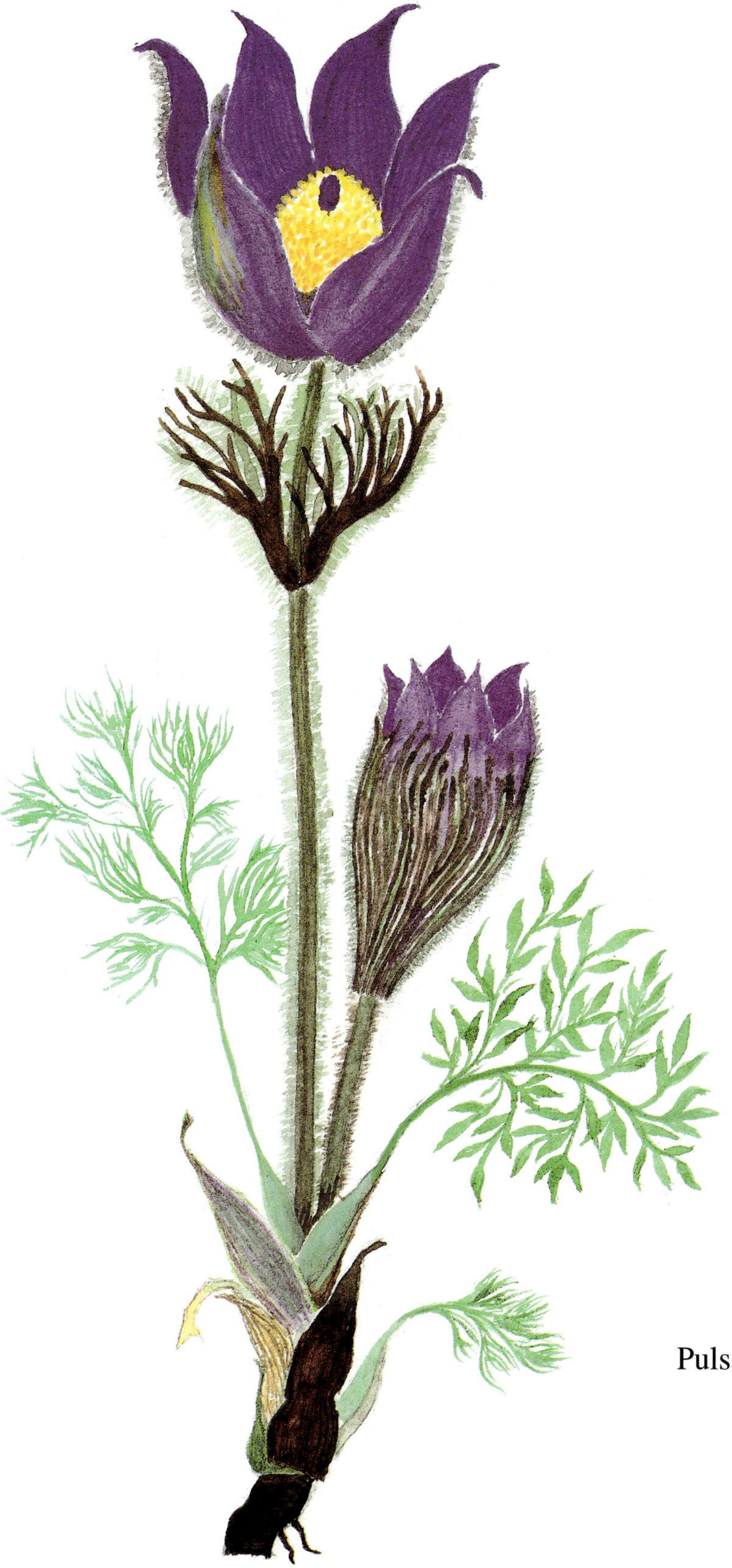

Pulsatilla

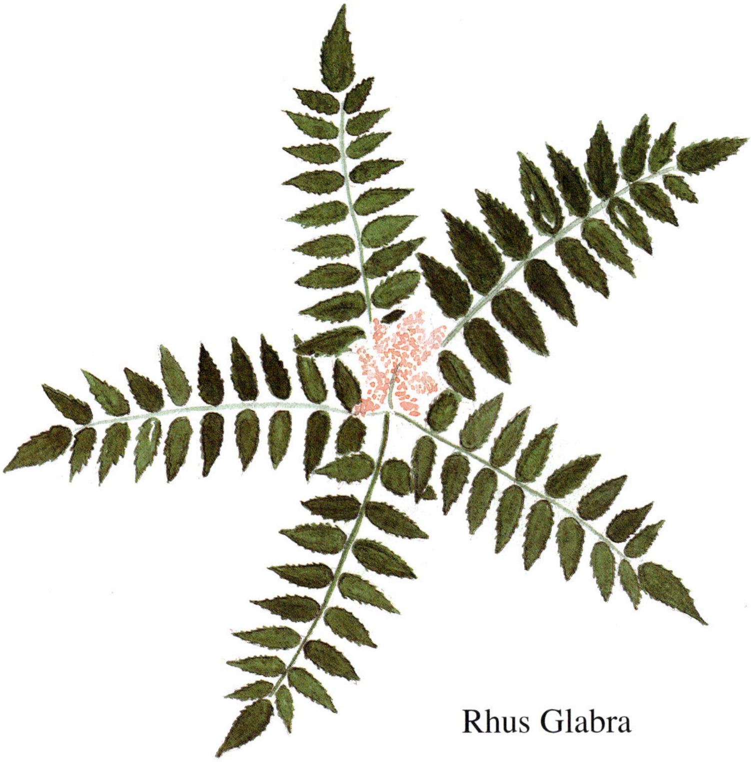

Rhus Glabra

Rhus Toxicodendron

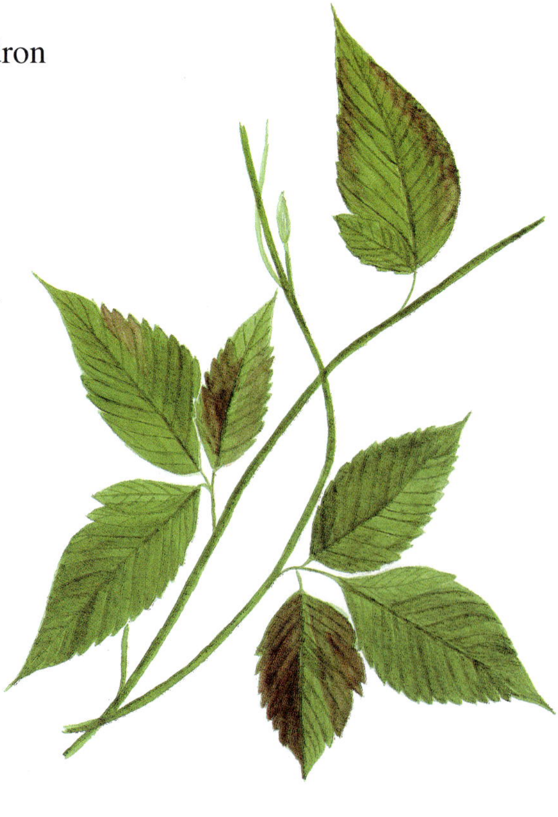

remedies, so that the patient neither catches cold nor develops asthma since prevention is better than cure.

Nux Vomica is also useful in the **treatment of leg cramps**. Given at the outset it offers instant relief. If the cramps are associated with symptoms like Belladonna, even then Nux Vomica, by itself proves to be curative. Regarding the cramps associated with Nux Vomica, there is some contradiction in that the backache becomes worse in the cold and the stomachache becomes worse from heat. The reason for this is that Nux Vomica contains many chemical compounds which behave differently on different occasions. Nux Vomica contains Belladonna and Cuprum, so some of the symptoms of Nux Vomica may aggravate from heat.

Nux Vomica has proven to be the best general remedy for the **treatment of common day-to-day leg cramps**. It is also very effective in the **treatment of sleeplessness**. For example, Nux Vomica is the **best alternative for drug addicts** and people with the habit of taking sleeping pills. I often start the treatment of drug addicts with Nux Vomica. With some exceptions, all the patients have benefited from the treatment. Once, a young drug addict was brought to me by his parents. Obviously, they were very worried and dismayed. The patient was being treated for drug addiction with sleeping pills, yet he could not sleep even with heavy doses of hypnotic medicines. I advised him to take Nux Vomica 30 three times a day, and kept his sleeping pills with me. I assured him that if he could not go to sleep during the night, he could come and take the sleeping pills back from me in the morning. That night, for the first time in a long time, the patient enjoyed sound sleep. In the morning he told me that with sleeping pills, he could never have comfortable sleep, whereas with Nux Vomica, he had slept comfortably. His sleeping pills remained with me for a long time as a souvenir. Thus, Nux Vomica has proven to be a very useful medicine for **treating the side effects of drug addiction** and also for getting rid of the habit of using sleeping pills. If Nux Vomica alone is not fully effective, Chamomilla should also be given along with it. Together, besides acting as sedatives, they also dispel the ill effects of the addictive drugs.

Nux Vomica is the best remedy for **sleeplessness** resulting from a heavy workload, lengthy talking or some sort of mental anguish. Nux

Vomica is also an excellent antidote for the ill effects of coffee. By the grace of God, the people who lose sleep due to drinking coffee can instantly go to sleep with just one dose of Nux Vomica. The patient goes to sleep right away without a feeling of preliminary drowsiness.

**Morning dizziness** is a symptom of Nux Vomica. Probably, the patient did not get a good night's sleep and the mind was not properly rested, resulting in dizziness. In some sensitive individuals Nux Vomica 200 can cause sleeplessness. Generally nux vom 20 is more effective for sleep than Nux Vomica 200. One learns the proper use of the potencies from keen observations and long experience.

If the **nasal discharge solidifies** clogging both nostrils, it produces severe headache. The pain becomes worse on bending forward. The patient feels pressure inside the head. The **nose remains blocked** all the time. This condition is called a sinus problem. Nux Vomica 1000 given at night proves to be extraordinarily effective. By the morning, the patient sneezes a lot, expelling the liquefied nasal discharge and clearing the nose. There are some other possible remedies too for this condition. However, one should always start the treatment with Nux Vomica.

One symptom of Nux Vomica is that **in women, menstruation becomes irregular**. If the periods start earlier than the usual time, they become prolonged. However, if the periods start delayed, they stop relatively earlier. Bryonia also has a similar symptom, with the difference that in Bryonia, the menstrual irregularities become worse on movement. In Nux Vomica, the symptoms are not affected by movement.

In Nux Vomica, there is a feeling that the **uterus is prolapsing downwards**. There is a feeling of uneasiness in the bladder and one feels like passing urine frequently, but in small quantity. The patient develops **constipation**, which keeps alternating with diarrhoea. In Nux Vomica, the **haemorrhoids** itch a lot. The stools are rather small though frequent. The peristaltic movements of the intestines become slow. The stomach secretes an excessive amount of acid. However (unlike Pulsatilla), a Nux Vomica patient can digest oily food.

Nux Vomica is an excellent **appetizer** and an equally well appetite suppressant. Patients getting hunger pangs should be treated with Nux

Vomica. Many such patients can get an **asthma** attack due to hunger. Once they are treated with Nux Vomica, they do not get asthma.

In Nux Vomica, the **headache** begins mostly in the area above the eyes, getting worse on moving the eyeball. It feels like a stabbing pain. On going into sunlight or on opening the eyes in the sunlight, the headache intensifies. The headache aggravates in the morning and after eating food. Sometimes during the headache, the patient may also bleed from the nose. Severe constipation is common. The headache is also related to haemorrhoids. The patient cannot tolerate noise or touch. The mouth tastes bad. **In the morning, the patient feels nauseated** but does not vomit. After eating food, the **patient feels pressure and pain in the stomach**. The patient cannot tolerate even light pressure on the stomach. The lower part of the stomach appears swollen and heavy like a stone. **At the onset of an asthma attack, the cough begins a day before the stomach upset**. The chest rattles with the accumulation of secretions in the lungs. Other symptoms of Nux Vomica are a dry or suffocating type of cough associated with blood in the sputum, the **onset of headache and backache on coughing**, a burning sensation in the backbone which becomes worse at three or four o' clock in the morning, and relief of suffering on resting at noon time and on sweating. In Nux Vomica, **small sores develop inside the mouth**. The margins of the tongue become yellowish-white and fissured. The **gums become swollen**, are white and bleed. There is a feeling of being choked and pinching in the throat, which appears to be spreading to the ears.

There is an interesting symptom of Nux Vomica. Some **bad-natured and malicious persons** always backbite and keep finding faults in other people. Treatment with high potency Nux Vomica restores their normal thinking. They do not remain jealous of others either. However, it is not essential that every Nux Vomica patient be of jealous nature.

A Nux Vomica patient wakes up in the later part of the night and cannot go back to sleep again. He feels drowsy in the morning. He may feel **sudden weakness in the arms and legs**. The symptoms become worse after eating food, mental overwork, eating oily spicy food and in dry cold weather. The patient feels better in the evening, on taking rest, on being pressed locally, and in humid climate.

| | |
|---|---|
| Adjuvants: | Sulphur, Sepia |
| Antidotes: | Coffea, Ignatia, Cocculus |
| Potency: | 30 to CM |

# OPIUM
## (Dried Latex of the Poppy)

The Poppy plant is abundantly grown in Eastern countries like Turkey, Iran, Afghanistan and the Indo-Pak sub-continent. Its flowers can be of various colours. Its petals are very soft and tender. They easily fall and disperse with the wind and even light rain. The juice squeezed out of the capsule containing the seeds contains two alkaloids and many other chemical substances. Morphine is prepared from the shavings of the plant. In allopathy, Morphine, the most important component of Opium, is used as a hypnotic and as an analgesic for the quick control of severe pain. According to Dr. Hahnemann, it is more difficult to understand the effects of Opium in comparison to other remedies, because of its contrasting mode of action. A change in the amount of this drug produces opposing effects. For example, a small dose of Opium allays nausea and vomiting, while a larger amount induces nausea and vomiting. An Opium patient is insensitive, but on the contrary can be extremely sensitive too. In allopathy also, the effects of Opium have been divided into the primary and secondary type.

It is said that the initial action of Opium is to ameliorate the pain sensation, but after some time, the same patient becomes hypersensitive to pain and in fact experiences more pain than before.

Opium exhibits some of the symptoms of Arnica also i.e. a dry nature, the thickening of the blood (hyper-coagulable), and the tendency to clot. The Homoeopathic form of Opium, like Arnica, works as a blood thinner and helps in the dissolution of a clot already formed (anti-coagulant and thrombolytic). In particular, it is a must in the treatment of clotting of blood inside the brain (**cerebral thrombosis**). In case of **sudden rupture of the arteries in the brain** (cerebral haemorrhage) causing **unconsciousness,** prompt administration of Arnica and Opium given together in very high potency, works wonderfully well. In this situation, Arnica alone is not of much use. Arnica and Opium given together give a new lease of life to the blood. The patient starts to gain alertness, the body starts warming up and the coagulability of the blood becomes normalized.

As already mentioned, Opium is a strong hypnotic. The patient of Opium remains either asleep or drowsy. On the other hand, he may sometimes be unable to sleep altogether. In Coffea also the patient loses sleep and becomes hypersensitive. When unable to sleep, the Opium patient becomes hypersensitive, restless and confused. If the patient loses sleep due to Opium, then Coffea will induce sleep. If the patient loses sleep after drinking coffee, then Nux Vomica as well as Opium will help the patient go to sleep. People suffering from **severe constipation** with the dried up intestines and who have no feeling for opening the bowels, can be treated with Opium. Sometimes, the Opium patients can suffer from dysentery associated with severe gripes. The stools are very soft.

A typical patient of Opium is a **complete coward**. He is scared of the dark. His thoughts are fearful. He lacks comprehension so much so that he cannot even understand his own disease. He remains drowsy or semi-conscious. On beings startled, he feels **dizzy**.

Opium resembles Sulphur also. Sulphur stimulates the natural percepivity of the patient. Sometimes, even the true homoeopathic remedies fail to work as expected; a dose or two of Sulphur makes them effective once again. Opium also, reactivates the suppressed and inactive body defences. Moreover, a typical Sulphur patient also happens to be extremely lazy and a philosopher.

In Opium, the **muscles at the upper end of the throat become weak**. They **cannot direct the food to the gullet, which may then enter the nose or the windpipe and cause severe choking**. The person can even die. Opium plays a significant role in averting this tendency.

The Opium addict can be extremely insensitive and unresponsive to his own sickness. His mind remains preoccupied with all kinds of fears. He has to be subjected to treatment under duress.

Similarly, Opium produces dryness in the body. However, during a fever, the patient may sweat profusely, yet the fever does not subside. This is peculiar for Opium. There is frequent hot sweating as during the summer rains. It does not lower the body temperature. Rather, it makes the patient feel hotter.

An Opium addict loves to eat. He is ever hungry but continues to feel weak. In spite of overeating, he is thin and lean. The patient vomits frequently after injection of morphine. With homoeopathic Opium treatment, the patient feels better. Opium can also be a good remedy for **vomiting during the pregnancy** untreatable otherwise. In Opium, the patient continues to feel hungry even when nauseated. However, soon after taking the food he throws up. **Due to a slow-down of the digestive system**, the food stagnates in the stomach, causing **nausea and vomiting**. Later on, the appetite is completely lost. The patient cannot eat any more and becomes very weak. In this particular situation, Chamomilla may be found as effective as Opium in controlling the vomiting. **Seasickness** can be effectively treated with Chamomilla or Opium used alone or in combination.

In Opium, the patient feels cramps in his head, hands and feet. **The hands are shaky and numb**. Tonic convulsions / spasms of the extremities are not uncommon. The limbs may also shake. The pupils of the eyes become dilated and show no reaction to light.

In an Opium patient, the **headache begins at the nape of the neck**, which then spreads downwards to both sides of the neck. The entire head feels numb and heavy. The patient becomes intolerant to the slightest movement like the blinking of the eye. Therefore, he remains lying down completely still with his eyes closed.

**The sudden spasm of muscles**, wrenching of the hands and feet and **convulsions** of all types may be treated with Opium if other symptoms of Opium are also present.

Opium plays a very important role in treating **meningitis**, which usually affects children severly. A timely use of Opium can save the child from serious sickness. In this condition, it is difficult to make the correct diagnosis based on the apparent symptoms alone. A good homoeopath should be well conversant with these remedies beforehand for their effective use.

If, **out of fear** a patient starts **suffering from spasm of the muscles**, wrenching of the hands and feet or starts having **hysteria or epilepsy-like fits**, then Opium should be given in high potency.

The severe form of epilepsy arising out of fear and tending to be permanent can sometimes be cured with a single dose of Opium in very high potency. It must be remembered that Opium will be effective in the **treatment of epilepsy arising only out of fear**. The epileptic fits associated with Opium usually occur during sleep. They begin with a scream. The patient has nightmares about black objects, devil, fire or massacre. A strange type of fear sets in the mind of the patient. Sometimes, he feels as if someone is taking him away. If besides fear, the **mind becomes affected due to sudden joyful news** leaving bad aftereffects, then the patient can be treated with Coffea besides Opium.

An Opium patient is given to gossiping and telling lies without any reason. Unfortunately, the patient does not realise this himself but continues in this bad habit.

**Lead poisoning** causes gripe and colic in the abdomen. A single dose of Opium can immediately relieve the colic. However Opium is not of much use in the treatment of chronic lead poisoning. It works only in the acute form of lead poisoning.

An Opium patient is always dozing. He has no special wish or demand. His pulse becomes slow. Generally, he is severely **constipated**. Sometimes, **out of fear**, he may develop **diarrhoea** passing dark offensive stools. The bladder becomes weak. The patient may have retention of urine or passes only scanty amounts. The hearing of the patient becomes unusually sharp. He can perceive noises from a great distance. The patient snores a lot and may even feel choked. The ailments become worse during sleep. His symptoms subside with cold drinks and on walking about.

In women, **periods may stop out of fear**. The **labour pains** may also stop during childbirth. The woman becomes **unconscious** and has convulsions. She may suddenly become unconscious or drowsy. Sometimes, she may even abort due to fear. Breathing becomes difficult. There is a sort of burning sensation inside the chest. During a severe bout of coughing, the face may become cyanosed interspersed with red spots.

In Opium, the patient is **insensitive to pain**. The nerve endings become functionally dead and unable to convey the true message of pain sensation. Thus, the wounds neither heal properly nor hurt. Homoeopathic Opium will rekindle the inner body response activating the natural defence system of the body.

| | |
|---|---|
| Antidotes: | Ipecac, Nux Vomica |
| Potency: | 30 to CM |

# PHOSPHORUS

Phosphorus is found in many different forms in nature. The most abundant form of Phosphorus is white Phosphorus, which is a highly inflammable and a fluorescent solid substance. On heating, white Phosphorus changes into a red coloured powder, which is used to make matchsticks.

Phosphorus is an important component of animal and plant life also used in traditional remedies to treat various diseases. The powder form is used to prepare the homoeopathic remedy.

Phosphorus is a profoundly active and powerful remedy. It is deeply related to the functioning of inner linings i.e. the mucous membranes, nerve fibres, glands and the brain. It also affects bones and bone marrow. It is one of the best remedies for the control of **red bleed (arterial)**. It has no effect on dark coloured bleeding (venous bleeding). Therefore, it should be considered as a treatment of arterial bleed only.

Phosphorus is used for the **treatment of tuberculosis and brain tumours**. However, one has to be very careful in choosing its potency. One should always start the treatment with Phosphorus 30 and then if necessary, the potency may be gradually increased. It is a top class remedy for treating **bone cancer**. It is also very useful in the treatment of asthma. If asthma does not respond to the commonly used remedies and the symptoms of Phosphorus are present, then by the grace of God, the patient will respond well to Phosphorus.

Generally, the external symptoms of Phosphorus patients have been stressed so much in homoeopathic literatures that homoeopathic doctors have started to pay extraordinary importance to these symptoms. Yet, if the internal symptoms are present, then, whether the external symptoms are present or not, the remedy works very well. It is said that a Phosphorus patient is skinny and tall. He has conical fingers and possesses an artistic mind. The patient is of extremely fair complexion, has blond hair and light coloured eyes. He happens to be tender and sensitive. Obviously, it is very difficult to find a person with all these features and characteristics. Furthermore, in some countries, one will rarely encounter such a person. Even if such a person is found, he may not necessarily be of the Phosphorus constitution. A Phosphorus patient should not be identified based on his physical appearance rather; the identification should be based on the constitution of the patient. One must definitely keep in mind the sensitive nature of the patient. Phosphorus can be recognised on the basis of the behaviour of certain diseases. For example, in certain diseases of women, the hands and feet become cold. The patient loses the courage to fight the disease and the body temperature falls sub-normal. All these are the symptoms of Phosphorus. It does not matter if the patient is black or white. Sometimes, the patient's **hands and feet become cold** in the diseases of the bones, chest and kidneys. Since these are the symptoms of Silicea also, therefore treatment by alternating Phosphorus with Silicea benefits the patient more.

One of the symptoms of Phosphorus is the red bleed whereas in Sulphur, the bleeding is dark. In women, during their period, **bleeding of a bright red colour before the actual period** is due is a specific symptom of Phosphorus. The discharge of Phosphorus is usually acidic. The **leucorrhoeal discharge is also excoriating**. The **diarrhoeal stools are acidic** to the extent that they cause blisters on the skin.

Phosphorus also resembles Natrum Mur and Bryonia. In Bryonia, **crusts form on the lips**, which fissure at their edges due to severe dryness. Phosphorus also exhibits these symptoms. Some symptoms of Platinum may also be present i.e. the patient becomes aloof and thinks himself superior to others. The Phosphorus patient may remain aloof simply being honest and straightforward. However, the patient is not arrogant, like Platinum. The Platinum patient thinks of himself as special and despises others. The Phosphorus patient is very kind and polite to others. His gentle nature makes him extraordinarily sensitive, which may sometimes cause certain diseases. Sometimes, when alone fear of death overcomes him or he may become mentally agitated. He feels as if something is creeping inside his body.

Many of the Phosphorus ailments ameliorate with heat, while the stomach and the head feel better in the cold. Because the pressure inside the head is already high, application of heat will make the headache worse. The main difference in the **headache** of Phosphorus and that of Belladonna is that the Belladonna patient feels comfort on lying down, whereas the headache of Phosphorus aggravates by lying down. Therefore, the Phosphorus patient keeps his head elevated while lying down. In Belladonna, the headache is associated with cramps, whereas in Phosphorus the headache is without cramps. Cold things improve the stomach complaints, while hot things cause vomiting. In a child the ingested milk, warms up in the stomach after a little while and causes vomiting. This symptom is similar to Aethusa.

Phosphorus is closely related to the nerve fibres. It also affects the visual mechanism of the eye. The patient sees many colours. The patient sees a green halo around the light and also notices red and black spots. When someone becomes **suddenly blinded due to unexpected shocking news**, he should be treated with Phosphorus.

Phosphorus is also an effective treatment for **baldness and dandruff**. These conditions are usually treated with Acid Phos. However, if the nerves become highly sensitive then Phosphorus is better. Phosphorus strengthens the hair and prevents hair loss. Thin blond hair considered to be the symptom of Phosphorus, are in fact due to the weak hair roots. It is the weakness of the hair follicles that make the hair soft and silky. Such kind of hair is a symptom related to Phosphorus. Skin problems arise due to lack of pigmentation. **Albino** children, i.e., the children with clear white skin as found in some forms of leprosy, are an example of Phosphorus. Thus, Phosphorus can be used in the treatment of albino children. Phosphorus is connected with the diseases in which the skin looks raw and the hair is unhealthy, regardless of the skin colour of the patient. Some of the symptoms are also found in Natrum Mur. For example in Natrum Mur, the hair becomes lifeless and split at the end. However, the skin neither becomes raw nor loses its normal lustre.

In Phosphorus, the **vision becomes foggy**. Besides Phosphorus, a green halo around the candlelight is found in Opium also. Opium can also afflict and paralyse the optic nerve. Phosphorus is useful in the treatment of many **eye diseases**. The Retina of the eye contains cones and rods. The cones are triangular in shape and are responsible for colour vision. They split the light into various colours. The rods help differentiate between white and black colours. If the retina becomes damaged or the optic nerve transmitting the message becomes weak, then the eyes cannot register various colours i.e. the person becomes colour-blind.

**Gradually progressive blindness** leading ultimately to complete blindness is a symptom of Phosphorus. This symptom is also found in Causticum. Many other symptoms of Causticum and Phosphorus also resemble each other.

The Phosphorus patient feels very thirsty. He feels comforted by drinking cold water. However, when the water becomes warm in the stomach, it induces vomiting. **Severe uncontrollable nausea developing after surgery** can be effectively treated with Phosphorus. Yellow spots develop on the abdomen, chest and parts of the neck, apparently due to a pigmentation disorder. This is in fact due to the weakness of the suprarenal glands. Phosphorus is extraordinarily effective against the kidney diseases.

Phosphorus is widely effective against the **diseases of the mouth**. When the gums become diseased and there is light red offensive bleeding from them, then Phosphorus is the most effective remedy in this condition. Phosphorus is the foremost remedy to stop bleeding. If, after **childbirth, bleeding continues for a long time** and smells putrid, Phosphorus often works. **Infections and tumours of the uterus** can also cause bleeding. Sometimes, the bleeding is without any bad odour, at least in the beginning of the bleed. Phosphorus is useful for this condition aswell. The **Hoarseness of the voice** is also a symptom of Phosphorus. Besides Phosphorus, Carbo Veg, Causticum, Borax and Coca are also well-known remedies for a hoarse voice. In Carbo Veg, like Phosphorus, the patient loses his voice in the evening, but the condition improves in the morning. In Causticum however the throat is hoarse in the morning and becomes better in the evening. In Phosphorus, irritation of the throat causes **coughing**. The cough starts either on laughing or on talking loudly, causing inflammation of the throat. Sometimes the cough starts due to itching of the throat. The phlegm dries up and sticks in the throat causing discomfort and more itching. For this problem, Rhus Tox and Hepar Sulph, depending upon the symptoms of the disease, can be useful remedies. The uneasiness and restlessness of Phosphorus is due to the increased nerve sensitivity. This symptom is found in almost all the diseases of Phosphorus. The symptoms become worse in the presence of strangers. The mind needs rest and cannot handle extra burden. Thus, the nerves become extraordinarily sensitive. Weakness is a common symptom of Phosphorus. Phosphorus acts slowly against the chronic diseases, while in acute diseases it acts fast. For the **joints of the hands, arms, elbows and the feet, becoming suddenly infirm**, Phosphorus can be useful.

Sometimes, the patient may be **restless during sleep**. The sleep is shallow. He frequently wakes up without any particular reason. This is due to mental anguish. Here, Phosphorus happens to act very fast. **Thunderous clouds make the symptoms of Phosphorus worse**. Sometimes, the symptoms of the disease begin to appear before the weather changes. Phosphorus patients can perceive such changes in weather, which cannot be detected with the most sensitive scientific instruments. Their suffering begins before the actual change in the weather takes place.

One symptom of Phosphorus is that climbing up the stairs makes the patient feel worse. However, this symptom per se is not related to any particular remedy.

Besides Natrum Mur and Nux Vomica, Potassium Permanganate is also an antidote of Phosphorus. Potassium Permanganate is very good in the **treatment of extraordinary hypersensitivity**. It is often used to prevent the numbness of extremities.

**Severe nasal catarrh**, which can only be treated with Phosphorus, but if not treated on time will become chronic. The mucous membranes of the nose become weak. Still, the treatment would be Phosphorus. The ill effects of Potassium Permanganate and Phosphorus on the throat and mucous membrane, i.e. the inner linings, are the same, however, the two are not identical with respect to their symptoms related to nervous system. Therefore, Potassium Permanganate cannot be used as an antidote of Phosphorus in all situations.

Phosphorus is an excellent treatment of fatty degeneration of the liver and other parts of the body. Failures of the liver and kidney, as well as fatty degeneration of the heart muscles, are the characteristic symptoms of Phosphorus. Phosphorus also protects from the ill effects of drinking. Phosphorus is very sensitive with respect to its action on the nerves. The liver is the smallest but most active yet silent chemical-manufacturing factory in the world. Almost five thousand chemicals are directly manufactured by the liver, while the rest are synthesised by various organs through the mediation of chemicals released by the liver. **Cholesterol** is also produced by the liver. The liver converts the normal fat into cholesterol. In some people, there is a familial tendency of overproduction of low-density of lipo-proteins LDL by their liver. Cutting down the fat in their diet will not help in lowering their blood cholesterol level. It is this type of cholesterol i.e. LDL which causes occlusion of the coronary arteries and predisposes to heart attack. Phosphorus normalises the function of the liver concerning the production of LDL and thus lowers the level of cholesterol in the blood.

Phosphorus is very effective in resolving nasal polyps, relieving blockage of the nose. The polyps and adenoid glands block the nose, forcing the child to breath through the mouth. The sense of smell becomes affected. The nose may bleed also. In the presence of such tendencies, Phosphorus could be useful in the **treatment of swollen uterine glands** in women.

In Phosphorus, the stomach problems and headache get better in cold weather. If the **bleeding starts due to high blood pressure**, Phosphorus helps to stop the bleeding. Once, a friend of mine developed a severe nosebleed in the middle of the night. I went to see him and found a pool of blood on the floor, as if a goat had been slaughtered. He was also bleeding into the mouth. I administered Phosphorus and Millefolium together, into his mouth, which was full of blood. Within fifteen minutes, the bleeding stopped and he went to sleep comfortably. Phosphorus is very effective in controlling unusual wound bleeds. The patient finds relief with cold and the bleeding stops by application of cold water. During a **headache due to severe hypertension**, there is a serious **danger of cerebral haemorrhage**. In this condition, cooling the head helps. However, it is absolutely essential to continue the treatment with Phosphorus in order to completely prevent this tendency forever.

Phosphorus is exceptionally effective in the **treatment of bladder and prostate cancers**. Against **bone cancer** also, Phosphorus has proven to be very effective. Once I treated a patient who had been given all types of radiation with Phosphorus 30. I told the patient to let me know of his condition after one month. After this time he told me that he was not losing weight any more and his appetite had significantly improved. Previously the patient's bones had become very weak. He could not walk or even stand on his legs and he had to use crutches. Within three months, his health improved so much that he walked without any support. The patient remained healthy for about eight years therafter, later developing brain cancer. By the grace of God, he was cured of the brain cancer also and lived for another fifteen years. Cancers have a tendency to recur therefore a cancer patient should be treated continuously. One must be very cautious in using Phosphorus because it is a very potent remedy. It should be avoided in high potency. Phosphorus is effective against cancer of the liver, bone, bone marrow as well as the lymphatic glands. One should always keep Phosphorus in mind while **treating the cancers of the throat, bones and bladder**.

One characteristic symptom of Phosphorus is that the **patient loses his voice due to ulceration in the throat**. In fact, the loss of voice is also a symptom of throat cancer. Thus if someone has an ulcer in the throat and loses his voice, treatment should be started immediately. If the treatment is delayed, the prognosis becomes gloomy and the cancer will become untreatable.

Sometimes, the muscles become flabby and the supporting tissues and membranes become weak. As after delivery, the muscles of the **uterus become flabby** and the **uterus tends to prolapse**. Furthermore, **hernia** and other similar conditions can develop. Phosphorus plays an important role in restoring organs to their original position by strengthening the musculature.

One symptom of Phosphorus (similar to that of Rhus Tox and Bryonia) is that initial movement causes discomfort. Later, the patient feels better. In Rhus Tox, the symptoms aggravate on lying down, and also at the beginning of the movement. Every time he changes his side, he feels uncomfortable. The Rhus Tox patient feels relief for a short while and then becomes rather more uncomfortable. The patient is restless. In Bryonia, the increase in the discomfort on movement is very prominent. This is the reason why in homoeopathy, Bryonia Alba 200 given in combination with Arnica 200, proves to be the best **treatment for fatigue following strong physical exercise**. In Phosphorus, particularly the patient's legs feel very heavy as he tries to stand up and walk, first thing in the morning.

Phosphorus is also a very effective **treatment for the generalised stiffness of the joints**. I have prepared two prescriptions for this

condition. If the **stiffness is on the left side of the body**, then Arnica, Lachesis and Ledum combined in 200, are very effective. This can be given to the patient repeatedly suffering from **chronic arthritis**. Despite the potency 200, they can be used three times during a day in the first week, twice a day in the second week and once a day during the third week. By the fourth week, when the full effect of the treatment becomes apparent, the patient will be found feeling surprisingly relieved and then fully cured of the disease. The second prescription is useful when the **pains are on the right side of the body** and the patient feels severe discomfort on movement and massage. In such a situation, Arnica, Bryonia and Causticum 200 are very effective. This triad is very effective for the **treatment of knee pain and the aches due to the sports injuries of the past**.
Phosphorus is an excellent remedy for **facial neuralgia**. Also, the following remedies are very effective when used in different combinations: Spigelia, Silicea, Phosphorus and Mag Phos. Phosphorus given in combination with Spigelia is a very good treatment in the neuralgia of the left side of the face. If the neuralgia happens to be on the right side, then Silicea along with Mag Phos proves very effective. Phosphorus also can be included in this prescription.

If the **men or women have been unable to have children due to heightened anxiety**, then Kali Phos and Phosphorus prove useful. Increased sensitivity of the nerves (premature ejaculation), in itself does not make a person sterile. However, the reproducing cells (the sperm cells and the egg) do not mature or become viable.

In Phosphorus, problems become worse on empty stomach. The **warts** (papillomata) tend to bleed. Sometimes, the warts fungate and look horrible, as in Nitric Acid. Bright red bleed is often a symptom of Phosphorus. The wounds bleed heavily. The wounds can apparently heal up only to reappear. **Bluish black spots** appear on the skin. The patient develops **jaundice** and feels cold in the evening. The patient feels rapid heartbeat while lying down on the left side. The pulse is fast but weak. The patient feels warm over the heart area.

The patient feels hungry immediately after eating food. The taste becomes sour. There is a tendency to vomit. The patient develops **stomachache**, which subsides on taking cold things. The **stomach becomes inflamed and painful**, more so on walking and putting pressure over it with the hands. The patient feels relieved by lying on the right side. There is pain and a burning sensation over the back, a feeling of heat in the area between the shoulders, numbness of the hands and fingers with a feeling of ants crawling, and a pain and burning sensation of the joints of the elbows and the shoulders.

In Phosphorus the **hearing** also becomes affected. The patient hears sounds echoing. The face becomes pale and bluish rings develop around the eyes. The jawbone becomes swollen and painful. **Sores develop inside the mouth**, which tend to bleed. Women develop muscular pains after washing clothes on cessation of their periods. The teeth also hurt.

The Phosphorus patient is very restless and anxious.

| | |
|---|---|
| **Adjuvants:** | Arsenic, Allium Cepa, Lycopodium, Silicea, Spigelia, Mag Phos |
| **Antidotes:** | Coffea, Nux Vomica |
| **Potency:** | 30 to 1000 and occasionally CM |

# PHYTOLACCA

## (Poke Root)

Phytolacca is prepared from the roots of a plant, the fruit of which is toxic when ingested in large quantity. The early symptoms of the toxicity are vomiting, diarrhoea and headache.

Phytolacca is a very important remedy. It resembles Mercury with respect to many of its symptoms. That is why it is also called Botanical Mercury. The diseases of Mercury become worse in the cold and humidity. At night also, the discomfort increases. In Phytolacca also, **backache** increases with cold and humidity. When the patient warms up in the bed at night, the pain intensifies further. All its ailments aggravate during the night. Both Mercury and Phytolacca are strongly connected to the diseases of the glands. Phytolacca acts as an **antidote to the toxic effects of Mercury**.

The feeling of pain and scraping of the skin over the sensitive area of the human body, where the skin is closely attached to the bone without the cushion of muscle or fat, is found both in Phytolacca and Mercury.

Both Mercury and Phytolacca are widely effective against **bone pain**. Eupatorium too is effective against **influenza** and **the fever associated with severe bone aches**. However, Mercury is the most important remedy for the treatment of bone problems. Mercury is very effective in the diseases in which the bones start to decay, with the formation of sinuses.

Phytolacca is very effective against the **lesions of the inner linings (mucous membranes), skin and throat as well as glands** that become hardened and have a tendency to produce pus. However, sometimes it becomes necessary to use Hepar Sulph or Silicea as its helpers. In Phytolacca, like Hepar Sulph, the **phlegm is thick and sticky**.

Phytolacca is the foremost remedy for the **treatment of syphilis**. It is also effective in **chronic syphilis and diphtheria**. **Chronic joint pains, including rheumatoid arthritis**, stiffness of the left shoulder and arm, a lightning type of migrating pain and the pain at the ankles and forefoot, are all the symptoms of Phytolacca. Phytolacca is also effective in the treatment of the cancer of the nose. The redness of the eyes, along with the flow of hot watery tears due to cold, a cough, sensitivity to light, a burning sensation with a feeling of sand in the eyes, the margins of the eyelids being hot, an abrased tongue and the feeling of a hot ball stuck in the throat, are all the symptoms of Phytolacca.

The Phytolacca patient often feels quite **dizzy**. He feels weak on getting up from the bed. The **headache** moves from the forehead towards the back of the head. The patient feels pressure in the eyes and the temples. The **headache becomes worse during the rain**. If there is itching on the head, accompanied with the formation of bumps and scabs, then Phytolacca can also be a good remedy.

Phytolacca is an exceptional remedy for breast-feeding women. If the **mammary glands become indurated and sensitive** with a tendency towards cancer, these women should be treated with Phytolacca without any delay. Besides Phytolacca, Bryonia, Belladonna and Conium can also be useful. In Belladonna, the mammary glands are not only hardened but also become red. However, in Bryonia, the glands harden, but there is no redness. Even the slightest movement is unbearable. In Bryonia and Phytolacca, the glands become stone hard. The milk of a Phytolacca woman is sour, poisonous and in clotted form. Breast-feeding the baby is very painful. The pain spreads throughout the body. (For details on Conium, please refer to the relevant chapter). Phytolacca is also useful for women in whom the **breast milk is either deficient of dries up completely**. Before and during the menstruation, the breasts become swollen and tender. In these women, the cold weather affects the mammary glands causing them to become painfully hard. The breast milk becomes thready like a spider web. If**, while breast-feeding, a women develops convulsions** and the pain spreads all over then Phytolacca is the treatment of choice. **Frequent menstruation and excessive bleeding** (menorrhagia) is also a symptom of Phytolacca. Usually these women develop a pain in the right ovary. In Phytolacca, the **stomach feels injured**. The vomitus is sticky. Phytolacca is also useful in the **treatment of nausea associated with pain** and a feeling of heat in the stomach, as well as **bleeding piles**.

Phytolacca is very useful in the **teething problems of the children**. Children clench their teeth forcefully leaving their marks on the tongue. Phytolacca ailments aggravate in humid and cold weather, during night and on movement. The discomfort subsides in dry, hot weather and on taking rest.

One form of Phytolacca called Phytolacca Berry is very famous in the **treatment of obesity**. I have treated several patients with it and have seen excellent results. Although Phytolacca is not as dangerous for the heart patients as Fucus, yet some patients with weak heart feel weaker while using Phytolacca. If so, Phytolacca should be immediately discontinued. Furthermore, the patients desirous of losing weight must, as a rule, be given Crataegus Q, which strengthens the heart. Fucus is more effective against obesity however it must be used with extreme care. As soon as the patient feels weakness of the heart, Fucus should be immediately stopped or there is a danger that the patient may have heart attack any time, which may prove fatal.

| | |
|---|---|
| Antidotes: | Belladonna, Meserium |
| Potency: | Usually 30 to 1000. CM as needed. |

# PICRICUM ACIDUM

## (Trinitrophenol)

Generally patients of acidic types are chilly and feel better in heat. However, in Picric Acid, patients are intolerant to heat and feel better in cold weather. Their ailments aggravate in hot weather, while the cold breeze feels very pleasant and soothing. Picric Acid is the drug of choice for this latter group. Picric Acid plays an important role in the **treatment of mental fatigue and general weakness**. Usually, the symptoms of mental fatigue appear in old age with the onset of **arteriosclerosis** i.e. the thickening, hardening and narrowing of the blood vessels going towards the brain and the resultant decrease in blood flow to the brain. Similar symptoms are also seen temporarily in "Brain Fag". The brain fag occurs due to a transitory spasm of the cerebral vessels decreasing the blood flow to the brain and is usually related to stomach upset. When a patient of arteriosclerosis develops stomach upset, the brain fag becomes more obvious. In brain fag, there is a sudden temporary loss of recent memory. For example, the patient forgets what he had eaten a few minutes ago and becomes angry with his relatives for not feeding him. He keeps on insisting that nobody does his work when in fact it has already been done. The patient is unable to recognise faces. **Loss of recent memory and retention of the old memory is typical of brain fag**. It is brain fag that is more pronounced in Picric Acid. There is no cure for the chronic mental deficiency resulting from arteriosclerosis. However, the severity of the symptoms may keep on fluctuating. If the symptoms like brain fag are not due to arteriosclerosis but due to some other temporary conditions, like poisoning and toxaemia, then the appropriate treatment can be readily effective.

The brain fag of Picric Acid closely resembles arteriosclerosis. Picric Acid is very useful in the treatment of frequent episodes of loss of recent memory. Picric Acid is beneficial for a **headache**, only if it is caused by prolonged mental overwork and a prolonged period of grief. Some students who are very hardworking, and are always **afraid of examinations develop permanent headache**. Picric Acid is an important remedy for these patients. Picric Acid is an effective treatment for headaches, no matter whether these are severe or not. Sleep comforts the Picric Acid patients.

In Picric Acid, the **eye muscles become weak** and the patient feels heaviness in the eyes. The feeling of dryness and heaviness and sand in the eyes, are very conspicuous. In Picric Acid, like Ruta, fine visual work hurts the eyes. The **strain of reading fine print hurts the eyes** also. When the muscles around the eyes become weak, this interferes with the performance of daily activities of life. Picric Acid is useful for relieving this weakness, as is Ruta. In Onosmodium also, the headache starts on reading fine print. The cause of this headache is different, though the end result i.e. the headache is similar.

Onosmodium is stated to be good in the **treatment of sexual weakness** of men and women. In particular, it is said to be very effective in treating some weaknesses of young men.

In the patient of Picric Acid, there is an increase of uric acid and phosphates and a decrease of sulphate. It is readily detectable on urine examination. There are several remedies whose symptoms are related to the lower half of the body, while there are some related to the upper part of the body. The homoeopathic form of Picric Acid relieves the heaviness of the lower part of the body. For the **weakness of the spine and the legs**, Conium and Phosphorus are also useful.

For all symptoms resulting from the **ill effects of grief** or emotional upset besides headache, Picric Acid is very useful. Furthermore, Ambra Grisea, Ignatia, Natrum Mur, Acid Phos and Silicea, are excellent remedies for relieving the ill effects of grief and sorrow. It is not difficult to differentiate them from Picric Acid.

Picric Acid is also very useful for the **treatment of pimples and acne**. For those who are **anaemic** and get tired of hard physical and mental work, Picric Acid is very useful. In a Picric Acid patient, the **headache** becomes less by lying down and on tightly tying the head. However, the headache becomes worse with movement, bending over and mental exertion. The patient feels comfortable in the open and cold air. However, in the humid weather, the pain increases.

| | |
|---|---|
| Potency: | 30 to 200 |

# PIPER NIGRUM
## (Black Pepper)

Piper Nigrum is prepared from black pepper. I have found it very effective against **sneezing problems** where the other well-known remedies had failed. It is especially beneficial to those patients who are allergic to black pepper. These patients have an outburst of sneezing as soon as black pepper is sprinkled on anything. The remedy is also effective in treating the problems of patients who sneeze due to reasons other than allergy to black pepper.

The patient of Piper Nigrum remains by nature sad and depressed. The patient cannot concentrate on anything. His thoughts become scattered. The patient is startled by the slightest sound. He feels severe pain and burning in the eyeballs as if they are about to explode. If there is itching in the nose and sneezing also, then Piper Nigrum should be used. The Piper Nigrum patient has a **tendency to bleed from the nose**. His lips are dry, his head feels heavy and there is pressure over his temples. There is **pain and burning sensation in the tonsil area of the throat**. The patient feels very thirsty. The stomach is full of gas. The patient may also suffer from severe intestinal colic.

There is **burning inside the bladder and along the urethra**. The bladder appears full and distended. There is difficulty in passing urine. The patient, despite a constant urge, cannot urinate. Piper Nigrum is very useful in alleviating this condition. In all ailments of Piper Nigrum, the feeling of pressure and burning is common.

A Piper Nigrum patient also exhibits the **symptoms of heart disease**. There is pain in the chest, provoking cough. The heart beats very fast. There is difficulty in breathing. The patient feels pain over the heart area. Sometimes the pulse feels slow and interrupted. As lactating mothers produce much more milk than the need of their baby, Piper Nigrum is very **useful in reducing the formation of milk** in such women.

| | |
|---|---|
| Potency: | up to 30 |

# PLATINUM
## (Platina)

Platinum is very famous for the treatment of diseases of arrogant women. However these days, this drug is used less frequently. Maybe, in the old days there were more arrogant women than now. Nowadays times have changed, and one rarely finds women who are proud and arrogant i.e. who consider themselves superior to everyone else. Women belonging to rich families, who are brought up with a silver spoon in their mouth, consider themselves above everyone else. Such women are a typical example of Platinum constitution. Platinum is by far a more expensive element than gold. It is strange but understandable that Platinum induces an artificial feeling of richness and makes even poor women proud and arrogant.

The Platinum patient **thinks himself far superior and of very high status**. He becomes irritated about minor things and despises others. Considering himself to be the most important person, he remains always fearful of danger to his life. This state of his mind changes him physically also. The patient is always scared that something harmful is going to happen to him.

In a Platinum patient, the heart beats fast, the limbs tremble and soon, fear of death overtakes him. The patient is a **religious fanatic**. The female patient thinks of herself an alien. All these are the symptoms of insanity, which ultimately leads to more severe form. The **sexual trends** of Platinum resemble those of Hyoscyamus. The patient has spasm of muscles with convulsions. The **convulsions** slowly become worse, affecting the muscles. The skin becomes numb. The bleeding is of dark reddish colour. The nose bleeds in the form of dark clots. There is cramping at the root of the nose, which is very painful. The affected area feels caught in a vice. The patient feels a neuralgic type of pain on the face. The bones feel insensitive.

If the **ovaries become inflamed**, and the patient has been unable to conceive for a long time and there is heightened sexual urge without any apparent reason, then Platinum may be kept in mind to treat this condition.

If the **sterility** is due to an excessive leucorrhoeal discharge, then Borax is the remedy of choice. In Platinum, the **symptoms of other diseases of the uterus** are also found i.e. hardening of the uterus, the tendency to develop fibroids and the downward sagging of the uterus with excessive bleeding. The bleeding is usually dark in colour, with the formation of blood clots. The menstrual bleeding starts before it is due. This symptom is very common. However, if the other symptoms of Platinum are present, then Platinum will prove to be a promptly effective remedy.

**Stomach conditions** like excessive formation of gas and nausea, are also common in Platinum. The patient feels very uncomfortable and restless. The motions are intermittent and small. The patient feels exhausted.

In Platinum, the symptoms of the disease become worse in the evening and on sitting as well as standing. The symptoms improve with movement and on walking.

| | |
|---|---|
| Antidote: | Pulsatilla |
| Potency: | 30 or higher |

# PLUMBUM METALLICUM

In Latin, the metal lead is called Plumbum. Some paint used to decorate the houses contains lead. Even after the paint dries, the lead particles remain suspended in the air. Those who are allergic to lead will develop an allergy as soon as they enter a room treated with lead-containing paint. They will develop **severe abdominal pain** as if the abdomen is tightly squeezed. Even if the patient is not allergic to lead, a severe type of abdominal pain will benefit from Plumbum.

A special symptom of Plumbum is related to the gums i.e., **a blue line (lead line) appears on the gums below the teeth.** It darkens with the passage of time.

Plumbum is the best **treatment for muscular spasms**. Besides this, if the **hand becomes paralysed** resulting in **wrist drop** (which may be due to an excessive use of the hand for writing), and the patient has the basic symptoms of Plumbum, then Plumbum acts extraordinarily fast against this condition.

A Plumbum patient is often very slow and lazy. He **appears somewhat mentally as well as psychologically deficient**. When questioned, the patient either responds after a pause or just repeats the question. Plumbum is ideal for the treatment of delayed response. Sometimes while deeply lost in his thoughts, a person may not listen to a lightly uttered question, but will become aware of the question a little later, when his mind receives the message recorded earlier and wakes him up. Then he will ask what the matter was. Although a delayed response should not only be taken as a sign of Plumbum ailment, nevertheless, a Plumbum patient always reacts slowly. In fact, his perception of pain is also very slow and delayed. Therefore, there is always a danger that by the time such a patient comes to realise the pain, he may have already been seriously hurt. Luckily, only full-fledged Plumbum patients exhibit this symptom. A Plumbum patient understands the matter, but it takes time to register in his mind. The nerves carrying the pain sensation become slow in transmitting the pain message. Sometimes, this slowly progressive sensory loss may end in **complete loss of sensation**. The skin becomes numb. The feet and other parts of the body may gradually become insensitive and lifeless. When the disease progresses further, the patient becomes physically weak and is ultimately reduced to looking like a skeleton covered with loose skin.

A special symptom of Plumbum is that the **painful part of the body ultimately becomes wasted**. This symptom is also found in other kinds of paralyses. Fevers causing paralysis, such as typhoid etc., weaken the affected part but this weakness is not due to the pain. Typhoid sometimes paralyses the legs or arms but there is no pain associated with it. However, in Plumbum, there is always some pain in the part that is paralysed. In such a situation, immediate treatment with Plumbum should be started. Plumbum is also very useful in the **treatment of sciatica**. If other symptoms of it are also present then one must always treat the patient with Plumbum first. Whenever the limbs become flabby, painful and weak due to paralysis, then Plumbum will be found to be an effective treatment.

Piano players often develop **paralysis of the finger joints**. Their fingers become weak and frail. For this condition, two remedies are very famous, i.e. Plumbum and Curare. Curare is an extremely dangerous poison causing **paralysis**. Rhus Tox is a very effective remedy for the rapidly developing ill effects of paralysis. When used in the beginning of the disease, it immediately produces a positive response. However, if the use of Rhus Tox is delayed then it does not fully benefit the patient unless combined with Sulphur. Rhus Tox is relatively weak and a slow acting treatment. In contrast to Rhus Tox, Plumbum is a strong and a long-acting homoeopathic remedy. Treatment by alternating Sulphur with Rhus Tox increases the effectiveness of Rhus Tox. I alternate Rhus Tox with Sulphur. Sulphur activates the immune body system, while Rhus Tox cures the paralysis. By the grace of God, many chronic patients of **polio** have benefited greatly from this prescription. Rhus Tox is deeply related to paralysis. Although homoeopathic doctors do not usually use it for the treatment of chronic paralysis, although, it is a very useful remedy provided it is alternated with Sulphur.

The Plumbum patient suffers from severe **constipation**. The stools are hard, rounded and difficult to be excreted. Often, ulcers form in the rectum. The rectum may need to be evacuated digitally or with instruments. The reason for the problem is that the circular muscle fibres in the wall of the intestines become paralysed and lose the strength to push the faecal matter onwards. This paralytic condition slowly becomes worse and the constipation becomes more severe and chronic. Such constipation should be patiently treated with Plumbum, over a long period. Full results of the treatment show up in about fifteen days of the treatment. Those diseases that develop slowly, must respond to the treatment relatively slowly. However, sometimes the homoeopathic treatment may produce immediate response, e.g. the **relief of griping pain and spasmodic pain in the abdomen**. In homoeopathy, the effects of a poison which appear immediately can be cured equally fast by treatment with the homoeopathic potency of the same poison. In Plumbum, due to the **paralysis of the bladder wall**, the patient loses strength to void urine, resulting in retention of urine. Urine continues to collect in the bladder and then excreted drop by drop (retention with overflow). This is not related to the prostate; rather the condition is due to the paralysis of the bladder wall. The symptoms of the two diseases (bladder weakness and enlarged prostate) are obviously different. Urinary stoppage is not necessarily due to only one cause. When **urination stops after delivery of a child**, then Causticum happens to be the most ideal treatment. If this condition develops after an operation, then Strontium Carb is better. Plumbum also can be effective if the kidneys stop functioning due to sudden shock. Plumbum stirs up the kidney function.

One symptom of Plumbum is that whatever kind of food is taken, it produces acidity in the stomach, leading to severe vomiting. Usually the partially digested food with the gastric secretions passes on to the small intestines within three hours. If the stomach fails to empty itself within this period, then the food starts rotting in the stomach. This produces **acidity** and foul smelling belches. Acidity in the stomach can also be caused by decreased peristaltic movement of the intestine and the resulting stasis. Plumbum is the best remedy in this condition.

In Plumbum, the **vomited material is either dark** in colour or greenish and is sometimes mixed with blood. The function of the stomach and liver becomes deranged. The stomach feels full and heavy. The belly button becomes retracted.

Plumbum is famous for the gradually **progressive weakness of the muscles** (progressive muscular dystrophy). There are two to three different remedies useful in this disease. Opium and Kali Phos are also good remedies for this disease. When treating with Kali Phos, the dose should be increased gradually. In progressive muscular dystrophy, the neurons in the central part of the brain responsible for the voluntary control of the muscles start to die. There is no known cure for this disease. The patients slowly become more and more weak and often die before attaining the prime of their youth. Even if they remain alive, their life is very miserable. Progressive muscular dystrophy being a hereditary disease, sometimes all the children may be affected. No definite cure has yet been found for the disease. However, the patients obtain some relief with homoeopathic treatment.

Occasional **rapid heartbeat** (tachycardia) along with convulsions, benefit from Plumbum. For a sudden feeling of the heart being squeezed, Cactus Grandiflora is the best remedy.

Plumbum is said to be capable of treating the bad habit of **cheating and dishonesty**. If this is true, then it should be used freely throughout the world!

Plumbum is a good remedy for the treatment of chronic kidney diseases associated with **loss of albumin and sugar in the urine**. Plumbum improves the function of the kidney tubules and helps retain both the albumin and the sugar.

The symptoms of Plumbum also resemble those of Opium. In **apoplexy**, there is sudden rush of blood towards the head, which can result in cerebral haemorrhage. The face becomes congested with blood, and the pupils of the eyes become dilated. These symptoms often lead to death. Arnica and Opium given in high potency at the onset of the symptoms proves very useful. It is also necessary to treat the patient of Plumbum with high doses of Plumbum. Both Opium and Plumbum show their effects at the same time. Dr. Kent states that the treatment should first be started with Opium and later Plumbum should be added to the treatment. This is correct because the initial symptoms of the disease resemble those of Opium.

Two other remedies are also considered very useful in the treatment of apoplexy. If there are multiple red bleeds, then Phosphorus is better but Alumina is also famous for the treatment of this condition.

**Painful severe cramps of the legs** in the evening, which get relieved on movement and by application of local pressure, can possibly be treated with Plumbum. A lightning type of undulating pain is a symptom of Plumbum, which is also found in Causticum and Caulophyllum.

With regards to cold and heat, the nature of Plumbum resembles Psorinum i.e. the patient is very sensitive to cold. He keeps himself covered with a blanket even during summer. Like Arnica, the head of the patient is warm and there is a tendency to form blood clots.

Often, **blisters develop between the toes of the feet**. Besides Plumbum, Sulphur is also very useful for such boils. If **gangrene** develops in the fingers or toes, or knots form in the feet, then also Plumbum will be effective if the patient is of the constitution of Plumbum.

Plumbum is also very good for the treatment of the swelling of the glands beneath the tongue (sublingual salivary glands). The tendency towards **severe body jolts and locking of the jaw, the paralysis of the muscles in the wall of the windpipe and the food pipe (oesophagus)**, resulting in the entry of the food into the air passage and choking due to water or food entering the windpipe or nose, are all the symptoms of Plumbum. Symptoms of many other remedies related to paralysis are also found in Plumbum.

Sometimes, the **severe abdominal colic related to Plumbum leads to a tendency towards delirium**. The patient feels as if a painful ball is moving from the throat up, towards the brain. The hair become dry, pupils constrict and the eyes become yellow. Sometimes, the patient may suddenly become unconscious and blinded. The face becomes pale, the cheeks wrinkle, and the skin becomes greasy and shiny with the formation of dark brown spots.

In Plumbum, the symptoms aggravate at night and with movement, while they ameliorate with local pressure

| | |
|---|---|
| Antidotes: | Alumina, Petroleum, Platinum |
| Potency: | 30 to 200, 1000 or even CM |

# PSORINUM

## (Scabies Vesicle)

Psorinum is prepared from the sinister material obtained from the skin lesions of chronic psoriasis. Psorinum is a vastly effective and powerful remedy. Regarding its efficacy against various diseases, Psorinum is similar to Sulphur. However, with regards to sensitivity to heat and cold, it is just the opposite of it. Sulphur by nature is very hot, whereas Psorinum by nature is very cold. If a patient shows all the symptoms of Sulphur but is cold by nature, then Psorinum will be the ideal treatment instead of Sulphur. Both Sulphur and Psorinum produce powerful effects on the skin and the glands. In both, the excretions stink and the body appears unclean and filthy as if the patient has not taken a bath for a long time. Sulphur and Psorinum are topnotch homoeopathic remedies for the **treatment of severe skin diseases**, which have become suppressed due to the use of strong, forceful allopathic treatment, and are now adversely affecting the intestines and the inner linings. In these conditions, Sulphur and Psorinum are both equally important. These skin diseases exhibit similar symptoms, though they react quite differently to heat and cold. Irrespective of cold and heat, Psorinum proves to be very effective against certain dangerous diseases not amenable to Sulphur, for example, the **cancer of the root of animal horns**. It is a very dangerous type of cancer killing the animal within few days. Many a time, a single dose of Psorinum 1000 will, by the grace of God, cure the disease, although it is considered incurable.

A Psorinum patient feels very cold and likes to cover himself with a quilt. However, when the patient becomes a little warm in the bed, itching starts. Despite some similarity in the mode of action between Psorinum and Sulphur, both differ widely from each other in their nature.

A unique totally unrelated feature of Psorinum, not shared by any other remedy including Sulphur, is that strands of the **hair in young children start turning grey**. I have yet to see a remedy better than Psorinum in the treatment of this condition. Soon after the treatment with Psorinum 1000, every week for a few weeks, black hair starts to grow from the roots. The upper part of the hair that has become grey cannot become black again. But the newer, lower part of the hair grows as black. I do not know with any certainity if Psorinum could also be helpful in turning the colour of grey hair of advanced age back into black. On rare occasions it has been seen that after becoming grey due to ripe old age, hair starts growing black again. I myself have seen many women whose hair turned black after becoming grey due to old age. God only knows the functioning of this mechanism. If a homoeopathic doctor could find a sure shot remedy by which the grey hair of old people could turn black, then that doctor might become the richest person in the world. I invite everybody to do more research on this project using Arnica and Psorinum. It is possible that this prescription may work in old people of cold constitution.

The skin diseases of Psorinum resemble those of Graphites. In both of these, the **eczema** is marred with scabs, underneath which very foul smelling pus is formed and the eczema continues afresh. In Psorinum, the **foul smell from the wounds** is distinctly more pronounced than Graphites and other remedies. It is simply unbearable. There is **severe itching** in the wounds, which bleed on scratching. The skin becomes dry and dirty. Scaly bumps develop over the entire body that are resistant to healing.

In Psorinum, the **eyelids are swollen and sticky**. The margins of the eyelids become red and swollen, as in several other remedies. If the disease becomes worse and the eyes become disfigured, Alumina or Alumen can prove to be ideal remedies, especially Alumina, which is very powerful and effective in this respect. If the **eyes become inflamed** and develop lumps, then Aesculus would be better than Alumina. Most of the eye diseases can improve with these or similar remedies. Sometimes, the **eyelids swell** and turn outwards, exposing the inner red surface (ectropion). The eyes look dreadful. The **eyelashes start to fall**. For all these symptoms, Psorinum, Hepar Sulph and Alumina are very high-rated remedies.

In Psorinum, the patient suffers from recurrent **nasal cold**. The nose gets blocked. Despite blockage of the nasal passages, thin yellowish-green fluid runs from the nose, slightly relieving the burning sensation. In view of the changing forms of the influenza virus, Psorinum remains effective only for a short while and then loses its effect. The reason is that the symptoms of the disease keep on changing. Therefore, it is not possible to depend on one or two remedies alone for the entire treatment of catarrhal diseases. It becomes imperative to change the treatment when the symptoms change.

Psorinum is the remedy for people of cold constitution. It acts rapidly against the diseases caused by cold. Furthermore, Psorinum has the capability to surface the suppressed diseases out. Even if Psorinum cannot cure the patient, it helps the physician in treating the patient with other remedies by exposing the symptoms related to a particular remedy. One should not be afraid if Psorinum became ineffective after being effective for a short while, this does not mean that the diagnosis was wrong. It is a characteristic of Psorinum that it is effective for a short while and then becomes ineffective. However, after a while, if the patient is put back on Psorinum again, it picks up its previous effectiveness.

A Psorinum patient is always hungry, especially **at night.** Characteristically, hunger wakes him up in the latter part of the night. Food makes the patient feel better. A Sulphur patient does not feel hungry at night or in the morning, however, after sunrise, around 11a.m., the patient feels extremely hungry by way of severe craving in the stomach.

In Psorinum, the **headache** alternates with nasal catarrh. In this condition, Bryonia and Rhus Tox are also effective. In Psorinum, the **cough** is dry. Phlegm does not form at all. Usually such a cough is very troublesome. At the beginning of the disease, Aconite, Belladonna and Arsenic benefit the patient. However, these remedies do not offer a permanent cure. For symptoms developing later, some other remedies should be looked for. It is important to keep a constant watch on the patient and then change the remedies as frequently as the symptoms change. However, the remedies conforming to the patient's constitution usually cure the patient permanently. These need not be changed.

In Psorinum, **sores develop at the angles of the mouth**. The **tongue and the gums feel painful** constantly. The teeth become loose and start to shake. Often due to some kind of severe infection, despite the fact that the gums have become diseased, symptoms of pain, inflammation and fever do not develop. Bacteria erode the gums from the inside. Similar symptoms are also found in Baptisia i.e. there is severe throat infection, to the extent that the tonsils start to necrose, yet the patient does not feel any pain.

Sometimes, a Psorinum patient experiences a sudden urge to pass stools. The slightest delay may result in soiling the clothes.

The **constipation** of Psorinum resembles that of Bryonia and Graphites. Sometimes, despite loose motions, there is difficulty in excretion of the faeces, because the peristaltic movements of the intestines become sluggish. The symptom of difficulty in excretion of the faeces is also found in Alumina, China and Nux Moschata. In the **diarrhoea** of Psorinum, the stools contain undigested food particles. Moreover, the patient urinates frequently. It is a symptom of weakness of the urinary bladder and is not due to diabetes.

Psorinum is very effective against certain diseases of the **prostate**. Psorinum is also effective against **cancer of the prostate**, though, for this disease, Silicea CM is the most effective remedy. During the last few years, Silicea CM has been tried for the treatment of prostate cancer and found to be very effective. After treating with one dose of Silicea CM, the benefit may stop. The remedy may then be repeated after a short interval. However, it should not be repeated without reason. In the treatment of cancers anywhere in the body, if necessary a high potency of Silicea can be repeated sooner. However, while the first dose is still effective, the second dose should not be given unnecessarily. Generally, Psorinum is beneficial in the treatment of weakened heart muscles, severe pain which is relieved by lying down and **inflammation of the covering membrane of the heart** (pericarditis). One symptom of Psorinum is that the pulse is very weak and difficult to feel.

Psorinum is beneficial in the treatment of women's diseases only if the symptoms of feeling cold and the foul smell of the discharges are conspicuous.

In Psorinum, sexual urge decreases and there is a complete loss of libido. This symptom is found in Graphites also. Apparently, by nature, Psorinum is a cold and dry remedy, yet the body temperature rises very high in the fever of a Psorinum patient. A patient sweats as if steaming. Despite sweating, the patient's body temperature does not subside. The patient experiences **scary dreams**, feels very thirsty and cannot go to sleep due to unbearable itching.

The Psorinum diseases become worse with cold and during the change of weather. A whiff of cold air becomes unbearable to the patient. Eating food gives only short relief. In the open air, the cough and itching subside.

| | |
|---|---|
| Adjuvants: | Sulphur, Alumina |
| Potency: | 200 or higher. Sometimes, the first dose produces its effect after nine to ten days. Therefore one should wait at least that long to see its effect. |

# PULEX IRRITANS

Pulex Irritans is very important for the treatment of urinary diseases and women's problems related to the uterus. The patient of Pulex is very short-tempered and easily provoked. The patient develops headache in the frontal area with the feeling that his eyes are really big. The face is wrinkled, showing signs of premature ageing.

There is metallic taste in the mouth. There is a feeling of hair sticking in the throat. The patient feels unusually thirsty especially when suffering from headache. The patient's breath has an offensive smell.

Stomach upset is associated with severe nausea, vomiting and diarrhoea. The stools smell offensive. The abdomen is distended with gas.

**Urinary symptoms** are very important. The patient needs to pass urine frequently, though the urine is scanty. The patient needs to rush to the lavatory, lest he wets his clothes. There is pressure on the bladder and a burning sensation along the urethra. Sometimes, the urine may stop altogether, causing severe discomfort in the urinary bladder. The urine smells offensive. In women, the **discomfort and irritation in the bladder before the onset of the menstrual period**, the late onset of the period, excessive salivation in the mouth and severe vaginal burning, are exemplary symptoms of Pulex to be treated with Pulex.

There is an **excessive amount of vaginal discharge** which is very odorous and stains the undergarments yellowish green. These stains are difficult to remove even with a lot of washing. The backache resembles that of Oxalic Acid. The skin smells. The patient feels better on sitting and lying down. The discomfort increases on walking, and is felt more on the left side of the body.

One characteristic of Pulex is very important whether its other symptoms are present or not, i.e. Pulex is extraordinarily effective in controlling the sudden urge to urinate (urgency). The patients wake up frequently in order to urinate. The remedy decreases the frequency and significantly prolongs their sleep. It reduces the bad smell of urine and clears its colour.

Pulex is very useful in the treatment of women's **cancer of the uterus and liver**. It restores the functioning of the internal lining of the uterus. If chronic inflammation of the uterus (endometritis) and the inflammation of the ovaries prevent pregnancy, then the treatment with Pulex over a period of few months can reasonably brighten the chances of conception.

| | |
|---|---|
| Potency: | 200 or higher. |

# PULSATILLA
## (Wind Flower)

Pulsatilla is prepared from a plant (wind flower), after grinding it into a powder form. In allopathic remedy, the powder has been used for eye diseases only. However, in homoeopathy, Pulsatilla is one of the most widely used remedies.

In Pulsatilla, the mental and physical symptoms keep interchanging. The Pulsatilla patient is very mild natured, weeps easily and is a coward. This temperament is more common in women. Therefore, this remedy is known as a **ladies' medicine**. The pulsatilla patient is kind towards everyone, starts crying over minor things, remains still and silent, and is very sensitive to trivial matters. When the patient thinks that his ego has been hurt, he feels very insulted and gets irritated. The patient has a very suspicious nature and is extremely sensitive with regard to self-respect. He gets perturbed over petty matters. He always suspects that someone is insulting him. Yet, the patient is neither aggressive, nor violent rather, he becomes very sad, depressed and dejected. He cries a lot and becomes superstitious. Such patients may become **religious fanatics**. In particular women suffer from such type of fanaticism. Since women keep suppressing their anger, their emotions ultimately turn into religious fanaticism that is evident from their thoughts and their conversation. For example, they may strongly believe that a particular food is harmful for human beings and it is the cause of their downfall. Such imagination is typical of Pulsatilla. Pulsatilla is an antidote for the symptoms resulting from the bad effects of Lycopodium, which make a person so shy that he is afraid of his own shadow.

Often, Pulsatilla women **hate to get married**. When a woman hates marriage without any evident psychological reason, she should be treated with Pulsatilla.

Pulsatilla is also related to the **disorders of the stomach**. The patient cannot digest oily food laden with fat. Eating a little bit of cream or butter can upset the stomach. Either these patients develop a strong dislike for fatty food or they will simply not be able to digest it. This symptom is also found in Carbo Veg and some other remedies.

In Pulsatilla, the **patient does not feel thirsty**; however, drinking cold water soothes the patient. The patient likes to eat cold food. The stomach problems aggravate in the morning and the mental anguish in the evening. Usually fits of **depression and sadness** begin in the evening. The evening time is hard on these patients. A cold breeze and light movement comfort the patient. The discomfort increases on entering a heated room. The feeling of cold inside becomes more pronounced by going into a heated place. This is very strange but interesting to note that apparently the patient's body is warm but deep inside the patient feels very cold, and on entering a heated room, the feeling of cold further aggravates.

Sulphur acts as an antidote to Pulsatilla. Other than the symptoms of a burning sensation in the hands and feet, the symptoms of Pulsatilla are dissimilar to those of Sulphur. Over treatment with Sulphur should be treated with Pulsatilla and the overdose of Pulsatilla should be treated with Sulphur.

For **psoriasis** appearing in the form of circular sunken brown specks, Pulsatilla is very effective. In Pulsatilla, the veins may become distended and engorged with blood, over any part of the body. The blood may also clot inside. A spider web of small veins is formed, which may become inflamed (phlebitis). Usually, this problem appears in the calves of the legs during pregnancy. The subject of varicose veins has already been discussed under Aesculus. If, in addition to the above symptoms, a patient also has the tendency to develop varicose ulcers, then Pulsatilla will prove to be very effective.

Pulsatilla is also very effective in the **treatment of catarrhal diseases**. Pulsatilla cures chronic catarrh and diseases of the inner linings. Chronic catarrh usually involves the chest producing thick phlegm. The treatment with appropriate remedies can cure this problem fast, by the grace of Allah. Since the catarrhal diseases resemble each other very closely, it is very difficult to differentiate between them. If the **nose becomes blocked**, one immediately thinks of treatment with Pulsatilla. However, several other remedies also, have this symptom, as already detailed in different chapters of this book. Despite the blockage of the nasal passage, the nasal discharge continues to some extent. Nux Vomica and Coccus are also useful for the treatment of this condition. One should always be on the lookout for a remedy according to the constitution of the patient.

Like Calcarea Phos, Pulsatilla is also very important in the treatment of girls reaching adulthood. Pulsatilla is very effective in the treatment of complete cessation or delayed onset of girls' periods resulting from submerging their feet in cold water. Pulsatilla women hope for the periods to commence every month, but do not have them. Pulsatilla is also stated to be very useful in the problems associated with the **menopause**. When used in combination with Lachesis or Belladonna, Pulsatilla produces excellent results. At menopause, usually, the patient feels as if hot air is being blown onto her face. The face becomes red. In women suffering from **anaemia**, excessive menstrual bleeding dilutes their blood further, i.e. they become more anaemic. Pulsatilla being the best treatment for blood deficiency, when it is given to anaemic women it will stop their periods. However, after a few months when the blood deficiency has been corrected, normal menstrual periods resume automatically. Pulsatilla will not let the periods start unless the anaemia is corrected. Even in the absence of anaemia, Pulsatilla can offer immediate cure for dark, scanty menstrual bleeding.

In Pulsatilla, the patient feels pain in the shoulders and the back. A strong local pressure reduces the severity of the pain. Similarly, sleeping on a hard surface also relieves the back pain.

In Pulsatilla, the **headache** is like migraine. The pain is usually on one side, over the temple and the same side of the face. A special symptom of Pulsatilla is that one side of the body is warm while the other side is cold. The difference in temperature on the two sides can be easily felt by touch of the hand. The face is red hot on one side while it is cold and blanched on the other side, as if devoid of blood. This prominent symptom makes the diagnosis of Pulsatilla very easy. Therefore, besides other features of headache, this may be a leading symptom of Pulsatilla. However, this symptom is not a must in every pain. Even if this symptom is not present, Pulsatilla can still be used provided that its other symptoms are present.

In Pulsatilla, the symptoms related to eyes are very common, such as **multiple styes**. Pulsatilla works very well on the styes. The discharge from the eyes is very thick. Eyelid margins become swollen and sticky. In young children, "pink eye" develops. There is swelling of the conjunctiva and symptoms related to the nose and throat appear like Natrum Mur. Natrum Mur is the chronic of Pulsatilla, so if the symptoms happen to be of Pulsatilla but the patient does not respond to Pulsatilla, then Natrum Mur may be used instead.

Pulsatilla is also the best **treatment for ear diseases**, such as the infection of the ear, discharge of sticky and stinky material from the ears and hardness of hearing. Once the nasal cold has affected the ear, the Pulsatilla patient tends to torment himself furthermore and starts crying due to pain to the extent of complete helplessness and despair. However, if the earache is associated with anger, then the patient should be treated with Chamomilla instead of Pulsatilla.

In chronic nasal catarrh, there is a feeling of **dryness** inside the nasal passages. The secretions become dry and encrusted causing a constant mild pain. Pulsatilla relieves this condition.

In Pulsatilla initially the nasal secretions are whitish but soon become yellowish and offensive. The **sense of smell** either decreases or is completely lost. In the morning, coughing brings out a lot of sputum. It turns into a **dry cough** by the evening. In chronic catarrh, the nose may also bleed.

Nosebleed is also related to menstruation. If **menstruation stops and the nose starts to bleed**, then Bryonia should be used instead of Pulsatilla. If the nose bleeds during menstruation, then Pulsatilla should be used.

In Pulsatilla, the symptoms of **allergy** become severe in the evening. However, in Natrum Mur, the situation is just the opposite. In the morning, particularly around nine o' clock in the morning, the allergy becomes much more severe. If sneezing ensues when the patient goes from a cold to a warm room, the remedy is Pulsatilla. However, if sneezing ensues after going from a warm to a cold room, then Sabadilla, Silicea or Natrum Mur should be used.

The Pulsatilla patient suffers from insomnia and has difficulty in sleeping. Furthermore, the patient has feeling of shortness of breath and suffocation. If the disease is not properly treated, it can turn into asthma. When the **allergy changes into asthma**, then Pulsatilla can also be the effective treatment. Silicea is the chronic of Pulsatilla. In case a fever does not subside with Pulsatilla and the patient feels hot, or similarly, if certain infections do not respond to treatment with Pulsatilla despite their symptoms being of Pulsatilla, then in this situation, the patient should be treated with Silicea. In my experience, Silicea has often been effective. In the beginning, I did not treat such patients with Silicea; then I realised that since Silicea is the chronic of Pulsatilla, it is possible that Silicea may be effective even though the disease has not responded to Pulsatilla.

Pulsatilla is an excellent **treatment for mumps**. It prevents the migration of the diseases to other sites. If not treated appropriately, the disease may seriously afflict the reproductive organs. Such patients are then rendered sterile forever. In such cases, the first treatment of choice is Abrotanum. If Abrotanum is ineffective, Pulsatilla should be used. One similarity between these two drugs is that the aches and pains keep shifting from one location to another. Abrotanum pains keep shifting all over the body. However, the Pulsatilla pains migrate in a particular direction i.e. either from left to right or from right to left. This symptom is also found in Lac Caninum, whose pains migrate rapidly. In Abrotanum, it is mostly the nature of the disease that changes into another disease. For example, if **lung cancer** spreads into the bone then the remedies of a migrating nature should be considered, Abrotanum being one such remedy. However, the most effective remedy is Phosphorus. Whether the **cancer has started in the bones** or has spread to the bones from somewhere else, in both cases Phosphorus is the best.

In Pulsatilla, **stomach ailments** such as irritation, sour belches and distension of the abdomen with gas, etc. start within a few hours of eating food. In Nux Vomica, the ailments aggravate on an empty stomach. The patient finds some relief on taking food, but the discomfort returns in an hour or so.

The Pulsatilla patient has a dry mouth yet does not feel thirsty. The liver produces an excessive amount of bile, which regurgitates into the mouth with nausea. Oily food causes distension of the abdomen and **diarrhoea** consisting of greenish, watery stools (more so at night). Soft stools, yet **constipation**, are typical of Pulsatilla. Despite the repeated urge of going to the lavatory, the patient does not feel fully relieved. There is a similar feeling in Nux Vomica also. However, in

Nux Vomica, the stools are hard like stone. In women, the constipation sometimes resembles that of Graphites. In this case, the stools are like large hard masses. Like Pulsatilla, Graphites also is famous for alleviating a deficient menstrual flow. However, Graphites suits the cold constitution, while Pulsatilla suits the hot constitution patients. If the constipation reaches the point where it cannot be relieved by Pulsatilla, then it can often be relieved with Silicea. In case Silicea also fails, then Veratrum Album could be effective. Patients who suffer from constipation often develop **piles**. The piles are often very painful. However, if the pain over the piles is relieved by lying flat on a hard surface, it is a specific sign of Ammonium Carb and it is not a symptom of Pulsatilla. If there is severe burning on the piles, then Arsenic and Kali Carb are better than Pulsatilla. Paeonia is very famous for the treatment of continuously painful type of piles. However, when the constitutional symptoms are those of Pulsatilla, then only Pulsatilla will be effective.

If a person feels like urinating, but urinates very little and there is a burning sensation and irritation, then Pulsatilla may be useful. In Pulsatilla, sometimes the urine is mixed with blood. One of its symptoms is that while sleeping on his side, the patient may not need to get up to pass urine throughout the night. However, if he sleeps flat on his back, he gets up frequently for urination during the night. Such children who happen to **wet their beds at night** may be helped by tying a big knot in the waistband of their pyjamas, preventing them from sleeping on their back. This tactic works mostly in the Pulsatilla type of patients. Moreover, Natrum Mur and Kali Phos 6X combined are also very useful for treating this condition in children.

For the treatment of **involuntary passage of urine during coughing, sneezing or laughing** (stress incontinence), Pulsatilla is very useful. In case the patient wets the bed soon after going to sleep, then Causticum 200 or Sepia 200 are better. If a person cannot manage to ease himself while sitting for however long but urinates immediately on standing up or walking (due to sudden pressure on the bladder), then this is typical of Bryonia. In Rhus Tox, the patient feels like passing urine while sitting, but as soon as he gets up and walks the feeling is gone. In short, all these remedies function within their own spectrum of symptoms.

The Pulsatilla patient feels comfort on movement. From this point of view, Pulsatilla partially resembles Rhus Tox. Functioning in the presence of dampness is similar in both. Both Pulsatilla and Rhus Tox are useful in the **treatment of catarrhal conditions** developing due to careless exposure to wet weather. Besides other remedies, Dulcamara is also well known in the treatment of conditions related to changing weather, especially so if the change in the weather includes dampness.

Pulsatilla is also very useful in the controlling the **tendency to abort in women**. Often instead of a foetus, a lifeless lump of flesh grows in the uterus. Pulsatilla dissolves this lump of flesh. In this condition, there is severe abdominal cramping during menstruation. If such pain is only occasional then Pulsatilla is useful. However, if the episodes are frequent, then Natrum Mur should be given preference, as it is the chronic form of Pulsatilla. Young girls experiencing this type of pain in their early adulthood can benefit from Calcarea Phos also. Pulsatilla is also very useful in the treatment of the **downward sagging tendency of the uterus** (i.e. prolapse). For this, there are several other useful remedies, whose symptoms would of course need to be identified.

Some women develop milk in their breasts in the absence of pregnancy or delivery of a child. Pulsatilla is very useful for treating this condition. Besides Pulsatilla, Mercurius and Cyclamen are also very useful. Pulsatilla often benefits mothers who suffer from a **shortage of milk production** in their breasts. If after the delivery, the placental remains and blood are not fully excreted, then Pulsatilla helps in their expulsion from the uterus. Pulsatilla is a **strong clearing agent of the uterus**. However, the remedy benefits only if it is used before the development of the puerperal fever. Once a fever develops, then only Silicea or Sulphur and Pyrogenium will be effective.

Pulsatilla 200 is reknowned for **correcting the position of the child inside the uterus**. It also invigorates the labour pains during the delivery of a child. Some doctors routinely start giving Pulsatilla at the beginning of the ninth month of the pregnancy. This has produced significant results. However, after the onset of the labour pains, a combination of Mag Phos and Kali Phos works much better than Pulsatilla in facilitating the delivery. The tablets are dissolved in water and then sipped at intervals.

Pulsatilla is very useful in the **treatment of crookedness of the vertebral column (scoliosis)** as it strengthens the muscles around the spinal column and equalizes their tone and strength on both sides. In children, the spinal column can become crooked giving the **appearance of hunchback** and loss of height. Pulsatilla is useful in correcting this deformity and dwarfism. In a Pulsatilla patient, the painful limbs start to contract and become weak. For example, if there is a chronic pain in the leg, the leg becomes short and slender. Similarly, the painful leg and the arm start to shrink.

During an **attack of malaria**, if the patient exhibits the **stomach symptoms** of Pulsatilla, Pulsatilla will work very well. The Pulsatilla patient often does not feel thirsty. However, during malaria, the patient feels unusually thirsty before the onset of severe chills and then the thirst disappears as soon as the fever develops. In the presence of this symptom, the patient must be treated with Pulsatilla. In Pulsatilla, there is a neuralgic type of pain on the right side of the face. The lower lip becomes thick due to swelling. These symptoms usually become worse during the evening. The patient also develops a dry cough in the evening and at night.

The problems of Pulsatilla aggravate with heat and on eating oily food. The symptoms are relieved on movement, in the open air and on eating cold food. When the hands burn hot and the feet are very cold and vice-versa, then Pulsatilla could well be very useful.

| | |
|---|---|
| Adjuvants: | Kali Mur, Lycopodium, Sulphuric Acid |
| Antidotes: | Coffea, Chamomilla, Nux Vomica |
| Potency: | 30 to 1000 or even CM in certain conditions |

# PYROGENIUM

Pyrogenium is prepared from the putrid matter obtained from decomposed meat, which is deadly poisonous. On ingesting decomposed meat, either a person catches high fever, becomes disorientated and then dies, or keeps suffering from its ill effects for a long time.

Pyrogenium has been so frequently referred to in this book that the reader may think that he has already read about it. Here, it is described briefly.

In a Pyrogenium patient, the discharges are extremely foul and poisonous, producing high fever, even death. It is a very powerful panacea for **puerperal sepsis** i.e. the fever developing after childbirth due to the infection and putrefaction of the retained placental contents in the uterus. It is extremely effective in curing this dreadful and potentially fatal condition. If Sulphur 200 is used in combination with Pyrogenium 200, it works even better.

Like Arsenic, it can also be of use in the **treatment of influenza complicated by severe weakness and restlessness**. Arsenic and Pyrogenium given together work much better in invigorating the weakness. The same prescription stands high in the **treatment of diarrhoea and dysentery associated with foul smell**. All sorts of **catarrhal fevers** associated with chills, putrefaction and restlessness can be satisfactorily treated with Pyrogenium, Bacillinum and Natrum Mur. In Pyrogenium, like Phosphorus, there is intense thirst for cold water. The cold water soon becomes warm inside the stomach and induces vomiting. The Pyrogenium patient is very cold deep down to the bones, yet likes to drink cold water. In this condition, Pyrogenium should be mixed with Phosphorus.

Pyrogenium is also useful in combating **bad breath**. If the patient also feels very cold, then Psorinum should be added to Pyrogenium.

I have found the combination of Pyrogenium 200 and Typhoidinum 200 very useful in the treatment of all **typhoid** patients. My late father also used Pyrogenium in the treatment of typhoid. Most probably it is he who invented this particular combination. In addition to Pyrogenium and Typhoidinum, Kali Phos 6X and Ferrum Phos 6X should be given seven to eight times a day. If a patient passes odorous stools, then Baptisia 30 should also be included, seven to eight times a day.

Pyrogenium is also effective against **malaria**, which is untreatable with common remedies. The patient feels severe chills and is restless like Arsenic and the discharges are extremely foul smelling.

In cattle also, Pyrogenium 200 and Sulphur 200 are equally effective in the treatment of puerperal fever following retention of the placenta and its infection.

Pyrogenium is also useful in the **treatment of inflammation of the kidneys (nephritis).** Once it becomes known that the patient had previously suffered from puerperal fever, causing damage to the kidneys, Pyrogenium will be found very effective.

Another symptom of Pyrogenium is that in spite of the high fever, the **pulse rate** is relatively slow. This conflicting type of heart rate is typical of Pyrogenium.

If the symptoms of Pyrogenium already mentioned are present, then Pyrogenium may be useful in the **treatment of all kinds of skin diseases** of the patient. Pyrogenium being basically related to the venous blood, the patient may develop **piles**, which can become infected and then putrefied. Pyrogenium is also useful in the treatment of a resistant type of offensive vomiting. If the constitutional symptoms of Pyrogenium are present, then broncho-pneumonia and other infections of the lungs can also be satisfactorily treated with it.

| | |
|---|---|
| Adjuvants: | Bryonia, Sulphur, Arsenic, Typhoidinum, etc. |
| Potency: | 30 to CM |

# RADIUM BROMIDE

Radium Bromide is prepared by dissolving room air in solvent after having radiated the room with 1,800,000 rads of Radium Bromide (inside the clinics for radiotherapy). It seems hard to believe that such a solution works. Yet, it is a fact. In homoeopathy, the working of a remedy is an extremely fine mechanism, undetectable in the physical sense.

Radium Bromide is commonly used in the **treatment of pimples, acne and boils**. Some homoeopathic physicians use it for the expulsion of a dead foetus from the uterus. It is also used in the prevention and **treatment of cancer**. Radium Bromide should never be forgotten while treating chronic types of **boils and abscesses**.

Radium Bromide protects against the **ill effects of radiation**. For this purpose it is used in potency CM alternating with Carcinocin CM on a weekly basis for a few months. Because radiation affects gradually, so, would Radium Bromide and Carcinocin bring about the necessary defensive body response in a gradual way.

Symptoms get better in the open air and on constant movement, taking a hot bath and lying down.

| | |
|---|---|
| Antidotes: | Radium Bromide and Carcinocin can be used as antidotes for each other. But it is more important to control the dangerous effects of radiation. One should not depend on just one antidote. |
| Potency: | 30 to CM |

# RHUS GLABRA

Rhus Glabra is prepared from the extract obtained from the leaves and stem of a particular plant. **Its most important function is to dispel the bad smell from all the discharges from the body**, including the smell of faeces. I have tried it on many people. Some young men who were sick of their own body smells, benefited significantly with Rhus Glabra. Some were completely cured. Rhus Glabra **improves the function of gastro-intestinal tract by controlling the inflammation and healing the ulcers of the intestines**. The gut is cleansed and the patient stops passing foul gases.

One symptom of Rhus Glabra is **bleeding from the nose**. The patient sweats profusely, the odour being extremely foul. The patient starts feeling weak due to excessive sweating. In his dreams, the patient finds himself flying in the air. Rhus Glabra is supposed to be the antidote of Mercury. It is usually used in the form of Mother Tincture. However, I have found it more effective and useful in potency 6X and potency 6X.

| | |
|---|---|
| Potency: | Mother Tincture Q or 6X<br>Biochemic 6X |

# RHUS TOXICODENDRON

## (Poison Ivy)

Rhus Toxicodendron is better known by its short name, Rhus Tox. It is prepared from a wild plant called 'bichhoo booti' (poison ivy). Its poison produces severe intractable itching. The patient contracts high fever. The appetite is lost. There is nausea and severe headache. The glands become enlarged inside and out. Sores develop inside the mouth and on the tongue. In 1798, a French doctor accidentally found out that this particular poison cured a serious skin disease of a patient. The doctor subsequently tried this in the treatment of various skin diseases, paralyses and joint pains and found it very useful. For homoeopathic use, the leaves of the plant are ground in the humid season.

Rhus Tox is indispensable for homoeopathic doctors. It is used in the treatment of many diseases.

The most important symptom of Rhus Tox is **burning and inflammation** leading to the **formation of large blisters**. In fact, the largest blisters associated with skin disease are found only in Rhus Tox. In Anacardium and Cantharis, blisters are also found but they are relatively small. Rhus Tox benefits the **burn's patients** immensely. It must be given at once and in high potency. Besides this, Rhus Tox is highly beneficial in the **treatment of paralyses**. Right-sided paralysis (hemiplegia) gets better with Rhus Tox and Sulphur used alternately. Even if the patient does not show the whole spectrum of Rhus Tox symptoms, he could still benefit to some extent.

When the **vision of one eye is being affected** as a result of severe physical strain or continuous mental overlay and the heart is also under stress, a dose or two of Rhus Tox benefits immediately. In this condition, either there are dancing shadows before the right eye or the right half of the field of vision is lost.

Rhus Tox is very beneficial in the **treatment of neuralgias** that become worse with rest and get better on movement. The severe burning sensation does not let the patient rest. He remains restless and does not find comfort in any position. Movement seems to offer comfort to begin with but the pain soon returns. Light movement and light exercise are comforting while strenuous exercise can be dangerous.

If the symptoms match completely, Rhus Tox can relieve **headache as well as all other body aches**. Whenever Rhus Tox is the constitutional homoeopathic remedy, the patient will enjoy sound sleep in no time, with no anguish or restlessness any more. I have observed it so many times. Some patients will even 'complain' that the night was too short since they previously used to toss and turn all night!

Another symptom of Rhus Tox is **mild chronic inflammation of the bladder or the kidneys** resulting in the **frequent passing of urine** at night. The patient cannot sleep much. He remains restless. Frequency of urination is not always due to diabetes. Similar symptoms are also found in Phosphorus. The patient wakes up at night for no apparent reason. Even if the patient looks healthy he does not feel like going to sleep. He may wet himself unknowingly at night. Unexplained frequency of urination associated with restlessness will most probably benefit from Rhus Tox.

If skin diseases are forcefully suppressed with allopathic medicines, then the disease process may affect the lining of the uterus, mucous membranes or the glands. Sometimes, the condition may become very serious. If the pancreas is afflicted, then the patient can develop severe **diabetes**. A single dose of Rhus Tox in high potency may immediately cure the patient. No doubt, it will forcefully surface the suppressed eczema on the skin. Once, in view of some resemblance of the symptoms, I treated a diabetic patient with Rhus Tox in high potency. All of a sudden, his entire body became riddled with eczema but his diabetes was cured. On further questioning, it was found that the patient had suffered from a serious kind of eczema in the past that had been suppressed with strong medication and the diabetes had come on later. In this patient, Rhus Tox cured the diabetes, but the eczema returned. Unfortunately, some of these patients do not feel happy to be rid of diabetes but rather take the recurrence of the eczema too seriously. In fact, if they continue their treatment patiently using Rhus Tox, their skin disease would also be cured. No doubt, the eczema would flare up in the beginning but eventually disappear gradually.

In Rhus Tox, the eczema is of the weeping type. Once an afflicted lady came to me. She suffered from severe **weeping eczema.** She was even unable to cook food. Her husband and children were also dismayed. I treated her with Rhus Tox 1000. With the first dose, the eczema flared up and then in a few days, the watery discharge started becoming less. On the second dose, after a week, the reaction was less pronounced. In three to four weeks, her hands were looking completely healthy, devoid of any signs of eczema. In my experience, I have found it surprisingly effective and beneficial. To my knowledge, there is no substitute for Rhus Tox. If the symptoms are of Rhus Tox, then Rhus Tox and nothing else will have to be administered. Rhus Tox symptoms are very closely related to humidity. In the rainy season, when it is also hot, its symptoms become aggravated.

Rhus Tox is also very useful in the **treatment of malarial fever**. It becomes even more effective if used alternately with Bryonia right at the onset of symptoms. Prevantative use of Arnica 1000 will induce the natural body response against malaria. I invite the readers to study Arnica, Arsenic and Natrum Mur also, with reference to malaria.

Rhus Tox is also useful in the **treatment of fevers other than malaria** such as fevers of remittent nature or continuous ones. Such fevers make the patient physically exhausted. The patient feels restless, chills and dryness of the tongue. He is sensitive to cold. The pivotal symptom, is still the persistent restlessness and aching of the entire body

Rhus Tox is very useful in the **treatment of cellulitis**. This inflammatory process involves the glands, the outer surface of the skin and the inner linings (mucous membranes). The patient feels pain and tightness. Rhus Tox should also be used in the **treatment of endometritis** i.e. the inflammation of the inner lining of the uterus. It may possibly treat the underlying condition of the uterus and surface it to the skin. Sulphur 200 and Pyrogenium 200 can significantly overcome the disease. When given alternately with Rhus Tox, they offer complete cure, by the grace of God. Rhus Tox can be useful in the treatment of all skin conditions associated with the formation of blisters filled with clear fluid, blood or even pus, provided the burning sensation is prominent.

Rhus Tox works extremely well in the **treatment of infantile paralysis (Polio)**. At first, the child contracts a high fever, which is followed by the gradual onset of **paralysis**. If someone has previously suffered from polio in early childhood or his leg starts becoming weak, then Rhus Tox should be started without any delay. Rhus Tox works much better when used alternately with Sulphur. Sulphur is also very effective in the treatment of paralytic conditions. Thus, a combination of the two is obviously much more useful. Some **polio** patients have actually been completely cured with this prescription. Sometimes, the whole body becomes numb for a short while then the numbness disappears automatically. However, if there is any sign of associated weakness, Rhus Tox must be given immediately. It seems to work very well. The **gradually progressive paralysis** of chronic and profound nature may be treated with Causticum. Causticum is not a remedy for immediate effect only. In Causticum, the process of paralysis sets in early, soon after exposure to the cold. When noticed, the patient feels that the paralysis happened suddenly. Partial or localized paralysis of a few muscles responds better to Causticum. In particular, it has no match with regards to its effectiveness against right-sided facial palsy. Traditionally, Causticum is famous as the ideal remedy for **paralysis of the face**.

In Rhus Tox, the paralysis affects mostly the right side, though its use is not restricted only to the diseases of the right side. Nevertheless, there are some other remedies much stronger and more effective than Rhus Tox for conditions affecting the left side of the body, such as Lachesis and Ledum, which work wonders when given along with Arnica. Additional use of Cadmium Sulph 30, three times a day, makes the prescription even more effective. If there is still no favourable response, then Sulphur and Rhus Tox should be used alternately.

The Rhus Tox **headache** resembles very much the headache accompanying fevers. If the symptoms of the patient resemble one particular remedy, then that remedy alone should be used. If the symptoms are non-specific, then Rhus Tox may often be found useful. Generally speaking, in Rhus Tox the head feels heavy. The headache begins at the forehead and then spreads backwards to the nape.

In Rhus Tox, blood flow to the face and head increases. The skin becomes red, swollen and tender, associated with intense itching. Thick scabs form all over the area of eczema.

Out of the lists of eczemas, the one most responsive to Rhus Tox is the **eczema in children affecting their scalp.** However, it must be remembered that the body may react to Rhus Tox violently. Once it gets better, then Rhus Tox may be repeated in a few days. If the eczema does not respond, then some other homoeopathic remedy should be sought. This is not an easy task. Such a condition may in fact be cancer of the skin, which should be treated with Carcinocin 1000 and Radium Bromatum 1000, once a week for one to two months. Similarly, Graphites and Psorinum given alternately may prove very useful in the treatment of resistant forms of eczema.
Rhus Tox is also very useful in the **treatment of eye infections** i.e. redness with the discharge of pus (pink eyes) especially in the humid weather. The pain gets worse on moving the eye or by pressure. Warm tears flow out of the eyes.

The **sores and blisters inside the mouth** that look raw and red can be treated with Rhus Tox, if the symptoms match completely with Rhus Tox. The taste of the mouth is metallic as if one is tasting torch batteries. The **tongue becomes red and looks bruised**. Blisters form at the mouth and the chin. The **tonsils become inflamed and enlarged**. The throat hurts and swallowing becomes obviously difficult. Rhus Tox is very useful in the **treatment of inflammation of the oesophagus with the above symptoms** (oesophagitis).

Rhus Tox is also useful in the **treatment of typhoid**. The fever affects the mouth adversely. The gas produces rumbling sounds in the abdomen. The abdomen becomes distended with gas. The patient tries to **belch** the air out unsuccessfully, nor can he pass flatus naturally. It is an extremely troublesome situation. Rhus Tox and Colchicum both may prove useful in easing this situation.

Sometimes, as a **result of lifting or carrying heavy weight, the muscles of the pelvis and the muscles at the back may become badly stretched or strained**. Women can develop the tendency of the uterus to prolapse. Rhus Tox happens to be the ideal and indeed the best remedy for this. However its beneficial effect is not limited to only the uterus. Severe muscular strain or sprain in any part of the body can be effectively treated with Rhus Tox and Millefolium.

Another symptom of Rhus Tox is that the **voice becomes hoarse** due to severe soreness of the throat. The voice improves on starting to talk. The more the person talks, the better the voice gets. In fact, such persons can make long speeches although they suffer later.

In Rhus Tox, the cough is very troublesome and severe. There is a **constant irritation inside the throat and trachea**. Rhus Tox can offer quick relief.

Rhus Tox is very effective in the **treatment of a failing heart** resulting from the overstretching and **enlargement of the heart**. A similar condition in athletes responds only to Rhus Tox. The patient has the **feeling of numbness and increasing weakness of the left upper extremity**, secondary to the weakness and dysfunction of the heart. Rhus Tox once again is the number one remedy for this condition. Lachesis and Arnica should be given for a few days. If these are not effective, then a few doses of Rhus Tox must be given. After that, Lachesis and Arnica combined should be started again.

Rhus Tox is also very useful in the **treatment of severe strains and sprains of the back** due to faltered muscles and ligaments of the back. It may also be very useful in the **treatment of chronic sprains of the ankles** if other remedies have not been of avail.

In women especially, restlessness and constant movement of the legs during sleep may be due to suppressed eczema or itchiness. Treatment with Rhus Tox will offer immediate relief of the discomfort though the suppressed skin disease may surface to the skin.

**Urticaria** may be found in many kinds of fevers. The Rhus Tox type of patients, tend to develop urticaria during a malarial attack.

Rhus Tox is also very effective in the **treatment of shingles** (Herpes Zoster). One type of Herpes is the result of sexual promiscuity. The Herpes Zoster is related to the inflammation of the nerves. Rhus Tox can be of significant avail if the skin lesions of the patient exude lot of warm watery fluid.

| | |
|---|---|
| **Adjuvants:** | Bryonia, Calcarea Fluor, Phytolacca |
| **Antidotes:** | Anacardium, Croton, Grandelia, Mesereum, Graphites |
| **Potency:** | 30 to 200 or very high potency. |

# RUMEX CRISPUS

## (Yellow Dock)

Rumex Crispus is extremely useful in the **treatment of cough** arising from the irritation and itching in the throat. There is one continuous stream of phlegm from the nose and throat down to the larynx, trachea and chest. The phlegm may either be thin, or very thick and tenacious. Rumex is commonly stated to be associated with a cough producing a lot of phlegm, although, sometimes, it may be associated with a dry cough. It is not right to only consider phlegm to reach the diagnosis of Rumex. In fact, Rumex can work very well in a dry cough that becomes persistent. According to Dr. Kent, Rumex is associated with a severe, dry cough. The cough is of a spasmodic type. There is a feeling of rawness inside the throat and trachea (windpipe) provoking cough. The cough is associated with pain at the breast bone (sternum). The patient gets severe spasmodic coughing shortly after going to sleep. He may sometimes not be able to sleep. The patient may unknowingly wet himself during a severe bout of coughing.

Sometimes, inflammation or infection results in the production of a copious amount of phlegm. Such a patient is described of phlegmatic nature. In Greek medicine, patients are ascribed to be of various natures, including bilious, phlegmatic, asthmatic and melancholic. The Rumex patient will produce a lot of phlegm, if he is of phlegmatic nature. But another patient showing symptoms of Rumex who is not of phlegmatic nature may not produce any phlegm at all. The nature of the patient works as a guideline for arriving at the correct diagnosis. This should be understood with reference to the classical medical definition, otherwise one may be confused.

Rumex is also useful in the **treatment of many abdominal problems**, such as excessive gas and rumbling in the abdomen. Usually **severe diarrhoea follows nasal catarrh**. The patient contracts sudden, severe and painless morning diarrhoea, making him leave the bed abruptly. The stools are copious, watery and of dark colour. The stomach feels heavy up to the throat after taking food. There is pain in the left side of the chest. The patient cannot eat meat. The belly aches more on movement and on talking.

In Rumex, the tongue becomes excoriated at its margin and is coated with a thick, yellowish crust. There is **itching** over various parts of the body, especially the legs. Small pimples form over the legs. On exposure to the cold air and while changing one's clothes, the itching becomes more severe.

A Rumex patient is very weak. He is extremely irritable and not able to comprehend very much. He suffers from a light continuous type of headache, affecting the forehead and the right side of the head. The headache becomes worse on sneezing. The patient is extremely sensitive to the cold air. He sneezes a lot. The nose runs profusely. Symptoms become worse in the evening and at night. The cough begins usually at 11p.m. whether the patient is awake or asleep. Another symptom of Rumex is the **hoarseness of voice**. Excessive amounts of thick phlegm make speaking difficult. There is a feeling of a lump sticking in the throat, which does not get better even on swallowing and hawking.

**Joint pains** are also not uncommon in Rumex. The joint pains of Rumex get worse from the cold. In Calcarea Phos also, the cold aggravates the joint symptoms.

Rumex symptoms aggravate on movement, as in Bryonia. However, in Bryonia (unlike Rumex), the patient is not very sensitive to the cold air.

| Potency: | 30 |
|---|---|

# RUTA GRAVEOLENS
## (Rue-Bitterwort)

Ruta is derived from a herb called Rue-Bitterwort. This herb has also been utilised in many other conventional medicines. Its seeds have also been previously used to neutralize the ill effects of many poisons. The homoeopathic remedy is extracted after grinding the herb, including its root.

Ruta, like Arnica, is one of those remedies used in the treatment of injuries. It is especially useful in the **treatment of bone injuries**. When a part of the body is subjected to **unusually heavy pressure, load or pull and becomes stiff**, then Ruta (like Rhus Tox and Millefolium) can also be very useful. Regarding its effects on such injuries, Ruta resembles Rhus Tox a lot. The symptoms of Ruta aggravate from both cold and heat. Athletes who develop **heart problems** under severe physical strain may well be treated with Ruta and Aconite combined. In workers doing fine work, the **eyesight** becomes badly affected. The eyes feel tired, the eyesight becomes dim and there is a feeling of pressure and pain in the eyes, especially the left eye. The eyes quiver. Ruta may indeed be very useful in the treatment of this eye problem.

Due to heavy strenuous exercises undertaken over a long period, the **hearts of some athletes may become enlarged**. It is a very common notion that the heart once enlarged cannot revert to its normal size. In homoeopathy however, it is possible to control the size of the heart. The stretched out muscle fibres of the heart become elastic once again and retract to the original size. Ruta and Rhus Tox behave very similarily to each other in this respect.

Once **nerve fibres become injured**, common conventional nerve tonics are of no avail. Even Arnica may not be effective. However, Ruta and Rhus Tox are found to be extremely effective. Hypericum is also very useful in the treatment of the injury to the nerves. Accidental cuts on the bone during surgery can heal very well with Ruta. Ruta expedites the **healing of broken bones** (fractures) by revitalizing the outer coverings of the bone (periosteum). The combination of Ruta, Calcarea Phos and Symphytum proves very effective. Calcarea Phos works on the inner substance of the bone while Ruta and Symphytum invigorate the periosteum. In case the injury is fresh, Arnica 30 may also be included.

In general, Ruta is indicated in the treatment of patients who are not anaemic but who tend to bleed. Ruta is useful in the **treatment of various fevers**, neuralgias and a sub-normally functioning stomach. The Ruta patient is very sensitive and easily enraged. The legs feel weak and unable to carry the weight of the body. The limbs feel tired and painful; **especially there is pain in the back** (upper and lower parts, both). These are the salient features of Ruta. The severity of pain is easier on lying down flat, however generally the pain is worse with rest and better for movement. Rest aggravates while movement ameliorates the pain. There is **pain over the mastoid processes (the prominences behind the ears) and heaviness in the ears**. The facial bones hurt. The gums are sore and bleed easily. At about **midnight**, the **patient wakes up due to coughing**, tightness of the chest and heaviness. The trachea hurts as if physically injured.

Ruta has already been mentioned under **ankle sprains**. Ruta is no doubt very famous for the treatment of this condition. Ruta is also useful in the treatment of **pain in the bones of the feet** that makes walking difficult, the feeling of formation of sores on the feet, **wrist sprains,** as well as the **stiffness of the fingers.**

| | |
|---|---|
| Adjuvant: | Calcarea Carb |
| Antidote: | Camphor |
| Potency: | 30 to 200 |

# SABADILLA

## (Cevadilla Seed)

Sabadilla is renowned for the **treatment of persistent sneezes**. Sneezing may occur in the absence of a nasal cold. Some people are **allergic to grass and pollen** and contract a violent type of sneezing. After the sneezing is over, the nose does not run, showing that the cause is not a nasal cold but simply the irritation inside the nose. Some homoeopaths use Sabadilla in a very low potency. However I have found it useful in 30 potency. The Sabadilla patient is very sensitive to cold, and starts to shiver even when it is not very cold outside. Every cold object aggravates the symptoms. Most of the symptoms of Sabadilla resemble those of Lachesis, such as the pain shifting from the left to the right and the body feeling very cold.

Lachesis itself is the topmost remedy for **hay fever**, especially in the spring season. Sabadilla is also most commonly employed in the spring season (flowering season). Some people who have an allergy to the scent of flowers can benefit from Sabadilla. However, when the **sneezing is due to allergy in the autumn**, it will respond better to Allium Cepa. Lachesis is the chronic of Sabadilla, and Alumina that of Allium Cepa. One must remember to use a fast acting remedy for the treatment of a sudden acute illness. When the acute stage has been brought under control, then the long-acting remedies can be used. If a patient exhibits the symptoms of Sabadilla, he must be treated with Sabadilla. Once the patient becomes apparently cured, Lachesis 1000 (the chronic of Sabadilla) must be given without waiting for the next course of the illness. Lachesis 1000 should then be repeated in fifteen days. Thus the patient can be permanently cured. In case Sabadilla and other quick remedies similar to it, do not offer initial relief, then Lachesis may be used. In some patients, it offers rapid relief. In other words, Lachesis is not only used as a chronic remedy, it may occasionally also be used as a quick remedy. At times, just one dose of Lachesis may stop the sneezing immediately. Sneezing is a common symptom in different remedies, so it is important to take a note of other symptoms as well. Mostly, all of the above remedies (Sabadilla, Lachesis, Allium Cepa) seem to work and do not disappoint the treating physician.

Sabadilla itself has the capability of treat certain chronic illnesses, like **chronic nasal catarrh** blocking the nasal passages.

It is very strange that some Sabadilla patients believe that a certain part of their body is extraordinarily large compared to the others. I have also seen such patients, who said that their face was badly swollen, while actually, this was not the case. This symptom is typical of Sabadilla. Based on this symptom, if the patient is treated with Sabadilla, then his other symptoms may also be cured. I remember one such woman patient, declared untreatable according to doctors. She insisted that one of her cheeks was badly swollen. When treated with Sabadilla, her other symptoms also disappeared by God's grace. When an idea gets riveted in the mind, it helps in identification of the disease and the appropriate remedy. A Sabadilla patient comes to believe that his ribs or legs have become bent or his limbs are wasting; he just cannot forget about it.

The presence of certain strange ideas and superstitions helps in arriving at the proper diagnosis rather easily. In Thuja, the **patient believes that he is made of glass** and naturally brittle. It is said that one such patient used to walk with utmost care, lest he fell down and broke. He was taken to a psychologist. To make the patient believe that his idea was false, the psychologist slapped him on his face, assuming that he would realise his thinking was wrong. However, the patient fell down and died on the spot. God knows best if this story is true or false. If it is true, then the patient must have been a perfect patient of Thuja!

In hay fever, there is a constant irritation inside the throat. The **presence of worms inside the intestines** produces irritation over or inside the nose, provoking sneezing. No wonder Sabadilla is the useful treatment for intestinal worms. Although Dr. Boericke though did not mention this effect in the chapter on Sabadilla he has mentioned it in his repertory under the heading of remedies for worms. **Sabadilla seems to be deadly to worms of the intestines**. Persistent itching at the nose, around the lips or at the palate area indicates the presence of worms in the intestines. The projection of the intestinal conditions outwards on the skin is only natural. For example, a stomach upset may show up as blisters in the mouth. Intestinal worms and nasal catarrh can be cured with just one remedy i.e. Sabadilla. Stannum is another good remedy against the intestinal worms, which simply melt away under its effect. The Sabadilla itch is mostly at the palate. Wyethia causes a similar pain at the palate area instead of itching. If the pain at the palate becomes shifted to the back of the throat, provoking a troublesome cough, then Nux Vomica is better. In regard to **nasal catarrh** Sabadilla behaves like Arsenic, except for the absence of a burning sensation.

There are conditions related to certain homoeopathic remedies, in which the patient feels very hungry while ill. In Sabadilla also, the patient feels very hungry in between sneezing.

In Sabadilla, the **patient suffers from dry cough, bellyache** and difficulty in breathing. He does not feel thirsty at all. The Stomach feels empty and there is a craving for sweets. The patient feels better on eating hot food, while cold drinks aggravate the symptoms. There is a feeling of heat, burning and something creeping on the skin. The skin becomes extremely dry and begins to split, especially under the toes. **Chronic infection around the toenails** is yet another symptom of Sabadilla.

The patient has a feeling of **something being stuck in the throat**, which he keeps trying to swallow. This is a chronic type of complaint which becomes worse in the cold. The tongue feels as though it is burning.

In Sabadilla, the children tend to suffer from **diarrhoea**. The abdomen feels as if it is being cut with a knife. Periods are delayed in women, and there is stabbing sensation in the ovaries. The uterus tends to sag downwards, as in many other homoeopathic remedies.

| | |
|---|---|
| **Adjuvant:** | Sepia |
| **Antidotes:** | Pulsatilla, Lycopodium, Conium, Lachesis |
| **Potency:** | 30 |

# SABINA

## (Savine)

Sabina is frequently used in the diseases of the women. Except for the menstrual symptoms, its overall picture resembles Pulsatilla. Its symptoms aggravate from heat. In Pulsatilla, the menstrual bleeding is scanty and interrupted while in Sabina it is excessive. The **bleeding tendency** is not limited to the uterus. The **nose and kidneys can also bleed**. Sabina is very useful in the **treatment of excessive menstrual bleeding** along with the generalized tendency to bleed. The patient is **prone to abort in the third month of pregnancy**. Sometimes, the women develop **small knots (cysts or tumours) in the ovaries, barring pregnancy**. In this condition, Sabina helps to cure the cysts of the ovaries and also promotes conception.

Sabina is also useful in the **treatment of bleeding piles**. It is also very beneficial in the **treatment of kidneys becoming painfully inflamed,** associated with the passage of blood in the urine. Thus, it resembles Pareira Brava. In Sabina, the kidneys are inflamed all over, causing constant localised pain (not colicky). In Pareira Brava, the pain radiates downwards along the ureter into the bladder. The stones from the kidneys may get lodged in the urinary bladder. In Sabina, the patient has a **constant urge to pass urine**. The act of urination does not relieve the urge however. The quantity of urine passed is scant as in Cantharis.

Sabina is certainly indicated and useful, in the **treatment of discharges resembling gonorrhoeal diseases** in both sexes. Even if there is no active gonorrhoea and the patient is apparently well; if the discharge resembles that of gonorrhoea, Sabina will be very effective.

In Sabina, the patient may experience **labour-like pains, even in the absence of pregnancy**. The uterus contracts and bears down as in labour. This pain results in the loss of pregnancy (abortion/miscarriage). Another symptom of Sabina is **prolonged excessive menstrual bleeding**, so much so that the period-free gap may be very short. The colour of the blood is bright red. The patient becomes anaemic due to excessive loss of blood. The blood obviously becomes of light colour due to dilution.

Violent pains through the uterus and the ovaries associated with genital itching are best treated with Sabina. The pain is not steady, rather it continuously moves upwards or downwards. Most of the experienced homoeopaths are of the opinion that Sabina is the **best remedy to prevent abortion**. In my experience, Caulophyllum is also very effective (see under Caulophyllum).

When combined with Calcarea Carb and Murex, Sabina becomes more effective in the **treatment of prolonged menstrual bleeding, diseases of the uterus, and the tendency to form fibroids**. This prescription also prevents against the tendency to abort. If the placental attachment of the foetus becomes detached, threatening abortion, then the immediate use of Sabina will obviate the loss of foetus. If the periods are followed by copious corrosive and offensive leucorrhoea and heightened sexual urge, then Sabina should be used. Sabina also exhibits sign of polyp formation with a tendency to bleed, often present at the back or thighs (natal cleft). They may prove quite dangerous.

In Sabina, the patient tends to bleed though not suddenly and profusely. In Millefolium, the bleeding is as if a tap has been opened. This difference must be kept in mind.

Sabina is also useful in the **treatment of gout**. One very peculiar feature of Sabina is that during the attack of gout, the bleeding stops altogether. As soon as gout is under control, the patient starts to bleed again and vice versa. Gout symptoms aggravate in a warm room. The joints become swollen, red and shiny. There is a feeling of burning in the chest. The taste of the mouth becomes bitter and the belly hurts. The patient may suffer from sudden headache, which subsides only slowly. The face and the head become congested with blood. The teeth hurt on chewing food. The abdomen feels full. The patient may also remain **constipated**.

| | |
|---|---|
| **Adjuvant:** | Thuja |
| **Antidote:** | Pulsatilla |
| **Potency:** | 30 |

# SANGUINARIA
## (Blood Root)

Sanguinaria is derived from the word Sanguine, which means having the colour of blood or mixed with blood. The word Sanguine fully reflects the nature of the remedy. The face of a Sanguinaria patient becomes red and hot. Burning hot and redness are its peculiar features.

In Sanguinaria, the **headache begins at the nape** and then becomes localised in the right temple area or in the right eye. **The pain localised in the left eye is indicative of Spigelia**. The ailments of Sanguinaria are due to blood disorder while those of Spigelia result from hypersensitivity of the nerves. Their nature is thus obviously different. In Sanguinaria the painful area throbs, while in Spigelia, the pain is of lightning nature. In Sanguinaria, like Lachesis, sleep aggravates the symptoms.

In Sanguinaria, the headache is associated with severe nausea, which causes further aggravation. On vomiting, the patient feels much better. In Sanguinaria, the palms of the hands and the feet feel burning hot. The patient keeps the feet out of the bed. In Pulsatilla, these symptoms pertain only to women. However in Sanguinaria, the symptoms affect men and women equally. Sanguinaria is a relatively short acting remedy. Thus, it is not of much use in chronic diseases, except those of the chest, e.g., tuberculosis. In **tuberculosis**, it has proven to be very effective and long acting.

In Sanguinaria, the patient feels a lot of **discomfort in the trachea and the upper respiratory passages**, on coughing and even on talking. The patient feels as if a ball of air is stuck in the throat. He feels relieved on its expulsion.

Sanguinaria is effective in the **treatment of tuberculosis and other chronic chest diseases** by way of relief of the symptoms, but it does not offer complete cure. Sulphur, Silicea and Graphites have the capability to cure **tuberculosis**, though the treatment is usually begun with the milder type of remedies, Sanguinaria 30 being one amongst those. High potency Sanguinaria is not usually required.

Sanguinaria is the complete **antidote for the allergy to the smell of roses**. In Sanguinaria, the headache sometimes recurs every seven days.

Other symptoms of Sanguinaria being present, it can be very useful in the treatment of left-sided pain as well. **Frozen shoulder, pain and stiffness of the right side of the neck and the upper back** respond very well to Sanguinaria. However, Sanguinaria is not of much avail in the treatment of pain resulting from external injuries. Rather it is the optimal remedy for deep-seated, internal diseases.

In Sanguinaria, the face of the patient always stays red. The patient develops headache on improper eating and on eating spicy, oily food. The **stomach feels burning**. The discharges are **acidic**. The patient feels **nauseated**. The vomiting, being strongly acidic, can corrode the throat. Sanguinaria is significantly effective in the treatment of extremely severe acidity of the stomach, if other symptoms of Sanguinaria are also present. The appetite increases. However, when the disease progresses further, the stomach fails and vomiting sets in. Then though still feeling hungry, the patient does not like to eat.

Sanguinaria is also useful in **treating the asthma secondary to the hyperacidity of the stomach,** besides Nux Vomica. The stomach bloats with gas. The patient may get sudden severe **diarrhoea,** like Croton, Aloe and Podophylum. Sanguinaria may be of use in the **treatment of diarrhoea beginning on the sudden cessation of nasal cold**.

In Sanguinaria, the **menstrual bleeding and leucorrhoea** are very offensive. Sanguinaria is used in the **treatment of menopausal symptoms** as well as premenstrual nausea and severe abdominal pain.

During **coughing**, the patient feels a **hissing sound in the throat** that wakes him up. The patient feels better on sitting up. This cough is related to the stomach. The symptoms of Sanguinaria become worse upon sleeping, resting and after eating fruit. The person feels better on movement and sitting up in the bed.

| | |
|---|---|
| **Adjuvant:** | Antimonium Tart |
| **Potency:** | 30 or higher as needed |

# SECALE CORNUTUM
## (Ergot)

Ergot, a dreadful poison, has been used since ancient times in labour, despite the fact that its slightest overdose can prove extremely dangerous. The general health of the woman can be seriously affected and she may suffer from some sort of serious internal problem throughout her life. There is no known cure for such complications so far.

Ergot has a constricting effect on the arteries and other tissues of the body, resulting in serious life-long illnesses. A woman overdosed with Ergot suffers from continuous dark coloured vaginal bleed. The body becomes thin and wasted. The skin becomes dark and contracted. The limbs can become paralysed. The patient cannot tolerate heat. He/she likes to be in the open air and cold. As in Arsenic, the patient feels very restless and a burning inside. The difference is that the Secale patient feels hot inside though the body feels cold to touch. The hands and feet may become ice cold, yet, the patient feels hot and under fire, putting the feet out of the bed. Whereas, in Arsenic, the patient feels severe burning inside, and the body may not be cold. He feels better in the heat and likes to keep himself covered and still feels cold, although his body may be warm on the outside. He feels better with hot fomentation i.e. external heat seems to suppress his feeling of heat inside. Concersely a Secale patient feels comfortable with cold applications. Even if it is very cold outside, he feels hot. Sometimes, it may be very difficult to distinguish Arsenic from Secale due to similarities of symptoms. They are also complimentary. In other words, they can compliment each other, if used one after the other.

On proving, it was discovered that Secale works better on patients of thin and lean build. Obese people are rarely Secale patients. This is why the remedy is described to be ideal for the patients who are thin, lean and rather emaciated. Their skin is dry, shrivelled and very unhealthy. As already mentioned, every Secale patient does not have to be so. It can also be effective in obese people. Additionally, Secale patients exhibit violet coloured spots or red spots with bluish hue. It is the **bluish tinge or the cyanosis**, which is important. These spots are indicative of diminished blood supply to that part of the body, such as the legs, calves, hands and wrists, especially over the superficial bones.

In Secale, there is a **tendency towards the formation of chronic sores and ulcers**, which can turn into gangrene, on further deterioration. For example, a simple cut on the finger may not heal. Instead, the wound becomes infected and the process of infection may gradually spread upwards. It smells terrible. The affected part can become rotten leading to the need for amputation through the joint, or the infection can spread beyond the joint, turning the rest of the limb gangrenous as well. In homoeopathy, by God's grace, there is treatment available for gangrene. I myself have treated many such patients successfully. By God's grace, none of them needed amputation, whereas, the doctors had definitely made the diagnosis of gangrene and advised surgery for them. The first sign of recovery is change in the colour of the affected part, which starts becoming pinkish instead of a dark colour. Secale and Arsenic are both very useful in the **treatment of gangrene**. Addition of Arnica further adds to their beneficial effect.

In Secale, a feeling of burning sensation everywhere, affecting the nose, the throat, as well as the upper respiratory passages.

In Secale, the **bleeding**, whether from the uterus, the nose or from any wound or cut, is of dark colour. This means that the bleeding is of venous origin. In the treatment of patients rapidly advancing towards death, whose blood has become thick, dark and cyanotic, Secale must be remembered and put to use.

Secale in homoeopathic form is very useful in the treatment of internal diseases of women such as **ulceration of the uterus**, causing continuous dark vaginal bleeding interrupted with short periods of dark coloured and offensive smelling discharge. The discharge contains dark blood clots that putrefy. Secale is very important and a very effective treatment for this condition as well as against the risk of formation of gangrene inside the uterus. General symptoms of Secale being present, it will cure the abortive tendency of the patient also. When treated with Secale for a month or two, the uterus recovers completely and becomes capable of carrying the foetus to full term.

At the time of childbirth, if the uterus is contracting to push the baby down, but the mouth of the **uterus (cervix) becomes tightly contracted**, the child cannot be born. In this condition, Secale must be used without delay, otherwise immediate surgery would be required to save the life of the patient. If left untreated with Secale and without immediate surgery, the patient would die in agony. Secale can also cure the pain and the excessive dark coloured bleeding from the uterus after delivery. Sometimes, the **breasts shrink in size during pregnancy** and an insufficient amount of milk is produced. Secale will restore the normal amount of lactation, which is enough to feed the baby.

Another symptom of Secale is that the **urine is rather black**, resembling the urine of Terebinthina. In Terebinthina, the black colour is due to the excess of protein in the urine, resulting from damage to the kidneys. Terebinthina is very effective in this situation. In Secale, the black colour is not due to an excess of albumin in the urine; instead, it is due to the mixture of blood from the dark coloured vaginal bleed.

In Secale, a patient of **pneumonia** can develop gangrene in the lungs (necrotizing type of pneumonia), which must be treated with Secale. Timely use of Secale works profoundly and offers immediate beneficial effect. Wherever there is a tendency of sores and ulcers to become necrosed and gangrenous, be it in the stomach, lungs or anywhere else on the mucous membranes, Secale must be an essential part of the treatment in all these conditions.

In Secale, **cramps and tightness** are common, and may be localized to the soles of the feet, calves or a part of the upper extremities. If other symptoms of Secale are also present, then Secale will provide immediate relief of the symptoms. It is also very useful in the treatment of neuralgias (the lightning type of pain along the course of the nerves). These pains are very troublesome. These pains get better on covering the affected part of the body.

**Insanity** is also common in Secale. The patient becomes delirious and violent. Being out of his mind, he exerts his utmost even if he is physically weak. It becomes really difficult to control him in this situation.

In Secale, the **stools are black** and smell stinky. The patient is unaware of his diarrhoea. The body becomes extremely cold and weak, yet he feels hot inside and does not like to be covered.

Secale is also useful in the treatment of **Asiatic cholera**. As in Camphor, the body becomes extremely cold, although the patient feels warm and uncomfortable inside. In Camphor, the body is cold but the patient does not feel cold inside.

In Secale, the patient may have **paralysis of the legs or any one particular part of the body**. The paralysis may also affect one side of the body with no special predilection. It may affect the right or left side. Without wasting time on the diagnosis of the paralysis, if the general symptoms of Secale are present, it should be used without delay. In Secale, whatever part of the body is affected, it feels numb with a burning sensation. The cramps and tightness always become worse at night. The patient feels better in the open air. The symptoms become worse in heat, with hot fomentation and before the onset of periods. Camphor and Opium annul the effects of Secale.

| | |
|---|---|
| **Adjuvants:** | China, Arsenic, Aconite, Belladonna, Pulsatilla |
| **Antidotes:** | Camphor, Opium |
| **Potency:** | 30 |

# SENECIO AUREUS

## (Golden Ragwort)

Senecio is commonly used in the treatment of gynaecological problems of young girls. During early adolescence, the periods may become irregular on exposure to the cold. If not treated properly in time, the condition may last throughout their life. In addition to Calcarea Phos, Senecio is also famous in the treatment of this condition. Young girls do not usually complain out of shyness. They may be careless in taking a cold shower, submerge their feet in cold water, remaining wet and exposed after a shower or walking in the wet weather with naked feet. This can result in serious irregularity of menstruation. All these symptoms can be treated with Senecio.

**Bleeding** is the hallmark of Senecio. The patient bleeds from everywhere, especially the areas where the mucous membranes and the skin join (junctional areas).

There are important urinary symptoms associated with Senecio. There is a constant burning pain along the urethra and continuous urge to pass urine. Senecio is also famous for the treatment of arthritis. For the kidney pain of Senecio, Pareira and Berberis work as adjuvants. However, if other symptoms of Senecio are present, this alone may be curative.

The headache is not very severe but stuns the patient. Sometimes the patient feels sharp pain in the left eye, radiating to the left temple area. There is a lot of sneezing and a burning sensation in the throat. The teeth become very sensitive. There is pain on the left side of the face. The inside of the mouth, palate and throat become dry, causing difficulty in swallowing.

The **griping pain in the abdomen** disappears after passing stools. Thin watery stools may also contain some hard faecal matter. The u**rine is very scanty** and of dark colour. It may be mixed with blood or pus. The children may also suffer from irritation of the bladder, causing frequent burning urination. The patient may also develop headache and pain in the abdomen.

Young girls may experience irritation of the throat, chest and bladder **before the onset of periods**. These symptoms become relieved after the periods finish. In case the periods stop and the patient starts bleeding from the nose, then Senecio may be found useful.

**Displacement of the uterus**, burning urination or stoppage of urine, **severe inflammation of the kidneys** and fever with chills are all the symptoms of Senecio, to be treated with Senecio.

Senecio illnesses become worse at noon and at night. The patient contracts **common cold** in the open air. The symptoms ameliorate with the onset of menstrual bleeding. The patient feels better if his attention is diverted.

| | |
|---|---|
| **Potency:** | 30 to 200 |

# SENEGA
## (Snake Wort)

Senega is an allopathic medicine used for the treatment of chest diseases for over 100 years. It has been a constant component of the conventional therapy for chronic cough, tuberculosis and other chest diseases. No doubt, it helps in the initial stage of treatment however, its prolonged use can be dangerous. The diseases that initially improve become worse later on. On the other hand, the homoeopathic treatment with Senega can cure all these conditions, without any fear of harm. Senega has also been found useful in the treatment of cardiac asthma.

Senega is very closely related to **pleurisy** and has been successfully used in its treatment. Pleura are the outer covering of the lungs, which when inflamed is called pleurisy or pleural pneumonia. Its effectiveness against pleurisy is well established. At times, it may not prove that effective in human beings due to a wrong diagnosis, but in the case of cattle, Senega has always worked as a sure shot remedy for pleurisy. In the cattle, the symptoms of an ailment are persistently universal and unlikely to change. So, if it works in one animal, it would certainly be found useful in other animals also.

In most of the **lung diseases**, the sputum is very sticky and copious. With the aggravation of **tuberculosis**, the sputum becomes more copious. Senega offers a significant relief of phlegm, although it does not provide complete cure.

The chest pain associated with Senega becomes worse on taking rest. The cough increases on movement, especially the cardiac asthma becomes much worse on movement. The patient does not like to be moved during an attack of asthma. It is particularly useful in the treatment of tuberculosis of the larynx. The extremely sticky sputum is very difficult to expel even on repeated coughing. Senega has been successfully used in the terminal stage of tuberculosis also. According to some homoeopaths, if the patient is of Senega constitution, it can cure his left-sided facial palsy, also. A Senega patient by nature is very quarrelsome.

| Potency: | 30 to 200 |
|---|---|

# SEPIA

## (Inky juice of Cuttle Fish)

Sepia is considered to be ideal for the treatment of women of slender build and narrow pelvis. The body may be rather toughly built. This however is not the only essential feature of a Sepia patient. It is also related to the **diseases of the liver and the uterus**. Once the symptoms of the disease have become manifest, Sepia may be used even in the absence of the constitution described above. It is important to keep the important symptoms in view, rather than the external appearance of the patient. The specific symptom of Sepia is the **absence of sexual desire** and lack of the emotions of love and affection, so much so, that an affectionate mother suddenly becomes indifferent to her child as well as her husband. Her social circle begins to shrink. She may even have the tendency to **commit suicide,** or she may become partially insane. In fact, these conditions develop as a result of having silently suffered over a long period. People around her do not notice it. To them she looks normal. The pressure keeps on building up, only to finally gush out like lava. Now, the patient has a full-fledged Sepia picture. She does not pay attention towards her husband and children, which is the natural result of pressure building up. In fact, she has completely broken down inside and is sick of everything.

In Sepia, the liver is the most affected. Any kind of uterine dysfunction will result in a variety of complications, both during pregnancy and after childbirth, which are accompanied by liver dysfunction. **She hates everything that in fact she should have liked**. The hate and indifference make her feel frightened and this further aggravates her sickness.

Another salient feature of Sepia is the formation of a dark, saddle-shaped mark over the bridge of the nose like two wings of a bird. In view of this sign alone, like so many other homoeopaths, I have also treated many patients with Sepia, to no avail. This particular sign is often indicative of liver dysfunction. But Sepia becomes effective only in the presence of liver derangement in a person of Sepia nature. Otherwise, some other remedy will be required. Sepia proves to be very effective in the treatment of the afore-mentioned sensitive type of woman, lacking emotions and showing the typical pigmented mark on the nose and the face.

Liver dysfunction ultimately leads to jaundice. Some women, **during pregnancy**, may **develop dark marks on their face**. The **face loses its healthy glow**. In Sepia, this sign may become apparent even without pregnancy. **Light Brown specks** form with black dots in the centre. This is typical of Sepia. Whitish or light brown spots can also form over the body, indicative of a liver problem. In homoeopathy, these are called **liver spots**. Brownish yellow spots are indicative of and responsive to Phosphorus and Sepia. White spots can be treated better with Merc Sol or Calcarea Carb, etc.

In Sepia, the patient tends to be **constipated**, more so during pregnancy. She cannot effectively pass stools, due to the weak propulsive power of the intestines. Such a woman also faces **difficulty during childbirth due to the weakness of pelvic and abdominal muscles** i.e. she cannot push the child with full force. In the presence of its other symptoms, Sepia will facilitate the birth of the child. If it fails, then Caulophylum and Gelsemium may be helpful.

In Sepia, the stomach feels empty and the patient feels extremely hungry. However, the appetite and weakness do not get better after eating food. If this type of woman also tends to have **prolapse of the uterus** or weakness of the muscles of the back, then Sepia will offer immediate relief. Sepia has been found very effective in the **treatment of vomiting of pregnancy**, as long as the patient is that of Sepia. Other characteristic features of Sepia are the vomiting of milky white material and **whitish leucorrhoeal discharge**. The taste of the mouth and smell are also affected.

Sepia also can be useful in the treatment of herpes if other symptoms of Sepia are also present. Sepia offers immediate relief of headache associated with vomiting of bitter contents. Provided that the patient is of sepia constitution; Sepia can cure every **eye condition** and most of **skin conditions** of the patient. Skin diseases, in general are common in many remedies, however if the overall picture is of sepia type then sepia would be useful.

In Sepia like Sulphur, the discharge is purulent and stinky. Nasal secretion is of green colour. Associated degradation of the skin and mucous membranes can also get better with Sepia.

A Sepia patient is mostly **constipated**. Sometimes, the patient gets **diarrhoea**, passing lot of whitish sticky mucus. Mucus may also be passed along with hard stools as well as **dysentery**. The stools smell foul. The associated **piles** also are very painful. The patient passes blood in the urine. **Retention of placenta** (after childbirth) can be a source of many serious complications. If Pulsatilla becomes ineffective, then Sepia may help. However, Pulsatilla and Sepia can only be effective before the onset of the infection (i.e. **puerperal sepsis**). Once the infection develops, Sulphur and Pyrogenium 200 happen to be the best standard remedy.

During lactation in Sepia woman menstruation usually ceases, while they are irregular in Calc Carb. The vaginal discharge of a Sepia woman is acidic in nature, causing neuralgic pain.

Moderate physical exercise aggravates the symptoms of Sepia while t strenuous exercise offers relief.

In Sepia, the **hands and feet tend to be numb**. **Malarial fever** of unpredictable timing may be made to behave more timely with Sepia therapy. In addition, the diagnosis as to the most appropriate treatment needed may also be established. If the patient is of Sepia constitution then Sepia itself will affect the cure.

The **eyesight becomes weak**, due to weakness of the eye muscles. Black spots (floaters) seem to be dancing before the eyes. The eyes become inflamed due to the general weakness and the diseases of the uterus. The eyelids become swollen and baggy. Lumps form behind the ears, near the neck. In some patients, yellow spots may form on the skin. The tongue is coated white. Taste of the mouth is salty. The patient relishes sour things and feels extremely weak and exhausted. The patient becomes **nauseated** at the smell of food; more so while lying on the side.

| | |
|---|---|
| **Adjuvants:** | Natrum Mur, Nux Vomica, Phosphorus |
| **Potency:** | 30 and higher. In psychiatric patients, it should be given in CM potency |

# SILICEA

## (Silica – Pure Flint)

Silicea or Silica is an element naturally present in sand and certain stones. It is widely distributed in the entire world. This element, along with clay, became the first building block for the creation of life. No wonder it is present in each and every living cell. Through the work of some renowned homoeopaths, Silicea has been found to possess many qualities. Silicea has never been used as a remedy except in homoeopathy. Its symptoms and signs have been discovered on homoeopathic proving, over a long period. Silicea is one of those remedies in which proving is a very slow and time consuming process. On proving, it has been found to be a profoundly active remedy, capable of working for a long period of time.

**Silicea cannot tolerate the presence of any foreign material in the body**. It stimulates the body defences to react against any foreign body and expel it as soon as possible. If the foreign material happens to be inanimate, then Silicea initiates the process of pus formation around it. The pus formed creates a soft resilient medium like Mobil oil, through which the foreign body gets expelled gradually and softly without further injury to the soft tissues. If the foreign body happen to be animate, such as bacteria, viruses or intestinal worms, etc., then Silicea provokes an appropriate body response. This process is definitely more effective than the conventional antibiotic therapy. Silicea may simply kill the germs and worms, liquefy them in the form of pus or just expel them through the different natural orifices.

In some diseases, Silicea has little or no effect on the patient, such as the typhoid fever. Similarly, in certain cases of blood poisoning (toxaemia and septicaemia) it may not be as effective as Sulphur and Pyrogenium, which are definitely much superior. Now, after long experience, we have come to know the diseases where Silicea will be definitely effective, as well as the conditions where something else would be more appropriate. For certain deep-seated illnesses of a grave nature, requiring the activation of a very specific response on the part of the body, the physician has to work hard in order to find the most appropriate remedy, keeping in mind both the nature of the disease as well as the remedy. The powerful defence system of the body is very intricate and individually designed to combat hundreds of thousands of illnesses. The system is like a great powerful factory beyond the comprehension of not only ordinary people but also the expert scientists. Silicea, despite appearing wideranging and powerful, has yet to overwhelm the natural defence system or even match it.

Generally speaking, Silicea is very effective against **contagious disease, boils and abscesses.** Similarly, it provokes a surprisingly strong reaction against inanimate foreign objects entering the body. For example, Silicea is extremely **effective in the expulsion of a retained nail, fishbone or shotgun pellets in the body**. Here, it works in two ways. When given in low potency, it gradually increases the local blood flow, kills the germs and produces pus. The process of healing of the **boils and abscesses**, which normally takes seven to ten days to get ready to burst open, may be completed in two to three days. Moreover, the pain is relatively less and much less pus is formed. The hole through which the pus exudes is also small and insignificant. On the same lines, Silicea helps the **expulsion of a needle,** piece of metal or stone retained in the body. The process is very intricate and yet to be understood but the practical examples are so obviously true. Once, an eminent surgeon told me that one of his patients had swallowed a needle, which became stuck in his intestines. Obviously, it was dangerous to remove it surgically. The surgeon had heard about the efficacy of Silicea and decided to use it. After a while, the needle showed up on the surface of the skin, without injuring the internal organs. The path adopted by the needle was the shortest towards the skin surface. There was no damage inflicted to the linings of the intestines, or the fat inside the abdomen. The method by which Silicea performs this harmless function cannot be conjectured by human intellect and imagination, but the observation is too weighty and hard to be denied. Once when I was in Rabwah, a large irregular piece of glass got stuck in the foot of a child, deep to the bone. The foot became extremely swollen and the doctor refused to remove it surgically. The child was treated with Silicea 6X for a month. At first, the swelling started getting less and then the large piece of glass started to gradually emerge from the skin. It was then safely removed with forceps.

Due to the use of contaminated water in Africa and Sindh province of Pakistan, quite commonly a **worm enters the body**, which can be very dangerous. It starts growing in length like a tape. It then shows up like a cotton ball under the surface of the skin, which may grow up to the size of a football. The leg may grow to the size of the foot of an elephant. This is why this condition is called elephantiasis. A Waqf-e-Jadid missionary Homoeopathic doctor named Nisar Maurani, a convert from Hinduism, successfully made use of Silicea in the treatment of this disease. He observed that Silicea 6X simply dissolves the worm inside the body and thus obviates the need for surgery. Surgery can in fact be very dangerous. If the worm is not completely removed and is severed or accidentally cut into pieces, every piece will then rapidly grow into a new worm, wherever it deposits in the body. This is potentially fatal. Local experts in Africa extract it by rolling it on a thorn or a matchstick. The worm may be hundreds of feet long. If it gets severed during this process, all the hard work goes in vain. Be it Sindh or Africa, Silicea works equally well everywhere. It dissolves the worm and lets it be extruded through a minute hole.

Sometimes, a **fishbone gets stuck in the throat** and is difficult to remove. Once, I confronted a similar situation myself. I tried to remove it but failed. Then, I took Silicea 6X. Within a few hours, the fishbone came out with an act of a mild cough. I have found it effective in children too. With rare exceptions, Silicea is always effective.

When given in high potency, **Silicea dries pus**. **Large abscesses** thus gradually regress and disappear. Pus does not form with the use of Silicea in high potency. Pus formation is usual with Silicea used in low potency. One must understand the dual role of Silicea, which obviously is under the control of the natural defence system of the natural human body. In **tuberculosis**, Silicea in high potency plays the role of expulsion of the germs by way of formation of pus. It cannot kill the tuberculous Bacillus however. In case the germs happen to settle in the vicinity of an artery, then Silicea may result in rupture of the artery and cause severe haemorrhageing, which may prove fatal. Therefore, the physician has to be very cautious before embarking on the use of Silicea 6X or 30 even. In general a, low potency works rather slowly and mildly and thus prevents against any serious reaction. According to Dr. Kent, whether given in low or high potency, Silicea is dangerous to the patients of tuberculosis. So, as far as possible it should be avoided but if it needs to be given at all, only potency 30 should be used. It is neither too high, nor too low.

Silicea is incompatible with some remedies and should never be mixed with them. For example, it is incompatible with any form of Mercury, so Silicea and Mercury should never be given together. Hepar Sulph is similar to Silicea in some respects and similar to Merc Sol in others. It must always be used in between the usage of Silicea and Mercury. It serves as a bridge between the two remedies. Sometimes, Silicea works in an unexpected way, for example, a patient has infection in the root of a tooth, but is not aware of it. If by chance, he is treated with Silicea, his jaws will start swelling up and the tooth will become loose. At this stage, he should take Hepar Sulph (the antidote for Silicea). He will be relieved of the pain immediately and will also know for sure that he had an infection in the root of the tooth. A suitable homoeopathic remedy then can be administered to help restore the tooth.

A general symptom of Silicea is that the patient feels very cold. His hands and feet remain cold. This symptom may however be deceiving and hinder the way to proper treatment. In general, the patients suffering from infectious fever (septicaemia) have very hot hands and feet. Many a physician will then treat them with Pulsatilla instead of Silicea. Obviously, it is of no avail. The real diagnosis of Silicea is that before the onset of fever, the hands and feet become cold. As the temperature rises, the symptoms of Pulsatilla manifest. It must be remembered that Silicea is the chronic of Pulsatilla. Sometimes, the body of a patient is fiery hot, including the hands and the feet, but he needs to be treated with Silicea instead of Pulsatilla. It happens very commonly in the treatment for severe **infection of the tonsils**. Some of these children who are wrongly treated with Pulsatilla instead of Silicea may lose their life.

A Silicea patient is by nature, apprehensive of failure i.e. job or exam. Particularly school children have this problem. For example, many people who in spite of being able to drive efficiently, repeatedly fail in the driving test, in spite of having reasonable knowledge and practice of driving. Similar fear is also found in some other homoeopathic remedies. Therefore, Silicea is often forgotten. Nevertheless, administration of Silicea 6X along with Kali Phos can produce wonderfully positive results.

Some **wounds and ulcers become indolent** and resistant to healing. If the patient exhibits the symptoms of Silicea, then Silicea can activate the healing process of this dormant condition, by way of formation of pus. After the pus comes out, the wound becomes dry, leaving a very inconspicuous scar.

Silicea is extremely useful in the **treatment of enlarged body glands in women**. It is very effective against the common **skin infections such as pustules, blisters and abscesses**. Ugly looking pubertal acne often responds very well to the treatment with Silicea 30 and Kali Bromide. It can often cure the stubborn type of acne. The treatment should continue for at least a month, and then repeated on and off, as needed.

One should never forget using Silicea for infection causing the formation of pus, in any part of the body. **Excessive sweating of the feet** in Silicea resembles Sulphur. In Sulphur, the feet remain warm, sweat and feel burning. In Silicea, the patient feels cold, yet sweats excessively on his feet.

In Silicea, the **headache begins in the nape of the neck, commonly in the morning**. Thus, it is different from the headache of Gelsemium. Both Silicea and Gelsemium are of mild, cold nature. In Silicea, the headache may shift to the front of the head, forehead or even the eyes. If this symptom is evident, then the treatment should be Silicea. The headache begins in the morning and continues till late night.

In Silicea, sometimes, the lower part of the body is dry, while the upper part is sweaty. In Calcarea Carb, it is only the head that sweats. In Rhus Tox, the upper part of the body sweats, except the head. In Silicea, the ailment begins in a very timely manner and finishes on time (periodicity). The symptoms can recur however. The symptoms aggravate on the rise of the new moon.

In some **children, asthma** becomes more severe with the appearance of the new moon. This is typical of Silicea. Certain kinds of fevers, irregularity of the menstrual cycles and epilepsy is also **related to the moon.** Most of the ailments of Silicea last seven days.

In Silicea, besides the nape, the **headache is mostly on the right side of the head**, resembling Mag Phos (for details, please refer to Mag Phos). Silicea is also very useful in the **treatment of severe and troublesome eczema over the scalp**. However, the treatment should be combined with Psorinum and Graphites, which will definitely ameliorate the chronic eczema. These remedies should be given in potency 1000 and repeated alternately. In **psoriasis** too, the patient has to be given Psorinum, Sulphur, Silicea and Graphites one after the other. The disease being very deep and serious cannot be controlled with one or two remedies.

Sometimes, children develop blood naevi (haemangioma) in the form of **raw-looking blood-filled blisters**. If the patient is of cold constitution, then by Allah's grace, Silicea will be very useful. Otherwise, Ferrum Metallicum would be the first choice, which has also been found to be useful in the treatment of large birthmarks.

Silicea is very beneficial in the **treatment of dangerous and deep-seated illnesses of the glands**. It is capable of softening and reducing the size of the glands. Calcarea Fluor, Baryta Carb, Phytolacca and Causticum may also be useful. If the glands at the jaws, in the neck and in the armpits start growing rapidly and the patient is of cold constitution, then Silicea must be used. If Silicea does not offer any relief, then the condition is probably cancer. In this condition, Silicea alone will not benefit. This patient should be treated with Sulphur CM. When the patient starts feeling cold with the treatment of Sulphur, then one dose of Silicea CM should be given. As long as the symptoms of cold or heat do not change, the treatment should not be changed either.

Silicea is also useful in the **treatment of ulcers of the cornea**. Corneal ulcer is difficult to treat, but if the patient is of the constitution of Silicea then Silicea would work extraordinarily well. (For other similar remedies, please see under Calcarea Fluor).

Tonsillitis associated with catarrhal conditions is found in many homoeopathic remedies. Silicea will only be successful if this is a constitutional remedy. Silicea, like Calcarea Fluor, can also be useful in the **treatment of brittle teeth**.

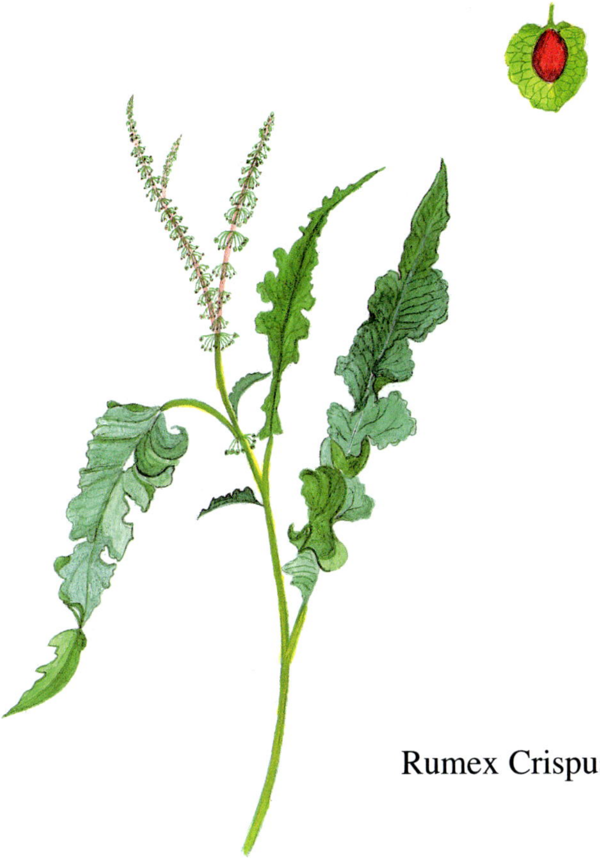

Rumex Crispus

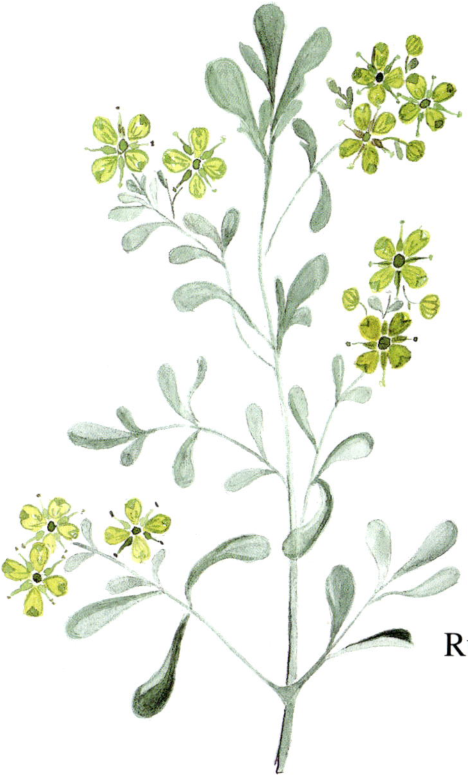

Ruta Graveolens

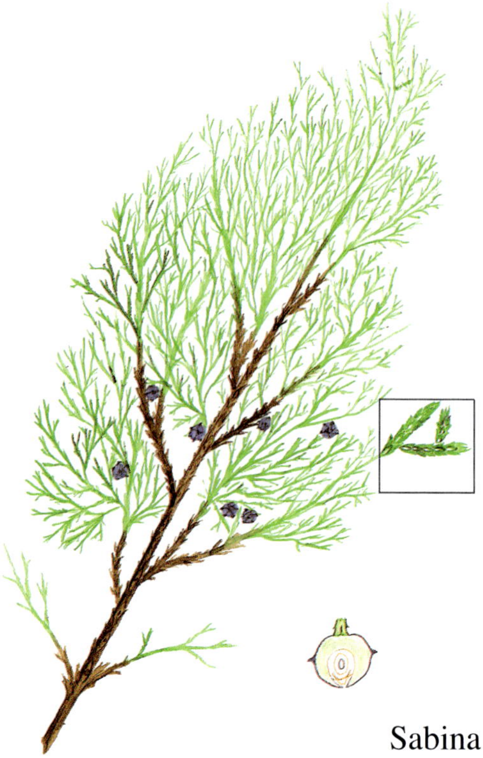

Sabina

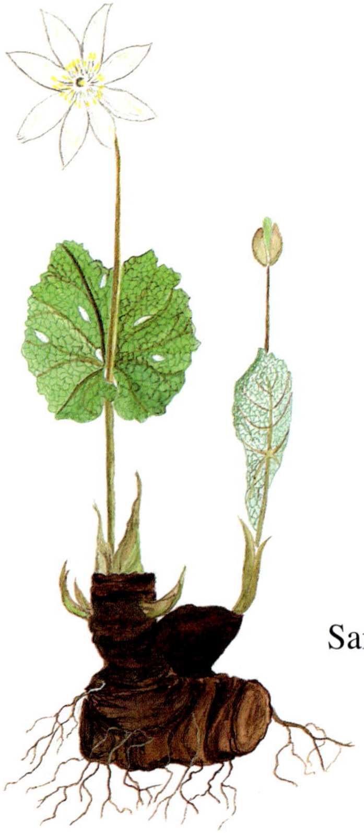

Sanguinaria

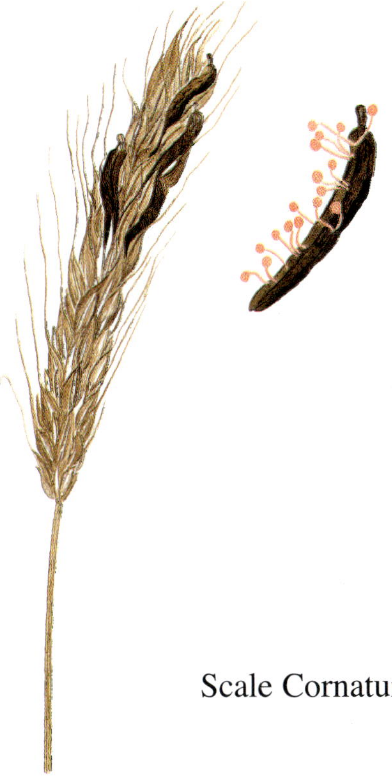

Scale Cornatum

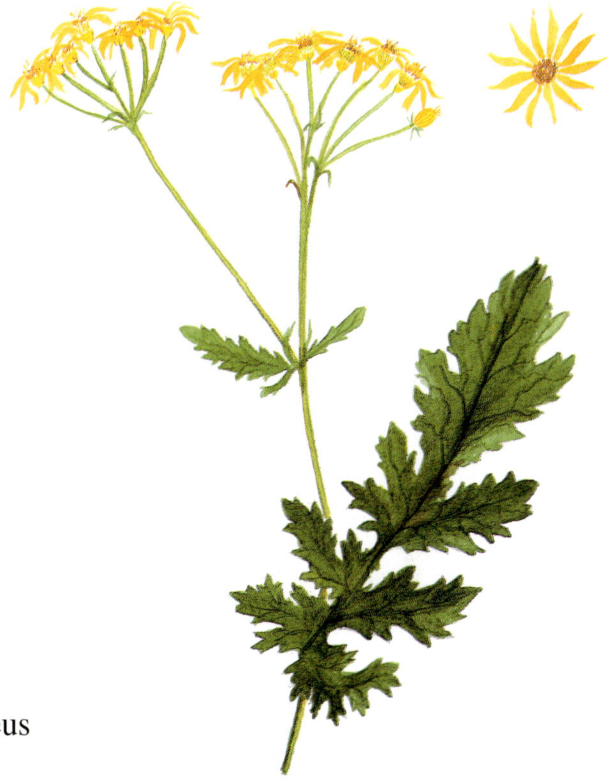

Senecio Aureus

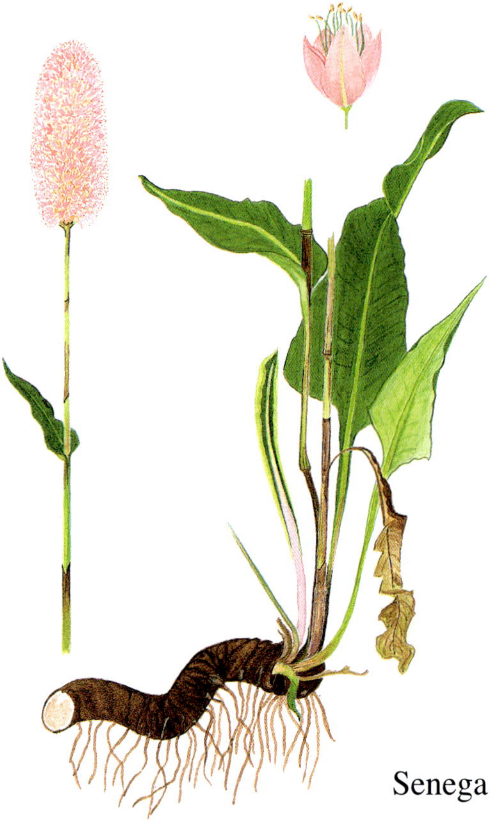

Senega

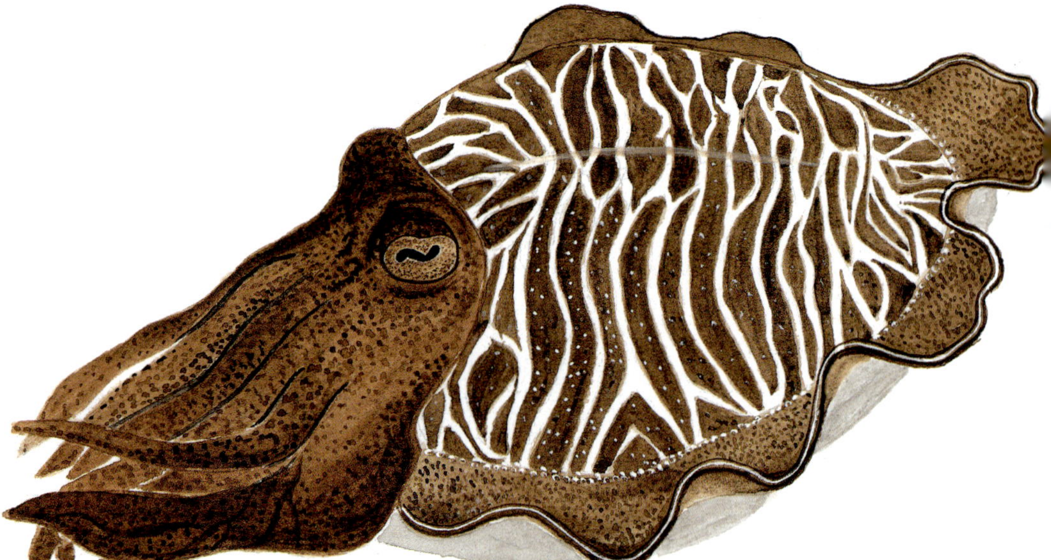

Sepia

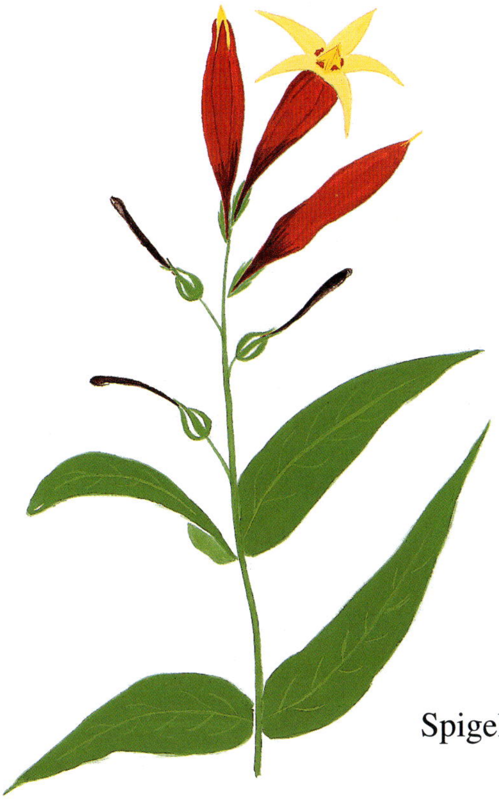

Spigelia

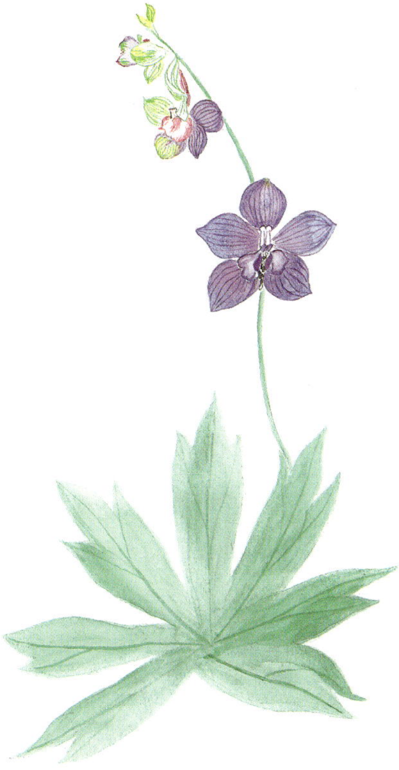

Staphysagria

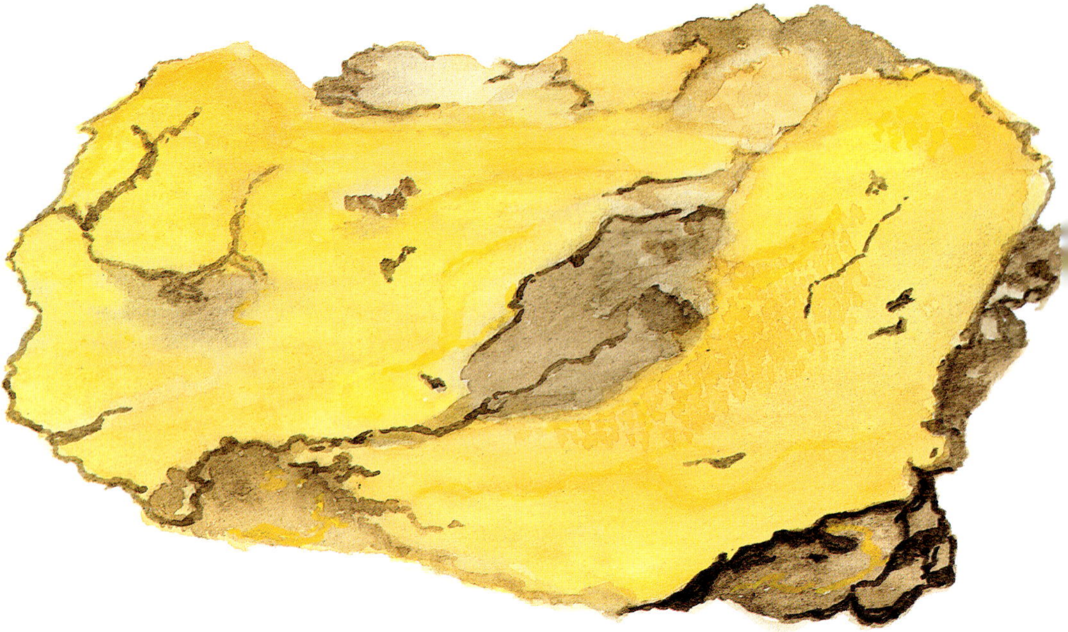

Sulphur

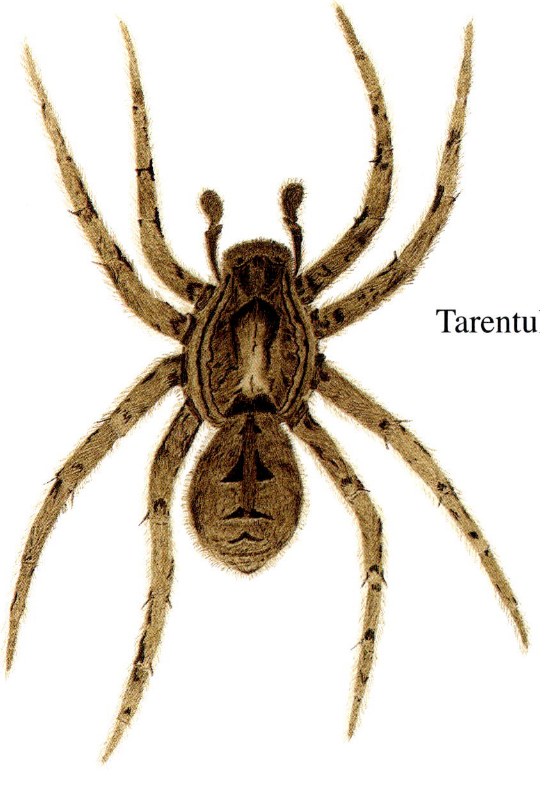

Tarentula Hispania

Veratrum Album

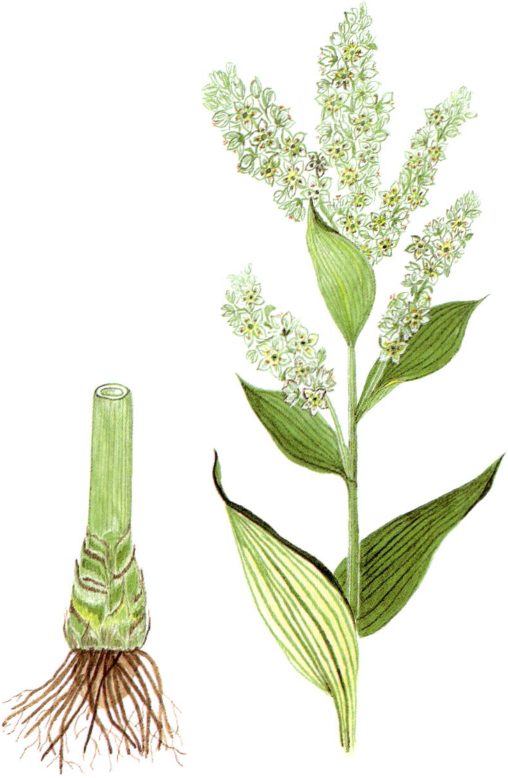

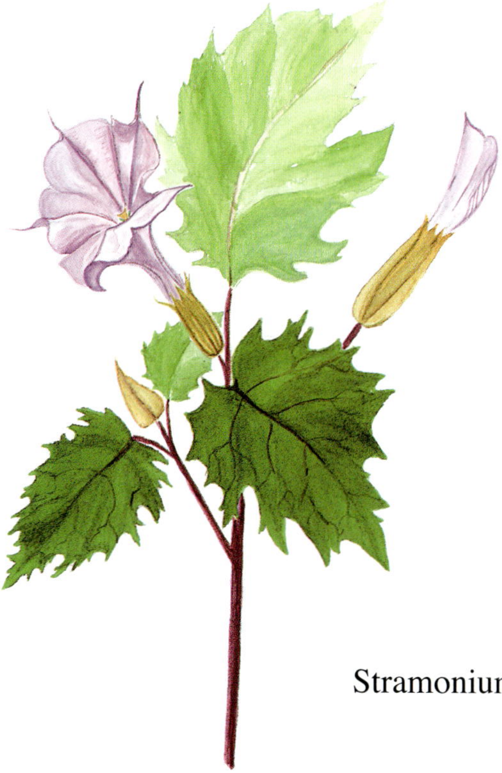

Stramonium

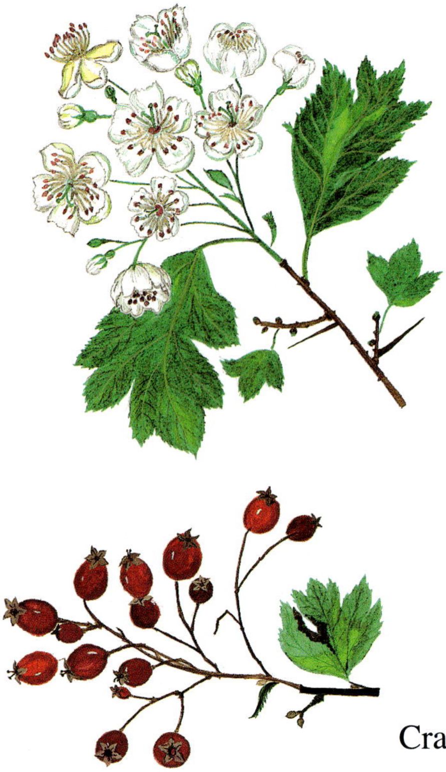

Craetigus

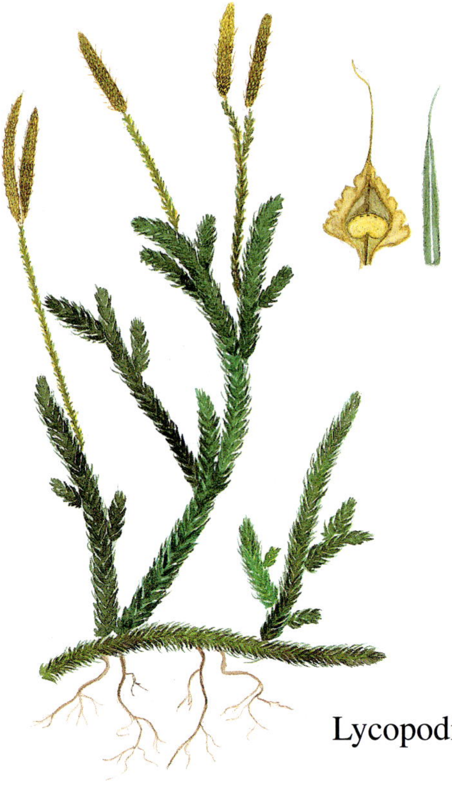

Lycopodium

In most homoeopathic literature, Silicea is not mentioned as the **treatment for acute inflammation of the throat**. It is only described for chronic illnesses of the throat. This is incorrect. In fact, Silicea is capable of curing the acute **infection of the tonsils** (quinsy) associated with fever. Simultaneous use of Kali Mur, Ferrum Phos and Calcarea Fluor 6X will help the **fever** subside rapidly, by the grace of God. If the fever does not come down on the first day, it will gradually subside in two to three days.

A patient of Silicea feels cold, yet likes to drink very cold water. He wants to eat ice or put ice in all the drinks. In some homoeopathic literatures, it is mentioned that a Silicea patient hates to take meat or if he likes meat at all, he likes to eat it cold. My own vast experience does not support this notion. Most Silicea patients do not in fact, dislike meat.

Silicea is also very useful in the **treatment of chronic diarrhoea**, which may be due to tuberculosis or unclean and unhealthy food (as the food sometimes available in refugee camps). In chronic diarrhoea or **dysentery**, besides Sulphur and Croton, Silicea may also be useful, provided that the patient's body remains cold. During a world war, a homoeopath used Silicea very successfully in the treatment of diarrhoea. At another occasion, Silicea did not benefit. The reason is that the diseases adopt different nature in different kinds of weather and epidemics, and will obviously need different remedies to treat them.

Some of the Silicea symptoms resemble those of Kali Carb. Both are of cold constitution. Silicea works extremely well in the treatment of sexual diseases (like Kali Carb). If the patient wets his bed due to cold, this can also be treated with Silicea.

Sudden **cessation of periods in women**, especially young girls can be effectively treated with Silicea, provided the patient also exhibits other symptoms of Silicea, so much so that it can effectively cure even the epilepsy resulting from the cessation of periods.

Silicea is also very useful in the **treatment of asthma**. Fever during asthma can best be treated with Silicea. Silicea given after the asthma attack is over will prolong its effectiveness and will stop the tendency towards asthma in the future.

Silicea is the **treatment of epilepsy** if the patient is of cold constitution and if the epilepsy is preceded by an aura originating at the abdomen and then affecting the brain. One should never forget using Silicea for the treatment of epilepsy occurring in the early part of the lunar month.

In Silicea, the **tongue hurts, as in gout, and is swollen**. One part or other of the tongue keeps hurting constantly. Blisters form over the gums. Silicea also relieves the **hiccuping resulting from stomach upset**. Nux Vomica and Ignatia are also very useful in the treatment of hiccups.
In Silicea, there is a tendency towards **nausea and vomiting**. The general symptoms of Silicea being present, Silicea can also cure the **liver dysfunction**. The patient dislikes hot food, but loves to eat it cold.

Sometimes, **children develop severe constipation** and strain hard. In these children, Silicea and Veratrum Album are very useful. (For detail, see under Veratrum Album).

Silicea is also useful in many **urinary problems**. If the urine contains pus as well as blood, or there is frequency of urination due to an irritable bladder or the urine contains particulate matter settling in the bottom of the container, then Silicea will be beneficial.

The **oxalate stones produced in the kidneys**, which are not amenable to any other treatment, may be excreted in the urine by using Silicea 6X. These stones are usually not visible in the x-rays. The diagnosis is mostly based on the severe pain (renal colic). Oxalate stones are more common in the areas where the food gets contaminated with minute stone particles. My pupils in homoeopathy have widely used Silicea in the treatment of these stones in Afghan refugee camps successfully.

Sometimes, **cysts form in the lower part of the uterus**, which can rupture letting their sticky contents flow out. It is a pretty troublesome and disturbing condition. The **ovaries become inflamed** and may even produce pus. Small nodules form inside the uterus. Silicea is very effective in the treatment of all these symptoms if it matches the constitution of the patient.

Warts, inflammation and pain due to an **in-growing toenail** or **formation of the calluses** due to tight shoes can be treated with Silicea or Sulphur according to the overall symptoms of the patient. But some homoeopaths claim that the best treatment of an in-grown nail is the homoeopathic remedy prepared from a magnet found in Northern part of Australia.

| | |
|---|---|
| **Adjuvants:** | Thuja, Pulsatilla, Fluoric Acid |
| **Potency:** | 30 or higher as needed, to be used with extreme caution. |

# SPIGELIA
## (Pink Root)

Spigelia is prepared from a plant called pink root. It is renowned for the treatment of neuralgic pains affecting the left side of the body. It is also of great value in the **treatment of joint pains**. Patients suffering from **chronic multiple joint pains** become irritable and hypersensitive. Spigelia will be very useful in the treatment of these patients. Spigelia is highly effective in certain heart conditions, such as **inflammation of the outer covering of the heart as well as the valves of the heart, and rapid heartbeat** (tachycardia). Spigelia is of immense value for the treatment of left-sided facial neuralgia. According to the majority of Homoeopaths, Spigelia can cure any form of **neuralgic pain affecting the neck and the face**. Sometimes, the pain at the neck and shoulder becomes chronic. It feels better on application of hot fomentation. The Spigelia ailments become worse in cold weather, though the pain as such is of burning and lightning type, as if the affected part has been tied with hot burning wires. The patient feels hot up to the end of the nerves. Spigelia should not be forgotten in this situation. As far as possible, one should avoid having injections, etc. Injection therapy may suppress the condition, but the wrong choice of injection may inflict permanent, serious harm. Spigelia, when effective, needs no supplementation with injections. If Spigelia fails then one should look for other appropriate Homoeopathic remedies.

The **neuralgic pain of the eye** (ocular neuralgia) usually arises, on exposure to cold. The pain undulates along the course of the nerves. The Spigelia pains fleet around, over the entire body.

Spigelia is very useful in the **treatment of pericarditis as well as endocarditis**. Pericarditis means the inflammation of the outer covering of the heart, causing fever and tightness in the chest. Endocarditis means the affliction of the valves of the heart by bacteria, resulting in fever, difficulty in breathing and dysfunction of the heart.

The neurologic symptoms of Spigelia include a **weak memory**, general indifference, restlessness and confusion. The patient feels dizzy on getting up suddenly. The weakness may be due to increase or decrease of blood pressure, or due to the disturbance of the fluid level in the internal ear (labyrinth). Dizziness may sometimes be due to an ear infection. Despite severe pain, the patient is drowsy. The patient feels better on lying down with the head elevated. The symptoms of Spigelia become worse on bowing the head forward.

The aches and pains of Spigelia can affect the right as well as the left side of the body. Yet, Spigelia is considered ideal for the treatment of left-sided problems. Sanguinaria is considered useful for the problems related to the right side of the body. The headache amenable to treatment with Spigelia begins at the nape of the neck, and then shifts to the right or the left side of the head. It is associated with severe throbbing and is of undulating type. The pain may become localized to the forehead over the right or the left eye. During the pain, the head feels tightly tied. Sometimes, the patient starts having cold sweats due to the extreme severity of the pain or he may start throwing up. Such a patient should be immediately wrapped in a heavy quilt, given hot black tea and Spigelia be administered to them without delay.

Unusual high sensitivity to pain is found in Pulsatilla, Hepar Sulph, Chamomilla and Oxalic Acid. For details, please refer to the appropriate chapters.

In Spigelia, the pain is felt in the **substance of the nerve**. It is not due to inflammation or injury to the nerve. The pain is very severe and may be externally marked with red lines along the course of the nerve. It may probably be due to increased blood flow along the nerves. This symptom is typical of Spigelia. The red lines are visible only on the affected area. The pain may be of piercing type and touch is unbearable.

In Spigelia, the **eyes feel big**. The patient cannot focus the eyesight and sometimes objects look out of their actual place. The **pain in the eye** is associated with extreme pressure. The eye hurts on moving the eyeball. However, the eye is not red. Pain without redness indicates the neuralgic nature of the pain. One may feel dizzy on trying to move the eye.

The eyes water and are sensitive to light. The facial pain may involve the cheekbones, eyes, teeth and the temple areas. The pain becomes worse on bending forwards. Spigelia is also useful in the treatment of intestinal worms.

| | |
|---|---|
| **Antidote:** | Pulsatilla |
| **Potency:** | 30 or higher |

# SPONGIA TOSTA

## (Roasted Sponge)

This is a soft and porous sponge type of marine life. It usually clings to the rocks and stones in the sea. Once detached or severed, it settles to a new stony surface and starts growing rapidly. Thus a new sponge colony forms. When dead, it floats on the surface of the sea. Some people pick it up from there and sell it to make their living. On squeezing a sponge loses its water, which it reabsorbs on the release of pressure. This quality of sponge is permanent. Even if left as such for hundred years, it keeps its quality. The Sponge is of great domestic use, and besides this, it has been used in many remedies in a roasted form.

The homoeopathic remedy prepared from roasted sponge is useful in many diseases. Its use is mostly related to **asthmatic bronchitis and heart problems**. Cardiac asthma / cough is a condition in which the muscles of the heart become weak, swollen and flabby. The resultant failure of the heart muscles causes water logging in the lungs (pulmonary congestion), leading to shortness of breath. Spongia is the best remedy for this condition. In this type of cough, the breathing sounds like the sound of a saw. Spongia definitely benefits the cough arising from failure of the heart. No other remedy will be of avail in this kind of cough.

**Cardiac cough**, associated with the feeling of fear, rapid shallow breathing and the feeling of a failing heart, resistant to common remedies for asthma, will be benefited by Spongia significantly.

Spongia, by way of the associated fear, also resembles Aconite. In fact, fear is a very salient feature of **cardiac asthma**.

On waking up at night, the patient feels disorientated as to where he is and where the door/window is. This can happen in the patient's own house, supporting further the diagnosis of Spongia. This kind of **mental confusion** is very pronounced in Spongia, though it can happen in other homoeopathic remedies too. A **sudden frightful wake-up at night with anxiety** is a very salient feature of Grandiola and Arsenic, but disorientation as to where the patient is, besides

Spongia, also present in Phosphorus, Lachesis, Carbo Veg, Glonoine, Lycopodium and Aesculus. Whenever startled at night, a Spongia patient, will be disorientated.

Spongia is also very useful in **the treatment of chronic failure and enlargement of the heart**. Usually, the heart once enlarged does not return to its normal size. Spongia is one out of many possible homoeopathic remedies for this condition. Rhus Tox should be specially studied in this connection. Besides Spongia, Crataegus Q should also be used to strengthen the heart.

Spongia is by nature a hot remedy. The patient feels very hot and likes the open air. The symptoms become worse in a heated room and with touch and pressure. It also aggravates on movement, walking and bending over. A patient feels better in cold weather, except the cough, which becomes more severe.

Spongia is also useful in the **treatment of thyroid goitre**. The thyroid gland becomes enlarged but it is not hard. It is soft and resilient like a sponge. In Spongia, the **glands inside the uterus** also become swollen like a sponge.

Children whose glands are swollen and their body is flabby will benefit from Spongia. Some people have a double chin with soft skin hanging down. Spongia is said to benefit them.

There is an interesting sign in Spongia i.e., the **throat becomes sore on eating sweets and candy**. Spongia 30 will help relieve this condition. Sweets must be abandoned during the course of the treatment but may be tried again after a few days. If the sore throat returns, then Spongia 200 should be tried. A Spongia patient is very restless at night and unable to sleep soundly. He gets frequently **startled during sleep**. His symptoms aggravate at night. Moreover, he cannot sleep well during the day either.

Spongia is very useful in the **treatment of pericarditis** (inflammation of the outer lining of the heart) as well as the **infection of the heart** (endocarditis).

A Spongia patient becomes fatigued easily. There is **severe headache** due to increased blood flow to the head. The discharge from the eyes is very sticky. The nose feels blocked, though dry. **Blisters form inside the mouth.** The throat feels stuck with a needle, is dry and very painful. A hissing type of cough arises from the throat.

In Spongia, the patient feels extremely hungry and thirsty. The taste in the mouth is bitter. Menstrual bleeding decreases; preceded by severe **backache**, **increased appetite and palpitation of the heart**. The patient, during her periods, frequently wakes up at night. The cough can become relentless and turns into **asthma**.

The symptoms of Spongia aggravate on climbing the stairs and at about midnight. The patient feels better on coming down the stairs.

**Potency:** 30

# STANNUM METALLICUM
## (Tin)

Stannum is a metal used for plating of utensils. In homoeopathic form, it is not used much. In my own experience, I have found it very effective and important. It is quite useful in the **treatment of the terminal stage of tuberculosis of the lungs** and very useful in the **treatment of phlegmatic type of patients**. A daytime headache that gets better at night is very amenable to treatment with Stannum. However, its best use is in the treatment of chronic diseases of the lungs and intestinal worm infestation. Its use in the treatment of worms is not much mentioned in the standard literatures, though it is definitely referred to in the repertories. Stannum used over a long period, helps kill or dissolve the **intestinal worms** and then expel them. It needs to be used for at least a few months. Stannum is also an antidote of **lead poisoning**. It is also useful in the treatment of **blisters inside the mouth**.

In the areas where utensils are plated with tin, Stannum should not be forgotten when treating the gastro-intestinal symptoms in that population. In Western countries, tin plating is not in vogue, so it is not much used. However, food and beverages are preserved in cans lined internally with tin. So, wherever the food is consumed out of the cans, Stannum may very well be needed.

The metal "Tin" melts easily and its homoeopathic form helps liquefy phlegm for easier expulsion. In case the **lungs have become congested**, inflamed and become firm. Stannum will be helpful to treat this condition. Pains related to Stannum begin at sunrise, and then gradually keep on getting worse. The symptoms start subsiding as the day declines and disappear completely at sunset.

**Headache becoming worse in the sun** responds very well to Natrum Mur, Sanguinaria as well as Stannum.

Stannum has a peculiarity that exposure to the cold affects the nerves, in particular of the face, causing **facial neuralgia**.

Another symptom of Stannum is that the chest feels weak. The patient feels easily exhausted even on talking as if the chest has lost its strength. The **chest becomes weak** and the lungs feel lifeless, as a result of which the patient cannot even talk. Some of these patients are chronic sufferers of these conditions. They must be treated with Stannum in high potency, to be repeated every two weeks or so for a few months. The patient will be found getting better surprisingly fast. Stannum is very helpful in the treatment of symptoms of tuberculosis of the lungs.

Another symptom of Stannum is **nausea**, which can occur from the **smell of food being cooked**, as in Colchicum. The taste of the mouth becomes bitter. The stomach feels empty, accompanied by cramps (hunger pangs). The feeling of weakness is profound, especially in the chest. The patient finds it difficult to talk. He has **dry cough**, which gets worse on talking, laughing and singing. The patient always feels tired and feels progressive weakness. He is very sensitive to the change of weather. There is a tendency to palpitate and the heart starts beating fast even on slight exertion. The arms and legs quiver, feel heavy and have cramps. The thumbs get drawn towards the palms which is a prominent feature of Plumbum.

In Stannum, typically, the patient feels exhausted even while descending the stairs, whereas normally in most illnesses, people feel difficulty in climbing the stairs. Muscles at the **forearms and the hands feel tight and contracted** while writing and typing. Spasmodic twitching of the fingers is its salient feature.

In women, the **periods are more frequent and more copious** (menorrhagia). There is **irritation inside the uterus and a feeling of downward sag**. The discharge is pale yellow or whitish and watery, rendering the patient weaker.

In Stannum, light touch aggravates the suffering, while the deep pressure or lying down on a hard surface offers relief. The symptoms aggravate gradually and subside equally slowly. The headache, however, subsides fast.

| | |
|---|---|
| **Adjuvant:** | Pulsatilla |
| **Potency:** | 30 to 200 |

# STAPHYSAGRIA
## (Stavesacre)

Staphysagria is prepared from the seeds of a plant that resembles the grape vine, bearing violet or blue-coloured flowers. Since ancient times, the fruit of this plant has been used in the treatment of many diseases. Besides being employed in inducing vomiting, it was used externally as **local treatment for the itch, killing head lice** and on the warts. The homoeopathic form prepared from the plant seeds is called Staphysagria.

Staphysagria is a very important remedy related deeply to the functioning of the nerves. Once the patient is identified, otherwise untreatable diseases can be easily controlled. The Staphysagria patient is of a very sensitive but affable nature. Some sensitive types of patients cannot control their anger and jump onto opponent right away while others can control their anger. Some women of delicate nature, while outraged, become mute and do not say a word. They suppress their anger out of their good nature, but later on develop a **headache** and severe mental anguish. They remain extremely sad for a few days. The physical illnesses resulting from suppression of their emotions may become permanent. They suffer from periodic bouts of headache and stomachache or similar illnesses, the reflection of their suppressed inner state. Staphysagria is the best treatment for any sickness resulting from **suppression of anger, torment and humiliation.** Sepia is more effective in the treatment of depression resulting from the ill treatment from near relatives.

Staphysagria patients are of very sensitive nature. A mere light touch on a tiny wound can throw them into a convulsion, which is the natural result of hypersensitivity to nerves.

Their **haemorrhoids** are also very painful as well as their minor ailments. Being highly strung, they over-react to every little problem. People around them consider them as feigning sickness. These remarks make their condition worse and they start having **fainting attacks**. Such women must be treated with Staphysagria. Their other symptoms include **complete silence, sleeplessness, being tired, and mental depression, lack of comprehension, forgetfulness and**

**frequent urination due to irritability of the bladder**. Hearing as well as smell also gets affected. The fingertips are also very sensitive. The patient cannot even tolerate the slightest noise.

Skin signs are also common. **Eczema** develops on the scalp. It is painfully disturbing but without any boils or pimples. There is a feeling of severe pain. Staphysagria will always be found effective against these symptoms. Sometimes, **swellings and lumps** form along the nerves (neurofibromas) that are very painful.

In Staphysagria, the ganglia of the nerves are very sensitive and painful to touch and pressure but painless otherwise. This is due to hypersensitivity of the nerves.

In males, Staphysagria is useful in the **treatment of prostate problems**, such as enlargement of the prostate, causing difficulty in passing urine. Most, but not all prostate patients get better with common remedies. In others, one has to look for other causes. If the patient is of Staphysagria constitution, then certainly, Staphysagria will be useful. Prostate problems must be treated promptly or they can cause infection of the bladder and kidneys. Cancer of the prostate may also develop. **Cancer of the prostate** is very dangerous and often proves fatal. Silicea CM happens to be surprisingly effective in the treatment of the cancer of the prostate.

In relation to other homoeopathic remedies, Staphysagria has to be used in a proper order, such as Causticum first, then Colocynth and finally Staphysagria. Staphysagria is very useful in the treatment of certain intestinal conditions as well as the pain and discomfort due to the involvement of the small peripheral nerves.

In Staphysagria, the **headache** usually begins at the back and then spreads all over. **Warts** too develop on the scalp, especially the dry and tender type, which are sensitive to touch.

In Staphysagria, the patient feels chillness deep inside, with no sign of external quivering. Gelsemium like Staphysagria is also useful in the **treatment of internal quivering**. In Staphysagria, the women suffer from **toothache** during menstruation. The **teeth become dark and brittle**. Staphysagria is also useful in the treatment of sexual diseases of women as well as men. **Pain in the leg and backache** become worse in the morning and get better on resting at night.

| | |
|---|---|
| **Adjuvants:** | Causticum, Colocynth |
| **Antidote:** | Camphor |
| **Potency:** | 30 to 200 |

# STRONTIUM CARBONICUM

Strontium Carb is very useful in the treatment of complications developing after surgery. A surgeon must keep Strontium in his possession while performing surgery. It proves very effective in combating **postoperative shock** (surgical shock), which, if untreated, may lead the patient to a near death situation. Strontium also proves to be the panacea for the **shock resulting from severe accidental injuries** (post-traumatic shock).

In general, the routine use of Arnica 1000 works very well in the **treatment of shock associated with injuries**, but if the patient goes into **severe shock** due to an accident and looks lifeless, in this situation, Carbo Veg as well as Strontium can reverse the shock and revert imminent death as though by magic. Strontium Carb and Carbo Veg are antidotes to each other. Some doctors suggest the use of Strontium Carb in surgical shock and Carbo Veg for the shocks following accidents and severe illnesses. This is not a hard and fast rule, however. As a routine, Strontium Carb must certainly be considered in the **treatment of shock following surgery**. Often, it succeeds in restoring the life of a dying patient. The body starts warming up and the patient then sleeps comfortably. If Strontium Carb does not work, then Carbo Veg must be given. In shock where the defence system almost fails and body does not react and the patient is moribund, this situation demands Carbo Veg which brings the patient back to life. The defence system of the body is restored and the body starts responding to other homoeopathic remedies. However, Causticum is the best in **restoring the local tissue damage** due to shock. Arnica 1000 combined with Natrum Sulph 1000 should be used in the **treatment of injuries to the nape** or in a blow to the spine.

The human body has been provided with the capability of fighting any disease. The real challenge, however, is how to make use of it. The homoeopathic system offers a way to achieve it.

Strontium Carb is very good in the **treatment of eye conditions**. The aching of the eyes, redness, watering of the eyes, strain on reading and burning sensation of eyes can all be treated with Strontium Carb.

Another peculiar symptom of Strontium is that the patient has complete **aversion to meat**, but has increased appetite for bread.

**Chronic sprain of the ankle** and the related symptoms have already been discussed in detail under Arnica, Ledum and Bellis. If the condition becomes chronic and not treatable with common remedies, then Strontium Carb may also be the an effective remedy. Strontium Carb is also useful in the **treatment of muscular strain and sprains of the neck**, but it should be used in potency 30. Strontium Carb has also been described to be useful in the **pain at the right shoulder**. In a patient suffering from **Rheumatism associated with diarrhoea and cramps of the legs and feet as well as ice cold feet**; Strontium Carb, like many other homoeopathic remedies, may also be useful.

In Strontium Carb, the patient loses appetite and hates to eat meat. He does not relish normal food either. The diarrhoea becomes more profound at night.

The ailments related to Strontium Carb become worse during the change of weather and on remaining silent. The patient cannot tolerate cold at all.

| **Potency:** | 30 according to Bolerokto |
|---|---|

# SULPHUR
## (Sublimated Sulphur)

Sulphur is among those homoeopathic remedies that a homoeopath cannot do without. It is an extremely potent homoeopathic remedy, capable of combating infections and is also a topmost anti-psoric remedy (for details, see under Psorinum and Mercury). Like Psorinum and Mercury, Sulphur has the ability to bring out the deep psoric disease from glands to skin.

The human body's natural defence mechanism has the capability of handling all kinds of diseases. Consequently, it is the basic defence system that needs to be activated and strengthened. Sulphur works as a powerful antibiotic by motivating the natural defence system of the body. Sulphur is almost always needed in the **treatment of chronic infectious diseases** and toxaemic conditions.

Sulphur and Silicea behave differently in response to heat and cold. Despite this difference, while a patient is being treated with Silicea, occasional supplementation with Sulphur adds to the working of Silicea. It does not conflict with Silicea at all. Apart from Silicea, Sulphur augments the functioning of many other remedies as well.

Sometimes, the human body becomes habituated and addicted to certain things, which it cannot give up easily. Sulphur is a profoundly effective remedy against such habits and addictions. If a remedy, previously effective, becomes ineffective during the course of the treatment, then it should be discontinued for a while and Sulphur should be started. Sulphur will restore the effectiveness of the remedy once again. By nature a typical Sulphur patient is fearless and disorganized. He hates to take a bath. An Opium addict also hates taking a bath. A Sulphur patient is extremely untidy and smelly. The sweat from his armpits and his feet smells awful. The patient does not care for cleanliness at all. Ironically, despite being dirty, untidy and smelly himself, he cannot tolerate bad odours from others. This quality is basically found in all animals. For example, a lion can perceive the smell of a human being but does not care for the bad smell of his own den. This seems strange but is understandably natural. In some exceptions, a Sulphur patient becomes disgusted of his own smell and may start throwing up.

As long as he is moving around, a Sulphur patient feels okay. But as soon as he retires to bed and becomes warm, his sufferings become worse. This particular nature is common to Sulphur and Mercury both. Regarding the response to heat and cold, both are similar, but there are many other symptoms different from each other. For example, the mouth of a Sulphur patient is normally wet or completely dry, while the mouth of a Mercury patient is full of saliva. The smell of a Sulphur patient is similar to his natural smell, however much stronger. The discharges excoriate the skin. Leucorrhoeal discharge in both Sulphur and Mercury is also of similar nature.

A Sulphur patient may present with any possible form of skin disease such as **blistering, dry itching, wet eczema, scaling of the skin like fish, bleeding from the itchy area and boils of different kinds**, among other things. In short, any kind of skin disease associated with a burning sensation and other general symptoms of Sulphur will respond to the Sulphur treatment well. In skin diseases, even in the absence of all the symptoms of Sulphur, it will at least clearly demarcate the disease, which can then be treated appropriately.

In Sulphur there is a burning sensation on the scalp, in the eyes, the chest and the area between the two shoulders. The body seems to be on fire. There is a **burning sensation** on the **haemorrhoids** (piles), **skin blisters and in the stomach and throat.** Urination is also associated with burning which lasts for a long time afterwards. The **feet also burn at night**. The patient exposes his feet out of the bed in order to cool them, like in Pulsatilla.

In spite of being very hungry, some Sulphur patients can eat only a little. This feature is most pronounced in Lycopodium. A typical Sulphur **patient loses his morning appetite** completely. From the morning, up to eleven o' clock in the morning, there is no appetite at all. At eleven o' clock, the stomach feels empty. There is a strong craving for food. If not fed immediately, the patient may faint.

In Sulphur, the skin is very sensitive and easily grazed with the slightest friction. Sulphur is one of the best treatments for eczema, though not the only one.

In Sulphur patients, venous circulation is affected, resulting in **piles** (haemorrhoids). Under treatment with Sulphur, the piles first enlarge and itch before getting better. Nux Vomica helps control the swelling and the itch.

Sometimes, the veins of the legs become distended and tortuous, a condition called **varicose veins**. The blood stagnates and may then clot inside the veins (venous thrombosis). There are many homoeopathic remedies that can relieve this condition. Sulphur is certainly one of them.

Sulphur is also very useful in the **treatment of menopausal syndrome** i.e. hot flushes on the face and head, as well as pressure on the heart. Pulsatilla is also used in this condition, but I have not found it as effective as it is claimed to be. Pulsatilla combined with Belladonna proves to be much more effective. However, if the patient exhibits symptoms matching Sulphur, then Sulphur alone may bring about the cure.

As in Lachesis, the symptoms of Sulphur aggravate after sleep and the patient wakes up agitated. **Restlessness starts becoming worse in the latter part of the night**. This is due to mental anguish rather than being of a physical nature. The patient wakes up confused and restless. By eleven o' clock in the morning, restlessness affects the stomach. At night, the symptoms of Sulphur are aggravated due to the warmth of the bed and not merely by sleeping, as in Lachesis.

Sometimes, after the childbirth, the placenta remains partially retained in the uterus, inviting severe infection. There is nothing better than Sulphur and Pyrogenium to combat this infection. Sulphur 200 and Pyrogenium 200 may be useful in any **chronic infection and fever following a nasal cold** usually untreatable with common remedies.

Sulphur is also very useful in the **treatment of gout**. By taking Sulphur, sometimes the suppressed symptoms of gout may erupt. Being scared off, the patient may give up using Sulphur. In fact, the continued use of Sulphur will cure the gout completely. If Sulphur is withheld at this stage, the gout will become suppressed and predisposed to other deep-seated illnesses that may be hard to treat.

Like Silicea, in tuberculosis and chronic lung diseases, Sulphur should also be used with the utmost care for fear of provoking a severe response from that part of the body. The lungs, already weakened, may rupture. Sulphur exposes the causative organisms (tuberculous bacilli), out of the cells and their protective shells just as in Silicea. If bacteria are abundantly present and overwhelming, then the weakened body will not be able to cope with them. Rather it will be overcome with the disease. Silicea has the natural tendency to expel foreign bodies from the body, which may merely be a particle of sand, a retained bullet or a piece of glass. Silicia will provoke a severe body response in the presence of advanced and well-established tuberculosis, the patient may even die. It is the duty of every good homoeopath to avoid giving a very high potency Silicia to such a weak person. At the outset, a low potency should be administered and then as the body gets acclimatised, higher potencies may gradually be administered. Additionally, Stannum may also be used to build up the defensive capability of the body.

It should not be forgotten that a Sulphur patient is of a hot constitution and a Silicea patient is of a cold constitution. Calcarea Carb, unlike Silicea and Sulphur, helps form a protective shell of calcium around the bacteria which become imprisoned. It should be remembered that the administration of Sulphur immediately after the treatment with Calcarea Carb can cause severe complications. If Sulphur has to be given at all, Lycopodium must be used prior to its use. Sulphur also works well in the treatment of **shingles** (herpes zoster).

Sulphur is also useful in the **treatment of morning diarrhoea**. Dr. Kent has, however, warned against the use of Sulphur in treating morning diarrhoea in a patient of tuberculosis, because by suppressing the diarrhoea it will badly affect the lungs already diseased, resulting in serious consequences. The diarrhoea of a tuberculosiis patient should first be treated with milder remedies and then the attempt may be made to cure the tuberculosis.

Sulphur is also very useful in the treatment of measles. If the burning sensation and restlessness aggravate, but the typical rash does not appear and there is a fear that the disease could affect the internal linings, then besides Sulphur, Arsenic may also be used. In Sulphur, restlessness is not as profound as in Arsenic, though the feeling of intense burning is similar to Arsenic.

Sulphur, like a few other homoeopathic remedies, may also **control the side effects of vaccination**.

A Sulphur **patient is philosophical** in nature and some indeed happen to be so. If this desire amounts to a frenzy, then a dose or two of Sulphur in high potency will make them feel well. Some of them are "economic philosophers" who simply present economic schemes all the time, but do not do anything practical. Even if they put their scheme into practice, they lose all their assets. They are extremely lazy. They cannot put their heart into anything. They remain lost in their own ideas. These people should also be treated with Sulphur in high potency.
A Sulphur patient frequently suffers from **headache**, at least once a week. Unlike other symptoms of Sulphur, which get worse in a heated bed and a warm room, the headache gets better with the application of heat and hot fomentation.

They have flashing lights before their eyes. Sometimes, on lifting the head up, the patient sees stars. He may see spots of different colours before his eyes. Usually these symptoms occur before the onset of **headache**. Sulphur given at the outset will prevent the headache. Sulphur is also useful in the **treatment of eczema and chronic itching** as well as chronic cold associated with a **bad smell from the nose**. The patient is aware of this bad smell himself, whereas normally he is not aware of his own smell.

Sulphur is also very useful in the treatment of neuralgic pain on right side of the face. Sulphur is also a good homoeopathic **remedy for the lips becoming fissured and ulcerated**. Sulphur can also be helpful in the **treatment of chronic enlargement of the glands,** as well as the **serial enlargement of the neck glands both on the right and left side**.

If other symptoms of Sulphur are present, then it can also **cure swollen gums and loose teeth**. If only one tooth hurts, then some other remedies should be looked for, instead of Sulphur.

**Flatulence and distension of the abdomen with gas** can benefit from many remedies, though a precise remedy is difficult to find. In case other remedies have failed, Sulphur may be useful, especially if the gas is offensive.

Sulphur is very important in the **treatment of cholera**. During an epidemic, Sulphur should be used extensively as a preventive measure. Sulphur 200 once a day for a few days can protect against cholera in the absence of other common remedies. Sulphur alone may suffice. Sulphur is very deeply related to cholera.

Sulphur has a profound effect on the **prostate gland**. For a better result, it should be given combined with Thuja. If other symptoms of Sulphur such as foul smelling sweat from the feet and armpits, symptoms of the scalp, hands and feet, do not resemble that of Sulphur, then Sulphur will not be effective. In other words, the mere presence of urinary symptoms is not enough to necessitate treatment with Sulphur.

Sulphur is beneficial in the **treatment of sexual weakness in men as well as in women**. It is also very effective in the **treatment of infertility in women**.

The mental symptoms of Sulphur are pronounced: a **weak memory**, difficulty in concentrating, a **headache** getting worse on lowering the head, **constant recurrent headache,** and **dandruff causing the hair to fall,** are also indicative of Sulphur.

A Sulphur patient feels pressure and a burning sensation over the area of the heart and breathing becomes laboured. The patient likes to be in the open air. He feels suffocated at night, with a feeling of pressure on the chest. The Sulphur ailments become worse on resting, standing up, by the warmth of the bed, on taking a bath and in the morning. The patient feels relieved by lying on the right side and in hot weather.

In people working in **coal mines** or related to the coal industry in any way, Sulphur is a very useful and essential remedy to **prevent the diseases of the lungs**.

| | |
|---|---|
| **Adjuvants:** | Aloe, Psorinum, Aconite, Arnica, Stannum, Pyrogenium and Thuja, etc. |
| **Potency:** | 30 and higher |

# SULPHURICUM ACIDUM

## (Sulphuric Acid)

Sulphuric Acid contains Sulphur, which affects the human defences deeply. During indigestion, the Sulphuric acid contained in the stomach produces Hydrogen Sulphide gas, with its typical foetid odour. Every acid in the body has certain basic properties, which affect the patients accordingly. Every kind of hyperacidosis can result in a sudden severe disabling weakness of the body. Sulphuric Acid is the ideal homoeopathic remedy for **hyperacidity in the stomach**. By studying Sulphuric Acid, one can easily understand how the imbalance of different elements in the body results in different kinds of symptoms and signs. Sulphur is such a strong remedy that it produces a burning sensation on the body from the head to the toes. The addition of an atom of hydrogen converts it into Sulphuric Acid, which has a different nature from that of Sulphur. Its patient suffers in both the heat and cold.

One symptom of Sulphuric Acid is that the patient quivers all over. This is not due to the cold, but is a spontaneous response on the part of the body. Bleeding is of dark colour. **Dark blood oozes from under the nails and the junctional areas where the skin and the mucous membranes** meet (like the bleeding from snakebite). The bleeding being in the skin, tends to surface externally.

Sometimes, spontaneous red spots appear on the skin (petechiae). These spots may also be dark coloured, raw looking and ugly. A strange kind of skin condition can also develop on the face making it difficult to diagnose. Such type of haemorrhage occurring internally is found in Sulphuric Acid, but may be found in other remedies too.

Sulphuric Acid is useful in the **treatment of many skin diseases**. If the nature of common remedies is known, it is definitely beneficial. Some of the symptoms of Sulphuric Acid resemble those of Sulphur, such as profuse morning diarrhoea.

Some of the Arnica symptoms are also shared by Sulphuric Acid, such as bruised feeling with pain, weakness and feeling of cold. Haemorrhagic spots develop on the skin. The spots may be darker in colour or bluish. Unlike Arnica, the blood percolates to the surface of the skin, forming haemorrhagic blisters that then spread. These are indicative of a serious unexplained deep illness. Sulphuric Acid is very effective in treating this condition. If other symptoms of Sulphuric Acid are also present, a dose or two of Sulphuric Acid may suffice. A Sulphuric Acid patient becomes easily exhausted mentally and his circulatory system may be disturbed due to the slightest carelessness. Serious blood disturbance may also result. Boils develop on the skin. The patient feels very weak. His facial complexion is not normal. He becomes hypersensitive. The aches and pains intensify gradually and then suddenly get better. Potentially serious and chronic diseases developing due to an excess of Acid Sulph may sometimes abruptly get better without leaving any long lasting ill effects.

The **discharges of a Sulphuric Acid patient are acidic as well as corrosive in nature**. Hyperacidity in the body (acidosis) may be accompanied by a feeling of sudden severe weakness when eating food. The patient sweats profusely. Mere eating food can tire the patient. A lightning type of pain swings from one side to the other. Some patients may actually enjoy this experience, which is a peculiarity of Sulphuric Acid. The **headache** and body aches intensify gradually and then stop suddenly. **Hearing loss progresses slowly** and does not return quickly which is rather different from the overall picture of Sulphuric Acid symptoms. Hearing returns in due course of time after the pain, pus and bad odour from the ear have been gone awhile. Sometimes, secretions from the nose can block the ear from the inside and affect the **hearing**. Other symptoms of Sulphuric Acid being present, this condition is well within the domain of Sulphuric Acid. Toothache goes on gradually getting stronger, and then ends suddenly without leaving any aftereffects. **Sores and ulcers form inside the mouth and the throat**, causing difficulty in eating. Children may not be able to suck milk. Sulphuric Acid is extremely useful in the treatment of this condition. The stomach begins to fail due to the effects of hyperacidity. The **breath is extremely foetid and pungent**. Usually, people get constipated on eating acidic things, but the Sulphuric Acid patient develops **diarrhoea** instead. For example Oysters, (a kind of sea-shell) as well as raw and sour fruit, can cause diarrhoea for which Sulphuric Acid is still the treatment of choice for such patients who have **abdominal pain**.

In women who see **dreadful dreams during their periods**, one should, besides other appropriate remedies, also remember Sulphuric Acid (for details, see under Arnica and Arsenic).

Sulphuric Acid may be the ideal homoeopathic remedy to treat women who cannot conceive due to excessive menstrual bleeding, if the patient is of a Sulphuric Acid constitution. In reality, there are innumerable causes of **infertility**. To find the correct remedy is a very laborious job. This subject has been touched upon under the chapters on Pulsatilla, Caulophyllum, Sabina, Calcarea Carb, Ashoka and Gossypium.

In Sulphuric Acid, the patient feels weakness of the back. He wishes to keep lying down. He finds it difficult to stand up or sit down. Slow walking offers some relief. The patient sweats in the morning, which is usually due to some tuberculous matter in the body.

Sulphuric Acid is the best remedy in alcoholics. In Europe, there are many, who are given to regular drinking, which unfortunately kills them eventually. Treatment with Sulphuric Acid works wonders. A drop of Sulphuric Acid should be diluted in a whole glass of water, which should be divided into three doses to be taken in one day. Many alcoholics who were considered incurable, recovered within a week of this treatment, and never touched alcohol again. In the field of remedy, there is nothing better than this therapy.

| | |
|---|---|
| **Adjuvant:** | Pulsatilla |
| **Potency:** | Mother tincture Q |

# TARENTULA HISPANIA

## (Spanish Spider)

Tarentula Hispania is an extremely poisonous form of spider found in Spain. Its bite causes intense burning all over the body. The homoeopathic remedy is prepared from the extract of this spider. Its effect on the urinary system resembles that of Cantharis, which is similarily produced from the poison of a fly. It produces severe scalding along the urethra. The kidneys become inflamed. Urine comes in the form of drops like molten copper.

In Tarentula, the **intense burning sensation affects the entire body, but the genitals even more so**. It is associated with restlessness and weakening of the heart. In Cantharis however, affliction of the heart is not essential. In Tarentula, the **patient has a special aversion to black, red and green colours**. Tarentula, in high potency, can cure this condition even after it has become chronic. As a matter of principle, for sicknesses of a chronic and well-established nature, the homoeopathic remedy should be given in a high potency, though in general, it is safe practice to start the treatment in 30 potency.

In Tarentula, one symptom is similar to Hysocyamus. In Hyoscyamus, even the most modest young girls, while out of their minds, subconsciously talk in a vulgar way whereas normally they are not vulgar at all. In Tarentula, however, there is a tendency towards obscenity in the normal state of mind. By hook or by crook, the patient is bent upon fulfilling his sexual desires. Such patients need to be treated with Tarentula in a high potency.

In Tarentula, the body starts wasting and emaciating so much that the patient is reduced to a mere skeleton as if destroyed by termites. This in fact is the nature of Tarentula i.e. on being bitten by the spider; the flesh of the victim liquefies so that it may be easily devoured by it. In other words, the poison of the Hispanic spider melts and liquefies the flesh. Thus, if anybody suffers from wasting of the body, even if other symptoms of Tarentula are missing, he should still be treated with Tarentula.

The Tarentula patient is **hypersensitive to cold**. He feels severe **restlessness in the legs** before going to sleep. This symptom is also present in Argentum, Lycopodium and Arsenic.

The symptoms of Tarentula ailments are strictly periodic and timely. For example, if the patient has been afflicted on a Monday, then the next episode will also be on Monday. Sometimes, the sickness returns exactly after two weeks. Strict periodicity of the symptoms is peculiar to the venoms of animal origin. For example, the diseases resulting from snakebites are common in the spring. This well-known tendency is often quoted in time-old stories. The truth is that the snake does not bite the same person every year. There is only reactivation of the old snake bite wound, although the person feels as if he was bitten by the snake again. Lachesis is the best homoeopathic treatment for such patients and must be given in high potency.

The exact timing of the recurrence of the symptoms of a Tarentula bite does not relate to a year or a month. Rather it is referable to days or a week.

By the Grace of God, the relapsing type of malaria, which returns every week or fortnight may also be cured with Tarentula, if other remedies have failed. A Tarentula patient is extremely thirsty, bad-tempered, evil natured and cunning. He keeps on planning dangerous wicked schemes to harm others. A Tarentula woman is extremely cunning and can harm others with her evil designs. Her conversation is very threatening. She sees **strange faces and has visual hallucinations of animals, demons, ghosts and other horrible figures**.

The **restlessness and burning** of Tarentula is similar to that of Arsenic. Burning of the hands and feet reminds one of Sulphur. **Aversion of certain colours**, especially red, resembles the aversion to red by the fighting bulls in Spain. They hate the colour red and rush to attack anything red.

Arsenic neutralizes the ill effects of Tarentula. At the same time, if Tarentula fails to relieve a condition, Arsenic can be used instead.

Tarentula ailments aggravate in the cold. Some of its symptoms resemble those of Sulphur. Tarentula can be very effective in the treatment of burning of palms and soles as well as the burning sensation inside the uterus of hysterical women.

A Tarentula patient believes in his mind that people neglect him. So, he keeps on preparing schemes to avenge his torment. A **person as cunning as a fox** and somewhat insane should be treated with Tarentula in high potency. Even if not actually sick, a Tarentula patient can feign any type of illness. He will confine himself to bed and make excuses to seek attention. His real sickness is deep internal unrest, which is different from Arsenic. The Tarentula patient rubs his head on the pillow out of anxiety. He is wild and beyond himself. He cannot open the eyes. Hypersensitivity to light results in a headache over the temples and the nape.

Like in Natrum Mur, a Tarentula **patient feels as if being lightly hammered over his head**. **The eye symptoms are mostly on the right side**. The vision becomes blurred and weak, associated with discharge from the right eye. There is **severe pain in the right ear**. The cold settles in the right nostril from where it erupts periodically. The **throat also hurts on the right side**. **Aversion to food**, thirst for cold water and nausea are specific to Tarentula. Inflammation of the throat may also show itself externally.

The Tarentula patient suffers from **severe type of chronic constipation** making him restless and apprehensive. He tosses about in the bed and rubs his head on the pillow. The severe constipation may sometimes not even be relieved by laxatives or an enema.

**Due to persistent grief and anxiety, a patient may contract diabetes**. In such a situation, associated with aching of the arms and legs, Tarentula is very useful. It may not just offer temporary relief but may even result in a complete cure.

Tarentula is very useful in the **treatment of renal colic** caused by urinary stones or inflammation. If there is a severe pain in the loin area above the hip associated with plentiful urine, a **burning sensation along the urethra** and a feeling of a sudden spasm, then perhaps Tarentula is the most ideal treatment.

Tarentula can also cure the **severe internal itchiness and burning sensation** in women. Formation of fibroid tumours in the uterus, tilting or sagging of the uterus, its prolapse and unbearable heaviness, are all the symptoms of Tarentula.

Tarentula is also intimately related to the tightness of the trachea. Hoarseness of the voice, a constant stinging sensation in the throat and heaviness of the voice are symptoms of Tarentula.

Tarentula may be extremely useful in the **treatment of heart condition and asthma,** if other symptoms of Tarentula are also present.

In Tarentula patients, large abscesses or even carbuncles can form on the back of the neck and above the shoulders on the right or left side. **Carbuncles usually form in diabetic patients**. Other symptoms of Tarentula being present, it may offer a complete cure for this condition.

In general, a Tarentula patient has **numbness over the limbs**, generalised weakness and burning sensations, restlessness and severe pain over the extremities. **Pain in the legs** is the most pronounced, as well as unbearable burning on the skin and intolerance to light pressure. Sometimes, the patient may not even tolerate the weight of clothing around him.

There is pain over the hip joints, especially at night. In Tarentula, the symptoms become worse at night. The entire body itches and burns. On walking, the patient feels pain over the thighs as if tightly tied with a bandage. **Paralysis of the legs** is also a prominent feature. On movement, the patient feels pain and discomfort over the back, while the **headache** feels better.

**Convulsions** are a prominent feature of Tarentula. Its other symptoms being present, Tarentula may also cure **epilepsy** once and for all.

| | |
|---|---|
| **Adjuvants:** | Cuprum, Mag Phos usually in potency 30 |
| **Antidotes:** | Lachesis, Cantharis |
| **Potency:** | 30 to 200 |

# TUBERCULINUM

## (A Nosode from Tubercular Abscess)

Tuberculinum is prepared from the material obtained from tuberculous lesions. Dr. Burnett has done most of the research on this remedy and others have significantly benefited from his experiments. Dr. Kent also has given a lot of importance to this remedy. Its basic nature must be well learnt so that its efficacy may be availed not only in the treatment of tuberculosis but also in some other diseases. It is a nosode i.e. the remedy prepared from the extract of a toxic, putrid matter. On repeated dilution and purification, the original toxic/poisonous substance does not exist except just as a memory in the form of a subtle power. Yet, it can be used to treat the original disease or its like.

The nosode should not be used in potency less than 200 or better still, it should be used in higher potencies. Potency 1000 is better. Dr. Kent has claimed that any person treated with Tuberculinum 200, 1000, 10 000, 50 000 and finally CM (two doses of each potency at long intervals) will never contract tuberculosis, even if he lives among TB patients. Tuberculinum or some other nosode may be needed to treat latent tuberculosis. This will enhance the action of other homoeopathic remedies. Tuberculinum produces a profound bodily reaction so that the previously ineffective homoeopathic remedies are rendered effective. Preliminary treatment with Tuberculinum helps the treatment to be more effective.

Tuberculinum is an anti-psoric remedy. In general, skin diseases are called psoric diseases. Malaria and all other fevers, which after being temporarily suppressed have the tendency to repeatedly relapse every second or third day, can be usefully treated with Tuberculinum. Some doctors use Tuberculinum during the malarial fever also. They call it a malarial antidote.

A symptom of Tuberculinum is that like Thuja and Arnica, the **patient likes to change places constantly.**

One must remember that the patients of tuberculosis and syphilis may become insane in the advanced disease. But there is a difference between their insanity. The tuberculosis patients usually become insane because of the constant severe headache and deep-seated lesions inside the chest. In syphilis, the entire body of the patient is studded with sores and ulcers, which can even dissolve the bones. The bridge of the nose settles down due to the decay of the nasal bones. Syphilis also affects the brain directly, and thus makes the patient completely insane. The **insanity due to tuberculosis is associated with the tendency of violence and aggression**. Sometimes, the patient may become altogether mute. Sometimes when insane, even women weakened internally by Tuberculosis may show great strength. Their mind becomes excited and leads to violence. Nevertheless, they are usually of a calm nature. Tuberculinum given in high potency can save them from becoming insane.

According to some homoeopathic doctors, Calcarea and Tuberculinum are very deeply related and may be used as a substitute for each other.

In Tuberculinum, the muscles become very weak and flabby. This sign is well pronounced. In a child suffering from tuberculosis, who has the tendency of **prolapse of the rectum at the time of defacation**, one should not forget to use Tuberculinum. It may also prove useful in the treatment of prolapse of the uterus or the tendency of prolapse of the rectum in men as well as women.

**Periods are frequent and prolonged** and may be associated with pain. One should not forget using Tuberculinum in the treatment of this condition along with the other homoeopathic remedies.

A **dry persistent cough** that is not necessarily the result of a nasal cold is very common in the patient of Tuberculinum. Pulsatilla may also decrease the severity of this cough.

**Ringworm** (i.e. formation of circle of minute spots) may affect the scalp and cause loss of hair. This is called **Alopecia**, in which bunches of hair fall in the form of circles. Both Tuberculinum and Bacillinum are useful in the treatment of this condition. According to Dr. Burnett, the basic cause of alopecia is tuberculosis and he suggests that anybody with this condition must be treated with Bacillinum or Tuberculinum. Picric Acid is also a very effective treatment for alopecia and ringworm.

Another salient feature of Tuberculinum is the **jerking of the muscles** during sleep. This, of course, can also be treated with many other remedies.

In Tuberculinum, the patient starts showing symptoms of the disease before its acute onset. Tuberculinum has often been used in the treatment of chronic rather than acute diseases. Chronic diseases, if untreated, may be transmitted to the next generation. Tuberculinum can, however, be effective in the treatment of acute illnesses.

In most of the poor countries of Asia and Africa, malaria is very common. The face of the patient becomes pale yellow and without normal glow. Diseases of the lungs; cough and asthma etc., are very common. Tuberculinum can effectively uproot asthma because tuberculous diseases ultimately result in asthma.

In some desert areas where pneumonia, tuberculosis and malaria are prevalent, sudden cooling of the temperature predisposes to pneumonia that weakens the lungs. It is no wonder that the lungs contract tuberculosis in these areas easily. In such malarial regions, such as the Sindh province of Pakistan, Tuberculinum is not only useful but is an essential part of their treatment.

**Malaria fever** is usually associated with headache and vomiting. A tuberculosis patient who has previously suffered from malaria may develop a headache that can be treated with Tuberculinum.

Body ache, feverishness and an overall state of despair is also a symptom of Tuberculinum. A condition called **hydrocephalus**, in which the head of a child keeps on growing and is not amenable to treatment with common homoeopathic remedies anymore, may well be treated with Tuberculinum given in a high potency. This produces a positive reaction which other common remedies should have shown, but failed to do so.

Most of the abdominal symptoms of Tuberculinum resemble those of Sulphur, such as **profuse morning diarrhoea and sometimes alternation of dysentery, diarrhoea and severe constipation**. They are all intestinal problems. If these conditions are not treated with Tuberculinum on time, the patient may become untreatable. He develops ulcers inside the intestines, resulting in constant oozing of blood. This condition can however, be treated with Tuberculinum given over a long period.

| | |
|---|---|
| **Adjuvants:** | Calcarea Carb, China, Bryonia, Sulphur, Thuja, Syphilinum may also be found useful after treatment with Tuberculinum |
| **Potency:** | 30 to 200 or very high potencies as required |

# VERATRUM ALBUM
## (White Hellebore)

In Veratrum Album, the patient feels extremely cold from head to toe. It is one of the most effective treatments of **cholera.** Dr. Hahnemann advises its use even before the onset of a cholera epidemic. In the effectiveness against cholera, it is comparable to Camphor and Cuprum. In Veratrum Album, the stools are exuberant, rendering the patient extremely weak.

A prominent feature of Veratrum is that the patient **feels extremely cold** yet is drenched in cold sweats from head to toe. Similar symptoms are also found in Camphor, though the stools are scanty. In Veratrum Album, the stools are watery and exuberant, causing severe dehydration which may even lead to death.

**Cramps in the legs** are an essential feature of Veratrum Album, Camphor and Cuprum as well as of cholera.

A rather contradictory symptom of Veratrum Album is dryness of the gastro-intestinal tract. It is an extremely effective **treatment of diarrhoea,** as well as for **severe constipation**. Severe chronic constipation, associated with a feeling of weakness and cold sweats can well be treated with Veratrum Album. Veratrum Album can still be useful even if the weakness and cold sweats are absent. In severe constipation, Veratrum Album 30 should be used two to three times a day. It gradually softens the abdomen by alleviating the dryness of the intestines. It is recommended however that prior to the treatment with Veratrum Album, severe constipation may better be relieved with an enema or glycerine suppositories. This will soften the dry voluminous stools which are otherwise impossible to pass naturally. Veratrum Album, like Carbo Veg, may also be tried in the treatment of cold sweats associated with severe irreversible shock and impending death.

The Veratrum Album patient happens to be irritable and is easily provoked due to the constant feeling of cold. If he is kept warm all the time, he becomes mellow, showing that the irritability is not his nature.

Some Veratrum Album patients are **religious fanatics**. They talk loudly and rapidly. At some times, they may be extremely talkative, and at others absolutely silent. During the period of silence, they become extremely depressed and have the tendency to commit suicide. A suicidal tendency is found in many other remedies. In rare instances, Veratrum Album can also be used to treat the suicidal tendency.

**Premenstrual tension** and **sadness** in young girls may well be cured with Veratrum Album. If untreated, this condition is likely to result in life-long mental illness. There is no smile left on their faces. The physician should remember well that the feeling of extreme cold is the most important indication for the use of Veratrum Album.

There are many inconsistencies in the constitution of Veratrum Album, such as the fact that the head is not cold even though the rest of the body may be ice-cold. Sometimes, the head feels submerged in ice especially at the scalp and the nape, quite unlike Sulphur. In Sulphur, the top of the head feels burning hot. In a Veratrum Album patient, in spite of feeling extreme cold, the patient likes to drink cold water. Fruits produce gas in the stomach. Despite the feeling of nausea and vomiting, there is a feeling of scraping inside the stomach and the craving for food.

| |
|---|
| **Potency:** 30 to 200 |

# ZINCUM METALLICUM

## (Zinc)

Zinc is a very important **neurotropic remedy** (i.e. the one that works on the nervous system). It seems to be the best remedy for patients who have become mentally exhausted due to chronic illnesses, and whose body has been rendered incapable of reacting to bring diseases out to the surface.

During an epidemic of infectious diseases like measles and smallpox, the appearance of skin signs, such as rashes, helps the diagnosis. In a patient of Zinc, these signs fail to appear on the skin, although the disease process has already afflicted the body internally. The homoeopathic form of Zinc helps to project these diagnostic skin signs.

During **paralytic conditions** of chronic and resistant nature, when the patient is treated with Zinc, it will set up a state of neurological provocation and reaction showing that the body is being prepared for a defensive stance. Zinc helps to express the suppressed symptoms and signs of diseases, infectious as well as neurological. This reaction is absolutely necessary to save the patient's life but may be extremely disturbing to him. In case Zinc needs to be administered to provoke the mind and body reactions, the patient <u>must be warned</u> beforehand. Dr. Kent has devised a humorous story about Zinc. He has suggested that a homoeopathic doctor should visit a Zinc patient who has paralysis, very fast on horseback and then also return equally as fast after giving him the treatment. The reason for this is that since Zinc provokes an immediate brisk tingling response so swiftly that the relatives of the patient might think that the doctor has poisoned the patient and rush to attack the doctor. After this abrupt tingling, the nerves begin to recover and the paralysis disappears. Then the relatives will run to thank the doctor. I have also Zinc on such patients. The patients did evidently show a brisk response though not of the severity described by Dr. Kent. As a matter of principle, I warn my patients that the <u>severe nervous response</u> is the first sign of the cure to follow.

Another characteristic sign of Zinc is the fidgeting of feet. Women usually keep their feet exposed out of the bedding and keep rubbing them against each other. Some patients may continually shake their legs. Any person exhibiting this sign and then falling sick must be treated with Zinc. Once the constitution of the patient is recognised to be that of Zinc, all his illnesses will respond to Zinc.

Nux Vomica, being completely opposite to Zinc, should never be given with it even though both have similar effects regarding the treatment of nervous tension In homoeopathy, two remedies of a similar nature may sometimes annul each other, or being incompatible may result in a severe bodily reaction. In case a patient needs to be treated with Zinc but has already been given Nux Vomica, then Camphor or Sulphur must be administered to neutralize the effects of Nux Vomica before he is given Zinc.

The **late onset of menses** and scanty menses are suggestive of Zinc. Unless they are treated with Zinc, some young girls may be predisposed to certain uterine and nervous conditions for life.

Zinc poisoning **slows down the digestive system**. Food gets digested extremely slowly. The appetite vanishes. Food rots in the stomach. Vomiting sets in due to acidity. The patient becomes constipated. Even the bladder function becomes slowed down. Bowel and urinary symptoms coexist. In contrast, Mercury produces its symptoms by way of irritation and intensity. There is a burning sensation during urination and after. Similarly, in dysentery, the patient keeps on feeling the gripes and tenesmus, even after having passed the stools. The Zinc patient has to sit down while passing urine; he cannot pass urine while standing. On the contrary, a Causticum patient can pass urine only while standing, whereas by sitting, the urination either stops or becomes obstructed. Some of the patients have to be pulled backwards so that they may begin to pass urine.

The face of a typical Zinc patient is pale and wrinkled. He always feels cold. Prior to the affliction of his mind and loss of memory, the patient first repeats the question and before answering. A slight sudden noise makes his body tremble. When a Zinc patient develops paralysis, he starts to look prematurely old. However a Zinc patient does not exhibit these signs in his youth whereas in Sarsaparilla and

Agaricus, a patient appears to be old at a very young age. In Sarsaparilla, even children look old.

Some of the Zinc patients, like those in Apis, may scream during sleep due to the excitability of nerve fibres in the brain. Symptoms of Apis are easily identifiable. In their absence, Zinc should be started without any hesitation. Once again, the relatives of the patient must be clearly warned that the tendency to scream may become aggravated before it gets better, slowly but surely.

The symptoms of Zinc include profuse sweating, severe nausea and vomiting. The heart sinks. All these symptoms do not manifest at the same time. Sometimes, it is the gastric symptoms, which appear first, while at other times the limbs or the heart become affected first. If the progressive slowing of the intestinal activity is suspected on the basis of a change of bowel habits, Zinc must be started without hesitation. If the diagnosis has been correct, then the condition may be completely cured. Sometimes such a patient starts vomiting as a reaction to Zinc. This is a good sign indicating that Zinc has reverted the slowly progressive intestinal paralysis (ileus). Initial severe reaction to Zinc therapy is temporary, but must occur, before the restoration of health. However, severe reactions may also be noted during the treatment from the improper homoeopathic remedy or potency, with serious consequences. In homoeopathy, every untoward serious reaction should not be considered a prelude to a successful outcome because the condition may sometimes keep becoming serious with no sign of improvement.

Zinc is also useful in the **treatment of spinal meningitis**. If remedies like Bryonia, Belladonna and Gelsemium etc., stop working, then Zinc will prove to be very beneficial. Zinc has also proved successful in the **treatment of tubercular meningitis**. During an epidemic of meningitis, Zinc 200 taken once or twice a week, proves to be a very good preventive measure.

Zinc is also very useful in the **treatment of many eye diseases** such as progressive swelling and heaviness of the eyelids, chronic redness of the eyes associated with the dimness of the vision and the affliction of the optic nerve (optic neuritis). Zincum Sulph is an excellent **treatment for cataract**. I once treated one ninety-year-old man with fairly advanced cataract. The surgeon had refused to perform surgery on him due to his age. I gave him one dose of Zincum Sulph CM. Surprisingly, within a few months, his cataract had disappeared completely. He lived many more years afterwards without recurrence of the cataract. Zinc is the best homoeopathic remedy in the prevention of cataract due to degenerative materials being deposited in the eye lens. However, once the cataract process is well-advanced, it should be treated by surgery. If Zinc is administered while the cataract is half-way towards maturity, it will neither disappear nor mature for surgery. Patients at this stage should be left alone, so that their cataract may mature and be treated with surgery.

The combination of Calcarea Fluor 6X with Zinc proves much more beneficial. Eye drops of Cineraria Maritima Sussex are also very useful. A drop in each eye, three times a day, helps resolve the cataract quite fast. In general, Zinc Sulph 200 is used once or twice a week. If given in CM potency, it should not be repeated before one month and stopped after one repeat.

Zinc 200 is very useful in abating the formation of the whitish membrane appearing inside the eye. In the eyelids, sometimes **eyelashes start growing inwards (Trichiasis)** and prove quite troublesome. Usually this is treated surgically. But after an operation, another hair can still grow inwards and this may continue to happen. Its permanent cure is Zincum Sulph. I have found it very useful in Potency 200. Zinc also cures **Pterygium** obviating any need for surgery.

When dizzy, a Zinc patient always thinks that he will fall on the left side. Tossing the head around and sinking it into the pillow is also a symptom of Zinc. Zinc is also considered to be useful in the treatment of involuntary movements and tremors of the head and hands (senile tremors).

Like Kali Bichrome, a Zinc patient feels pressure and pain at the root of the nose. The gums start receding from the teeth in zincum. Pressure on the gums relieves the discomfort. Children with weak nerves cut their teeth with difficulty. They keep on shaking their feet or rub them against each other due to restlessness. During swallowing, the muscles of the throat hurt. The stomach burns on eating sweet things. Besides this, the patient has a tendency of nausea, vomiting and hiccups. A Zinc patient has the habit of eating in a rush, indicating impatience. The stomach feels distended with gas.

The patient has pain in the lower part of the back, intolerant to local pressure. Reproductive organs also become affected in men as well as in women. The testicles feel drawn upwards. Women become sexually overexcited and the breasts feel swollen and congested. Menstrual flow increases at night. All these symptoms aggravate during their periods.

Zincum Met is also useful in Varicose veins and Chilblains i.e. redness and swelling of toes due to extreme cold which may result in frostbite and loss of toes. This can happen to mountaineers who walk continuously on snow in severe cold weather.

# REPERTORY

## AND COMMON DAILY ILLNESSES AND THEIR TREATMENT

# An Important Note about the Repertory

In this Repertory, there follows a detailed account of some homoeopathic remedies. An illness may be located under different remedies, and similarly a homoeopathic remedy can be useful to treat many different illnesses.

In the Materia Medica, reference has been made to the important remedies. If a reader goes through one chapter carefully he may be satisfied there or he may find a pointer leading to other remedies.

The new approach adopted in the Repertory would hopefully save a lot of time, and the reader should be able to understand why the repetition, as it may seem, was necessary.

**In the name of Allah, the Gracious, Eve r Merciful**

# Some Common Daily Ailments and their Treatment

Following is a list of some diseases, which may be acute or chronic, encountered in daily life:

**List of Topics:**

# Cold, Catarrh and Fever

Experience gained through day-to-day use of homoeopathic remedies proves that if the cold symptoms are effectively treated in their initial stages, then, by the grace of God, the patient can be saved from the serious complications of nasal catarrh. As soon as there is a feeling of cold inside the nose, either Camphor 30 or a lower potency should be given immediately, or Aconite in whatever potency it is available. Aconite 1000, by the grace of God, also proves to be very effective.

If the face is flushed and there is a throbbing type of headache, then Belladonna 1000 and Arnica 1000 should be added to Aconite. Two doses, half an hour apart, will work extremely well. If the sickness has well-advanced, then Bacillinum, Diphtherinum, Influenzinum and Oscillococcinum 200, all four combined, given once a day for 3 days or as needed, will prevent further deterioration of rhinitis and the development of fever and asthma. If the condition does not come under control, then the symptoms should be reviewed closely and treated accordingly.

If the coryza is associated with excessive sneezing, then in addition to the above, one must use Natrum Mur 200. If the patient suffers from fever in spite of that, the following remedy should be adopted:

Kali Phos + Ferrum Phos + Kali Mur + Silicea + Calcarea Fluor 6X combined.

If the fever still does not subside, then Sulphur and Pyrogenium 200 together should be used twice a day for a few days, or proceed according to the symptoms of the patient as follows:-

The watery secretions from the nose and feeling of cold are common to Gelsemium, Silicea, Natrum Mur, Psorinum and Kali Carb. In Kali Carb, the patient suffers from backache in the latter part of the day at three or four o'clock in the afternoon, while in Natrum Mur the backache lasts all day, from morning till evening. Pulsatilla and Apis can both be useful if the symptoms become worse from the heat. In both, the thirst becomes less and the nasal discharge is rather thick and yellowish. However, a Pulsatilla patient is of a mild nature while that of Apis is very irritable, feels a stinging type of strong wavy pain in the muscles, passes less urine and has inflammation of the kidneys.

Kali Bichrome is much more useful in the treatment of the chronic, stubborn type of nasal catarrh. The nasal discharge is thick, thready and sticky. There is pain at the root of the nose also.

In the spring, Sabadilla helps combat hayfever and severe episodes of sneezing due to allergies. Conversely, for allergies in the autumn that are associated with sneezing, a clear watery discharge from the eyes that does not cause itching, and a cold affecting the ears, Allium Cepa would be more appropriate than Sabadilla.

In a condition where a burning watery discharge flows from the eyes, into throat and the chest during sleep causing itching and coughing, Euphrasia should be used.
To cure the allergy of the spring, Lachesis 1000 is very beneficial. It should be used after relief from the allergy has been obtained with Sabadilla. It should be given in well-spaced intervals, over several months.

During humid weather or at any time when the weather changes rapidly, Dulcamara proves to be the best remedy for nasal catarrhs and for skin conditions. In such a cold, the nose is blocked though the watery discharge continues to flow lightly.

In case the patient feels weak, restless and has a burning sensation (alleviated with heat), then Arsenic would be the best treatment. If he feels nauseous at the smell of food, then it is a symptom of Colchicum.

For the "cold" conditions of diabetic patients, Natrum Sulph, Kali Sulph and Natrum Phos combined, besides other helpful remedies, should be administered two to three times daily. If the body and bones ache severely, then Arnica and Eupatorium combined will prove to be very beneficial.

Patients who suffer from chronic cold with thready discharge, will benefit from Kali Bichrome, as well as the combination of Coccus Cacti and Hepar Sulph.

If the patient develops a sore throat due to the cold, the following remedies should be used:

- ☆ Baryta Carb + Gelsemium (if there is no thirst, the mouth is dry and the head feels heavy)
- ☆ Arnica + Aconite + Causticum + Belladonna from potency 30 to 1000 for any kind of throat condition that is associated with congestion, swelling and pain in the throat. Sometimes, this combination in potency 1000 works extraordinarily fast. Two doses, 30 minutes apart are often enough.
- ☆ Baryta Carb + Belladonna + Causticum for Rhinitis and sore throats.

  Sometimes, Causticum may need to be replaced by Kali Mur, according to the specific symptoms.

If the sore throat is associated with a watery discharge from the mouth and there is an offensive smell, then one should try to find a remedy in Mercury compounds.

**Important Note:** A detailed study of any of the afore-mentioned remedies in this chapter would provide further clarification of the diseases discussed.

**Remedies**

Alumina
Arum Triphyllum
Aurum Metallicum
Bromium
Calcarea Carbonica
Capsicum
Carbo Vegetabilis
Carboneum Sulph
Cistus
Coccus
Guaiacum
Hydrastis
Kali Bichrome
Medorrhinum
Mercurius
Natrum Carbonicum
Nitric Acid
Nux Vomica
Phosphorus
Psorinum
Pulsatilla
Silicea
Thuja

# 2. Cough

If the patient is frightened due to a sudden attack of coughing associated with a dry mouth and throat, he should be treated with Aconite 1000, Arsenic 1000 and Belladonna 1000, two doses repeated at half hourly intervals and then at a longer intervals, as needed. For the associated constant restlessness, one should try Arsenic. A patient in need of Arsenic, whose dry cough and sneezing gets worse in the heat, should be treated with Arsenic Iodide, which is also useful in the treatment of anaemia.

Bromium is ideal for the treatment of the dry cough associated with enlargement of the glands under the jaw (sub-mandibular glands) and tonsils, and dizziness becoming worse on lying down.

Bryonia 200 is very useful in the treatment of nasal catarrh, beginning in the spring. If the patient develops whooping cough, spasmodic cough and asthma in this particular part of the year, Drosera 200 becomes imperative. Drosera ailments aggravate in humid weather.

If Belladonna does not work, then Calcarea Carb should be used. Remember that the Belladonna patient is not anaemic, while a Calcarea Carb patient happens to be anaemic.

Calcarea Sulph is useful in the treatment of patients of hot constitution who have a dry or productive cough with a tendency for pus formation in the throat.

Ignatia is very useful in the treatment of cough in those girls who become easily offended and are of hysterical nature.

The cough in a Rumex patient is extremely resistant and dry in nature. There is intense irritation in the throat. The cough becomes worse on lying down. Chelidonium combined with Rumex will be extremely useful. If the treatment is still not effective, then Sulphur 200 should be alternated with Rhus Tox 200.

Spongia is useful for the treatment of cough due to cardiac asthma (associated with a sawing sound).

Any kind of dry cough precipitated by laughing or simple talking needs to be treated with Phosphorus. Phosphorus is also ideal for the treatment of tuberculosis and cancer of the lungs. Phosphorus should not be used in more than 30 potency in the first few months of treatment. Combined or alternated with Bryonia 30, it should be given three to four times a day. Besides that, a quarter teaspoonful of turmeric dissolved in milk or water is one of the best treatments for cancer of the lungs.

Kali Carb works best in chronic cough. The eyelids of a Kali Carb patient usually remain swollen. The patient suffers from backache which gets worse in the early morning at about three or four o'clock

Inflammation of the throat spreading towards the ears and associated with the feeling of pain at the navel should be treated with Plumbum 200 or Allium Cepa 30. This is also a quick acting treatment for earache due to nasal catarrh. If satisfactory relief is not obtained, then Chamomilla and Pulsatilla will be found very useful.

Dry cough in children who have worms in the intestines, and who are in the habit of scratching in the nose, will better off treated with China. Nux Vomica will be more useful if the patient also has hyperacidity of the stomach.

China is ideal for the treatment of dehydration, resulting from the loss of body fluids or repeated loss of blood.

Ipecac is ideal for the treatment of the cough associated with nausea (but without vomiting). The chest rattles due to accumulation of phlegm in the chest.

A dry cough due to pressure on the throat and which worsens during sleep will respond better to Lachesis.

For the dry cough that becomes worse at night in children of extremely angry and stubborn nature, Chamomilla is ideal.

**Remedies**

Alumina
Antimonium Tart
Argentum Metallicum
Ignatia
Ipecac
Kali Bichromicum

Baryta Carb
Capsicum
Carbo Vegatabilis
Causticum
Conium
Drosera
Euphrasia
Hepar Sulphuris
Hydratis
Hyoscyamus

Kali Carbonicum
Kali Iodide
Lachesis
Nux Vomica
Psorinum
Sanguinaria
Senega
Silicea
Stannum
Tuberculinum

# 3. Diseases of Tonsils and Neck Glands

As soon as tonsillitis (inflammation of the tonsils) starts, one should give Aconite 1000, Belladonna 1000 and Arnica 1000 together, to show immediate relief. Day-to-day throat problems should be treated with Silicea 6X, Ferrum Phos 6X, Calcarea Fluor 6X and Kali Mur 6X. In the case of fever, the treatment should be repeated after half an hour.

Some details on problems related to tonsils have been discussed under the heading of Cold, Catarrh and Fever. One should read these carefully. If there is a fever, a bad smell from the breath and swelling of the throat causing difficulty in swallowing, then Baptisia alone may suffice.

Formation of pus in the tonsils along with the swelling of the uvula must be treated with Kali Bichrome.

For the tonsils that have become badly swollen and hard, are spotted with pus here and there, with dryness of the throat and severe burning sensation; with pain radiating to ears on swallowing, then Phytolacca is very important.

Baryta Carb is very useful in the treatment of current or old infections of the tonsils, in which the tonsils remain enlarged and hardened from the previous illness.

For an extremely offensive smell coming from the mouth, study the Mercury compounds to find suitable remedy.

For the seriously dangerous conditions of the throat, remember Tarentula Hispania in view of its physical and psychological effects. It should be studied carefully.

Use Nitric Acid for the treatment of severe pain in the throat and for jagged mouth ulcers associated with offensive saliva.

Bromium has previously been described as a treatment of catarrhal inflammations. It should be reviewed carefully regarding treatment of tonsils also.

Severe inflammation of the throat, the feeling of something being stuck, fever, and a pungent body smell are indicative of Hepar Sulph.

Syphilinum 200 or 1000 is very beneficial in every kind of throat infection when used at the beginning of the symptoms. The following may also be of use:

- Phytolacca + Baptisia + Kali Mur + Calcarea Fluor + Silicea 30 in combination, given three times a day. If the throat is very painful, then Silicea may be substituted by Hepar Sulph.

OR

- Phylotacca + Baptisia + Hepar Sulph + Carbo Veg 30 combined, three times a day.

Chronically inflamed tonsils resistant to everything else should be treated with Influenzium 200 + Bacillinum 200 + Diphtherinum 200 and Oscillo Coccinum 200, all four combined to be given once, or at the most twice a day, for three consecutive days during the severity of the illness.

**Remedies**

Alumen
Baryta Carb
Calcarea Carbonica
Guaiacum
Lac Caninum
Lachesis
Lycopodium

# 4. The Treatment of Infants and Young Children

Children commonly suffer from catarrhal illnesses, throat problems and ear diseases. They consequently contract fever every evening. Their body temperature may go on steadily rising or abate suddenly. This condition may prove fatal.

The standard routine formulary is as follows:
Aconite + Arnica + Arsenic + Belladonna 200 once or twice a day

Or

Ferrum Phos + Silicea + Kali Mur + Calcarea Fluor + Kali Phos 6X, four to five times a day.

If no benefit is obtained, then please refer to the appropiate chapter on these remedies to find the appropriate remedy. During the epidemic season, one should study under the chapters on infectious diseases. The child cannot express himself, so it is important for the physician to be extra vigilant in studying the symptoms carefully, to find a suitable remedy promptly.

**Remedies**

Allium Cepa
Alumina
Bryonia
Calcarea Phos
Chamomilla
Colocynthis
Ipecac
Natrum Muriaticum
Nux Vomica
Podophyllum
Veratrum Album

# 5. Diarrhoea, Dysentery, Constipation, and Acute and Chronic Diseases of the Intestines

Intestinal diseases may become complicated in many different ways i.e. frequent bleeding due to deep ulceration of the large gut (colon), various kinds of constipation and dysentery, cancer of the liver, cancer of the intestines, and diarrhoea of acute or chronic nature. In short, any complication may develop in the intestinal diseases. Naturally, it is very difficult to encompass them in the repertory. However, a list of the most important ones is laid down below. Under these headings, frequent reference has been made concerning other remedies too. A careful study of the following, a few times, will help in remembering them and to arrive at the correct diagnosis of the patient fairly easily.

**Remedies**

Abrotanum
Aconitum
Aethusa
Aloe
Alumen
Alumina
Apis
Apocynum
Argentum Nitricum
Arnica
Arsenicum
Baptisia
Baryta Carb
Belladonna
Bryonia
Calcarea Carb
Calcarea Carbonica
Calcarea Fluor
Cantharis
Cuprum
Dioscorea
Dulcamara
Ferrum Phos
Fluoricum Acidum
Gelsemium
Graphites
Hepar Sulph
Ipecacuanha
Iris Tenax
Kali Carb
Kali Mur
Mag Phos
Magnesia Carbonic
Mercurius
Millefolium
Natrum Muriaticum
Natrum Sulphuricum
Nitric Acid

Capsicum
Carbo Animalis
Carbo Veg
Carcinosin
Ceanothus
Chamomilla
Chelidonium
China
Cholesterinum
Cina
Colchicum
Colocynthis
Croton
Nux Vomica
Opium
Oxalic Acid
Phosphorus
Plumbum
Podophyllum
Psorinum
Silicea
Sulphur
Thuja
Tuberculinum
Veratrum Album

# 6. Disorders of the Stomach

Disorders of the stomach need special attention because any kind of stomach disorder, be it transient or chronic, can deeply affect the functioning of the entire body. The most commonly used remedies in the treatment of stomach disorders are:

| | |
|---|---|
| Absinthium | Gratiola |
| Aesculus | Hydrastis |
| Alumina | Ipecac |
| Ammonium Carb | Iris Versicolor |
| Argentum Nitricum | Kali Iodatum |
| Arsenic Iodide | Kreosotum |
| Arsenicum Album | Lac Defloratum |
| Asafoetida | Lachesis |
| Bismuthum | Lycopodium |
| Capsicum | Mercury |
| Carbo Animalis | Muriatic Acid |
| Carbo Veg | Nat Mur |
| Chelidonium | Nat Phos |
| China | Nux Vomica |
| Cimicifuga | Phosphorus |
| Colchicum | Phytolacca |
| Colocynthis | Plumbum |
| Conium | Pulsatilla |
| Crotalus | Rhus Toxicodendron |
| Cyclamen | Sanguinaria |
| Dioscorea | Sulphuric Acid |

From the above, the study of only a few will suffice; the rest of the remedies may be found under their respective headings. Ulcers of the stomach and the intestines can also be effectively treated with powdered unripe banana. The raw banana should be dried first and then powdered, to be taken three to four times a day. Even if not fully dried, the unripe banana may also be utilised. Besides that, liquorice may also be useful. A small piece of liquorice may be chewed between the teeth.

# Diseases of the Eye

Inflammation of the eyes should be immediately treated with Aconite and Belladonna combined, in any potency. If there is no immediate relief, then refer to the following chapters where eye diseases have been specifically mentioned:

Aesculus
Aethusa
Alumina
Apis
Arnica
Conium
Euphrasia
Gelsemium
Hepar Sulph
Millefolium
Psorinum

All the above remedies are of immense value. A physician would find most eye diseases covered in these remedies. However a more detailed treatment of some of them is described below.

When the blood vessels of the eyes become weak and cannot tolerate even slight pressure, the eyes remain permanently congested and red; some doctors call it piles of the eyes. In this situation, Aesculus 30 is the best. If untreated, there may be a danger of losing the eyesight. Aesculus is also useful in the treatment of nodular swellings resulting from chronic inflammation of the eye. Sometimes, the eyelids become swollen and inverted (inside out) exposing the deep red surface and look horrible. The eyelashes start falling out. In this condition, Psorinum, Hepar Sulph and Alumina are extremely useful.

In Aethusa, the eyes are hypersensitive to light and the margins of the eyelids become swollen. The eyeballs roll from side to side and become drawn downwards.

In Apis, there is puffiness and whole of the eye becomes swollen, looking like raw meat. Both Euphrasia and Belladonna resemble each other in the redness of the eye and its severity. In Euphrasia, the watery discharge is very corrosive.

Belladonna is also useful in the treatment of high eye pressure. Gelsemium is also significantly useful, in reducing the pressure. Calcarea Phos 6X and Gelsemium 6X combined are useful in Glaucoma. Sometimes, the eyes produce a watery discharge which becomes yellowish when the infection becomes chronic. Calcarea Carb is useful in this condition. In weakness of the eyes resulting from tiredness and pressure, Calcarea Carb is useful, but Onosmodium is more effective for tired eyes.

Carbonium Sulph is the ideal treatment for infections of the eyelids. When the eyes become sore and sticky, or there is a thready pustular discharge, or swellings form over the eyes which are itchy and burning, then Carbonium Sulph should be given if other remedies do not help.

Eczema of the eyelids, the feeling of heat, heaviness and discomfort, watering of the eyes mixed with beads of pus, swelling of the eyelids, hypersensitivity to light, weakness of the eyesight and colour blindness, are all the symptoms and signs of Carbonium Sulph. Steady progressive drooping of the eyelids (ptosis) and green spots before the eyes need to be treated with Causticum.

Extreme sensitivity to light, watering and dizziness (getting worse on lying down) are suggestive of Conium.

Yellowness of eyes, dark rings around them, a burning sensation in them, stabbing pain, blurring of vision, the progressive weakness of the eyesight, the tendency to bleed and photophobia, are all the symptoms of Crotalus.

Redness of the eyes along with the formation of ulcers, pimples and blisters on the eyelids are the symptoms of Croton. Other symptoms of Croton are flashes of lightning and stars before the eyes, dark spots appearing on stooping, pain, engorgement of the eyes with blood as if sand particles are causing inflammation in the eyes and severe discomfort on carrying out fine eye-work, like in Ruta. If, on doing fine eye-work, the head hurts instead of the eyes, then Onosmodium is more useful.

For the drooping of the eyelids resulting from paralysis, one should study Agaricus, Plumbum, Senega and Causticum. Tiny spots found on the cornea are a specific sign of Senega.

Silicea is very useful in the treatment of corneal ulcers. Calcarea Fluor is also deeply related to eye ailments. The pain in the eyes on sudden exposure to cold should be treated with Spigelia. For further details, please read under Spigelia.

Neuralgic pain in the eye responds very well to Lac Felinum which is prepared from cat's milk. Pain in the eyes, redness, watering, increasing discomfort on opening and closing the eyes and pain on reading, should ideally be treated with Strontium Carb.

If the symptoms are more marked in the right eye, such as blurring of vision, or weakness of the eyesight with discharge, then Tarentula should be used. When dark spots appear before the eyes, and there is dimness of the eyesight on opening the eye, with piercing pain and burning, then Natrum Carb should be used.
Besides the above, the following chapters should also be studied:

Argentum Nitricum
Aurum Metallicum
Baryta Carb
Borax
Calcarea Fluor
Calcarea Sulphurica
Chininum Ars
Cicuta Virosa
Cocculus
Crotalus
Cuprum
Cyclamen
Glonoine
Graphites
Hydrastis
Kali Carb
Lachesis
Ledum
Lilium Tig
Lycopodium
Medorrhinum
Mercurius
Millefollium
Muriatic Acid
Natrum Carb
Natrum Phos
Natrum Sulph
Nitric Acid
Phosphorus
Pulsatilla
Rhus Tox
Sanguinaria
Senega
Sulphur
Zincum Metallicum
Zincum Sulph

# 8. Tuberculosis and Other Lung Diseases, like Asthma and Cancer, etc.

Chest diseases have been described to be of three forms i.e. cancer, asthma and tuberculosis including pneumonia. Any patient with a chronic chest problem should be treated with increasing potencies of Bacillinum or Tuberculinum to build up the resistance of the lungs. The usage of these remedies is described in detail under their respective chapters. With this treatment, deep-seated ill effects of tuberculosis are eliminated and there no longer remains a danger of contracting tuberculosis in the future. For further details, one should carefully study Bacillinum and Tuberculinum to find the descriptions of their relationship with diseases of the glands also.

To cure and completely uproot the cancer of the lungs, the best treatment is Phosphorus and Bryonia used alternately and Carcinosin in high potency i.e., CM. The treatment should be given in a few doses with an interval of seven to ten days, and then wait for the results.

The treatment of asthma related diseases of the lungs is somewhat complicated, because they are related to a gonorrhoeal background which may have been passed on from generation to generation in a suppressed form. These patients do not apparently suffer from any significant urinary problem but suffer from frequently recurring asthma which makes life miserable. Such patients should be treated with Thuja CM as a preventative measure. If Thuja does not produce any significant beneficial effect after four doses given weekly, then Tuberculinum should be used.

The following instructions are very useful for a patient of asthma. The most important thing is the prompt treatment of any nasal catarrh or throat condition, because asthma usually results from the complications of these two illnesses. A correct and prompt treatment of cold and throat conditions will preclude asthma. If the cold and throat problems are forcefully treated with strong allopathic medicines, one may develop asthma as a consequence. The patient then needs to be given antibiotics again and again, and he suffers from asthma repeatedly. Nasal catarrh should be immediately treated with Influenzinum, Bacillinum, Diphterinum, and Oscillococcinum once a day for two to three days. By God's grace, the catarrh is permanently cured. For a sore throat, the following combination should be used in a low potency, i.e. 6X, showing immediate effect. These are also useful to abate the fever associated with sore throat;

Ferrum Phos + Kali Mur + Calcarea Fluor + Silicea + Kali Phos

This prescription has proven very useful in the treatment of children. Nevertheless, one should avoid taking sour or very cold things. Particularly fizzy and sour drinks eg Cola, etc. are very harmful. If the throat condition is not controlled with these and it remains swollen, then one should give Chelidonium, Coccus Cacti and Hepar Sulph 30 combined usually work well.

If the asthma is due to the weakness of the heart, then Spongia proves to be the best remedy. The cardiac asthma amenable to Spongia is associated with a sawing sound during breathing. Where the cause of the problem is the weakness of the heart, one should refer to the chapter on Diseases of the Heart.

The use of Bryonia and Phosphorus has already been mentioned in the treatment of cancer of the lungs. There is another medicinal aid, which is not homoeopathic but works as a good supportive therapy and that is turmeric. A quarter teaspoon of turmeric mixed in milk or water, given four times a day, has often proven to be an excellent treatment for cancer.

The diseases of the lungs and the intestines resulting from the suppression of skin diseases need to be treated with Sulphur, Psorinum and other remedies used for skin diseases. For further details, please refer to the chapter on Skin Diseases.

# 9. Skin Diseases

The subject of skin diseases is spread throughout the important diseases and remedies. It is impossible to sum them up in one place, in a repertory form. Reference to skin diseases has been made under all the important remedies, such as Psorinum, Sulphur, Bacillinum, Tuberculinum, Variolinum and Mercury compounds etc.

The latent form of skin diseases has been described to be the cause of suppressed restlessness. This is a good guide for a physician to treat this condition. With regard to skin diseases, the study of the infectious diseases is advised. Once again, I must say that it is impossible that the entire list of skin diseases be produced in one place in a repertory form. For the guidance of all the physicians, the following remedies are given:

Agaricus
Anacardium
Anagallis
Anthracinum
Anthrakokali
Apis
Arnica
Arsenicum Album
Arsenicum Sulph
Berberis
Bovista
Croton Tiglium
Dolichos
Graphites
Hepar Sulph
Hydrocotyle
Lachesis
Mercurius
Petroleum
Radium Bromide
Rhus Tox
Sepia
Silicea

# 10. Diseases of the Heart

For the prevention of the danger of a heart attack, Crataegus Q should be used regularly, and which can be continued indefinitely without the fear of any complications. Aconite, Belladonna, Arnica, Lachesis, Spongia, Spigelia, Berberis and Carduus Marianus should also be studied:

Adrenalin
Arsenicum
Aurum Metallicum
Cactus
Carbo Veg
Digitalis
Kalmia
Laurocerasus
Lilium Tig
Millefolium
Naja
Phosphorus
Plumbum
Psorinum
Rhus Tox

# 11. Diseases of the Gall Bladder and Diabetes

Pain in the gall bladder and the biliary colic associated with intense burning and discomfort should be treated with Belladonna in a high potency, one or two doses repeated ten to fifteen minutes apart. This will, with God's grace, help relieve the pain. After the initial treatment of Belladonna, once the pain gets better, the treatment should be continued with Sulphur and Lycopodium intermittently for a permanent cure. Both of these have a profound effect on the bile. Bile is a yellowish green secretion produced in the liver. It is very important for the digestion of food. The tendency of stone formation in the gall bladder is due to the altered quality of bile (cholestrosis).

Chelidonium is also very useful in the treatment of gall stones. The pain usually radiates to the back. The pain of Berberis spreads around, in all directions. China is also useful in the treatment of pain related to the gall bladder. The prolonged regular use of Natrum Sulph dissolves the gall stones.

If the gall bladder pain is associated with sugar in the urine, the urine being abundant in quantity and milky white in colour, then the most appropriate treatment is Argentum Metallicum. In Kali Carb patients, the gall bladder problems arise from diabetes. The urinary bladder is irritable and hypersensitive to pressure.

The patient, who suffers from slowly progressive mental weakness and is also diabetic, may sometimes be completely cured with Acid Phos. If the diabetes is due to prolonged anxiety, and there is a severe stinging type of pain at the gall bladder, and the legs and arms feel slightly achy, then Tarentula will be found very useful. It does not only offer temporary relief, but by the grace of God, it can offer a complete cure. Similarly, if the patient develops carbuncles over the shoulder areas, a very serious condition, then again Tarentula would be very useful.

# 12. Common Disorders of the Uterus, Cancer and Uterine Bleeding

The chapters relating to the following remedies should be carefully studied for various **Common Disorders and Cancer of Uterus**:

Actaea Racemosa
Alumen
Argentum Met.
Arsenic Iodatum
Belladonna
Bryonia
Calcarea Ars
Calcarea Carb
Calcarea Fluor
Calcarea Phos
Camphor
Carbo Animalis
Carbo Veg
Carcinosin
Caulophyllum
Coccus Cacti
Conium
Ferrum Phos
Gelsemium
Kali Carb
Kali Mur
Kali Phos
Kali Sulph
Murex
Nux Vomica
Psorinum
Pulsatilla
Pyrogenium
Sabina
Senecio Aureus
Sepia
Silicea
Spongia
Stannum
Sulphur
Tarentula Hispania

For **Uterine Bleeding**, the following remedies should be studied carefully.

Ammonium Carb
Antimonium Crude
Arnica
Arsenic
Baryta Carb
Cantharis
Graphites
Hamamelis
Hydrocotyle
Hyoscyamus
Kali Carb
Kreosotum
Lachesis
Lilium Tig
Millefolium
Natrum Mur
Phosphorus
Platina
Sabina
Secale Cor
Senecio Aureus
Sulphur
Sulphuric Acid
Zincum

# 13. Infertility, Abortion / Miscarriage Homoeopathic Remedies for Common Problems associated with Pregnancy and Childbirth

Sepia is considered to be a very effective treatment for infertility. The diagnosis for Sepia must not be based on the physical constitution of the patient alone. Unless the constitution of the patient exactly matches that of Sepia, it will prove to be of no use. If the constitution of the patient only resembles that of Sepia (rather then completely matching it), then Kali Phos will be found more useful than Sepia.

Sexual weakness resulting from nervous tension as well as the tendency to abort repeatedly (habitual abortion), can be effectively cured with Kali Phos. If there is a risk of miscarriage in early pregnancy, then Viburnum Opulus Q, ten to fifteen drops dissolved in small amount of water, used regularly in the first and second month of pregnancy is considered to be more effective. Sabina is given in the third month, while Kali Carb is given in the fourth and fifth month. Kali Phos can, however, be given every month.

An abortion threatened by a fall or an accident must be treated with Arnica 1000 before the appearance of symptoms. The addition of Kali Phos to Arnica will be much more beneficial. Caulophyllum 200 also is very effective prophylactially. Once the bleeding starts (threatened abortion), then Ferrum Phos must be added to Kali Phos. Likewise, Millefolium and Phosphorus together can avert the abortion.

Sometimes, the baby is malpositioned in the uterus, posing a threat to normal delivery; Pulsatilla is usually very useful in the correcting the position to normal. If it fails, then Kali Sulph, which is the chronic of Pulsatilla, should be tried. Kali Sulph strengthens the uterus against the tendency to abort. Kali Sulph is useful in every type of leucorrhoeal inflammation and burning sensation. Uterine prolapse, and pain and pressure in the womb are best treated with Kali Sulph, provided other symptoms of Kali Sulph are present.

In Kreosotum, the typical sign is bleeding. The slightest pressure, like the simplest touch during an eye examination, can cause bleeding.

Likewise, the uterus tends to bleed easily resulting in continuous menstrual bleeding.

In Ledum, the periods are frequent and profuse; the colour is bright red. If other symptoms of Ledum are also present, then Ledum alone can cure most of the problems related to the uterus.

Lilium Tig is more useful in the treatment of women of hysterical and explosive nature, who have problems related to the uterus and the heart. Their mind is occupied by all kinds of doubts, fear and anxiety. They feel as if the uterus and other pelvic organs are prolapsing downwards, all of which they unknowingly try to support manually. In such patients, their periods begin before their regular time and are scanty and offensive, containing dark blood clots. The bleed intensifies on movement and subsides on resting and lying down.

The main features of Merc Sol are sharp stinging pain associated with burning sensation, excessive menstrual bleeding, pain in the abdomen, corrosive vaginal discharge (leucorrhoea). These symptoms are worse at night. There is morning sickness, scalding urination, feeling better by washing with cold water. Merc Sol will also be useful to avert the tendency to abort in early pregnancy due to the weakness of the uterus, by strengthening the uterus so that it may safely hold and nourish the foetus.

After marriage, some women may develop irregularity of periods, pelvic pains and nervousness, and should be treated with Medorrhinum.

Periods lasting much longer, pain and cramps in the lower part of the abdomen and excessive bleeding are the main symptoms of Millefolium. If all the three symptoms are found together, then Millefolium, by God's grace, instantly relieves the condition, with rare exception. Likewise, Millefolium will allay the threat of abortion where bleeding starts due to slight movement and stops on resting. Millefolium is also very useful in treating varicose veins of the legs that develop during pregnancy. If Millefolium is given at this time, it will stop the progression of the disease. When a woman starts having fits of epilepsy and spasms due to the stoppage of her period, or the period starts due to excessive physical exertion, in this condition Millefolium is also useful.

Kali Carb is very beneficial in treating a myriad of weaknesses that develop after childbirth. Natrum Mur is also very effective in the restoration of health.

If a fever develops after childbirth, this (puerperal fever) can be treated with Sulphur and Pyrogenum combined. Pulsatilla helps in expulsion of the remaining placenta and blood clots.

Irregular periods, the irritating type of leucorrhoea, premenstrual tension, the bearing down type of pain, heaviness in the morning and excessive burning in urination are all indications for Natrum Mur.

Natrum Carb is ideal for the treatment of infertility resulting from chronic leucorrhoea. A Natrum Carb patient is of a cold constitution, has continuous leucorrhoea and cannot conceive. If these symptoms are found together, then through the Grace of God, Natrum Carb alone would be very effective in curing the infertility.

Pulsatilla, Ashoka and Gossypium Q are also excellent remedies for infertility. Other appropriate remedies should also be employed, depending on the associated symptoms e.g. if the uterus feels as if out of place, then Natrum Phos could be useful. The hands of the patient of Natrum Phos, like that of Psorinum, remain very cold. In Natrum Phos, some symptoms also resemble Pulsatilla. During menstruation the hands and the feet are especially cold in the morning.

## General Instructions Concerning Pregnancy And the Facilitation of Childbirth

Ferrum Phos, Calcarea Phos and Kali Phos 6X started twice a day in the third or fourth month of pregnancy serve as a very useful tonic for both the mother and the baby. The treatment must be stopped for a week or ten days after every one to two weeks. Continuous use of these is not advisable.

At the onset of labour pains, Kali Phos and Mag Phos 6X dissolved in warm water should be administered every one to two hours for eight to ten times a day. The first three doses should be given every half hour and then at prolonged intervals.

One dose of Arnica 1000 should be given before delivery and one right after the delivery. For the fever developing after delivery, Sulphur and Pyrogenum 200 together must be given two to three times a day for the first few days. Once the fever starts subsiding, then once a day for three days. After that, once a day for two weeks. In my experience, there is no better treatment for puerperal fever than this.

If milk is not being produced after childbirth, then Bryonia and Phytolacca should be given together once or twice a day. They work wonders. They may be given in potency 30, three to four times a day.

**Depression** after childbirth (Post-partum depression) can be effectively treated with Ignatia 200 instantly. If however, the treatment falls short, then one dose of Natrum Mur 200 after Ignatia will make up for it.

For the phobia of going out, the treatment is Calcarea Carb 1000 once a week for three weeks.

Weak and ineffective labour pains should be treated with Pulsatilla 30, three to four times a day. If the position of the child is breech (the reverse of the normal position), then give Pulsatilla 200, one or two doses. For the transverse lie (the child lying sideways), Arnica and Caulophyllum 200 combined, given once a day for a few days is very useful. This combination also produces wonderful results in a serious and potentially fatal condition, Placenta Praevia, in which the placenta is attached near the opening of the womb

Further reference concerning the problems related to pregnancy and childbirth are found under Kali Carb, Caulophyllum, Causticum and Gelsemium. The following should also be studied carefully in their relative chapters:

Actaea Racemosa
Agnus Castus
Aurum Muriaticum
Borax
Ipecacuanha
Kali Bromatum
Phosphorus
Secale Cor
Symphori Carpus

# 14. Diseases related to Disorders of the Arteries and Veins

Transient as well as long-lasting diseases of the arteries and the veins, including traumatic and psychological disorders have been referred to under the following chapters:

| | |
|---|---|
| Aconitum | Cimicifuga |
| Alumina | Crataegus |
| Ammonium Carb | Cuprum |
| Arnica | Fluoricum Acid |
| Arsenic | Hamamelis |
| Aurum Metallicum | Lachesis |
| Belladonna | Millefolium |
| Bellis Perennis | Opium |
| Benzoicum Acid | Psorinum |
| Carbo Animalis | Pulsatilla |
| Carbo Veg | Strontia Carb |
| Chininum Ars | Sulphur |

Whenever patients suffering from Arterial or Venous disorders are seen, the above remedies should be studied. Symptoms of such patients would be found somewhere in these remedies.

Sometimes, the tendency of the arteries to rupture may be the consequence of suppressed skin diseases. For example, in Rhus Tox, the affected area tends to exude a watery discharge, even though the skin disease had apparently healed over twenty years beforehand. The recurrence of the varicose veins will need to be treated with Rhus Tox 1000 once or twice a week. Besides this, standard treatment with Aesculus, Fluoric Acid, Calcarea Fluor and Pulsatilla should be used.

# 15. Diseases of the Nervous System

A study of the following chapters will cover all the diseases of the nervous system:

Actaea Racemosa
Agaricus
Agnus Castus
Alumina
Argentum Nitricum
Argentum Met
Arnica
Carbo Veg
Causticum
Cocculus
Crotalus
Gelsemium
Hyoscyamus
Hypericum
Ignatia
Kali Phos
Mag Phos
Nat Mur
Phosphorus
Picric Acid
Plumbum Metallicum
Rhus Tox
Ruta
Silicea
Spigelia

# 16. Remedies Related to Superstitious Ideas/Dreams Lack or Excess of Sleep

**a. Remedies useful in cases of sleeplessness/related to the dreams:-**

Absinthium
Actaea Racemosa
Agaricus
Arnica
Belladonna
Calcarea Ars
Calcarea Carb
Carbo Animalis
Carbo Veg
Coffea
Drosera
Helleborus
Hyoscyamus
Kali Carb
Medorrhinum
Nat Phos
Natrum Mur
Nux Vomica
Phosphorus
Pyrogenium
Sabadilla
Sabina
Silicea
Stramonium
Sulphur
Sulphuric Acid
Tarentula
Thuja

**b.** Study of the following Remedies for cases of **Sleeplessness (Insomnia):**

Arsenicum Album
Belladonna
Cannabis Indica
Causticum
Chamomilla
Cocculus
Coffea
Crotalus
Ignatia
Kali Phos
Nux Vomica
Opium
Passiflora Q
Phosphorus
Picric Acid
Rhus Tox
Silicea

**c. For Excessive sleep or somnolence,** the following remedies would be useful:

Ferrum Phos
Gelsemium
Kali Bichrome
Nux Moschata

# 17. Drug Addiction

The discourse on different addictions will be found under the following remedies and careful study is advised:

Caladium
Cannabis Indica
Crotalus
Nux Vomica
Phosphorus
Plantago
Platina
Sulphur
Sulphuric Acid
Tabacum

# 18. Mental Diseases/Disorders

Treatment of mind-related problems is extremely complicated because the mind is subjected to all kinds of psychological trauma. Mention of other remedies will be found in the discussion of these particular remedies. The relevant remedies are as follows:

Aconitum
Actaea Racemosa
Aethusa
Arnica
Aurum
Belladonna
Calcarea Ars
Chininum Ars
Cyclamen
Glonoine
Graphites
Helleborus
Hydrophobinum
Hyoscyamus
Ignatia
Iodum
Kali Phos
Lac Caninum
Lachesis
Lilium Tigrinum
Medorrhinum
Merc Sol
Natrum Carbonicum
Natrum Mur
Nitric Acid
Nux Vomica
Opium
Phosphorus
Platina
Psorinum
Pulsatilla
Sepia
Silicea
Staphysagria
Stramonium
Sulphur
Thuja
Veratrum Album

# 19. Diseases of the Reproductive Organs

The treatment of diseases of the reproductive system is very difficult due to the wide range of the diagnostic spectrum. A reader would perceive that every remedy he reads is useful to his patient's illness. There are over a hundred remedies related to the functioning of the reproductive system. But except for one or two, the others may not be of any use to the patient. The list of the repertory is as follows:

Abrotanum
Agaricus
Agnus Castus
Alumina
Anagallis
Arsenic Album
Arsenicum Iod.
Baryta Carb
Bufo
Caladium
Calc. Carb
Calc. Fluor
Calc. Sulph
Calc. Phos
Camphora
Cannabis Sativa
Cantharis
Capsicum
Causticum
Chininum Ars
Clematis
Coccus Cacti
Coffea
Conium
Croton
Cyclamen
Ferrum Phos
Fluoricum Acidum
Gelsemium
Graphites
Gratiola
Hepar Sulph
Hydrastis
Kali Bichrom
Kali Carb
Kali Phos
Kali Sulph
Lycopodium
Medorrhinum
Mercurius
Natrum Mur
Natrum Phos
Natrum Sulph
Nitric Acid
Nuphar Luteum
Nux Vomica
Onosmodium
Origanum
Phosphoric Acid
Phosphorus
Platina
Pulsatilla
Sabina
Salix Nigra
Selenium
Sepia
Silicea
Spongia
Staphysagria
Sulphur
Tarentula
Thuja
Tribulus Terrestris
Turnera
Yohimbinum
Zincum

# 20. Prostate Gland

Enlargement of the prostate gland results in some distinct urinary symptoms and, at times, sexual weakness. The patient cannot completely empty his bladder. The urine stream becomes very weak and lacks full force. This may lead to interruption of flow. Soon after passing water, the patient feels like passing urine again. The frequency of urination is increased gradually, and the interval between urination is decreased. Sometimes, the interval is half an hour or less. The quantity becomes less and the patient is not relieved completely.

Frequent urination is not always necessarily due to the enlargement of the prostate but if it is, the treatment should be as follows.

If the frequency is considered to be due to the suppressed gonorrhoea, then it should be treated with Thuja. Start in a low potency and then gradually increase to CM potency. Thuja also affects the Prostate Gland. It allays the burning sensation in the urethra. Therefore, this should be considered the first remedy. Among other illnesses reminiscent of Thuja, Asthma is the most prominent. Similarly, the presence of skin warts indicates Thuja. The peculiar symptoms of Thuja include the burning sensation in the urethra with frequency of urination. Another specific symptom is the splitting of the urine stream into two, becoming one again on straining.

The other homoeopathic treatment for enlarged prostate is Silicea. Potency CM works the best. The only condition is that the patient is of cold constitution, and that the limbs feel very cold. Silicea works equally well on the cancer of the prostate and the bladder. Two to three doses of Silicea CM at intervals of seven to ten days, by God's grace, will be found significantly effective.

Another good remedy for an enlarged prostate is Clematis. It happens to work on the right-sided diseases, affecting for example, the right limb, the right testis and the right ureter (the channel carrying urine from the kidney to the bladder). The patient is always restless and wakes up to pass urine again and again. Severe thirst can be quenched with cold water. Clematis offers only temporary relief of the urinary symptoms, but does not cure them. It simply decreases the frequency.

Instead of going to the lavatory every few minutes, the patient needs to go to the lavatory every two hours or so. Still the feeling of passing urine may be very pressing. The patient has to run to the lavatory. It is thus necessary that the physician should look for other remedies besides Clematis, to uproot the disease.

With the use of Clematis, it has been observed that the patient starts passing urine freely, though frequently. It shows that the urine problem was not due to the prostate, rather it was due to a kidney or bladder infection. Clematis cannot cure the symptoms due to the prostatic obstruction.

Urinary problems in general are not always easily understood. The symptoms have to be analysed and properly evaluated before suggesting the appropriate remedies. The few distinctive symptoms should be well understood and remembered. It is not necessary that every remedy would prove effective. This is why it is very difficult to find the correct remedy. It is important to know the distinctive features of the illness. Otherwise, it is impossible for the physician to recognise the remedy for every illness.

Sometimes, the patient passes foul-smelling thick turbid urine indicative of an infection in urogenital tract i.e. the kidney, bladder, urethra, testes and uterus. Treatment should be started promptly and continued long enough to control the infection. The remedies most appropriate for this condition are: Thuja, Sulphur, Pyrogenium, Psorinum, Ferrum Phos, Silicea, Arsenic Album, Conium, Cannabis Indica, Phosphorus, Merc Cor, Sabal Serrulata, Staphysagria and Chimaphila. During the study of all these remedies, more may be found cross referenced, e.g. Medorrhinum etc.

# 21. Joint Pains (Arthritis and Rheumatism)

Various types of arthritis and rheumatism are described under the following:

Abrotanum
Actaea Racemosa
Agnus Castus
Apis
Apocynum
Argentum Metallicum
Arnica
Belladonna
Benzoicum Acidum
Berberis
Bryonia
Calcarea Carb
Caulophyllum
Causticum
Colchicum
Eupatorium
Guaiacum
Kali Carb
Lachesis
Lactic Acid
Ledum
Medorrhinum
Mercurius
Natrum Sulph
Phytolacca
Pulsatilla
Rhus Tox
Sabina
Sulphur

During the study of the above, the reader will also find the discourse on these diseases and their treatment using other remedies also.

# 22. Diseases of the Bones

Among the serious diseases of the bone are bone cancer and tuberculosis of the bones. Besides them, some serious diseases can also inflict deep and long lasting damage to the bone, such as typhoid and polio. The treatment of some bone diseases is very difficult though not impossible.

The structural abnormalities of the bones of a congenital nature, such as dwarfism and brittle bones need the right treatment and patience. Under the following chapters, necessary references will be found concerning these diseases and their suggested treatment:

Argentum Metallicum
Aurum
Asafoetida
Baryta Carb
Bryonia
Calc. Carb
Calcarea Fluor
Calcarea Phos
Eupatorium
Ledum
Medorrhinum
Mercurius
Nitric Acid
Phosphorus
Pulsatilla
Ruta
Sepia
Silicea
Staphysagria

After studying these chapters, one would come to know the other remedies. This would prove very useful.

# 23. The Treatment (Immediate and Long-term) of Accidents and Injuries

The study of the following remedies will, God-willing, be very satisfying to the reader:

Aconite
Arnica
Belladonna
Bellis
Calc. Fluor
Calc. Phos
Carbo Veg
Hypericum
Muriatic Acid
Opium
Ruta
Staphysagria
Strontia Carb
Symphytum

# 24. All Types of Paralysis

The following are useful in the treatment of paralysis, depending on the nature of the symptoms and their identity relevant to the particular remedies.

Aconite
Alumina
Argentum Nitricum
Arnica
Belladonna
Causticum
Cocculus
Conium
Gelsemium
Lachesis
Muriaticum Acid
Natrum Mur
Nux Vomica
Opium
Phosphoric Acid
Plumbum
Pulsatilla
Rhus Tox
Ruta
Secale Cor
Spigelia
Sulphur
Tarentula
Zincum

# 25. Physical Appearances and Homoeopathic Remedies

In literature on homoeopathy, frequent mention is made about the physique and appearance of the patient. Diagnosis of the disease cannot be based on such descriptions alone. Under the following remedies, however, there are good pointers for the make up and appearance of the patient:

| | |
|---|---|
| Baryta Carb | Kali Carb |
| Calc. Carb | Natrum Mur |
| Calc. Fluor | Phytolacca |
| Chininum Ars | Plumbum |
| Cholesterinum | Sepia |
| Graphites | Silicea |

# 26. Infectious Diseases

## Cholera

Sulphur is the best preventative treatment during a cholera epidemic. Sulphur 200 every day for two days and then twice a week saves one from contracting cholera. As soon as the symptoms of cholera appear, Camphor in a low potency can cure cholera altogether. Once the symptoms have started, especially the silent type of cholera, associated with large exuberant watery stools, causing severe dehydration and weakness leading to coldness of the body, can best be treated with Camphor. The most prominent indication for Camphor is nausea and vomiting, more so than diarrhoea.

Cuprum is also an extremely effective treatment of cholera especially the kind associated with severe abdominal colic and severe cramps in the hands and the feet, starting in the fingers and toes and then spreads upwards. This type of cholera is best treated with Cuprum. In the diarrhoea of Cuprum, the stools are scanty, frequent and associated with severe griping. The cholera associated with exuberant amounts of stools and severe cramps in the calves will respond best to Veratrum Album. The following remedies may also be of use:

Aethusa
Arsenicum Album
Carbo Veg
Podophyllum
Secale Cor

## Abdominal Colic in Intestinal Infections

This may be associated with the tendency of nausea and vomiting due to cholera or any other illness. It should be treated with the combination of Croton 30, Ipecac 30, Carbo Veg 30, Baptisia 30.

Nausea and vomiting that get better with drinking cold water is indicative of Cuprum. Cuprum is also effective in the treatment of mumps. Similarly, Cuprum is useful in the treatment of paralysis of a limb caused by typhoid fever. The other possible remedies are:-

Antimonium Crudum
Argentum Nitricum
Arsenicum Album
Colchicum
Colocynthis
Dioscorea
Iris
Nux Vomica
Pulsatilla
Sulphur

## Malaria

Please refer to the detailed accounts of malaria under the chapters of the following remedies. The reader may be directed to some other related remedies and symptoms under the same chapters:

Aconite
Arnica
Arsenic
Bryonia
Cedron
China
Chininum Ars
Eupatorium
Gelsemium
Ipecacuanha
Natrum Mur
Natrum Sulph
Nux Vomica
Psorinum
Pulsatilla
Rhus Tox
Tarentula
Tuberculinum

A careful study of these homoeopathic remedies will, God-willing, enable the reader to control malaria fairly well.

## Chicken Pox and Measles

By the time chicken pox or measles become visible, they may have already done enough harm to the body. Silicea, Kali Phos and Ferrum Phos help manifest the symptoms onto the skin. Allium Cepa as well as Arsenic and Psorinum may also be useful, depending upon the situation i.e. symptoms and signs of the sickness. Necessary reference has also been made under the following:

Antimonium Crudum
Antimonium Tart
Apis
Calcarea Phos
Malandrinum
Merc Sol
Pulsatilla
Sulphur

Euphrasia
Kali Bichrom
Variolinum

## Whooping Cough

In whooping cough, commonly used remedies are Drosera, Allium Cepa and Arnica. Other useful remedies are:

Belladonna
Coccus Cacti
Cuprum Metallicum
Hydrocyanic Acid
Ipecacuanha
Kali Carb
Senega
Tarentula

## Influenza

Sulphur and Pyrogenium have been found very useful in the treatment of influenza fever. Besides them, Influenzinum, Bacillinum, Diphtherinum, Oscillo Coccinum, Kali Phos, Ferrum Phos, Kali Mur, Silicea and Calcarea Fluor should also be studied.

Arsenicum Album
Bryonia
Carbo Veg
Dulcamara
Eupatorium
Gelsemium
Natrum Sulph
Rhus Tox

## Dysentery

Commonly used remedies are: Ipecac, Aconite, Kurchi, Dioscorea and Colocynthis. More has been mentioned under the following headings:

Aloe
Arnica
Arsenic Album
Bufo
Cantharis
Capsicum
Carbo Veg
Carbolic Acid
Colchicum
Gelsemium
Mag Carb
Merc Cor
Merc Sol
Nux Vomica
Phosphorus
Rhus Tox
Sulphur

## Plague

During an epidemic, when Mercury and Sulphur compounds are used, the disease will surface to the skin, sparing the glands and thus curing the plague. The following may also be found useful:

Arsenicum Album
Belladonna
Crotalus Horridus
Hydrocyanic Acid
Ignatia
Lachesis
Naja
Phosphorus
Pyrogenium
Rhus Tox
Tarentula Hispania

## AIDS

In AIDS, Silicea CM, Psorinum, Syphilinum and Pyrogenium prove to be very beneficial.

## Meningitis

In addition to Natrum Sulph, Gelsemium, Silicea and Apis, the following should also be studied:

Aconitum
Belladonna
Bryonia
Calcarea Carb
Cicuta Virosa
Crotalus Horridus
Cuprum Metallicum
Glonoine
Helleborus
Hyoscyamus
Mercurius
Nux Vomica
Opium
Zincum

# 27. Some of the Tested and Proven Prescriptions of Daily Use

- Aethusa 200 – students who get **confused in exam and forget everything**
- Argentum Nit + Aaethusa 200 combined for **fear of examination.**
- Lycopodium 200 for **lack of confidence and anticipatory fear as in public speaking.**
- Kali Phos+ Silicea 6x for **fear of failure in exam.**
- Pulsatilla 30 + Phosphorus 30 in **children seeking extra attention.**
- Phosphorus 30 + Aconite 30 + Opium 30 for **fear of going to school.**
- Staphysagria in **sensitive weepy children**
- Chamomilla 1000 for **stubborn ad irritable children.**
- Phosphorus 30 for **fear of being alone.**
- Arsenic+ Opium + Aconite 30 for **children who wake up startled in the night.**
- Natrum Sulph 1000 + Arnica 1000 useful for **head injury.**
- Opium 1000 or higher in **head injury or stroke with brain damage**
- Helliborus Niger for **after effects of head injury.**
- Aurum Met 200 in **postoperative nausea after gaining consciousness.** Phosphorous can also be given.
- Aconite CM (1 dose) better if given with Opium CM for **ill effects of fear and shock.**
- One dose of Arnica 1000 **before and after surgery** safeguards against possible complications.
- Pulsatilla for **indigestion after overeating eating fatty food.**
- Carbo veg for **indigestion after overeating carbohydrates.**
- Nux vomica for **rice and meat allergy.**
- Calc Carb for **egg allergy.**
- Chinimum Ars for **diarrhea after eating eggs.**
- Sulphuric Acid one drop in water three times daily for **giving up smoking.**
- Nux Vomica 200 for **ill effects of wrongly given injections.**

- Nitric Acid or single dose of Sulphur in high potency for **diarrhea after penicillin.**
- Kali phos 1000 one dose and few doses of Plumbum 200 for **poor memory.**
- Lachesis 1000 for **people of suspicious nature and also for fear of the unknown**.
- Arsenic 1000 (few doses) **for fear of death, fear of accidents, anxiety and generally disinclined to work.**